Diagnostic Neuropathology

Diagnostic Neuropathology

A PRACTICAL MANUAL

MARGARET M. ESIRI MA, DM, MRCPath

Clinical Reader in Neuropathology, The Radcliffe Infirmary, and
Senior Research Fellow, St Hugh's College, Oxford

D. R. OPPENHEIMER MA, DM, FRCPath

Formerly University Lecturer and Honorary Consultant,
Department of Neuropathology, The Radcliffe Infirmary, and
Fellow of Trinity College, Oxford

FOREWORD BY

L. J. RUBINSTEIN

BLACKWELL SCIENTIFIC PUBLICATIONS

OXFORD LONDON EDINBURGH

BOSTON MELBOURNE

© 1989 by
Blackwell Scientific Publications
Editorial offices:
Osney Mead, Oxford OX2 0EL
   (*Orders*: Tel. 0865 240201)
8 John Street, London WC1N 2ES
23 Ainslie Place, Edinburgh EH3 6AJ
3 Cambridge Center, Suite 208
   Cambridge, Massachusetts 02142, USA
107 Barry Street, Carlton
   Victoria 3053, Australia

First published 1989

Set by Setrite Typesetters Ltd, Hong Kong
Printed and bound in Great Britain by
William Clowes Limited, Beccles and London

DISTRIBUTORS

USA
   Year Book Medical Publishers
   200 North LaSalle Street,
   Chicago, Illinois 60601
   (*Orders*: Tel. 312 726−9733)

Canada
   The C.V. Mosby Company
   5240 Finch Avenue East
   Scarborough, Ontario
   (*Orders*: Tel. 416−298−1588)

Australia
   Blackwell Scientific Publications
   (Australia) Pty Ltd
   107 Barry Street
   Carlton, Victoria 3053
   (*Orders*: Tel. (03) 347 0300)

British Library
Cataloguing in Publication Data

Esiri, Margaret M. (Margaret Miriam)
   Diagnostic neuropathology.
   1. Man. Nervous system. Diseases
   I. Title   II. Oppenheimer, D.R.
   616.8

ISBN 0-632-01951-4

Contents

List of colour plates

Foreword

Textbooks of neuropathology, like people and microglia, generally appear in one of two forms: thin and lean; or fat and crammed. The former are designed to sketch the bare bones of the subject for the otherwise overburdened medical student. The latter, replete with minutiae, are addressed to the practitioner already experienced in the field.

Rarer are those books which fall between these extremes and in which the balance between the skeletal outline and a profusion of details has been carefully adjusted, and the mixture blended with art. The present manual, authored by Drs Esiri and Oppenheimer, fits the description. The writers, whose experience is based on the extensive neuropathological material examined at the Radcliffe Infirmary at Oxford, have combined forces to share their considerable, and complementary, skills. The product of this labour of love is an exemplary model of what a specialized textbook should be.

What does this book supply, and to whom is it addressed? Obviously it is too detailed for the medical student. The authors state that it is chiefly aimed at the apprentice in neuropathology and at the general pathologist with, as they say, 'an interest'. They view its purpose as largely practical rather than systematic. They are too modest by half; I should predict that by reason of its unusual features and because of the manner in which it has been conceived and executed it will find its place on the shelves of even the most seasoned neuropathologist.

This work, understatingly labelled 'a practical manual', but in which so much reflection and wisdom has gone into the making of it, has, first, all the requirements that make it a reliable guide. It is abundantly and clearly illustrated, contains many apposite diagrams and tables, furnishes selected references at the end of each chapter and provides a wealth of useful recommendations. These include the types of neural tissue to be secured and reserved after consultation of the clinical notes; discussions on the problems of brain biopsies and on the brain smear technique; a timely review of the immunoreactivities of brain tumours based on a wide panel of antibodies; precautions to be taken in slow virus diseases; and of course the expected tabulated lists of metabolic central and peripheral nervous system disorders. The clinical neurological correlations that can be established with the sites and the nature of the neuropathological changes, both gross and microscopic, or with the localization of selective cell losses are succinctly, but comprehensively presented. But perhaps the most innovative aspects are the special features that cannot usually be found in comparable texts: not only an emphasis on an interpretative approach that closely correlates the clinical neurological picture and the pathological findings but separate chapters on the aetiology of epilepsy, on the diverse neuropathology of the very young, on a large number of different malfunctions that may involve the central and the peripheral nervous systems and on which neuropathological data are often scanty or incomplete, even on sundry but relevant matters such as the ceremony of brain cutting, advice on how to avoid reporting delays, suggestions on the manner of reporting, and counselling on the relationships to be maintained with one's colleagues and one's laboratory staff. The candour with which the advice is given, and these points made, should endear both neuropathology and the authors to even the least sympathetic reader.

Thus the contents, spirit and tone of this manual belie the austerity of its title. The writing is cheerful, alert and graceful, not devoid of its wry touches — even where it examines some of the causes of head injury, when the reader will momentarily muse on the dangers attending the fall of coconuts in the groves of Papua. The authors persistently ask questions, often leaving them unanswered, but always pointing the way to further questions and, sometimes, to possible solutions. Bearing the fruits of personal experience, this book counsels a modesty which is becoming to a relatively esoteric specialty. But it exudes the pleasure of problem-solving and breathes the joy of neuropathology.

L.J. Rubinstein
University of Virginia

Preface

Some years ago one of the authors of this book, as a junior neuropathologist, was accustomed to receiving from outside sources a succession of more or less damaged and distorted brains and spinal cords. Some of these had been sliced and diced into unrecognizable fragments in the post mortem room. Some were accompanied by an inch-square section of an unidentified part of the brain stained with haematoxylin and eosin. Sometimes an undistorted, well-fixed brain arrived, accompanied by a good set of clinical notes which made it clear that the main site of the patient's disorder lay in the spinal cord or peripheral nerves.

The recipient of these tantalizing specimens spoke of his frustrations to a fatherly, much respected, senior colleague, who was duly sympathetic. But when the young man spoke of his intention of writing a little pamphlet giving guidance to general pathologists on the handling of material from neurological cases, he was met with an alarming display of mock rage. 'You must do no such thing!' the old man thundered. 'If the priests reveal the mysteries of their craft to the multitude, what will become of them? If we allow the general pathologists to discover how simple our work is and how lacking in mystery, they will start doing it themselves, and we shall be out of a job.'

On reflection, we think the old man's fears were exaggerated. Many pathologists, we know, regard the nervous system and its diseases with distaste, or even fear, and are only too happy to unload the neurological material that comes their way, leaving more time to pursue the subjects that interest them. Others — especially those facing specialist examinations — are not averse to rounding off their general competence with a course of simple neuropathology. Yet others — and it is from these that the priesthood is mainly recruited — positively enjoy the subject; and it would be both selfish and impolitic to erect barriers to their initiation.

Of the two authors of this book, one underwent a preliminary indoctrination in general pathology, the other in clinical neurology and neuro-anatomy. In the course of 15 years or so of collaboration, often in different areas of the neuropathological field, each of us has profited from the effects of the other's apprenticeship, to the extent of acquiring at least a rough grasp of what the other was doing and thinking, and

even, on occasion, offering useful criticism. In this, we think we have been more fortunate than many others.

With these and similar considerations in mind, we are presenting this book as a guide to neuropathological methods, aimed principally at apprentices in neuropathology and at general pathologists with, as they say, an interest. It consists partly of advice on how to avoid the embarrassment of being shown to have destroyed or thrown away the evidence which should have led to a diagnosis. It contains a certain amount of descriptive matter, which overlaps with the conventional textbooks of neuropathology; but it is not, and is not intended to be, comprehensive. On the other hand, there are places where we have included theoretical, or speculative, remarks, based on our own observations, on matters which tend to be neglected in standard textbooks of neuropathology. Nor is it systematic in the sense of being arranged in separate categories of disease — inflammatory, degenerative, neoplastic and so forth. The chapter headings correspond for the most part to the immediate questions facing the neuropathologist in the post mortem room, such as 'what had caused this patient's epilepsy?', 'why was he so weak?', or 'why, after what seemed to be a successful neurosurgical procedure, did he suddenly die?'

The title *Diagnostic Neuropathology* entails a brief explanation of what we mean by 'diagnosis'. In our view, to write 'multiple sclerosis' at the end of a post mortem report is not an adequate diagnosis, unless the report has expressed an opinion on how the patient's history, signs and symptoms are related to the lesions and to their distribution, severity and chronicity. Similarly, 'chromophobe adenoma of the pituitary' is an inadequate diagnosis unless the report gives an idea of the size, manner of growth and hormonal activity of the tumour, with a view of how it affected the patient's state, and why he is now dead.

We realize that our criteria for the adequacy of a diagnosis may seem too demanding of effort to some readers and too easily satisfied to others. If a line is to be drawn between 'routine diagnosis' and 'research', there is no agreed principle deciding where it should be drawn. In this book, we have proposed what seem to us reasonable standards for routine diagnosis, but make no claim to have arrived at a generally

Preface

Some years ago one of the authors of this book, as a junior neuropathologist, was accustomed to receiving from outside sources a succession of more or less damaged and distorted brains and spinal cords. Some of these had been sliced and diced into unrecognizable fragments in the post mortem room. Some were accompanied by an inch-square section of an unidentified part of the brain stained with haematoxylin and eosin. Sometimes an undistorted, well-fixed brain arrived, accompanied by a good set of clinical notes which made it clear that the main site of the patient's disorder lay in the spinal cord or peripheral nerves.

The recipient of these tantalizing specimens spoke of his frustrations to a fatherly, much respected, senior colleague, who was duly sympathetic. But when the young man spoke of his intention of writing a little pamphlet giving guidance to general pathologists on the handling of material from neurological cases, he was met with an alarming display of mock rage. 'You must do no such thing!' the old man thundered. 'If the priests reveal the mysteries of their craft to the multitude, what will become of them? If we allow the general pathologists to discover how simple our work is and how lacking in mystery, they will start doing it themselves, and we shall be out of a job.'

On reflection, we think the old man's fears were exaggerated. Many pathologists, we know, regard the nervous system and its diseases with distaste, or even fear, and are only too happy to unload the neurological material that comes their way, leaving more time to pursue the subjects that interest them. Others — especially those facing specialist examinations — are not averse to rounding off their general competence with a course of simple neuropathology. Yet others — and it is from these that the priesthood is mainly recruited — positively enjoy the subject; and it would be both selfish and impolitic to erect barriers to their initiation.

Of the two authors of this book, one underwent a preliminary indoctrination in general pathology, the other in clinical neurology and neuro-anatomy. In the course of 15 years or so of collaboration, often in different areas of the neuropathological field, each of us has profited from the effects of the other's apprenticeship, to the extent of acquiring at least a rough grasp of what the other was doing and thinking, and

even, on occasion, offering useful criticism. In this, we think we have been more fortunate than many others.

With these and similar considerations in mind, we are presenting this book as a guide to neuropathological methods, aimed principally at apprentices in neuropathology and at general pathologists with, as they say, an interest. It consists partly of advice on how to avoid the embarrassment of being shown to have destroyed or thrown away the evidence which should have led to a diagnosis. It contains a certain amount of descriptive matter, which overlaps with the conventional textbooks of neuropathology; but it is not, and is not intended to be, comprehensive. On the other hand, there are places where we have included theoretical, or speculative, remarks, based on our own observations, on matters which tend to be neglected in standard textbooks of neuropathology. Nor is it systematic in the sense of being arranged in separate categories of disease — inflammatory, degenerative, neoplastic and so forth. The chapter headings correspond for the most part to the immediate questions facing the neuropathologist in the post mortem room, such as 'what had caused this patient's epilepsy?', 'why was he so weak?', or 'why, after what seemed to be a successful neurosurgical procedure, did he suddenly die?'

The title *Diagnostic Neuropathology* entails a brief explanation of what we mean by 'diagnosis'. In our view, to write 'multiple sclerosis' at the end of a post mortem report is not an adequate diagnosis, unless the report has expressed an opinion on how the patient's history, signs and symptoms are related to the lesions and to their distribution, severity and chronicity. Similarly, 'chromophobe adenoma of the pituitary' is an inadequate diagnosis unless the report gives an idea of the size, manner of growth and hormonal activity of the tumour, with a view of how it affected the patient's state, and why he is now dead.

We realize that our criteria for the adequacy of a diagnosis may seem too demanding of effort to some readers and too easily satisfied to others. If a line is to be drawn between 'routine diagnosis' and 'research', there is no agreed principle deciding where it should be drawn. In this book, we have proposed what seem to us reasonable standards for routine diagnosis, but make no claim to have arrived at a generally acceptable system. We would like to think that in areas of neuropathology in which the dividing line between routine diagnosis and research is particularly ill-defined, our comments may encourage our readers to contribute to further knowledge by systematic study of their own material. Regarding research, we have worked on the assumption that the user of this book will have some research interests, which will be based on material acquired in the course of his diagnostic work. He will also probably be called on to do some teaching at graduate or undergraduate level. We would ask our readers to bear these points in mind if at times they feel that our recommendations are unduly fussy and demanding of time and effort.

This book will inevitably contain some errors in presenting the facts, and some questionable recommendations. We, the perpetrators, would be very grateful for the help of readers who take the trouble to point out our shortcomings. Magnifications accompanying illustrations in the book are, we believe, accurate to within 10%.

A working knowledge of the basic anatomy of the nervous system, including its wrappings, is assumed throughout. For those in doubt, the following works of reference may be recommended:

Brodal A. 1981. *Neurological Anatomy in Relation to Clinical Medicine*, 3rd edn. Oxford University Press, Oxford.

Carpenter, MD, Sutin J. 1983. *Human Neuroanatomy* (8th edn. of Strong OS, Elwyn A. *Human Neuroanatomy*). Williams and Wilkins, Baltimore and London.

For detailed descriptions of neuropathological states, we recommend:

Adams JH, Corsellis, JAN, Duchen LW (Eds). 1984. *Greenfield's Neuropathology*, 4th edn. Edward Arnold, London.

Russell DS, Rubinstein LJ. 1989. *Pathology of Tumours of the Nervous System*, 5th edn. Edward Arnold, London.

Burger, PC, Vogel FS. 1976. *Surgical Pathology of the Nervous System and its Coverings*. John Wiley, New York.

For more summary textbooks, we recommend:

Escourolle R, Poirier J. 1978. *Manual of Basic Neuropathology* (translated from the French by LJ Rubinstein). WB Saunders, Philadelphia.

Okazaki H. 1983. *Fundamentals of Neuropathology*, Igaku-Shoin, New York and Tokyo.

And for illustrated guides, the following:

Adams JH, Murray M. 1982. *Atlas of Post Mortem Techniques in Neuropathology*. Cambridge University Press, Cambridge.

Weller RO. 1984. *Colour Atlas of Neuropathology*. Oxford University Press, Oxford.

Barnard RO, Logue V, Reaves PS. 1976. *An Atlas of Tumours involving the Central Nervous System*. Baillière Tindall, London.

More specialized chapters, monographs and articles are referred to at the ends of the relevant chapters. In general, we have cited individual papers only when the information in them is not readily available in textbooks.

M. M. Esiri
D. R. Oppenheimer
Department of Neuropathology,
Radcliffe Infirmary,
Oxford, UK

Acknowledgements

For reading parts of the text, and in many cases providing illustrations, we express our thanks to Drs M. Al-Izzi, R. O. Barnard, J. V. Clark, P. Da Costa, L. Horton, J. T. Hughes, J. Keeling, D. McCormick, T. H. Moss, R. Menai-Williams, M. Rossi, A. Sheehan and M. Squier; and to Professors J. B. Cavanagh and B. Lake.

For invaluable assistance in the preparation of figures, we thank Miss P. Deacon, Miss J. Dyer, Mr D. Gardner, Mr J. Haywood, Mr G. Richardson and Mr D. Webster.

For preparation of most of the material used for photomicrography we are deeply indebted to the late Mr R. Beesley, Mr R. Cross, Miss P. Deacon, Miss H. Kidd and Miss M. Reading.

For permission to reproduce figures or tables originally published in other books or journals, we wish to thank the editors and/or publishers of the following:

Books

Autonomic Failure, Ed. R. Bannister, 2nd edn (1988), Oxford University Press, Oxford. (Figs 15.3, 15.5 and 15.6.)

Clinical Neurology, Eds M. Swash and J. Oxbury (1988), Churchill Livingstone, Edinburgh. (Fig. 14.4.)

Developmental Neuropathology, by R. Friede (1975), Springer, Berlin. (Table 21.1.)

Development of the Human Brain by F. Gilles, A. Leviton and E. Dooling (1983), PSG Publishing Company, Inc., Littleton, MA. (Table 21.2.)

Fetal and Neonatal Pathology, Ed. J. Keeling (1987), Springer, Berlin. (Figs 23.22 and 23.24.)

Gray's Anatomy, 36th edn (1980) Eds P. Williams and R. Warwick, Churchill Livingstone, Edinburgh. (Fig. 21.1.)

Greenfield's Neuropathology, 3rd edn (1976; Eds W. Blackwood and J. A. N. Corsellis) and 4th Edn (1984; Eds J. H. Adams, J. A. N. Corsellis and L. W. Duchen), Edward Arnold, London. (Figs 14.1, 14.16, 14.17, 15.1, 15.2, 15.8, 15.9, 15.11, 15.12, 15.13, 15.17 and 19.26.)

Handbook of Clinical Neurology, vol. 37 (1979). Eds P. J. Vinken and G. W. Bruyn. Elsevier/North Holland, Amsterdam. (Figs 20.2–20.4.)

Muscle Biopsy: a Practical Approach, by V. Dubowitz (1985), Baillière Tindall, London. (Tables 23.1 and 23.2.)

Pathology of Peripheral Nerve, by A. Asbury and P. Johnson (1978), WB Saunders, Philadelphia. (Fig. 22.2.)

Viral Diseases of the Central Nervous System, Ed. L. Illis (1975). Baillière Tindall, London. (Figs 17.12, 17.13, 17.14 and 17.16.)

Viral Encephalitis, by J. Booss and M. Esiri (1986), Blackwell Scientific Publications, Oxford. (Figs 10.2, 10.3, 10.4, 10.5, 10.21, 10.23, 10.25, 10.38, 10.39 and 10.40.)

Journals

Acta Neuropathologica, Berlin (Figs 13.30 and 13.34).

Brain (Figs 3.6b, 15.8a).

International Journal of Leprosy (Fig. 22.17).

Journal of Neurology, Neurosurgery and Psychiatry (Figs 3.27, 3.32, 7.24b, 15.1a, 22.5, 22.9 and 23.8).

Journal of the Neurological Sciences (Figs 10.4, 10.14, 10.15, 10.25, 12.23, 15.18, 20.7 and 23.31).

Neuropathology and Applied Neurobiology (Figs 2.20b and 19.14).

Quarterly Journal of Medicine (Figs 10.26, 10.28 and 10.30).

Chapter 1
The Post Mortem

This chapter is concerned only with points where the recommended procedures for neurological cases differ from routine methods.

Removal of the brain

The usual procedure is to reflect the scalp, and remove a cap of bone by a circumferential saw-cut. If this is carefully done, the dura will not be damaged, and will remain covering the brain. At this stage the superior longitudinal sinus is tested for patency either by opening it or more simply by running a fingertip along it and observing any movement of the contained blood.

If the brain is to be fixed by suspension from the basilar artery (see p.7), the dura is incised on each side and reflected medially, cutting through the bridging veins with scissors or knife (if they are torn, they may give rise to a false appearance of subdural or subarachnoid bleeding). The anterior attachment of the falx is divided, and the dura is reflected backwards. If fixation is to be by suspension from the dura of the vertex, the bridging veins are left intact, and the falx is divided with scissors both in front and behind, i.e. it is separated from the crista galli in front and from the tentorium behind.

The frontal lobes are gently lifted away from the floor of the anterior cranial fossa, leaving the olfactory bulbs attached to the brain if possible. The optic nerves, internal carotid arteries, pituitary stalk and oculomotor nerves are cut cleanly across close to the base, as they come into view. The tentorium is exposed, first on one side then on the other, by gently lifting the temporal lobes; and the attachments of the tentorium to the petrous temporal bones are cut with a sharp knife. The same cut will sever the roots of the trigeminal, facial and auditory nerves as they pierce the dura. It is important at this stage to retract the cerebral hemispheres as little as possible, as overstretching very easily results in tearing the midbrain (Fig. 1.1).

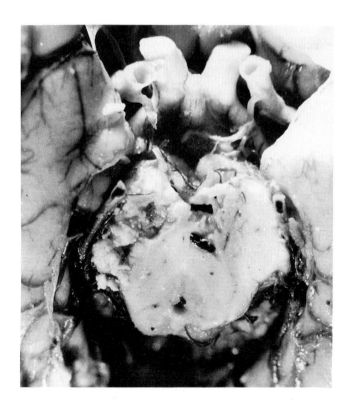

Fig. 1.1. Appearance, after formalin fixation, of a midbrain which has been torn during removal of the brain. (This happened to be a case of Parkinson's disease, in which the histology of the substantia nigra of the midbrain is of prime interest.)

In the gap which appears between the pons and the clivus, the abducent nerves are seen and cut. Not so clearly seen are the lower cranial nerves and the vertebral arteries, which are still holding the brain stem down. These must be cut, either with a knife or with long-bladed scissors, without damaging the lower brain stem. This can usually be carried out blind, but cutting as far as possible to each side. After the vertebral arteries have been cut the lower brain stem and upper cervical cord rise into view, and are cut across with the knife. All that remains to be cut after this is a number of bridging veins, including the great vein of Galen, which drains blood from the deeper cerebral grey matter into the straight sinus. During the whole performance, if the operator is holding the knife in his right hand, the brain should be supported by the left hand, and tension and distortion kept to a minimum. When the brain is free it should be placed, base upwards, in a suitably sized bowl rather than being laid on a flat surface.

There are many circumstances in which this routine has to be modified — too many, in fact, to be enumerated here. The most obvious ones are when the patient has undergone a neurosurgical operation. Often, of course, the neurosurgeon will welcome an invitation to come to the post mortem room and explore the outcome of his operation in person. In any case, it is important that the pathologist should have a clear grasp of what the surgeon has done, as well as of the clinical state before and after the operation. In cases where a ventriculo-atrial shunt has been carried out for the relief of obstructive hydrocephalus, it is best to explore the shunt mechanism before the cranium is opened. This entails finding the tube as it lies in the internal jugular vein (usually on the right side), cutting it, and testing the patency of the proximal and distal parts of the tube. Where there is a flushing device lying beneath the scalp overlying the burr-hole, a few squeezes should result in the escape of ventricular fluid from the proximal cut end.

In cases where high pressure in the posterior fossa has resulted in herniation of the lower medulla oblongata and cerebellar tonsils into the foramen magnum, the final severance of the brain from the spinal cord is hard to achieve without making an ugly oblique cut through the medulla itself; this, however, can usually be avoided by cautious manipulation. In any case, this cut, if it is performed from within the cranial cavity, will be an oblique one, reaching a lower level at the back of the cord than in front. If for some reason it is desirable to make a detailed anatomical study of structures near the junction of cord and medulla, it is best to make a *transverse* cut through the cord at the desired level before removing the brain.

Special care is needed in taking out *infants' brains*. Not only is the brain tissue itself softer and more friable but the leptomeninges are also very delicate; it is only too easy to drive an injudicious thumb through the cerebral cortex, or even to wipe a considerable area of cortex away from the rest of the brain. In some centres, the dangers of manipulation are reduced by removing the brain under water.

Preliminary inspection of the brain

If any serious anatomical study is contemplated, the brain should not be sliced before fixation. Because of the soft, soufflé-like consistency of the unfixed brain, it is impossible to make clean parallel cuts through it; when fresh-cut slices are fixed their surfaces are found to be irregular, wavy and pitted (Fig. 1.2). Unless a diagnosis is urgently needed, the examination of the brain at post mortem should be confined to significant surface features — in particular, features associated with brain swelling, such as flattening of cerebral convolutions and marks of tentorial or foraminal herniation (see p.9). Cautious palpation may disclose softenings due to infarction or tumour, or less often hardenings due to tumours, or to scarring, or to oddities such as tuberous sclerosis. Such hardenings are much more difficult to detect after fixation.

A firm diagnosis of *multiple sclerosis* (MS) can often be made without cutting into the brain, from the presence of clearly-defined grey patches on the surface of the pons, or on the cut surfaces of the optic nerves (Fig. 14.1).

The presence of frank pus in the subarachnoid space clearly calls for swabs and specimens for bacteriology. In cases of subacute or chronic meningitis the changes are generally far less striking, and to the naked eye may be identical with those of diffuse malignant spread. In case of doubt, a couple of wet films stained with, say, methylene blue and Gram's stain, will quickly make the distinction (for method, see p.70).

Blood in the subarachnoid space is best cleared away before fixation (see p.98), after noting where it seems to be coming from — a contused surface, or a ruptured aneurysm, or the exit foramina of the fourth ventricle. Aneurysms, in particular, should be dissected free of their surroundings while the vessels from which they arise are still supple.

In cases of proven or suspected *meningitis* or *encephalitis*, and in various other conditions, one may wish to collect samples of cerebrospinal fluid (CSF), preferably uncontaminated by blood. Clear CSF may be obtained, before removal of the brain, by aspiration with a hollow needle from an anterior or posterior horn of a lateral ventricle. However, if the hemispheres are swollen, this may be both ineffectual and disruptive. Ventricular fluid may be obtained from the fourth ventricle by gentle compression of the brain, and from the spinal subarachnoid space by tilting the lower spinal column upward after the brain is removed.

Dissection of the skull

After removing the brain, and noting any abnormalities in the dura at the base of the cranial cavity, the principal

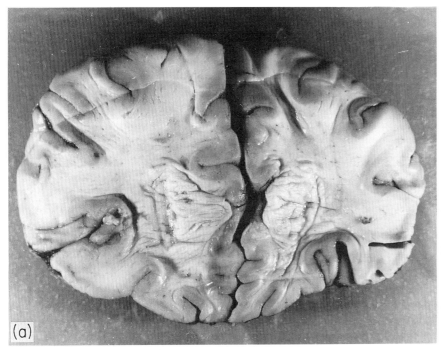
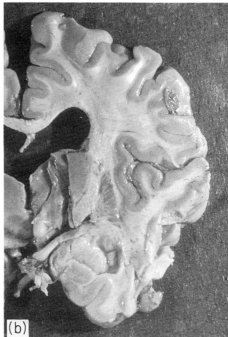

Fig. 1.2. Appearance, after fixation, of brain which has been sliced fresh.

venous sinuses (straight, lateral, sigmoid, superior longitudinal) are checked for patency. In cases of head injury the dura is stripped to reveal fractures at the base of the skull. For examining the internal carotid arteries, and at the same time the ear-drums and middle ears, a hammer and a 2 cm chisel are used. The chisel is applied to the floor of the middle cranial fossa at the point shown in Fig. 1.3; a sharp blow with the hammer will then display the middle ear and ear-drum, and the internal carotid artery lying within the carotid canal, whence it can be followed into the wall of the cavernous sinus. The frontal and ethmoidal sinuses (and after removal of the pituitary, the sphenoid sinus) are similarly opened and displayed.

A specimen containing the *pituitary* and portions of the second to sixth *cranial nerves*, including the gasserian ganglia, can be obtained with a de Soutter vibrating saw, applied in the planes indicated in Fig. 1.3. The block can be fixed and dissected at leisure, with the anatomical relations perfectly preserved. A more thorough examination of the *optic nerves* is desirable in cases with a suspected diagnosis of MS. For this, the simplest procedure is to remove the thin bony roofs of the orbits with bone forceps and nibblers, incise the soft tissues anteriorly, and cut carefully down until the eyeball is reached. The optic nerve is severed just behind the globe, and the remaining orbital contents are dissected away from the globe and from the bone of the orbit, back to the optic foramen. The specimen containing optic nerve, external ocular muscles, oculomotor nerve and ciliary ganglion, all embedded in fat, can be fixed for later dissection, with very little distortion.

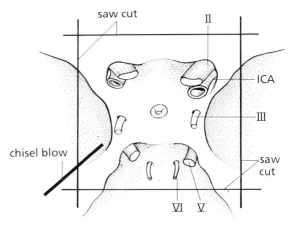

Fig. 1.3. Removal of sphenoid block, using the vibrating saw. For the anterior cut, the saw is directed downward and backward; for the lateral cuts, downward and medially; and for the posterior cut, forward through the clivus. If the cuts are deep enough, the block is easily detached. The thicker line on the left of the picture indicates the site where a chisel blow will expose the carotid canal and the middle ear, displacing the ridge of the petrous temporal bone backward. ICA = internal carotid artery; II = optic nerve; III = oculomotor nerve; V = trigeminal nerve; VI = abducent nerve. The block includes the pituitary gland, the cavernous sinus and the gasserian (trigeminal) ganglia.

Removal of the spinal cord

If this is to be performed in the post mortem room, the cord can be approached either from behind or from the front. For the *posterior approach*, the sacrospinal muscle mass is cleared away from neck to sacrum and the exposed vertebral laminae are sawn through, using either an electric vibrating saw, which is quicker, or a hand-saw, which is very much safer if the cord is not to be damaged. Directions for the saw-cuts are shown in Fig. 1.4. The cuts are directed forward and slightly inward, starting about 2 cm from the midline on each side. A rather narrower margin is adequate for the thoracic region. Provided that the spine is straight and symmetrical, the result will be that a bony strip, consisting of the vertebral spines and the medial halves of the laminae, will lift backward, leaving the spinal dura (theca) exposed. If the saw-cuts are too lateral, the bone will need to be cut away with bone shears — a safe but laborious procedure. If the saw-cuts are too medial, the saw will make its embarrassing way into the substance of the cord. If, as often

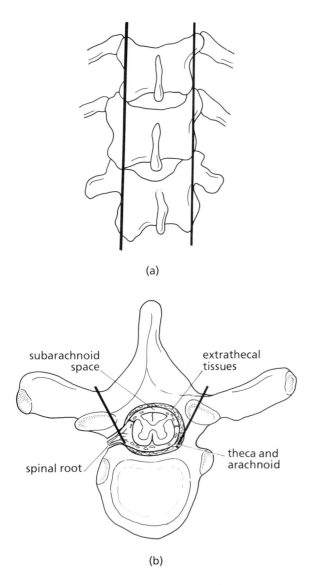

(a)

(b)

Fig. 1.4. Posterior approach to the spinal cord. The drawings indicate the position and angulation of the saw-cuts.

happens, there is some degree of scoliosis, there is a danger of entering the cord on one side while failing to enter the spinal canal on the other. If X-rays are available, they may help in avoiding this mishap.

When the theca is exposed, a decision must be made as to whether any *sensory ganglia* need to be examined (for instance, particular ganglia require to be looked at in cases of herpes zoster). These can be found in the intervertebral foramina by exploration with knife and nibbler, and left attached to the cord by their nerve roots. In a case of tabes dorsalis or of Friedreich's ataxia, several lumbar and cervical ganglia should be preserved. In extracting the cord, the main concern should be to avoid undue kinking, which alone can cause considerable damage. The lower end of the theca can be secured with artery forceps, and the cord lifted gently backwards, cutting nerve roots on each side from below upward. After extraction the cord must not be curled up or subjected to pressure. If its length makes fixation difficult, it should be divided into two or even three sections by clean transverse knife-cuts made after opening the dura; cutting the cord within the dura will cause damage by compression.

The other standard method of removing the cord is *from in front*, after clearing away the thoracic and abdominal viscera. If it is desired to examine the sympathetic chains, this is the moment to remove them. They come into view after stripping away the pleura and peritoneum, running up and down at the level of the exit foramina of the spinal nerves. Saw-cuts are made immediately in front of these, in a coronal plane. These cuts, if well placed, will expose the anterior surface of the dura as well as numerous nerve-roots and ganglia. This anterior approach is preferable if multiple spinal ganglia are wanted. It also entails less risk of damage to the cord than the posterior approach.

An alternative to both these methods, and one which is used routinely in Oxford, is to *remove the entire vertebral column* and extract the spinal cord after fixation. The approach is from the front. Oblique saw-cuts are made, separating the sacrum from the iliac bones, and through the vertebral ends of the ribs. The vertebral column is lifted forward, and separated from the skin of the back with a long knife. Finally, it is detached from the skull with knife-cuts through the atlanto-occipital joints. This involves inserting the sharp tip of a stout knife into these joints at just the right point and just the right angle. The manoeuvre requires skill and practice. The young pathologist, if in a hurry, is well advised to leave the joints in peace and saw blithely through the atlas vertebra. Little if any damage will result, except to the vertebral arteries. A broom handle, or similar piece of wood, is cut to an appropriate length and the upper end is tapered to fit tightly into the foramen magnum. The advantages of this method are that the time consumed in the post mortem room is much shortened, and the final dissection can be performed at leisure; the cord is kept safe from damage and distortion during fixation; and the resulting specimen includes all the spinal ganglia and both sympathetic chains, as far upward as the stellate ganglia, and the intravertebral parts of the vertebral arteries. The disadvantage, in some quarters, may lie in the need for a competent and cooperative post mortem room attendant.

Dissection of the neck

It is often desirable to study nerves, ganglia, muscles and blood vessels from deep in the neck. This is difficult if the skin incision is the one most commonly used in Britain — that is, in the midline from the larynx downwards. The alternative is a V- or U-shaped incision, running from the mastoid processes down to the upper end of the sternum. The skin flap is reflected upward, giving easy access to the anterior and posterior triangles of the neck. We recommend this approach for all cases of cerebral vascular disease, as it affords access to the *internal carotid arteries* up to their entry into the skull; also for cases with suspected peripheral neuropathy, in which the lower cranial nerves may be involved. The following procedure is suggested:

1 Expose the *sterno-mastoid* muscle, from which samples may be taken for transverse and longitudinal sections from the middle of its length, where the spinal accessory nerve penetrates its deep surface; then reflect the cut ends upward and downward.

2 Identify the intermediate tendon of the *digastric muscle*, which runs through a fibrous pulley attached to the hyoid bone (Fig. 1.5). The pulley is slit open, and the muscle is retracted by an artery forceps applied to the tendon. The anterior belly, going to the chin, and the posterior belly, going to the mastoid process in company with the stylohyoid, can be cleaned without damage to muscle tissue, and detached from their bony attachments and kept for histology if required.

3 Expose and explore the *carotid sheath*, which contains the common and internal carotid arteries, the internal jugular vein and the *vagus* nerve. Follow the vagus upward to the skull, and expose its *inferior ganglion*, which is a fairly conspicuous swelling. The glossopharyngeal and accessory nerves emerge close to the vagus; just behind these, lying ensheathed in loose connective tissue on the surface of the prevertebral muscles, is the *superior cervical ganglion* — the topmost, and much the largest, element in the sympathetic chain (Fig. 1.6). Following the chain downward, one comes to the middle cervical ganglion, and below this, just below the point where the *vertebral artery* disappears into the spinal column, is the *inferior cervical ganglion*, which is often fused with the *stellate ganglion*. In any case of autonomic failure, a portion of the vagus, including its inferior ganglion, and the superior cervical and stellate ganglia, should be examined histologically; if facilities for histochemistry are available, specimens of these may be deep-

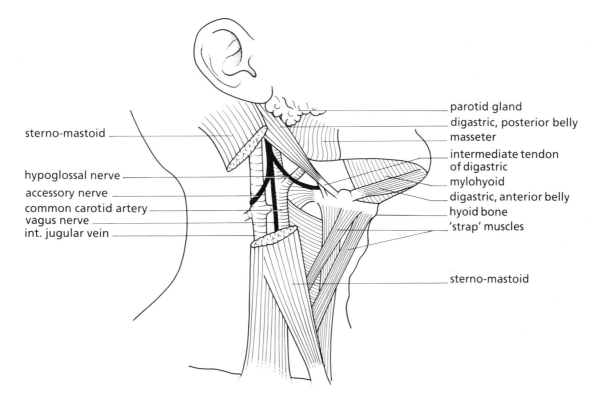

Fig. 1.5. Dissection of the neck. Relations of sterno-mastoid and digastric muscles with deeper structures. The submandibular gland and lymph nodes have been removed.

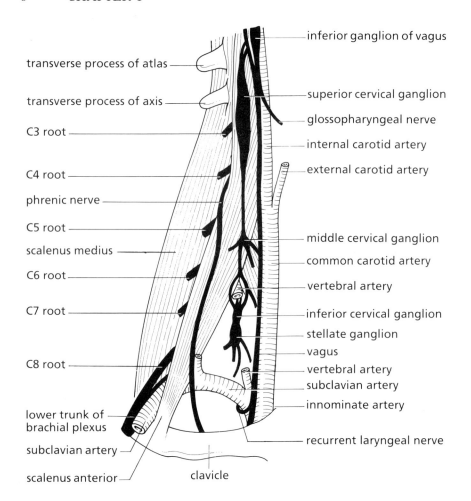

Fig. 1.6. Deeper dissection of the neck showing relations of the lower cranial nerves with the sympathetic chain and ganglia.

frozen. Since some cases of progressive autonomic failure suffer from laryngeal palsy, the *larynx* should also be taken for later dissection. Of the remaining cranial nerves, the *glossopharyngeal* is found running between the internal carotid artery and the internal jugular vein on its way to the pharynx, and the *hypoglossal* follows a similar course on its way to the tongue, looping around the internal carotid close to the inferior ganglion of the vagus.

4   Examine the *carotids*. In general, the common carotids are found to be free of atheroma; the trouble begins at the bifurcation, in particular at the bulbous lower end of the internal carotid, where turbulence is presumably at its greatest.

Muscles and nerves

In cases suspected of neuropathy or neuromuscular disease, the minimum requirements are the spinal cord, with anterior and posterior nerve roots, and samples of nerve and muscle from the neck and from proximal and distal parts of upper and lower limbs. For muscles innervated from the brain stem we recommend the *digastric* (anterior belly supplied by the trigeminal, posterior belly by the facial nerve), the

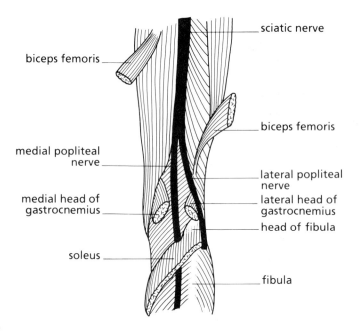

Fig. 1.7. Dissection of popliteal fossa.

sterno-mastoid (accessory nerve) and the *tongue* (hypoglossal nerve). In the choice of *nerves*, it is better to avoid those that are apt to be traumatized during life, such as the median nerve at the wrist and the sciatic nerve in the buttock. The main nerves of the *upper arm* — median, ulnar and radial — are better protected, and easy of access. For the *lower limb*, the femoral nerve is readily accessible in the abdomen as it emerges from the psoas muscle, and the medial and lateral popliteal nerves are easy to find in the popliteal fossa (Fig. 1.7). More distally, the *sural nerve* lies beneath the skin just behind the lateral malleolus (Fig. 1.8). This slender nerve, which is almost purely sensory, provides control material for sural biopsies.

For the *hand*, an incision such as that shown in Fig. 1.9 gives access to the muscles of the thenar and hypothenar eminences, lumbricals and interossei, as well as to the distal branches of the median and ulnar nerves. The short hand

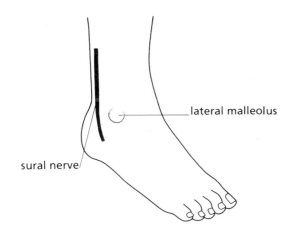

Fig. 1.8. Position of sural nerve.

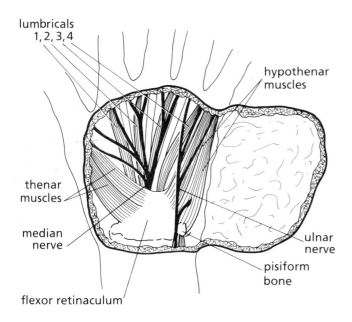

Fig. 1.9. Dissection of the palm of the hand.

muscles supply useful material for the study of motor endplates, and of muscle spindles, with which they are richly supplied.

In taking specimens of muscle it is important to take an adequate (3 cm or more) length, and to avoid trauma and distortion, so that accurately oriented transverse and longitudinal sections can be examined histologically. If part of a long muscle is taken, this should be from somewhere near the motor point, which is generally near the middle of the muscle belly.

Fixation of specimens

If the *brain* is to be fixed entire, it must on no account be left resting on the bottom of a hard container. Not only does this cause distortion, it also prevents the fixative from reaching the tissue where it is in contact with the floor. The most usual procedure is to *suspend* the brain in a plastic bucket, where it remains for at least two weeks. A hook or a loop of string is passed between the pons and the basilar artery, which is normally strong enough to support the weight of the brain *in water*, though not in air. If the basilar artery is diseased or damaged, pieces of string may be passed around two or more other basal arteries. An alternative, causing less distortion of the brain stem, is to suspend the brain topside upwards, by means of a few stitches passing through the dura of the vertex, which is left attached when the brain is removed. Whatever the method, suspension is from a loop of string running between the ends of the bucket handle. Plastic curtain hooks are preferable to pieces of wire or safety pins, which deposit rust, and are more apt to tear through the basilar artery. Once in its bucket, the brain should be left there, and not carried about, as minor accelerations may cause tearing of the artery.

If *biochemical* or *enzyme studies* are planned, selected portions of the brain can be excised at post mortem and put without delay into a low-temperature freezer. In some cases multiple sites in the brain may undergo biochemical investigation, and the results tabulated alongside the histological findings in the corresponding areas on the other side. The brain is cautiously bisected, passing a long, sharp knife through the corpus callosum and other cerebral commissures and splitting the hindbrain as near as possible to the midline. One-half of the brain is then frozen; the other half is either suspended in formalin or placed, resting on its medial cut surface, on a thick layer of cotton wool in a container, and periodically lifted and replaced over the next few days.

Diffusion of fixing fluid into normal brain tissue is rapid enough to ensure good fixation throughout; but this is not so when there are areas of *oedema*. Unless special precautions are taken, a swollen brain, when it is sliced, may contain areas (in particular the lentiform nucleus and centrum ovale) which are almost liquid, look like toothpaste and have a sour smell due to post mortem bacterial growth.

The most effective precaution is to make a slit in the corpus callosum, to ensure that the fixative reaches the interior of the hemispheres from the lateral ventricles. If one suspects blockages at the interventricular foramina, the insertion of a scalpel blade for a few millimetres in the midline between the mamillary bodies ensures access of fixative to the third ventricle. Another fixation artefact is attributable to leaving the brain unfixed at room temperature for many hours. The inner parts are invaded by gas-forming anaerobic bacteria, giving rise to the so-called Swiss cheese artefact (Fig. 2.18).

If the *spinal cord* is taken out at post mortem, it should be suspended in, for instance, a tall measuring cylinder filled with formalin, preferably with a weight attached to the theca at the lower end. This is because the theca tends to shrink longitudinally in the fixative, while the cord does not. As a result, the cord may buckle in many places and in the end look like a giant caterpillar. If the tall jar is not available no harm is done if the cord is divided by a clean transverse cut.

For reliable fixation of the whole *vertebral column*, there must be access of fixative to all parts of the subarachnoid space. This is hindered by tumours in the cord or elsewhere in the vertebral canal, and also by inflammatory exudates in the subarachnoid space. One precaution is to make a clean transverse cut through the whole specimen. This may be a necessary procedure if a fixing tank of sufficient length is not available. An alternative is to nibble away one of the thoracic spines and adjacent laminae, expose and incise the theca, and slit the underlying arachnoid before plunging the specimen into the tank.

Specimens of *muscle* and *nerve* should be laid, as soon as they are taken, on pieces of stiff card, on which their provenance is written with a grease pencil. They are left undisturbed for a few minutes, during which their natural juices congeal and act as a glue, thus preserving the orientation of the specimens. It is very difficult to obtain true transverse and longitudinal sections from specimens which have lain free in fixative. Pinning the specimens to a cork mat guards against later drift. This can be achieved using hedgehog quills, which, although not easy to obtain, do not rust.

Method for hydrocephalic children

Before examining the viscera, the skin is incised in the midline down the back. The incision is carried to the mastoid process on one side, then continued over the vertex to the opposite mastoid process. The anterior part of the scalp is reflected forward as far as the eyebrows and zygomatic processes. This entails cutting through the external auditory meatuses. The posterior part of the scalp is reflected sideways and the suboccipital muscles removed. Now the vertebral column is mobilized, cutting or sawing through the sacro-iliac joints and rib attachments. The column is dissected

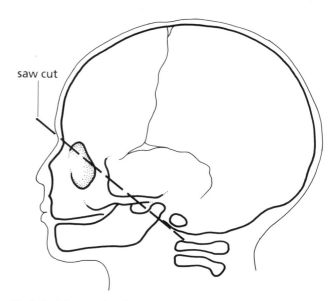

Fig. 1.10. Diagram showing direction of the saw-cut separating the vault of the skull from the bones of the face. Care must be taken to avoid damage to the eyeballs. The cut should barely graze the undersurfaces of the temporal lobes.

away from the soft tissues and displaced backward until the occipital bone immediately in front of the foramen magnum is exposed.

The orbital contents are dissected free from the roofs of the orbits and displaced downward. A saw-cut is then made in a plane passing from the orbital roofs to the angle between the occipital bone and the body of the atlas vertebra (Fig. 1.10). After this, the cranium and vertebral column, with their contents, come away as a single specimen, leaving the face and eyes behind. If the saw-cut is accurately performed, it may graze but will not seriously damage the lower surfaces of the temporal lobes. The subsequent reconstruction involves sewing up the scalp and stuffing it with some kind of wadding. If this is carefully done, the appearance of the child's head is often less horrifying than it was during life. Finally, the viscera are extracted backward and examined. The vertebral column is replaced with a length of wood.

The object of this manoeuvre is to avoid the usual combination of distortion and disruption attendant on the attempt to extract a hydrocephalic brain. For fixation, the vertebral column may be cut transversely below the level of a Chiari malformation (see p.252) of the cerebellar tonsils. If there is a meningomyelocele, i.e. a backward protrusion of cord, nerve roots and meninges through a defect in the bony column (spina bifida), this will be included in the specimen. For good fixation, formalin should be introduced into the ventricular system. This can be done with a large syringe and hollow needle, either through a fontanelle or through the exposed temporal lobes. Some caution is needed here as the blown-out cerebral hemispheres have a tendency to fall inward away from the skull.

Causes of death

The pathologist who has just completed a post mortem may be faced with two questions: (i) What was the patient's underlying disease? (ii) What was the immediate cause of death? The answer to the first may have been clear from the start; or it may take a couple of months to decide; or it may never be found. To the second question — why did the patient die when he did? — an immediate answer may be required, for a coroner's report, or for a cremation certificate. The finding of a blocked coronary artery, or of broncho-pneumonia, or of an intracranial haemorrhage, may supply a ready answer, but the pathologist is well aware that all these are compatible with continued life. On occasion, after reading the clinical notes, he may conclude that the principal cause of death was the patient's lack of desire to go on living. In such cases his answer to the coroner will be determined by common sense rather than by physiological expertise.

Sometimes the immediate cause of death is obvious from an inspection of the brain — in particular of the brain stem, in which the so-called vital centres are lodged. There may be a fresh pontine haemorrhage, or a thrombosed basilar artery. Commoner than either of these is some form of *internal herniation* causing distortion, haemorrhage or ischaemia in the upper or lower brain stem.

Tentorial herniation

This is the commonest type of herniation. It occurs at the tentorial opening, usually as a result of swelling of one or both cerebral hemispheres. The swelling may be caused by haemorrhage, or oedema, or tumour. Other causes of trans-tentorial herniation are compression from massive blood clots in the epidural or subdural compartments, and acute or subacute hydrocephalus from blocking of the flow of CSF through the ventricular system. The effects differ according to whether the space-occupying lesion is on one side or both, and whether it is in front or behind. When both hemispheres are affected the diencephalon — thalamus and subthalamic region — is thrust downward into the posterior fossa (see Fig. 2.8); at the same time the medial parts of the temporal lobes — unci and parahippocampal gyri — are thrust medially and downward over the tentorial edge, causing a mixture of downthrust and side-to-side compression of the midbrain and upper pons (see Fig. 2.9). At post mortem the visible effects of this sequence are (i) flattening of the cerebral convolutions, with diminution of the sub-arachnoid spaces, and (ii) deep grooving of the under surfaces of the *parahippocampal gyri* (see Figs 2.8–2.10). (Note that a shallow groove is normally present about 4 mm from the tip of each uncus (see Fig. 2.8a): it is caused by the edge of the tentorium, but does not indicate raised pressure.)

When cerebral swelling or compression is predominantly one-sided, grooving of the parahippocampal gyrus is deeper, and involves a greater area of the gyrus, on that side. The *mamillary bodies* are visibly displaced towards the opposite side. Not uncommonly, the midbrain is displaced strongly enough to cause bruising of the opposite cerebral peduncle from pressure against the free edge of the tentorium (see Fig. 2.10). During this process, branches of the posterior cerebral artery may be pinched on *either* side, causing infarction (usually haemorrhagic) of a large area on the inferior surface of the temporal lobe and of the visual cortex.

Bilateral swelling in the anterior part of the cerebrum results in backward displacement of the diencephalon, and herniation of the *unci*, which pinch the cerebral peduncles between them (see Fig. 2.9b). When the swelling is more posterior, the herniated parahippocampal gyri similarly pinch the tegmentum of the midbrain. A further effect of posterior swelling is that pressure is exerted on the upper surface of the tentorium. This reduces the amount of trans-tentorial herniation, but increases congestion in the posterior fossa. A common result is that a *foraminal* hernia is added to the tentorial one.

Foraminal herniation

The foramen magnum is approached from above by way of a conical basin, in which the lower medulla, flanked by the cerebellar tonsils, normally lies in a capacious bath of CSF, the *cisterna magna*. When increased congestion in the posterior fossa drives these structures downward, the bath empties, and unless the pressure is relieved herniation ensues. Medulla and tonsils are impacted in the foramen, and are moulded by the surrounding bone into a conical shape, which has given rise to the popular term 'coning' for the whole pathological process (see Fig. 2.15).

Clinical concomitants

The clinical concomitants of these two types of herniation are different. The cardinal signs of impending death from tentorial herniation are a lowering level of consciousness, rising blood pressure, stertorous or Cheyne–Stokes breathing, and loss of pupillary reflexes, leading to a fixed, dilated pupil, first on one side, later on both sides. This last feature has been attributed by some to compression of the oculomotor nerves by herniated unci; however, in most cases a more plausible explanation is that as the midbrain is forced downward, the oculomotor nerves become *kinked* as they cross the posterior cerebral arteries which, being teth-ered, cannot move downward. Such kinking can sometimes be observed at post mortem; but if the brain is fixed by suspension from the basilar artery, kinking occurs as a normal post mortem artefact.

Acute foraminal herniation, such as can occur from an

injudicious lumbar puncture in the presence of raised pressure in the posterior fossa, can be horrifyingly sudden in its effects. Breathing and heart-beat stop, and the patient is lifeless within seconds. When the process is more gradual, a common effect is the onset of pulmonary oedema, probably attributable to vagal irritation. This may give rise to a form of positive feedback, since impaired gas exchange causes hypercapnia and hypoxaemia, which in turn give rise to brain swelling.

Reverting to the coroner's question regarding the cause of death, we wish to record that the coroners with whom we have had dealings have been reasonable and kindly men, who wish to conclude their enquiries as quickly and painlessly as possible. In a case where poisoning is one of the possibilities, they will wait for the necessary investigations to be carried out. In a case of fatal road traffic accident, they will want a quick, easily intelligible report, rather than a detailed account of anatomical and physiological events following

Table 1.1. Recommended selection of specimens to be taken at post mortem, after consulting the clinical notes

Type of disease	What to take away
Primary brain tumours (most cases)	Brain
Dementia and psychosis (if no suspicion of CJD)	Brain‡
Epilepsy	Brain
Malformation of brain	Brain
Perinatal brain damage	Brain
Parkinsonism	Brain‡
Brain tumours with clinical evidence of spread via CSF pathways	Brain and spinal cord
Medulloblastoma	Brain and spinal cord
Meningitis	Brain and spinal cord*, serum, CSF
Encephalitis	Brain and spinal cord*, serum, CSF
CNS degenerations not affecting PNS	Brain and spinal cord
Myelopathies, all types	Brain and spinal cord
Multiple sclerosis	Brain and spinal cord†
Metabolic disorders	Brain, cord, peripheral nerves and ganglia‡
Degenerations involving PNS and CNS	Brain, cord, peripheral nerves and ganglia‡
Autonomic failure	Brain, cord, peripheral nerves and ganglia‡
Peripheral neuropathies	Brain, cord, nerves, ganglia and muscles
Myasthenia gravis	Brain, cord, nerves, ganglia and muscles
Motor neuron diseases	Brain, cord, nerves, ganglia and muscles
Head trauma	Brain, cervical spine
Cervical spondylosis	Brain, cervical spine
Cerebral vascular disease	Brain, heart, neck arteries
Vascular disease of cord	Spinal column, aorta
Friedreich's ataxia	Brain, cord, heart, sensory ganglia and nerves
Tuberous sclerosis	Brain, heart, kidney
Intoxications, including Reye's syndrome	Brain, cord, nerves, liver, kidneys‡
Congenital hydrocephalus	Brain and spinal column (see also p.8)
Hypopituitarism	Sphenoid block (see p.3)
Pituitary and parapituitary tumours	Sphenoid block
Ataxia−telangiectasia	Brain, spleen, lymph nodes, gonad, pituitary, sensory ganglia

* include specimens for microbiology.
† take optic nerves.
‡ consider keeping tissue for freezing.

CJD Creutzfeldt−Jakob disease.
PNS peripheral nervous system.

the injury. They may even be satisfied with the statement that the cause of death was a fracture of the skull.

We do not wish to moralize on these matters, but we would suggest that in such cases it would serve the cause of veracity, without causing unnecessary confusion, if the immediate cause of death was given as compression and distortion of the brain stem, with supplementary information on the causes of such fatal distortions. These causes may not be clear until the brain has been dissected, preferably after fixation; but fatal herniations at the tentorial opening and the foramen magnum are generally obvious if they are looked for as soon as the brain is taken out of the cranium. These are discussed in more detail in the next chapter.

Use of clinical information

Most pathology departments have a standard form on which the main post mortem findings and the final diagnoses are entered. Such forms usually have a space — sometimes regrettably small — for a summary of the patient's clinical history, along with details of relevant investigations. There is no need to dwell here on the general usefulness of such clinical summaries, or on the advantages of conveying as much relevant information in as few words as possible. It is worth pointing out, however, that the neuropathologist, unlike the general pathologist, is often faced with a delay of weeks or months between the post mortem and the cut-up, and may need to be reminded of the points on which he is expected to find an answer. Once the clinical notes have been returned to the Records Department it may be a little difficult to retrieve them. When cutting the brain from a case of MS it is irritating if one does not know whether the patient could walk or see, or hold an intelligible conversation. In short, the clinical summary should give clear indications of the problems to be solved (see Table 1.1).

In neurosurgical cases, it is usually prudent to keep hold of the relevant X-rays and computerized axial tomography (CAT) scans up to the time of cutting-up. In this and in many other respects, friendly relations with the neurosurgeons are of great importance.

Chapter 2
The Cut-up

Dissection of the fixed brain

A brain should be left soaking in formalin for 3 weeks or more. If it is sliced after a fortnight, no harm will be done, but the uneven colours seen on the cut surfaces usually betray incomplete fixation, and the inner tissues will not be ready for histological examination. Photography, too, will give unsatisfactory pictures. As it is advisable to have one's camera ready before starting on the dissection, a word on *equipment* will be inserted here.

We use a single-lens reflex 35 mm camera, with a 5 cm lens and extension rings for close-up photography. Using two camera backs, one can alternate readily between monochrome and colour film. The camera is mounted on a copying stand, with movable lamps on each side (Fig. 2.1), and kept close to the cutting-up bench.

Before examination, the brain should be washed in running water for at least 2 hours, and left soaking overnight. Many pathologists have lived to regret the casual attitude to formalin vapour of their earlier days. It is probably advisable to give the brain an extra wash after making the first cut into the ventricular system, especially if the specimen is hydrocephalic and contains a large reservoir of formalin. Formalin also affects the skin, and rubber gloves should always be worn when handling fixed tissues.

Superficial features

Features which may call for photography before slicing include such things as tumours, old infarcts, aneurysms, signs of tentorial or foraminal herniation, cerebral cortical atrophy (either generalized or localized, as in Pick's disease, Fig. 17.4), relative atrophy of the brain stem, as in ponto-cerebellar atrophy (Fig. 15.7), or hypertrophy, as in diffuse astrocytomatous infiltration (Fig. 12.3). Some dissection is needed before slicing in order to expose aneurysms of the middle cerebral artery, lying in the lateral fissure, or of the anterior communicating artery, between the two gyri recti.

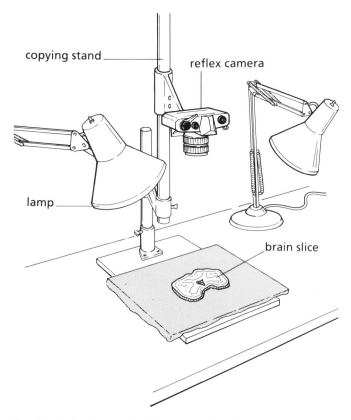

copying stand

reflex camera

lamp

brain slice

Fig. 2.1. A simple set-up for photography of specimens.

Key to Figs 2.2 to 2.6

Cerebral gyri

ang	angular
cing	cingulate
cun	cuneus
fus	fusiform (occipito-temporal)
gr	g. rectus
if	inferior (third) frontal
ilo	inf. lateral occipital
ins	insula
ip	inf. parietal lobule
it	inf. (third) temporal
lin	lingual
lo	lateral orbital
mf	middle (second) frontal
mo	medial orbital
mt	middle (second) temporal
occ	occipital gyri
ph	parahippocampal
post	postcentral (sensory)
pre	precentral (motor)
precun	precuneus
sf	superior (first) frontal
slo	sup. lateral occipital
sm	supramarginal
sp	sup. parietal lobule
st	sup. (first) temporal
trans	transverse (Heschl's)

Central grey matter

am	amygdaloid nucleus
c	caudate nucleus
cl	claustrum
gp	globus pallidus
hip	hippocampus
hyp	hypothalamus
lgb	lat. geniculate body
mam	mamillary body
p	putamen
rn	red nucleus
sn	substantia nigra
sub	subthalamic nucleus
t	thalamus

Central white matter

ac	anterior commissure
cc	corpus callosum
f	fornix
ic	internal capsule

Other features

aq	aqueduct
CALC	calcarine sulcus
CENT	central (Rolandic) sulcus
cereb	cerebellum
ch pl	choroid plexus
LAT	lateral (sylvian) fissure
lat vent	lateral ventricle
olf	olfactory tract
ot	optic tract
ox	optic chiasm
PO	parieto-occipital sulcus
vent 3	third ventricle

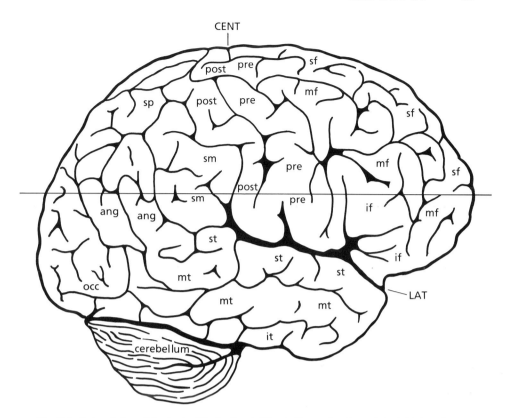

Fig. 2.2. Lateral view of the brain. The horizontal line indicates the plane of the initial cut for horizontal slicing.

This involves a little disruption of cortical tissue, of no great consequence, but one should watch out for local brown staining by blood pigments, i.e. evidence of earlier haemorrhages. Such superficial staining should also be looked for in the brains of epileptics, especially in the anterior temporal, orbital and frontal regions (Fig. 18.2).

The main *arteries* of the brain should be examined at an early stage. The *circle of Willis* is inspected before or after fixation, and its pattern noted (for normal pattern see Fig. 7.12). In cases of stroke, emboli may be found, the commonest sites being the bifurcation of an internal carotid artery, and the origin of a branch of a middle cerebral artery. Sites of atheromatous narrowing should be noted, and transverse scalpel cuts made in identified vessels to test for occlusion. If old or recent softenings are revealed in slicing the brain, an attempt should be made to relate these either to occluded arteries or to the border zones between arterial territories (see Chapter 7; Figs 7.11—7.20).

A special case calling for preliminary dissection is when there is a history of speech disturbance or hearing loss attributable to a cerebral vascular accident. The auditory cortex, consisting mainly of Heschl's gyri, and Wernicke's speech area, centred on the posterior third of the left first temporal gyrus, can be exposed by cutting the arachnoid covering the lateral fissure, and cleanly amputating the temporal lobe (Fig. 25.4; see p.380). After photography the temporal lobe may be replaced and sliced along with the rest of the cerebrum.

Slicing

The *first incision* is normally the one separating the hind-brain (brain stem and cerebellum) from the cerebral hemispheres. This should be made by a clean transverse cut across the midbrain, at right angles to the long axis of the brain stem (Figs 2.2–2.4). It is easier to see what one is doing after cutting the arachnoid overlying the cerebral peduncles. It is bad practice to make two separate oblique cuts through the cerebral peduncles, as this makes it almost impossible to examine the anatomy of the midbrain, tegmentum and subthalamic region.

It is customary to *weigh* the brain before slicing. If one wants to compare the weights of the two hemispheres — for instance, when one hemisphere is relatively swollen by tumour or oedema, or relatively shrunken from old trauma or infarction — they can be separated without damage by gently cutting through arachnoid attachments and making a midline incision in the corpus callosum from above, followed by midline cuts through the optic chiasm, hypothalamus, anterior and posterior commissures, and interthalamic connexus. The hemispheres can then be sliced together or separately.

For slicing, we use a long (40 cm or so), not too flexible, knife, a linoleum-covered cutting board, and pairs of L-shaped stainless steel guides, 1 cm and 0.5 cm thick respectively. In Oxford, two alternative planes of slicing are used: coronal and horizontal. For *coronal slicing* we make the first

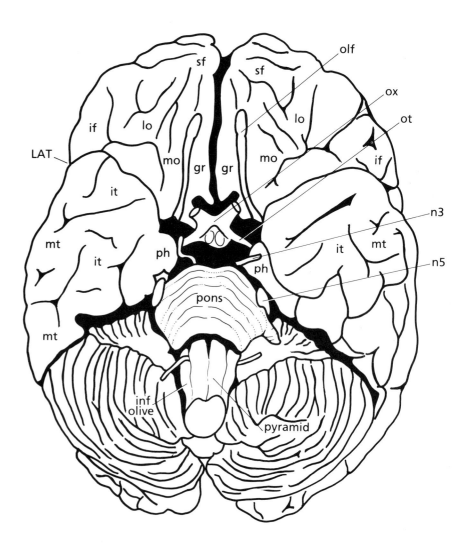

Fig. 2.3. Base of the brain.

cut through the mamillary bodies, passing through the anterior margin of the thalamus. The anterior part of the cerebrum is then placed, cut surface down, between a pair of centimetre guides, and successive slices taken at centimetre intervals and laid out, posterior surface upward, with the right side on the right. The procedure is repeated with the posterior part. For convenience in description, the slices are numbered; slices in front of the initial cut are A1, A2, A3, etc., progressing forward, and those behind it are P1, P2, P3, etc., progressing backward. Because of variations in size and proportions between one brain and another, the structures seen in slices A1 and P1 will be almost the same in all brains, the correspondence becoming progressively less in subsequent slices. When giving an anteroposterior *level*, the posterior aspect of the slice is referred to; thus the mamillary bodies are always level A1 (Fig. 2.5).

To produce accurate centimetre-thick slices, a little practice is needed. Assuming that the knife is held in the right hand, the blade is directed to the left and slightly downward, and the left palm holds the left side of the specimen down. If the blade is directed upward the knife will ride upward, and the slice will be too thick on the left. If the pressure exerted by the left hand is inadequate, the brain will ride upward, and the slice will be too thin on the left.

The alternative — *horizontal* — plane of slicing may be preferred, especially in cases which have undergone CAT scans during life, making possible a comparison between the actual and the radiographic slices. The usual initial cut is indicated in Fig. 2.2. From then on the procedure is as with coronal slices, except that rather longer cutting guides are required: 22 x 18 cm, say, as against 19 x 16 cm. The slices are laid out, upper surface upward, with the right side on the right. Figures 2.5 and 2.6 show the structures normally displayed in coronal and horizontal slices respectively.

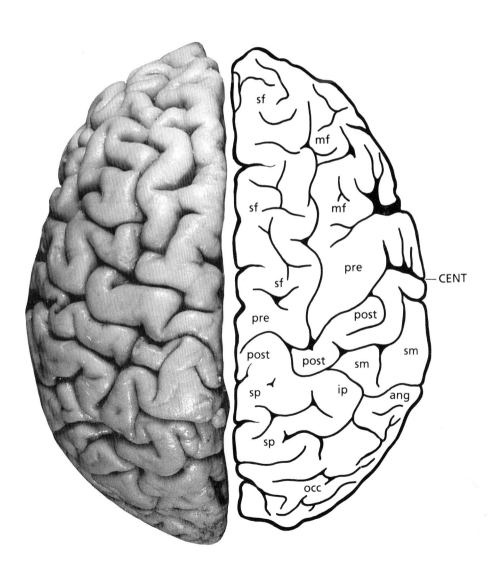

Fig. 2.4. Vertex of the brain.

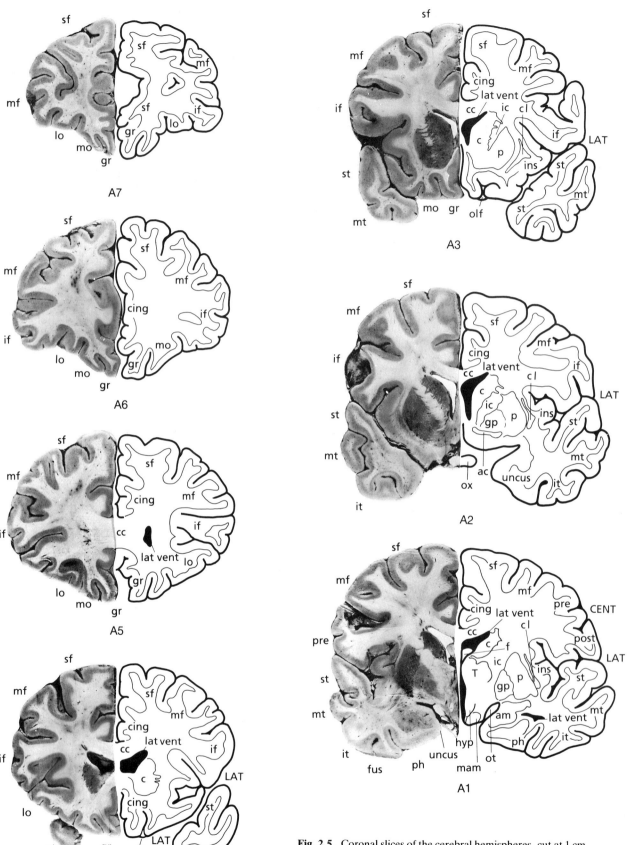

Fig. 2.5. Coronal slices of the cerebral hemispheres, cut at 1 cm intervals, from before backward.

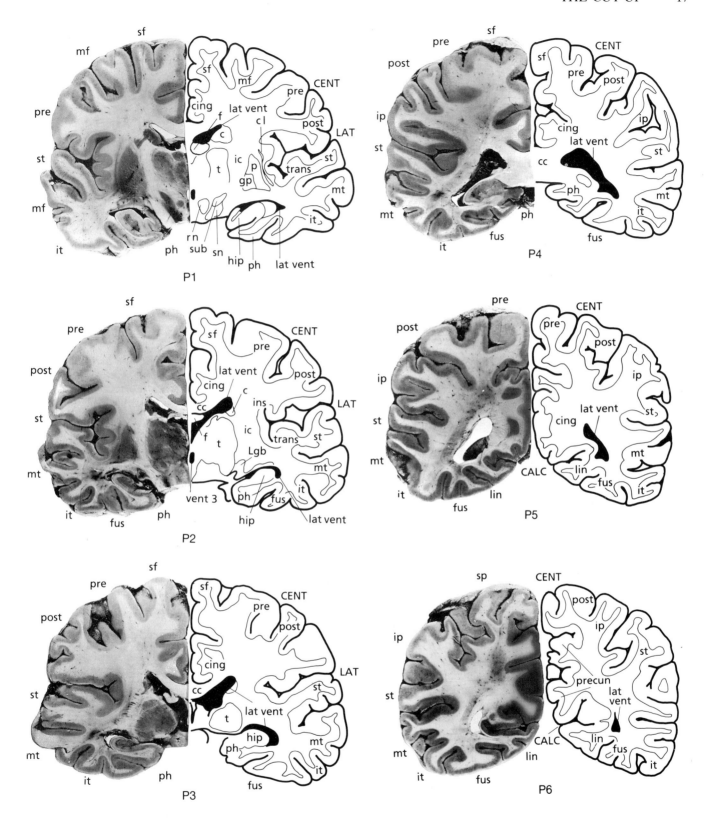

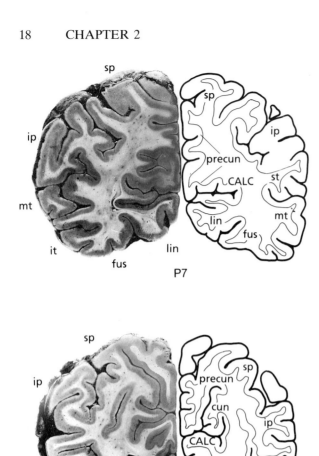

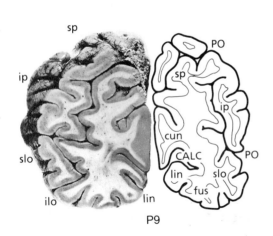

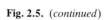

Fig. 2.5. (*continued*)

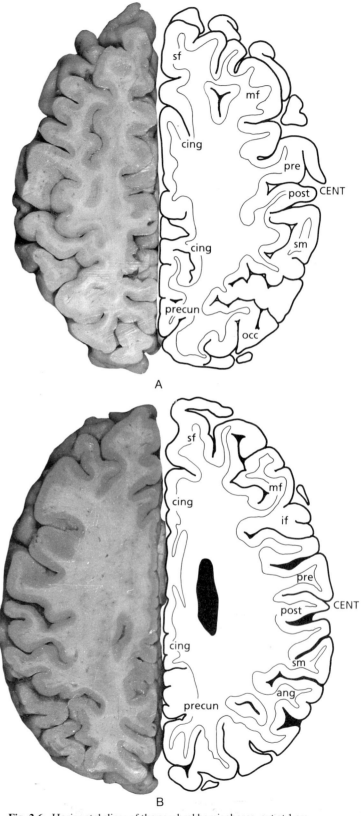

Fig. 2.6. Horizontal slices of the cerebral hemispheres, cut at 1 cm intervals, from above downward.

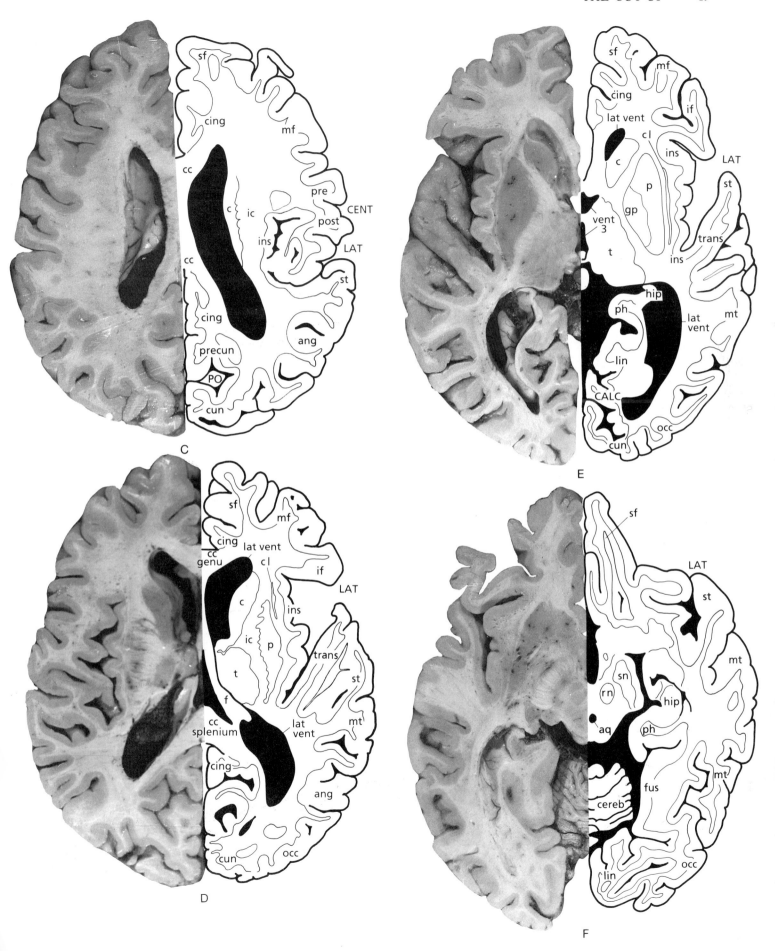

Nomenclature

Here we propose to digress on the subject of neuro-anatomy. Normal people forget, in the course of a few years or months, information which has been acquired purely for the purpose of an examination. This commonly includes the topology of the brain. Luckily relearning, when the need arises, is far easier than the initial learning. The apprentice in neuropathology need feel no shame if he has forgotten the difference between, say, the dentate nuclei and the dentate fascia; but it is incumbent on him, if his post mortem reports are to be of any value whatever, to relearn much of what he has forgotten. This will involve spending a lot of time over his first few brain-slicings, simply reminding himself of the relations of parts, and of their names.

The facts of neuro-anatomy are one thing; nomenclature is another. Professional anatomists enjoy meeting each other from time to time in order to change the terminology in current use. In this they resemble experts in tumour pathology, taxonomic botanists, and the promoters of new translations of the Bible. Although the new terminology is naturally superior to the old, this may create problems for outsiders using obsolete textbooks. In some cases, glossaries of old and new terms may help. A somewhat different problem arises with terms in common use which have no precisely defined application. An example is the word *brain*, which some people use as a synonym for *cerebrum*, while others (more correctly, we think) apply it to the whole of the intracranial part of the central nervous system. Another is *basal ganglia*, which is sometimes an alternative to *corpus striatum*, and at other times includes not only the caudate and lentiform nuclei but also the thalamus, hypothalamus, amygdala and subthalamic grey matter. We prefer the wider application. Even the terms *grey matter* and *white matter*, familiar as they are to laymen, are rather hard to define. Grey matter, of course, is central nervous tissue containing nerve cell bodies, whereas white matter is composed almost exclusively of axons, myelin and neuroglia. In the cerebral and cerebellar hemispheres and the spinal cord, the distinction is clear; but what of the brain stem? There is an analogy here with pork butchery. In a conventional joint, there is a clear separation of lean meat from fat; but what of streaky bacon? This is not mere pedantry. It is well known that what makes white matter white is myelin; but it is sometimes forgotten that there is plentiful myelin in grey matter. Hence the utterly false statement, seen in old textbooks of neurology, that MS is a disease of white matter. In fact, demyelination may occur throughout the CNS.

Regarding the terminology in this book, we have tried to remember, when two or more synonymous terms are in common use, to mention the synonyms (e.g. dorsal (Clarke's) nuclei; sensorimotor (Rolandic) cortex; pyramidal (corticospinal) tracts). For the terminology of the central cerebral grey matter, we use the following conventions:

Corpus striatum — caudate and lentiform nuclei, claustrum, internal and external capsules
Lentiform nucleus — putamen and pallidum (globus pallidus)
Striatum — caudate nucleus and putamen
Hippocampus we regard as interchangeable with *Ammon's horn*
Subthalamic nucleus we regard as interchangeable with *corpus Luysii*
Tegmentum and *subthalamic grey matter* can be used interchangeably; in practice, one or other is used according to whether the brain stem or cerebrum is being discussed.

Dissection of the hindbrain

After severing the midbrain, one can observe whether transtentorial herniation has taken place. The main visible signs of this are (i) grooving of the parahippocampal gyrus, on one side or both, and (ii) lateral compression of the upper brain stem (Fig. 2.9). For slicing the hindbrain, there are two commonly practised routines. The first (the one we normally follow) is to cut through the upper medulla at the level of the *lateral apertures* (foramina of Luschka) in a plane vertical to the long axis of the medulla, and continue the cut through the cerebellum. This displays the *fourth ventricle* at its broadest extent, the *dentate nuclei*, and the flocculi, uvula and nodulus of the cerebellum. Further cuts are made through the lower part of the specimen, using 5 mm guides, until it comes to an end. If the anatomy of the brain stem nuclei is of interest (as it very often is), wedge-shaped slices may give rise to later confusion. Figure 2.26 shows a series of hindbrain sections, stained for myelin.

In the upper part of the specimen, it is often the case that the upper and lower cut surfaces are not parallel, and the specimen is somewhat wedge-shaped, being thicker in the ventral than in the dorsal part. It should then be cut freehand, after taking 5 mm slices from the upper (midbrain) and lower (caudal pons) ends, making sure that each slice shows a complete transverse section of the pons.

The alternative routine may be preferred if interest is directed to regional differences between areas of the cerebellum. The cerebellum is separated from the brain stem by oblique cuts through the cerebellar peduncles into the fourth ventricle. Oblique cuts can then be made at right angles to the folia on the upper surface, and a midline cut will display the whole of the cerebellar vermis (Fig. 2.27). The brain stem is sliced at 5 mm intervals as before.

In slicing the brain, the knife may come across areas of gritty resistance. These may be due to calcification in the pineal gland and/or choroid plexus. Larger foci of calcification, up to the size of a date (so-called brain stones) occur, mainly in cases with endocrine disturbances, and have characteristic sites — in particular, the lentiform nuclei, thalami, and dentate nuclei. They are described and discussed on p.303.

Until the normal appearances of the slices are so familiar that any abnormality leaps to the eye, it is well to conduct one's inspection in a routine order. Apart from gross haemorrhages, large infarcts, tumours and malformations, the following must be noted:

Signs of brain swelling and herniation

Some of these — convolutional flattening, grooving of the parahippocampal gyri, and 'coning' of the medulla and cerebellar tonsils — will have been observed before slicing (see above, pp.2—9). Others are best seen at a later stage. One of these is an increased concavity on each side of the upper surface of the cerebellum. This is caused by downward pressure on the tentorium from the temporal lobes. In cases of tentorial herniation — even of mild extent — it is important to assess the degree of *diencephalic downthrust*. This can be done with a fair amount of accuracy by noting the position of the mamillary bodies (level A1) in relation to a line joining the lateral angles of the inferior horns of the lateral ventricles (Figs 2.7 and 2.8). Normally the mamillary bodies lie 1 or 2 mm above this line (Greenhall 1977). A severe downthrust brings them 5 mm or more below it.

Unilateral cerebral swelling or compression causes a shift of midline structures to the opposite side (Figs 2.9 and 2.10). At levels including the septum lucidum, this shift is easily measured by halving the distance between the lateral surfaces of the hemispheres, and noting the difference from the actual position of the septum. Other signs of a sideways

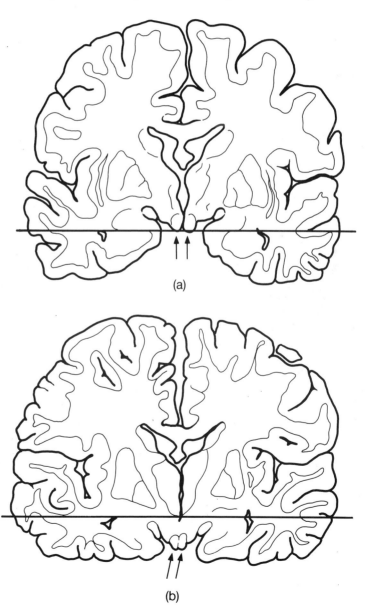

(a)

(b)

Fig. 2.7. The Greenhall line. At coronal level A1 a line between the inferior horns of the lateral ventricles normally lies above the mamillary bodies (arrowed). In the presence of cerebral swelling, the diencephalon, including the mamillary bodies, descends below this line. (a) Normal; (b) diencephalic downthrust.

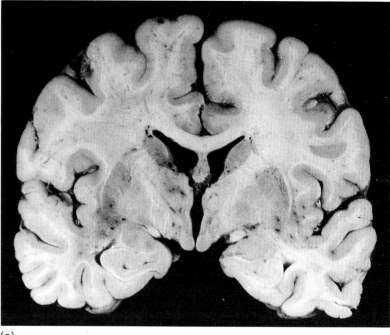

(a)

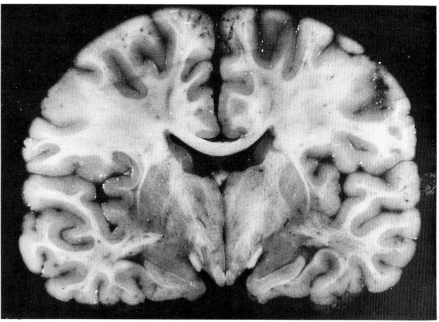

(b)

Fig. 2.8. Coronal level A1. (a) Normal. The mamillary bodies lie well above the Greenhall line. (b) Diencephalic downthrust in a case with bilateral cerebral swelling. (c — *facing page*) Downthrust in a case with right-sided haemorrhagic infarction due to phlebothrombosis. Note the midline shift to the left, herniation of the right cingulate gyrus, and bruising and grooving of the right parahippocampal gyrus (arrowed).

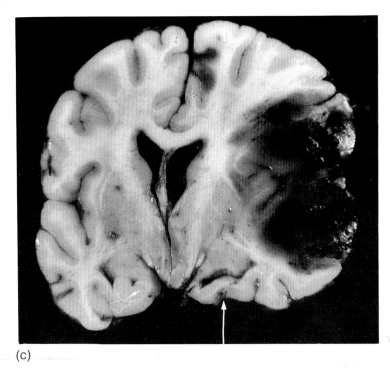

Fig. 2.8. (*continued*)   (c)

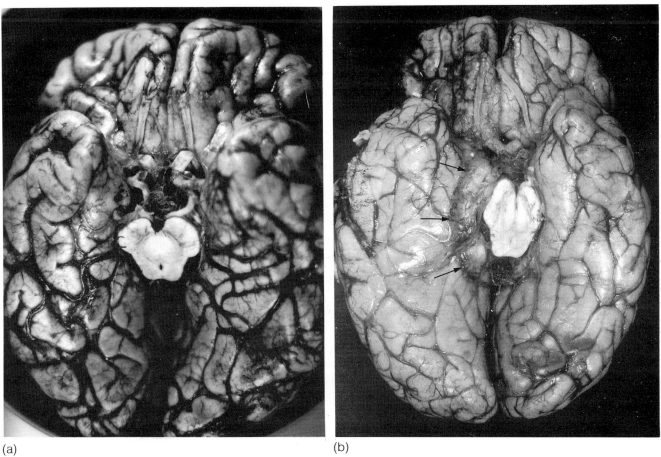

(a)   (b)

Fig. 2.9. Base of cerebrum after severing the midbrain. (a) Normal. (b) Showing effects of one-sided cerebral swelling. Same case as in Fig. 2.8c. The midbrain is laterally compressed and shifted to the left (right side of picture). The right parahippocampal gyrus is deeply grooved by the free edge of the tentorium (arrowed).

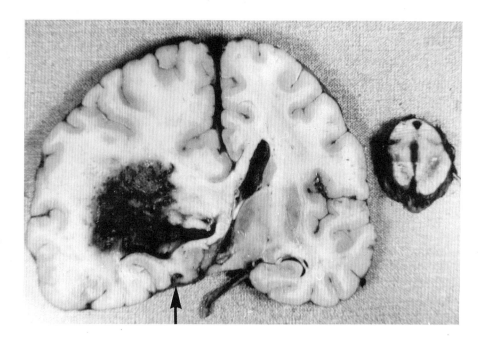

Fig. 2.10. Coronal slice, showing effects of a haemorrhagic tumour in the left cerebral hemisphere. Midline structures are shifted to the right, and there is a subfalcine herniation of the left cingulate gyrus, and bruising of the left parahippocampal gyrus (arrowed), as in Fig. 2.8c. The midbrain (on the right) shows lateral compression and a midline haemorrhage caused by distortion. The right crus (on the left) shows bruising from lateral pressure on the free edge of the tentorium.

shift are a grooving or indentation of the cingulate gyrus (Fig. 2.10) where it has come against the free edge of the falx cerebri. (Incidentally, there is no known clinical correlate of this type of subfalcine herniation.) Posteriorly, the falx comes close to the splenium of the corpus callosum: in front, the free edge of the falx lies a centimetre or more above the callosum.

Another type of herniation which is not often referred to, but which can be a very real threat to life, is an *upward* hernia through the tentorial opening. This occurs in the presence of tumours or haemorrhages in the posterior fossa, and can be precipitated by the sudden withdrawal of fluid from the lateral ventricles, or even, on occasion, by the turning of an osteoplastic flap, increasing the differential pressures above and below the tentorium. When the brain is cut, it will be found that the upper surfaces of the cerebellum, instead of being slightly concave, are convex, and display a distinct groove, caused by pressure on the free edge of the tentorium (Fig. 2.11).

The most important, i.e. the deadliest, effects of herniation are seen in slices of the brain stem. After a fatal tentorial hernia, the midbrain is distorted — mainly by lateral compression — and frequently haemorrhagic. The haemorrhages are usually symmetrical, mainly in the midline of the

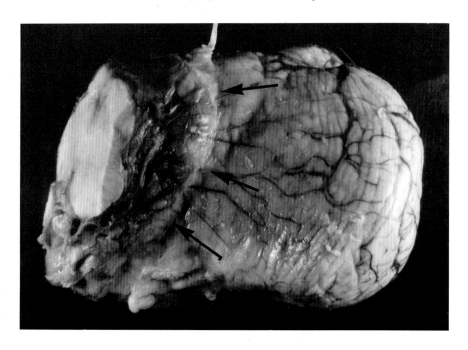

Fig. 2.11. Upward transtentorial hernia. A cerebellar tumour has displaced the brain stem upward, and the upper surface of the cerebellum has been grooved (arrowed) by the free edge of the tentorium.

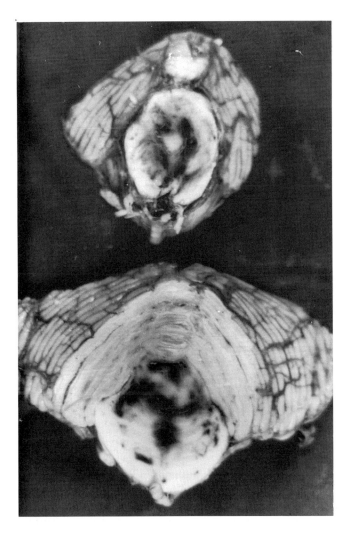

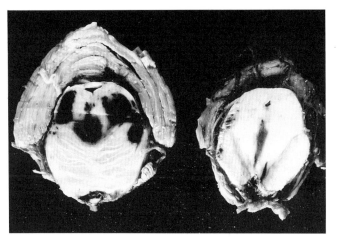

Fig. 2.13. Haemorrhages in the upper brain stem following an acceleration injury to the head, with 6 days' survival. There was a massive contusional haemorrhage at the right frontal pole, causing a shift to the left and a transtentorial hernia. The midbrain, on the right of the picture, is laterally compressed, and shows bruising from pressure on the free edge of the tentorium (compare with Fig. 2.10). There is a characteristic 'squeeze' haemorrhage in the midline. The upper pons, on the left of the picture, contains haemorrhages which were probably due to sudden stretching at the time of injury.

tegmentum, and may extend downward into the upper half of the pons (Fig. 2.12). This pattern differs somewhat from that seen in traumatic haemorrhage, which tends to affect one superior cerebellar peduncle (Fig. 2.13), or in primary spontaneous pontine haemorrhage, which is more disruptive but tends to spare the upper brain stem (Fig. 2.14). Lesions due to coning look rather different. The herniated tissue is softened and diffusely haemorrhagic, apparently as a result of mechanical compression of veins and capillaries, whereas the upper brain stem haemorrhages are attributed to stretching and tearing of intrinsic arteries (Fig. 2.15). Various causes of herniation are discussed in Chapter 11.

Fig. 2.12. Haemorrhages in the upper brain stem caused by distortion, with over-stretching of vessels, in the course of a tentorial hernia. Such haemorrhages are characteristically in or near the midline.

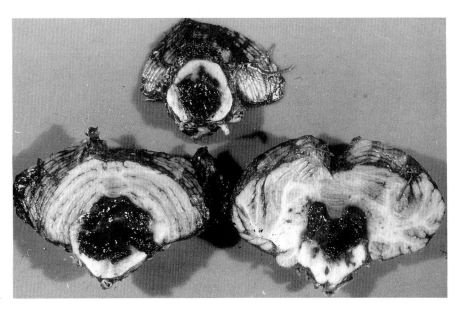

Fig. 2.14. 'Spontaneous' pontine haemorrhage, ploughing into the upper and lower brain stem and erupting into the fourth ventricle. The causes of such haemorrhages are not always clear, but some undoubtedly arise from vascular malformations.

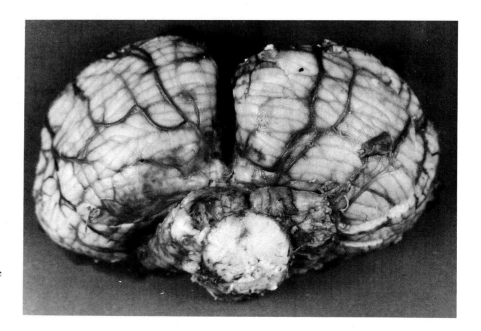

Fig. 2.15. 'Coning' in a case of acute brain swelling due to pneumococcal meningitis. The herniated cerebellar tonsils, and the ventral part of the lower medulla, are disrupted and haemorrhagic.

Appearance of the ventricles

The lateral ventricles may be larger or smaller than normal, or unequal. When they are larger than normal this may be due to loss of cerebral tissue, or to increased intraventricular pressure, which in turn is often due to an obstruction to the normal circulation of CSF. An account of the normal CSF pathways, and of the sites at which obstruction may occur, is given on pp.121–3. Briefly, the points to note in a brain with enlarged ventricles are these:

1 Whether the ventricles contain *blood*. Intraventricular bleeding can cause obstruction of the CSF pathway (for instance, in the aqueduct) by blood clots. Arterial bleeding will immediately expand the lateral ventricles, and may cause transtentorial herniation, resulting in compression of the aqueduct.

2 Whether the subarachnoid spaces between the cerebral sulci and in the basal cisterns are more or less capacious than normal. If more, there is a presumption of cerebral atrophy; if less, a block in the CSF pathway must be looked for.

3 Whether the ventricular dilatation affects the whole or only a part of the ventricular system; if only a part is affected, whether the difference can be accounted for by local atrophy or tissue destruction.

4 Whether the narrow places in the CSF pathway — the interventricular foramina, aqueduct, apertures of the fourth ventricle and cisterna ambiens (the subarachnoid space surrounding the midbrain) — are fully patent. Some of the causes of obstruction at these levels are mentioned in Chapter 8. The special case of the Chiari type 2 (Arnold–Chiari) malformation is discussed on pp.252–4; and some of the sequelae of perinatal injuries in Chapter 21, on pp.323–7.

The common causes of unduly *small* ventricles are external compression (e.g. by a blood clot or a meningioma), infiltrating or expanding tumours, and oedema. The last two may be combined, since some gliomas and some carcinoma deposits evoke an inflammatory type of response (Fig. 11.5). In this context, it is worth noting that adhesions often occur between apposed ependymal surfaces. Such adhesions are presumably congenital, and perfectly innocent. The *interthalamic connexus* is one such: and the tips of the

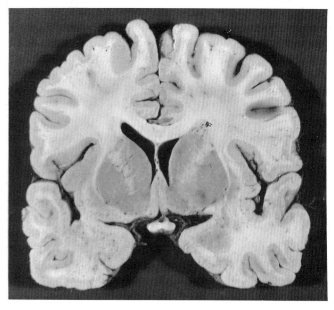

Fig. 2.16. 'Coarctation' of a lateral ventricle. Adhesions between the corpus callosum and the caudate nucleus, although of no pathological significance, sometimes gave rise to diagnostic errors when more reliance was placed on air ventriculography. Note that the midline is not displaced.

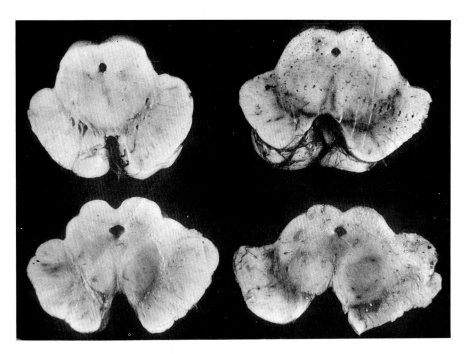

Fig. 2.17. Slices of upper and lower midbrain. On the right, normal pigmentation of the substantia nigra; on the left, loss of pigment in an advanced case of paralysis agitans (Parkinson's disease).

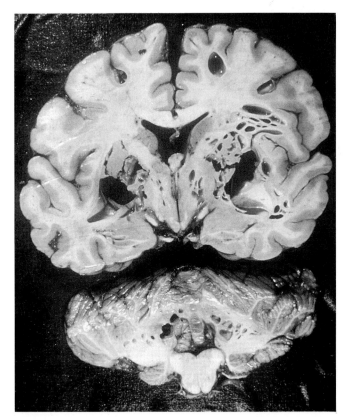

Fig. 2.18. 'Swiss cheese' artefacts in cerebrum and cerebellum, due to invasion by gas-forming organisms during the interval between death and fixation.

posterior horns of the lateral ventricles are normally obliterated to some extent, often asymmetrically. The same process often produces adhesions between the corpus callosum and the head of a caudate nucleus (Fig. 2.16).

Scanning for lesions

No cut-and-dried instructions can be given here. As would be expected, the more practice one has the easier it becomes to identify significant changes, and to ignore insignificant ones. Even practised neuropathologists, however, tend to refer to photographs and diagrams of normal structures and often need to settle doubts on naked-eye pathology by resorting to microscopy.

In scanning for lesions, the first guidance comes from the clinical notes. If MS has been suspected, one searches for plaques (see Chapter 14). If there was a parkinsonian syndrome, one looks for pigment loss in the substantia nigra and locus ceruleus (Fig. 2.17). If the patient was ataxic or dysarthric, special attention is paid to the pons, medulla and cerebellum. If he was blind, from other than ocular disease, the visual pathway, from optic nerves to visual cortex, should be looked at; and so forth.

It is important to learn — as soon as possible, in order to avoid wasting one's own and the technician's time — to recognize common *artefacts*. A few of these, such as 'Swiss cheese' artefact (Fig. 2.18) and toothpaste softening, have been mentioned above (pp.7—8). Common minor artefacts include pink haloes, a few millimetres in diameter, around small blood vessels. These are found, on microscopy, to contain bacteria, which have presumably left the bloodstream and proliferated at some time between death and diffusion of the fixative. They may be mistaken for small perivenous plaques of MS. Some doubts concerning the significance of colour changes may be settled by putting the cut slices back into formalin for a few days.

A change commonly seen in the cerebellum is a bluish discoloration of the cortex, often referred to as *état glacé*. It is believed to be due to post mortem autolysis, and is said to be commoner when there has been a delay between death and necropsy. Histological examination of the affected tissue shows dissolution of the cells of the granular layer, though the neighbouring Purkinje cells are unaffected (Fig. 2.19).

Patches of grey discoloration are commonly seen on cut surfaces in slices of the brain stem. These may even mimic plaques of MS. Histology shows no abnormality. We are at a loss to explain this phenomenon. Another form of discoloration is seen in slicing brain tissue which has been kept for many months in formalin. Here, the tissue has a dirty yellow hue for a distance of several millimetres inward from the exposed surfaces. Contact with blood clot in the storage jar inevitably causes dark discoloration of the tissue.

Fingertip palpation is a useful supplement to visual inspection. An area of fresh infarction may look almost normal,

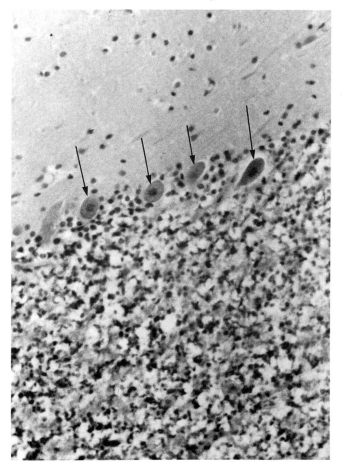

Fig. 2.19. 'Etat glacé'. The cells of the granular layer of the cerebellum show post mortem digestion. Purkinje cells (arrowed), though showing signs of agonal hypoxia, are preserved (×220).

though the softening and the demarcation from the adjoining arterial territory is immediately apparent on palpation. Oedematous white matter and diffuse astrocytoma may look alike, but the former is soft and slimy, the latter firm and dry. Owing to the hardening effect of formalin, the altered consistency of plaques of MS is hard to appreciate in fixed tissue; but in some conditions, such as globoid-cell and sulphatide leucodystrophies, fibrous gliosis of the affected tissue confers an almost wood-like hardness. In tuberous sclerosis the firm consistency of the tubers in the cerebral cortex, easily felt in the unfixed brain, is still just appreciable after fixation. A little caution is called for here. Many years ago, in the post mortem room, the author was rejoicing in having met his first case of tuberous sclerosis, until a colleague observed that the patient had been suffering from bronchial carcinoma. The 'tubers' were in fact secondary deposits.

Dissection of the fixed spinal column

In cases of peripheral neuropathy, particularly if this is complicated by autonomic disturbances, one may wish to examine parts of the *sympathetic chains*. These are easily identified after stripping off the remains of pleura and peritoneum overlying the sides of the vertebral bodies, up to the level of the stellate ganglia. They should be removed before beginning the dissection of the backbone.

The *tools* needed for the dissection are a metre of solid bench, a pair of strong vices, a stout knife, scissors and forceps, bone shears and nibblers, and a short handsaw and/or electric vibrating saw. The spinal column, fixed and well washed, is held dorsum upward in the vices, and the erector spinae musculature cut away. The laminae are sawn through and removed with the spinous processes as described on pp.3–4, with the same precautions against inflicting damage to the spinal cord. Spinal roots and ganglia are exposed at the desired levels, and dissected away from the bone of the intervertebral foramina. An artery forceps is placed on the lowest part of the theca, in the sacral part of the spinal canal, and the cord, enclosed in the theca, is gradually eased backward, cutting nerve roots with a sharp knife. During this procedure, there should be as little sideways or backward bending of the cord as possible. Although the cord is much firmer than before fixation, it is also more liable to crumble if it is bent, giving very unsatisfactory histological sections. Longitudinal stretching of the theca, on the other hand, is harmless.

For most of the distance (unless there is extrathecal tumour tissue) the theca will come away from the anterior wall of the spinal canal with only slight encouragement from the knife. In elderly subjects, however, dense fibrous adhesions are often encountered in the lower cervical region, the usual cause being *osteoarthritic and spondylotic changes*, with osteophytosis of the vertebral bodies and discs.

Cranial and spinal meninges

In the cranial cavity the dura mater consists of two layers, of which the outer layer is in effect the periosteum of the bone, and is continuous, via the various bony foramina, with the pericranium. Over the vault, the dura is relatively easily detached from the bone, as occurs in the formation of an epidural haematoma simply from the force of arterial pressure. The inner layer is closely bound to the outer layer over most of its extent, but leaves it at certain points to form infoldings such as the falx and tentorium. It is along these lines of infolding that venous sinuses occur. At the base, the dura is more firmly stuck down — densely so at and just below the foramen magnum. Below this the two layers separate, the outer layer becoming the periosteum of the spinal canal. The inner layer becomes the spinal *theca*, which is separated from the periosteum by a layer of loose connective tissue, containing fat and blood vessels. Until adhesions form, there is free movement between the theca and the bony canal, unrestrained by the spinal nerve roots, which lie loosely in the extrathecal space, and are covered with an epineurium derived from the theca.

The *arachnoid* membrane, though it is attached to the pial covering of the entire brain and cord, is everywhere in direct contact with the inner surface of the dura. Over the cerebral hemispheres, there is free gliding movement, checked only by dural folds and by bridging veins running between brain and dura. This presumably affords the brain some protection against the effects of accelerations. At the base, however, such a slipping plane would be useless because of the numerous nerves and blood vessels traversing the subdural space. Here, such movement as occurs is mainly in the subarachnoid space, and is checked by the excellent packing of the hindbrain within the posterior fossa.

In the spinal canal, as in the posterior fossa, the presence of numerous nerve roots would render a subdural slip-plane useless. The arachnoid, though easily stripped from the theca, only loses contact in peculiar circumstances, for instance, when a lumbar puncture is performed with a blunt or hooked needle. The subarachnoid space, however, is capacious, and the arachnoid is only loosely and intermittently attached to the pia of the cord, by the denticulate ligaments and the spinal nerve roots.

Movement of the cord relative to the bony canal — shown at its most impressive by gymnasts, acrobats and some dancers — is made possible by the elasticity of the cord tissue, and by the existence of two planes of movement, the epidural and the subarachnoid. In the presence of cervical osteoarthritis and spondylosis, the former is reduced or abolished. It has been suggested that this may have a bearing on the predominant patterns of cord lesions in MS.

In dissecting the spine, a note should be made of any dense fibrous adhesions met with during removal of the cord, and of any excrescences, tumorous or otherwise, projecting into the spinal canal. After the cord has been removed, the walls of the canal should be inspected and herniated discs identified. It is also worth making a midline saw-cut through at least the cervical part of the bony column, to reveal the ravages, if any, of cervical spondylosis — the degenerate discs and osteophytes, the obliteration or exaggeration of the normal cervical lordosis, and so forth (Fig. 2.20).

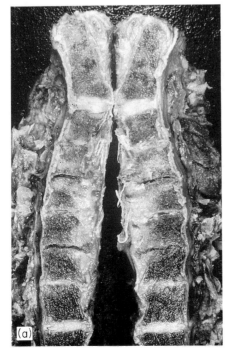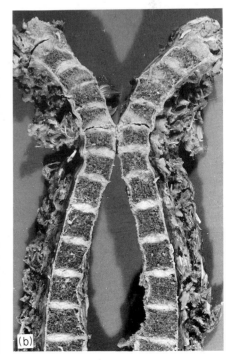

Fig. 2.20. Cervical spondylosis. The spinal cords have been removed after laminectomy, and midline saw-cuts made through the bodies of the cervical vertebrae. The specimens are displayed with the anterior longitudinal ligaments in the middle and the interior of the spinal canal at the sides. (a) From a man aged 80, with a sensory level at C6. The cervical spine has lost its normal lordosis. The C2−3 and T1−2 discs appear normal, but all the intervening discs are either narrowed or grossly degenerate. Detachment of the anterior and posterior longitudinal ligaments from the bone has resulted in the formation of osteophytic projections. Anterior osteophytes are relatively harmless, whereas posterior osteophytes become adherent to the theca, and narrow the spinal cord from before back. (b) From a woman of 83, with a long history of MS. Here the cervical lordosis is exaggerated. Discs C3−4 and C4−5 are narrowed. C4−5 is disrupted, and shows anterior and posterior osteophytes.

Examination of the spinal cord

If it is clear, from palpation, that there is more inside the theca than is accounted for by the cord and nerve roots, a transverse cut should be made before opening the theca. This may reveal pus, clear fluid, subarachnoid tumour, or a swollen cord. Otherwise, the theca can be slit open longitudinally, back and front, and peeled away from the arachnoid. The arachnoid itself should be delicate and transparent. It becomes somewhat thicker and more opaque in later life, and may develop a number of so-called *arachnoid plaques*. These are white, opaque, less than 0.5 mm thick, and often over 1 cm long (Fig. 2.21). Being composed of cholesterol they disappear completely in fat solvents. They are of no known pathological significance.

After the theca and arachnoid have been slit open, the front and back of the cord are easily distinguished by the pattern of surface vessels; behind, there are many small venous tributaries to the posterior spinal veins, whereas in front there is a prominent midline vein, accompanied by the anterior spinal artery. *Segmental levels* are most easily worked out by counting upward and downward from the first thoracic root, which is the lowest *large* root of the cervical enlargement.

Some yellow–brown staining may be seen in the leptomeninges (arachnoid and pia) at the lower end of the cord, and on the roots of the cauda equina. The pigment is *haemosiderin*, and the intensity of the staining is usually an indication of the number of lumbar punctures that the patient has undergone. More widespread brown staining (*superficial siderosis*) involving the brain, at least at the base, is due to intermittent small haemorrhages from a variety of sources. Blackish-brown discoloration of the pia covering the upper cervical cord and lower medulla is normal. The pigment here is melanin.

Acute and chronic meningitis

Purulent meningitis (i.e. pus in the subarachnoid space) is readily recognized. The more chronic forms, such as tuberculous or syphilitic meningitis or the mysterious noninfective chronic arachnoiditis, show less exudate, more discoloration, and conspicuous thickening of the leptomeninges (Fig. 9.16). This appearance may be mimicked in cases of diffuse spread of tumour through the CSF pathways.

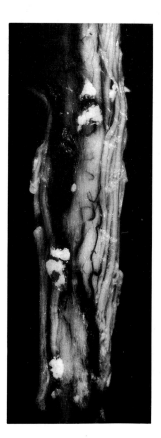

Fig. 2.21. Arachnoid plaques. These are thin white scales, embedded in the spinal arachnoid, especially in the lower regions. They are common in elderly subjects, and have no known clinical or pathological significance.

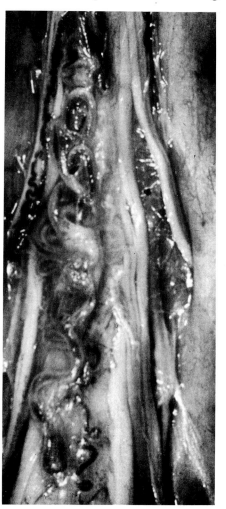

Fig. 2.22. 'Angioma' of the spinal cord. The posterior surface of the lower part of the cord is covered by an exceedingly tortuous, dilated, and thick-walled vein, clothed in thickened pia and arachnoid. (Courtesy of Dr J.T. Hughes.)

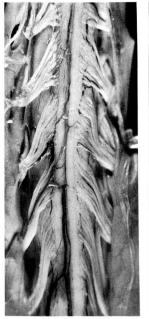 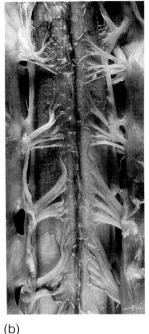 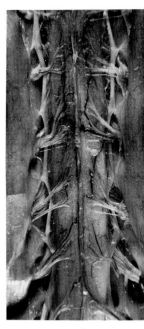

(a)   (b)   (c)

Fig. 2.23. Anterior roots of the cervical enlargement. (a) The roots are normal, but there is a shrunken, discoloured plaque of MS at the lower end. (b) Atrophic roots from a case of motor neuron disease. (c) Even more wasted roots from an old case of severe poliomyelitis.

Such spread is very characteristic of medulloblastomas, but rare with gliomas. It occurs with some carcinomas (especially of the breast and stomach), and is commonly referred to as 'carcinomatous meningitis' rather than the more correct *meningeal carcinomatosis* (Fig. 13.50).

'Angioma' of the spinal cord

In elderly patients with a history of progressive paraplegia, one may find a dilated, grossly tortuous vein overlying the back of the lower part of the cord (Fig. 2.22). This condition, sometimes referred to as 'angioma of the cord', is in fact the result of an *arteriovenous fistula* arising in or close to the vertebral column. Subjection to arterial pressure causes the posterior spinal vein to dilate, elongate, and develop a thick wall. This leads to changes in the substance of the cord, where venules undergo fibrous thickening and hyaline change, with eventual obliteration of the lumen. The cord tissue becomes ischaemic and undergoes patchy necrosis.

Spinal nerve roots

The proximal, intrathecal parts of the spinal nerve roots should be examined at an early stage, and histological blocks taken in cases with a history of neuropathy and/or diabetes. Samples of anterior and posterior roots can be taken from the cauda equina for transverse and longitudinal cutting; likewise, *sensory ganglia*, which are easily accessible in the sacral region. Anterior nerve roots are visibly wasted in motor neuron disease (amyotrophic lateral sclerosis) and after severe *poliomyelitis* (Fig. 2.23). Posterior roots are wasted, more in the lumbosacral region than higher up, in *tabes dorsalis* (Fig. 2.24) and *Friedreich's ataxia*. The spinal cord itself is wasted in Friedreich's ataxia, and in some long-standing cases of MS.

(a)   (b)

Fig. 2.24. Posterior lumbosacral roots. (a) Normal; (b) from a case of tabes dorsalis. The roots are wasted, and there is some meningeal fibrosis. The discoloration is probably due to traumatic lumbar punctures.

Swelling of the cord

Local swellings of the spinal cord (other than the cervical and lumbar enlargements) are attributable to *intrinsic tumour* (Figs 11.9 and 11.12), *syringomyelia* (Fig. 8.14) or inflammation. The commonest tumours are *gliomas* — epen-

dymomas, subependymomas, and astrocytomas (see Chapter 12). Deposits of secondary carcinoma are rare. The division of fluid-filled cavities, or syrinxes, into those lined with ependyma (hydromyelia) and those not so lined (syringomyelia) is probably somewhat artificial. The subject

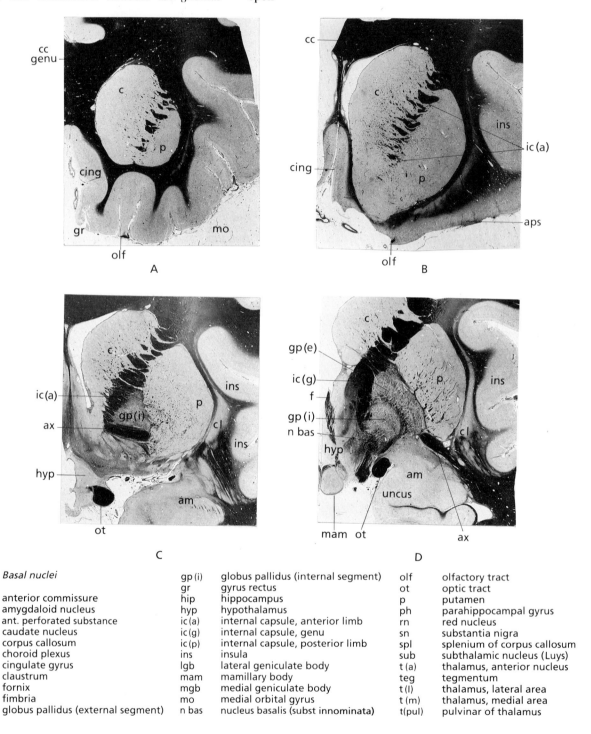

Key	*Basal nuclei*	gp(i)	globus pallidus (internal segment)	olf	olfactory tract
		gr	gyrus rectus	ot	optic tract
ax	anterior commissure	hip	hippocampus	p	putamen
am	amygdaloid nucleus	hyp	hypothalamus	ph	parahippocampal gyrus
aps	ant. perforated substance	ic(a)	internal capsule, anterior limb	rn	red nucleus
c	caudate nucleus	ic(g)	internal capsule, genu	sn	substantia nigra
cc	corpus callosum	ic(p)	internal capsule, posterior limb	spl	splenium of corpus callosum
ch pl	choroid plexus	ins	insula	sub	subthalamic nucleus (Luys)
cing	cingulate gyrus	lgb	lateral geniculate body	t(a)	thalamus, anterior nucleus
cl	claustrum	mam	mamillary body	teg	tegmentum
f	fornix	mgb	medial geniculate body	t(l)	thalamus, lateral area
fim	fimbria	mo	medial orbital gyrus	t(m)	thalamus, medial area
gp(e)	globus pallidus (external segment)	n bas	nucleus basalis (subst innominata)	t(pul)	pulvinar of thalamus

Fig. 2.25 (*and facing page*). Myelin-stained sections, taken at roughly 7 mm intervals, of the central part of the right cerebral hemisphere. The levels correspond with levels A3–P3 in coronal slices (Fig. 2.5).

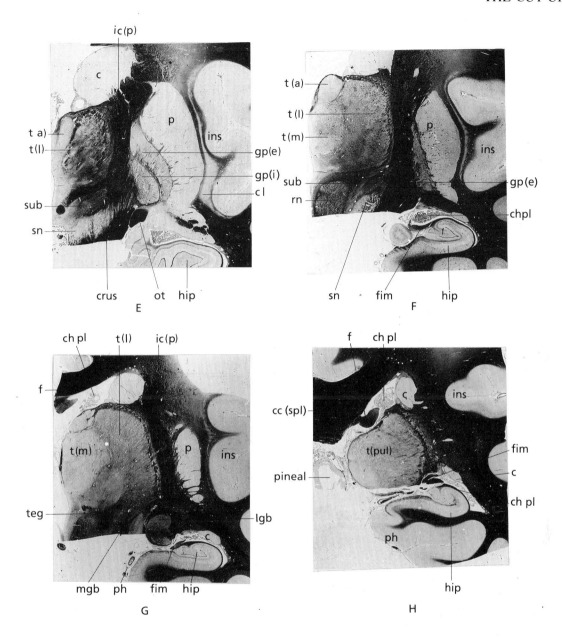

Fig. 2.25. (*continued*)

of the origin and pathology of these lesions is still an area of dispute (see p.127).

Examples of *inflammatory* lesions causing swelling of the cord are poliomyelitis (p.147), perivenous encephalomyelitis (p.154) and acute MS (Fig. 11.10). As the pia mater is somewhat inelastic there is a tendency for the lesion to extend itself upward and downward, producing the clinical state of 'ascending myelitis' (see p.168).

Segmental levels

The cords of paraplegic patients (other than those with MS)

will generally show a sharply defined locus of thinning or destruction, due to compression or to trauma. The segmental level of such a lesion should be determined (see below), and compared with the assessed sensory level recorded in the clinical notes. If the vertebral column is still available, the vertebral level of the lesion, which is numerically higher than the segmental level in the cord, should be ascertained.

In assessing segmental levels by reference to the vertebral column, it must be remembered that the first cervical nerve roots emerge below the occipital bone, *above* the first cervical vertebra; similarly, the seventh cervical roots emerge *above* the seventh cervical vertebra, the eight cervical roots appear between the seventh cervical and first thoracic vertebrae, and from there downward, each pair of roots emerges *below* the similarly numbered vertebra.

Close to the cord, the entering and emerging roots are split into a number of rootlets which form an almost un-interrupted series in front and behind. The cord segment is defined as the portion receiving and emitting the rootlets of a particular root — a rather imprecise definition, as the division between one set of rootlets and the next may be at different points on the cord in front and behind. In an adult, each cervical and thoracic cord segment measures a little over 1 cm from above down. Below this the segments are progressively shorter, so that the lower sacral segments are no more than 2 or 3 mm long.

If the vertebral column is not available, segmental levels may be worked out by counting upward and downward from the first thoracic segment. T1 is normally the lowest segment in the cervical enlargement, and the T1 roots are the lowest *large* nerve roots in that region. In case of doubt, two transverse cuts may settle the matter. The upper half of T1 cord segment has a typical 'cervical' appearance, with massive anterior grey horns; the lower half has a typical 'thoracic' shape, with slender anterior horns and well-defined lateral horns.

Transverse slicing

On transverse slicing of the cord, the following may be observed:

1 Areas of *softening* or even disruption. If these are not the immediate effect of trauma, they are probably due to infarction. Causes of infarction include: atheroma of the aorta, with occlusion of one of the major radicular arteries supplying the anterior spinal artery; surgical procedures in the posterior abdominal wall, with damage to an important radicular artery; compression of a nerve root carrying such an artery by tumours, especially neuroblastomas, lympho-mas, myelomas and secondary carcinomas (one of the commoner causes of '*malignant paraplegia*'); and fat or air *embolism*. In cases with inflammatory cord swelling, a common finding is a *plug of necrotic tissue* which has been forced upward or downward into the posterior white columns by pressure within a tightly stretched pia mater.

2 Well-defined *patches of grey discoloration*, unrelated to grey–white boundaries or to tracts in the white columns, or to areas of vascular supply. These can be confidently diagnosed as plaques of MS. They are more frequent in the cervical cord than elsewhere, and tend to affect the lateral columns more than the rest of the cord. In long-standing cases of MS, the outlines of the plaques may be blurred as a result of wallerian degeneration in long tracts.

3 *Grey discoloration* of such long tracts as are large and compact enough to be distinguished by the naked eye. It should be remembered that in wallerian (anterograde) degeneration loss of myelin from the affected tracts is a slow process; thus it may be several weeks before the effects of a hemiplegic stroke are reflected in naked-eye changes in the relevant corticospinal tract.

Bilateral degeneration of the crossed and uncrossed corti-cospinal (pyramidal) tracts is seen *below* the lesion after cord transection (p.95); in Friedreich's ataxia (p.244), and in most cases of motor neuron disease (p.236). Bilateral degeneration of upgoing pathways (posterior columns and spinocerebellar tracts) is seen *above* a cord transection and in Friedreich's ataxia, and of the posterior columns alone in tabes dorsalis. In Strümpell's *familial spastic paraplegia*, where it appears that the cells of origin are unable to maintain the vitality of very long axons, one finds pyramidal tract degeneration in the lower part of the cord, and posterior column and spinocerebellar tract degeneration in the upper part (see p.249).

Choice of blocks for histology

In some neuropathological departments a standard number of blocks, taken from standard sites, are embedded, sec-tioned and stained from every brain examined. We feel that this practice is unnecessarily wasteful of time, technical skill, materials and storage space. Ideally, in our view, each block, and each stain, should serve the purpose of answering one or more questions; thus, if the technician were to ask 'why did you take that block?' or 'why did you ask for that stain?' the pathologist should be ready with a satisfying answer.

Neuropathologists have been laughed at by general pathologists for demanding sections of extravagantly large size, requiring very expensive glass slides and coverslips. In return, general pathologists are mocked for examining sec-tions no bigger than postage stamps, stained with haema-toxylin and eosin, and labelled simply 'brain'. We do not wish to argue these points, apart from maintaining that there are situations demanding large sections, and that there should be technicians able to prepare them.

Freezing and embedding

In selecting blocks for histology there is an initial choice to be made between *frozen sections* and *paraffin or celloidin embedding*. If fat stains are required, frozen or cryostat sections are obligatory, since fat is dissolved away during the embedding process. Some of the most used metallic impregnations—for instance, Cajal's gold sublimate method for astrocytes, or the Weil–Davenport method for micro-glia — require frozen sections. For most other purposes, blocks are embedded, and the choice lies between paraffin and celloidin embedding.

Key | *Brain stem*

acc cun — accessory cuneate nucleus
ambig — nucleus ambiguus
ant — anterior horn (C.1)
aq — aqueduct
ch pl — choroid plexus
c teg — central tegmental tract
cun fun — cuneate funiculus (column of Burdach)
cun nuc — cuneate nucleus
dent — dentate nucleus
dors coch — dorsal cochlear nucleus
dors vag — dorsal vagal nucleus
fr pont — frontopontine tract
grac fun — gracile funiculus (column of Goll)
grac nuc — gracile nucleus
icp — inferior cerebellar peduncle (restiform body)
inf col — inferior colliculus (inf. corpus quadrigeminum)
inf ol — inferior olive
lat ap — lateral aperture (foramen of Luschka)
lat lem — lateral lemniscus (lateral fillet)
lat vest — lateral vestibular nucleus
loc cer — locus ceruleus (locus pigmentosus pontis)
mcp — middle cerebellar peduncle (brachium pontis)
med lem — medial lemniscus (medial fillet)
mgb — medial geniculate body
mlf — medial longitudinal fasciculus
mo nuc 5 — motor nucleus of trigeminal nerve
m vest — medial vestibular nucleus
n3 — oculomotor nerve
n4 — trochlear nerve
n5 — trigeminal nerve
n6 — abducent nerve
n7 — facial nerve
n8 — cochleo-vestibular (acoustic) nerve
n9 — glossopharyngeal nerve
n10 — vagus nerve
n12 — hypoglossal nerve
nuc 3 — oculomotor nucleus
nuc 4 — trochlear nucleus
nuc 6 — abducent nucleus
nuc 7 — facial nucleus
nuc 12 — hypoglossal nucleus
par pont — parieto-pontine tract
pyr — pyramid
pyr tr — pyramidal (corticospinal) tract
pyr x — decussation of pyramidal tract
retic — reticular formation
rn — red nucleus
scp — superior cerebellar peduncle (brachium conjunctivum)
sn — substantia nigra
sp nuc 5 — spinal nucleus of trigeminal nerve
sp tr 5 — spinal (descending) tract of trigeminal nerve
sp vest — spinal (inferior) vestibular nucleus
sup col — superior colliculus (sup. corpus quadrigeminum)
sup ol — superior olive
sup vest — superior vestibular nucleus
tr sol — tractus solitarius
vent coch — ventral cochlear nucleus
vent 4 — fourth ventricle

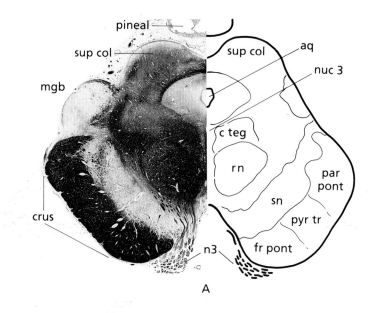

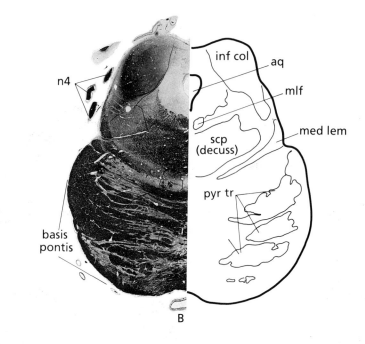

Fig. 2.26. Myelin-stained transverse sections of the brain stem. Intervals between sections are unequal, being larger in the pons and smaller in the medulla.

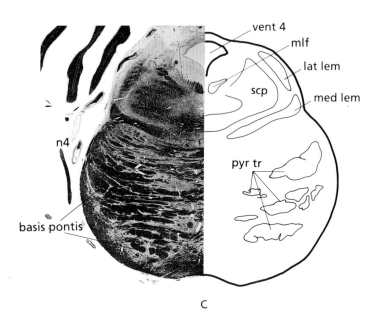

C

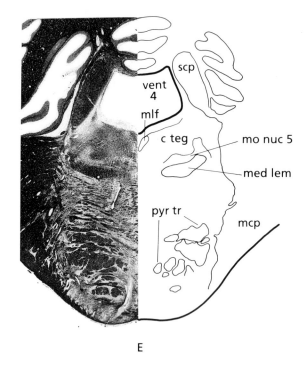

E

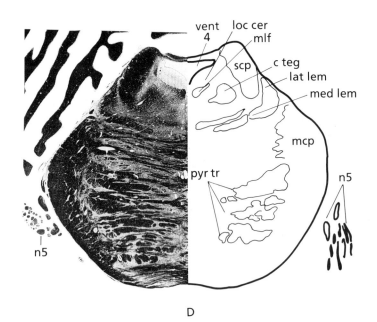

D

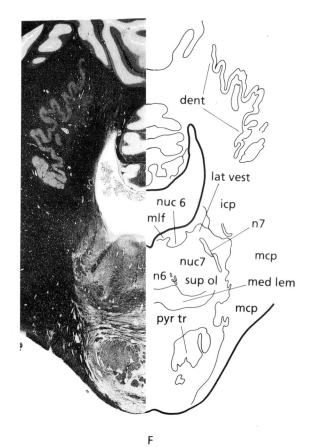

F

Fig. 2.26. (*continued*)

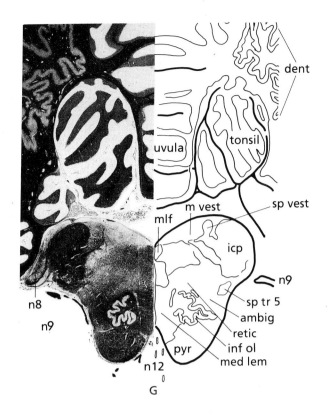

G

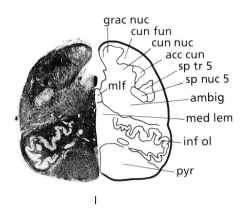

I

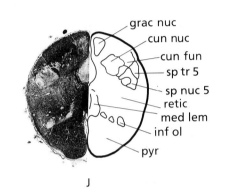

J

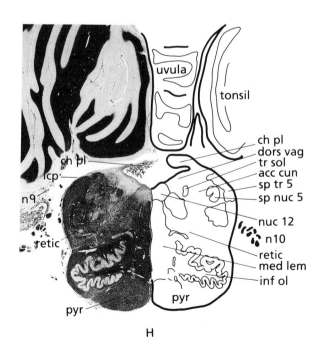

H

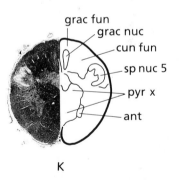

K

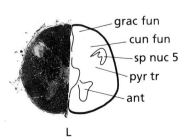

L

Key

ant	anterior lobe
D	dentate nucleus
l	lingula
mb	midbrain
med	medulla
n	nodulus
p	pyramis
post	posterior lobe
t	tonsil
u	uvula
1	primary fissure
4	fourth ventricle

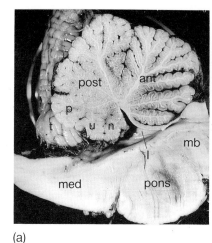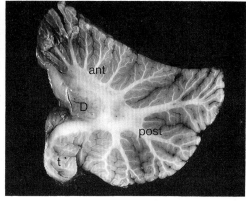

Fig. 2.27. Sections through the cerebellum: (a) in the midline, showing divisions of cerebellar vermis; (b) oblique, passing through the dentate nucleus.

(a)   (b)

Celloidin embedding has the following advantages:
1 Large sections are easier to handle than paraffin sections of comparable size;
2 Nissl-type stains for neurons, and haematoxylin stains for myelin, are generally clearer, more vivid, and thus more suited for photography than in paraffin sections. It is also claimed that there is less shrinkage of tissue during processing.

The main disadvantages are:
1 it is sometimes difficult to achieve perfect flatness of the section. This can be a drawback in high-power photography;
2 the process of embedding is slow, and the pathologist may have to wait several months for his sections;
3 the blocks, which are stored in dilute alcohol, deteriorate over the years, becoming very hard, and difficult to stain effectively when cut, whereas paraffin-embedded blocks last indefinitely;
4 nitrocellulose (celloidin) is an explosive substance, and the solvent is ether. The handling and storage of these materials entails certain hazards.

By and large, the disadvantages of celloidin outweigh the advantages, especially if the technician has acquired the skill needed for handling large paraffin sections. We currently use paraffin almost exclusively.

No rigid rules can be laid down regarding choice of blocks for embedding, except that some at least should be relevant to the probable diagnoses. For instance, blocks from the brain of a patient with parkinsonism must include the *putamen* (Fig. 2.25), *substantia nigra* (Fig. 2.26A) and *locus ceruleus* (Fig. 2.26D). In the case of an elderly patient with progressive dementia, in the absence of naked-eye lesions, samples of *cerebral cortex*, including a temporal lobe, must be looked at, as recommended on p.272. In a case of heart failure, or if there is reason to think there was cerebral ischaemia or hypoxaemia shortly before death, elements known to be particularly sensitive to hypoxia should be examined. These include the *thalamus*, *hippocampus*, and *Purkinje cells* of the cerebellum.

More often than not, the clinical notes and the naked-eye appearances provide one with a firm, or at least a provisional, diagnosis. When this is not the case, one may be reduced to scanning for lesions with the microscope. For this purpose there are certain useful blocks which include a number of different structures in a single section. For example, a block can be taken at level A1 (Figs 2.5 and 2.25D) which includes third ventricle, hypothalamus, mamillary body, striatum, pallidum, amygdala and insula. Similar blocks from P1 and P2 show anterior and posterior thalamic levels, medial and lateral geniculate bodies, and hippocampus (Figs 2.5 and 2.25E–G). A section taken at or just below the lateral apertures of the fourth ventricle shows the medullary pyramids, inferior olives, medial lemnisci, descending trigeminal tracts and nuclei, dorsal vagal nuclei, inferior cerebellar peduncles, cerebellar cortex and dentate nuclei (Fig. 2.26G and H). If interest is focused on cerebellar topography, the cerebellum should be severed from the brain stem (p.20), and sections taken of the midline and of one or both hemispheres, with a cut at right angles to the folia on the upper surface, passing through the dentate nucleus (Fig. 2.27a and b).

Routines for brain and cord

Routine histology on the spinal cord is carried out on transverse slices at various levels — for instance, one from the cervical enlargement (C5 to T1), two from upper and lower thoracic levels, and one from the lumbosacral enlargement (Fig. 2.28). The lowest block should include anterior and posterior nerve roots. These are liable to fall away from the cord during processing, but can be kept in place until the last moment by tying a piece of thread around the specimen. In cases of peripheral neuropathy, a bundle of roots, with the tip of the conus medullaris to distinguish between anterior and posterior aspects, is similarly wrapped. All specimens of cord and cauda equina should be clearly labelled with at least approximate levels, and inked on the

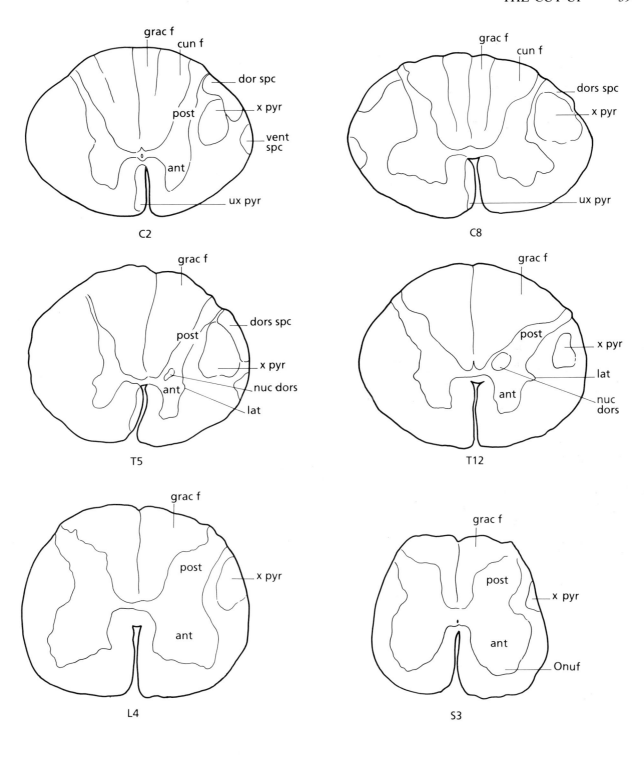

Fig. 2.28. Drawings of sections of spinal cord at levels C2, C8, T5, T12, L4 and S3.

Key

ant	anterior grey horn	nuc dors	nucleus dorsalis (Clarke's column)
cun f	cuneate funiculus (column of Burdach)	Onuf	nucleus of Onufrowicz
dors spc	dorsal (posterior) spinocerebellar tract	post	posterior grey horn
grac f	gracile funiculus (column of Goll)	ux pyr	uncrossed pyramidal tract
lat	lateral grey horn (containing the intermediolateral cell column)	x pyr	crossed pyramidal tract

surface opposite the one from which sections are to be cut.

In cases of MS, longitudinal sections may be desirable, in order to distinguish between normal, degenerate and demyelinated tracts. Either coronal or paramedian planes may be used; but the former, passing through both left and right sides of the cord, are somewhat easier to interpret.

Examination of long tracts

An important part of the examination of a diseased nervous system consists of tracing degeneration through the *long myelinated tracts* of the brain and spinal cord. For this, the most usual approach is to look for unnatural localized pallor in low-power views of myelin-stained sections. This negative, so to speak, impression of tract degeneration can be reinforced by stains which give positive evidence of myelin breakdown (for methods, see below). To avoid confusion, we propose to define 'tract' as a bundle of myelinated fibres of similar origin and destination, sufficiently large and homogeneous to be identified by low-power microscopy. In this sense, the optic radiation (running from the lateral geniculate body to the visual cortex), the medial lemniscus (running from the gracile and cuneate nuclei to the thalamus), the superior cerebellar peduncle (running from the dentate nucleus to the red nucleus and thalamus on the opposite side) and the middle cerebellar peduncle (running from the pontine nuclei to the opposite cerebellar cortex)

are *tracts*; whereas the spinothalamic pathway, running in the anterior quadrant of the spinal cord, being mixed with many other pathways, is not a tract in this sense.

The longest, and most famous, tract in the CNS is the *pyramidal* (corticospinal) tract. Its course is indicated in Figs 2.26, 2.28 and 2.29. This tract originates in the cerebral cortex on both sides of the central sulcus (not merely in the motor cortex, as is sometimes stated) and courses downward through the posterior limb of the internal capsule to the brain stem and beyond. In the internal capsule, it lies well behind the position ascribed to it in older anatomy textbooks. It occupies the middle third of the crus of the cerebral peduncle, the medial and lateral thirds of which terminate among the pontine nuclei. In the pons it is broken up into several bundles, which come together as the *pyramid*, from which the tract takes its name, in the medulla oblongata. At the junction of the medulla and spinal cord, most of the pyramidal fibres decussate (i.e. cross to the opposite side), and run downward in the lateral columns of the cord. A variable proportion, on one side or both, continues downward, as the uncrossed pyramidal tracts, and decussate at lower levels. The fibres terminate in the grey matter of the spinal cord, and exert an influence on the motor cells of the anterior horns. The more rostral fibres (the corticobulbar tracts) exert a similar influence on cells in the motor nuclei of the brain stem.

The pyramidal tract has traditionally been regarded as

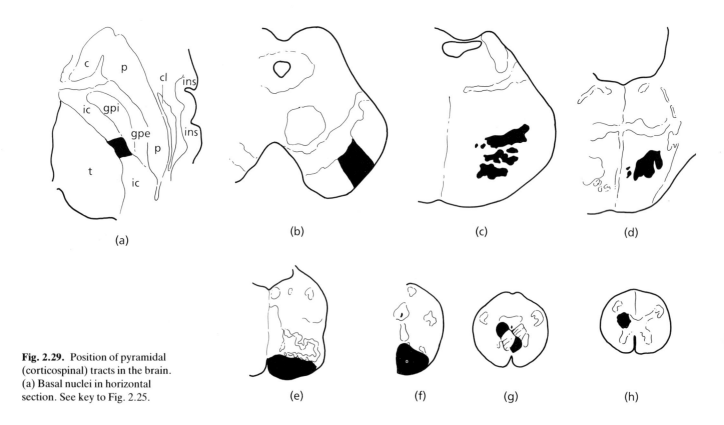

Fig. 2.29. Position of pyramidal (corticospinal) tracts in the brain. (a) Basal nuclei in horizontal section. See key to Fig. 2.25.

Table 2.1. Some myelinated tracts in the CNS

Tract	Origin	Principal destination	Conditions (other than MS) causing degeneration
Olfactory	Olfactory bulb	Pyriform cortex (uncus and parahippocampal gyrus)	Head injury, with avulsion of olfactory bulb (see p.94) Neurosurgery, with retraction of frontal lobe
Optic nerves and tracts	Retinae, with hemidecussation at chiasm	Lateral geniculate bodies	Retinal disease. Glaucoma. Ocular trauma. Orbital tumours Optic neuritis. Pituitary and parapituitary tumours (see Chapter 13) Methyl alcohol or clioquinol poisoning (pp.311, 313). Tobacco/alcohol amblyopia (p.310)
Geniculostriate (optic radiation)	Lateral geniculate body	Striate (visual) cortex	Cerebral tumours and vascular accidents Leucodystrophies (see Chapter 19)
Fimbria and fornix	Hippocampus	Septal nuclei and mamillary body	Mesial temporal sclerosis (see p.283). Cerebral tumours (see Chapter 12). Neurosurgery
Pyramidal (corticobulbar and corticospinal)	Pre- and postcentral cortex	(Via interneurons) contralateral motor nuclei of brain stem and cord	(Unilateral) cerebral trauma, tumour or vascular accident (Bilateral) cord compression. Motor neuron disease (p.236) Friedreich's ataxia (p.244). Strümpell's paraplegia (p.249) B_{12} deficiency (p.318). Toxins, including organophosphorus and clioquinol (Chapter 20)
Medial lemniscus (medial fillet)	Contralateral gracile and cuneate nuclei	Thalamus (nuc. ventralis lateralis)	Acceleration injuries (see p.92). Brain stem tumours (see Chapter 12)
Superior cerebellar peduncle (brachium conjunctivum)	Dentate nucleus	Contralateral red nucleus and thalamus	Acceleration injuries (p.92). Friedreich's ataxia (p.244) Progressive supranuclear palsy (p.248). DRPLA (p.248)
Middle cerebellar peduncle (brachium pontis)	Pontine nuclei	Contralateral cerebellar cortex	Pontocerebellar degeneration (see p.244)
Inferior cerebellar peduncle (restiform body)	Dorsal, accessory cuneate and vestibular nuclei: contralateral inferior olive	Cerebellar cortex	Cerebellar and spinocerebellar degenerations (p.244) Syringobulbia (p.127)
Solitary	Ganglia of facial, glossopharyngeal and vagus nerves	Nucleus of solitary tract	Peripheral neuropathies (Chapter 22) Multiple system atrophy
Cuneate funiculus (column of Burdach)	Cervical and thoracic sensory ganglia	Cuneate nucleus; accessory cuneate nucleus	Ascending, from lower spinal trauma or tumour Friedreich's ataxia and other system degenerations (Chapter 15)
Gracile funiculus (column of Goll)	Lumbar and sacral sensory ganglia	Gracile nucleus Thoracic nucleus	Peripheral neuropathies (Chapter 22). B_{12} deficiency (p.318) Carcinomatous radiculopathy (p.160). Tabes dorsalis. Toxins, including organophosphorus, clioquinol and vincristine (Chapter 20)
Dorsal spinocerebellar	Dorsal nucleus (Clarke's column)	Cerebellar cortex	Ascending, from lesions of lower spinal cord Friedreich's ataxia and other system degenerations (Chapter 15) Chronic meningitis and other causes of marginal degeneration of the spinal cord (p.131)

DRPLA dentato-rubro-pallido-luysian atrophy

the essential pathway for 'willed' movements. Since cases have been described in which interruption of the tract has not been followed by permanent hemiplegia, this view can no longer be treated as dogma; but it remains true that in most cases of hemiplegic 'stroke' the relevant pyramidal tract is found to have degenerated a few months later.

The positions of other important tracts are indicated in Figs 2.26 and 2.28. Some of the commoner degenerative conditions, in which individual tracts undergo progressive decay, are discussed in Chapter 15. Table 2.1 is intended to show the origins and destination of some of these tracts, along with some of the common conditions in which tract degeneration can be observed by low-power light microscopy. It is probably the case that not one of these tracts is 'pure', i.e. homogeneous in its origin and destination. The table merely indicates the *predominant* fibre composition.

In addition to those listed in the table, there are a number of conspicuous bundles of myelinated fibres, of mixed origin and destination, in which it is often possible to detect degenerative changes. These include: the *corpus callosum*, which is mainly composed of fibres connecting corresponding areas of cerebral cortex in the right and left hemispheres; the *anterior commissure* (Fig. 2.25C), similarly connecting the right and left temporal lobes; the *internal capsule*, which comprises not only the corticobulbar and corticospinal pathways but the many projections running from thalamus to cortex and cortex to thalamus; the *fornix,* which consists largely of fibres running from the hippocampus to the mamillary body and septal nuclei of the same side; the *lateral lemniscus* (lateral fillet), which contains auditory fibres on their way to the inferior colliculus and sensory fibres running to the thalamus; the *central tegmental tract*, with mainly descending fibres from the thalamus and other basal nuclei to the olives and other brain stem structures; the *medial longitudinal fasciculus*, which connects the nuclei of the third, fourth and sixth cranial nerves with each other and with the various vestibular nuclei; and the *inferior cerebellar peduncle* (restiform body), which carries the fibres of the dorsal spinocerebellar tract and its cranial equivalent, arising in the accessory cuneate (lateral cuneate) nucleus to the cerebellum, as well as fibres from the opposite inferior olive, and fibres running in both directions between the vestibular nuclei and the emboliform, fastigial and globose nuclei in the roof of the fourth ventricle.

In the spinal cord, the *posterior columns* (gracile and cuneate funiculi) are relatively pure, consisting of the central processes of primary sensory ganglion cells. The crossed and uncrossed pyramidal tracts, the dorsal spinocerebellar tracts, and less conspicuously the ventral spinocerebellar tracts, are tracts in the sense given above. The rest of the lateral and anterior white columns consists of a mixture of ascending and descending fibres, having various origins and destinations. The neatly defined 'tracts', so commonly illustrated in textbooks of neurology, are mainly the product of the passion for systematization of an older generation of German anatomists.

Loss of nerve cells

The other major preoccupation in the exploration of a sick brain or cord is the search for loss of, or pathological changes in, *nerve cells* in relevant areas. In general, the detection of cell loss is more troublesome than scanning for tract degeneration. It may involve careful (but often inconclusive) comparison with 'control' materials, or even cell counting in selected sites. It hardly needs saying that familiarity with the normal appearances is conducive to speed. In addition, there are two well-tried ways of making the task less formidable. One is the use of glial stains, which draw attention to foci of tissue loss or damage (see below). The other is to examine the efferent pathways serving the cells in question. For instance, loss of fibres in anterior nerve roots is a reliable indication of anterior horn cell loss; and loss of cells in a dentate nucleus is reflected in the superior cerebellar peduncle (Fig. 15.13).

Visual pathways

When there is a clinical history of *visual disturbances*, the reason for which is not readily apparent, it may be helpful to remind oneself of the anatomy of the visual pathways, the main points of which are shown in Fig. 2.30. It should be clear from this that a defect in the sight of *one* eye will result from a lesion in that eye or in its optic nerve. A defect in the temporal fields of *both* eyes points to a lesion affecting the fibres from the medial halves of both retinae. This may happen with a tumour such as an olfactory groove meningioma, lying just in front of the chiasm, or from one lying just behind the chiasm, such as a pituitary adenoma. A defect in corresponding areas of the visual fields of *both* eyes (homonymous hemianopia) indicates a lesion in the optic tract on the side opposite the field defect, or in the related lateral geniculate body, optic radiation or calcarine cortex. The optic radiation itself arises from cells in the *lateral geniculate body*, which is a detached part of the thalamus, situated just above the choroidal fissure at coronal level P2 (see Fig. 2.5). The fibres of the radiation at first run laterally and forward and then hook around the inferior (temporal) horn of the lateral ventricle; they then run backward, close to the lateral wall of the inferior and posterior horns of the ventricle. The fibres serving the *upper* halves of the visual fields reach further forward in the temporal white matter than those serving the lower halves of the visual fields; further back, they lie more ventrally, and pass underneath the ventricle to reach the lower lip of the calcarine sulcus on the medial surface of the occipital lobe. The fibres serving the lower halves of the visual fields pass over the ventricle to reach the upper lip of the calcarine sulcus (see Polyak 1957).

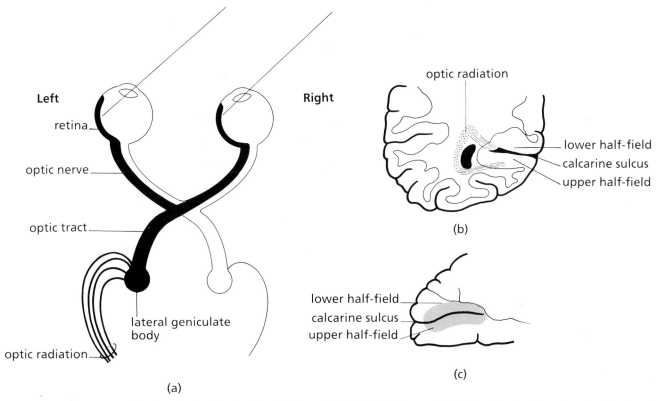

Fig. 2.30. Visual pathways. (a) Fibres involved in signalling light from the right side, falling on the left sides of both retinae. Note the direction of fibres of the optic radiation, originating in the left lateral geniculate body. (b) Coronal slice at level P6, showing the optic radiation lateral to the occipital horn, giving off fibres to the upper and lower lips of the calcarine sulcus. (c) Medial surface of the left calcarine area. Most of the visual cortex lies buried within the depths of the calcarine sulcus.

Fornix system

In recent years students of higher brain function have been increasingly interested in the *hippocampus−fornix 'system'*, lesions of which result in disturbances of memory formation (see p.369). The *hippocampus* itself is a rolled-up continuation of the cortex of the parahippocampal gyrus, lying in the floor of the inferior horn of the lateral ventricle (Figs 2.5, P1−P3; 2.25E−H; 2.31). The axons of the pyramidal layer collect to form a thin layer of white matter (alveus) immediately below the ependyma. They run medially and backward, to form a distinct white ribbon, the *fimbria*, which continues medially, at first backward and then upward, closely following the horseshoe-shaped line of the choroidal fissure. The two fimbriae meet under cover of the splenium of the corpus callosum between coronal levels P3 and P4, and become the *fornix*. The fornix continues in the line of the choroidal fissure, and runs forward in the roof of the third ventricle, slung from the corpus callosum by the septum lucidum. Between levels A1 and A2 it dips abruptly downward into the *septal area*, whence fibres pass to the septal nuclei and thalamus. The main body of the fornix runs down to end in the *mamillary bodies* at level A1. A conspicuous bundle (mamillothalamic tract: bundle of Vicq d'Azyr) runs hence to the *anterior nucleus of the thalamus* (Fig. 2.25E), which projects largely to the *cingulate cortex*, which in turn projects to *the entorhinal region* of the parahippocampal gyrus, leaving only a short step back to the hippocampus proper. Needless to say, the discovery of this circuit (the *Papez* circuit)) has given deep satisfaction to neurologists, who were looking for an anatomical substrate for the reverberating circuitry required by most theories of the mechanism of memory. Parts of this circuit are sometimes assigned to a vaguely defined 'limbic system'. See Brodal (1981), p.689.

Cerebral cortex

For sampling particular areas of cerebral cortex, reference should be made to labelled photographs of standard slices. If blocks of cortex are taken which do not include identifiable landmarks such as the hippocampus or basal nuclei, a note should be made of the side and level (coronal or horizontal) from which the sample is taken. The *visual cortex*, most of which lies within the lips of the calcarine fissure, is usually easily identified in both coronal and horizontal slices, by the presence of the white line of Gennari (Fig. 2.32). The *Rolandic (central) sulcus* is somewhat harder to identify, as it pursues a wavy course forward and downward from the vertex to the Sylvian (lateral) fissure (Fig. 2.2), and is

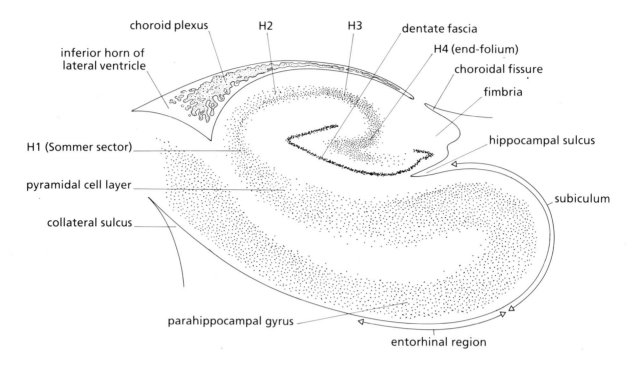

Fig. 2.31. The left hippocampus, in coronal plane passing through the lateral geniculate body (level P2).

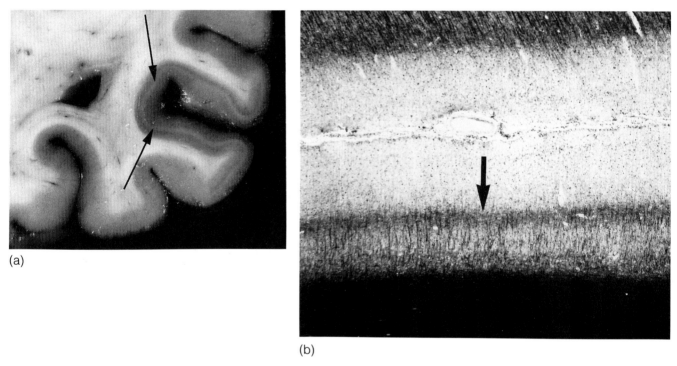

(a)

(b)

Fig. 2.32. Visual (striate, calcarine) cortex, (a) Naked-eye appearance in coronal section. The white line (of Gennari) is clearly visible (arrowed). (b) Myelin-stained section (×30). The line of Gennari (arrowed) is even more conspicuous.

liable to be cut at many different angles in routine slicing. In coronal slices, there will be some point between A1 and P4 where the cut is truly transverse to the central sulcus. Here, there is a striking difference of thickness between the pre-central (motor) cortex and the postcentral (primary sensory) cortex, the former being up to twice as thick as the latter (Fig. 2.33). Because the central sulcus runs forward and downward, the motor cortex will lie above the sensory cortex. In horizontal slices it lies in front of the sensory cortex. The difference in thickness is equally obvious (Fig. 2.6A−C). In some cases, it may be desirable to compare the cortex of different cerebral lobes in a single section. It is here that the temptation arises to put the technicians on their mettle by calling for sections of an entire hemisphere — for instance a block from level P1 or P2, showing not only basal nuclei and hippocampus but also large areas of frontal, temporal and parietal cortex.

Specimens, either for embedding or for frozen sections, should be marked (for instance, with a spot of Indian ink) on the side opposite that from which sections are to be made. When the specimen is more or less symmetrical, as in transverse sections of the brain stem and cord, it is advisable to have a consistent method of marking, so that sections are routinely made from *either* the lower *or* the upper surface. In this way one can be sure which is the left side and which is the right. If in a particular case one wishes to examine the other surface of the specimen, a nick can be made with a knife on the left side of the block.

Even when the case appears to be devoid of research interest, it is usually wise to keep the rest of the material until the histology has been examined and reported on. In complicated cases, it is often economical to make a few sighting shots, so to speak, before making one's final selection of blocks.

Storage of material

As it is difficult to be sure when interest in a particular case has subsided, or whether at a later date one may wish to take further samples for histology, it is desirable to have plenty of storage space, fitted with shelves, at one's disposal; failing that, to make a nuisance of oneself until one gets it. For brains and spinal cords, we find plastic paint-kettles, of some 4 litres capacity, with metal handles and tight fitting lids, convenient and relatively cheap. In these, tissue stored

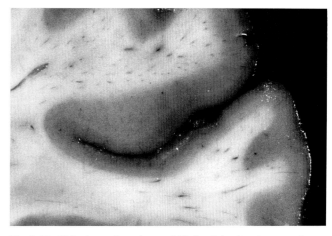

Fig. 2.33. Naked-eye view of central (Rolandic) sulcus in coronal section. The motor (precentral) cortex (above) is considerably wider than the sensory (postcentral) cortex.

in 10% formalin keeps well, and yields satisfactory histological specimens for several years. (An exception is the Weil−Davenport silver impregnation for microglia, which requires fairly fresh tissue.) Brain slices should be kept flat; distortions from folding quite soon become permanent. Spinal cords should be cut into three or more lengths rather than coiled up. It is useful to have a record of which specimens have been stored, and which discarded. We would also recommend keeping fairly meticulous records of photographs taken in the course of cut-ups, with an index enabling one to find the relevant illustrations for a particular condition without undue hassle, waste of time, and frustration. It is pleasant to be able to meet one's colleagues' requests for the loan of teaching slides, and at the same time display the efficiency of one's filing system.

Further reading

Brodal A. 1981. *Neurological Anatomy in Relation to Clinical Medicine*, 3rd edn. Oxford University Press, Oxford.

Greenhall RCD. 1977. *Pathological findings in acute cerebrovascular disease and their clinical implications*. D.M. thesis, University of Oxford.

Oppenheimer DR. 1984. Diseases of the basal ganglia, cerebellum and motor neurons. In Adams JH, Corsellis JAN, Duchen LW (Eds) *Greenfield's Neuropathology*, 4th edn. Edward Arnold, London, Chapter 15.

Polyak S. 1957. *The Vertebrate Visual System*. University of Chicago Press, Chicago.

Chapter 3
Histology

In dealing with most cases of vascular, neoplastic and inflammatory disease there are no great differences between the methods used by general pathologists and those of neuropathologists. Their methods diverge, however, in cases where detailed neuro-anatomical investigation is required — for instance, in dealing with 'degenerative' diseases or 'organic' mental disorders. Basic knowledge in these fields owes more to the researches of neurologists and psychiatrists, mostly French and German, working around the turn of the century, than it does to the great Virchow and his followers. Standing apart from these is the towering figure of Ramón y Cajal.

The following brief account of the histopathology of the nervous system is concerned mainly with features not present in other parts of the body.

Neurons

Neurons occur in many different shapes and sizes. Textbooks of histology regularly illustrate the larger and more flamboyant types (Figs 3.1−3.5), but sometimes fail to mention that most of the nerve cells in the CNS are small and unimpressive, and often hard to distinguish from glial cells in conventional cell stains. Fortunately, it is the larger and more spectacular types which are most often of interest to the neuropathologist. In general, these are recognizable (in well-preserved and well-stained material) by their prominent nucleoli and the flecks of Nissl substance in their cytoplasm.

Of the various pathological changes observed in nerve cells, the commonest is caused by ischaemia or anoxia. This, the so-called *homogenizing change*, is most readily observed in pyramidal cells of the cerebral cortex and hippocampus, and in Purkinje cells of the cerebellar cortex

(Plates 1.1−1.3). The whole cell shrinks; the cytoplasm loses its Nissl granules, acquires a glassy uniformity, and becomes eosinophilic. The nucleus is shrunken and uniformly basophilic, and the nucleolus disappears. The change is observable 12 hours or so after the insult. After a few days, the cell body is devoured by phagocytic microglial cells — a process rather pompously referred to as *neuronophagia* (Fig. 3.6). The cell processes — dendrites and axons — disappear; and at the sites where neurons and their processes (including myelin sheath) are lost, astrocytes react by laying down glial fibres (see below). In some circumstances dead nerve cells, instead of being absorbed, become impregnated with iron and calcium salts (ferrugination; Fig. 3.7).

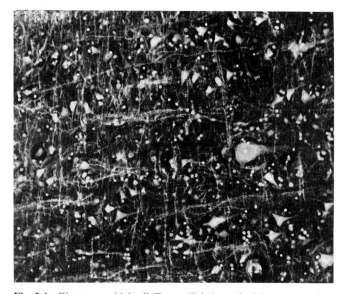

Fig. 3.1. Giant pyramidal cell (Betz cell) in layer 5 of the precentral gyrus. The pial surface is to the right. Klüver−Barrera, ×100.

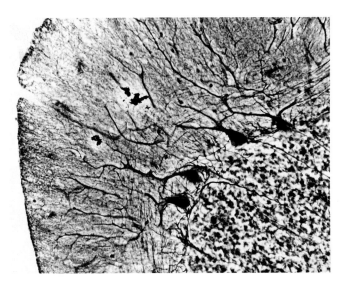

Fig. 3.2. Cerebellar cortex. Molecular layer, upper right; granular layer, lower right. Between them, the layer of Purkinje cells spread their dendrites in the molecular layer. Basket fibres are seen running in the deeper part of the molecular layer (cf. Fig. 3.9). Holmes silver, ×130.

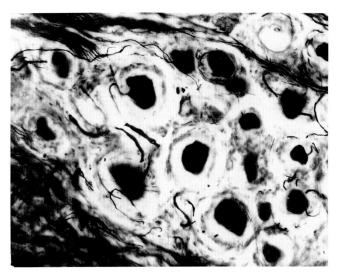

Fig. 3.4. Sensory ganglion cells. The cells have a single axon (often tortuous at first), which divides into two branches, one of which runs out to the periphery, while the other runs, via a posterior rootlet, into the posterior column of the spinal cord (cf. Fig. 3.27). Schofield silver, ×200.

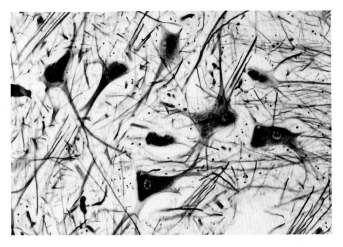

Fig. 3.3. Motor cells from the anterior horn of the spinal cord. The cells are large, with widely spreading dendrites. Holmes silver, ×250. Compare with Plate 1.5.

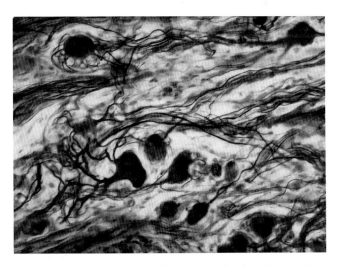

Fig. 3.5. Autonomic ganglion cells. They are of various shapes. Many are multipolar. Schofield, ×200.

Central chromatolysis is a non-lethal change undergone by neurons whose axons have been severed. It is thought to signify a state of increased metabolic activity directed toward the regeneration of the axon from its proximal stump. The process is most often seen in lower motor neurons — for instance, in the anterior horns of the spinal cord after a motor root or nerve has been interrupted by trauma or tumour. Here, in contrast to the homogenizing change, the nucleus and nucleolus are intact; but the whole nucleus is displaced towards the periphery. Nissl granules are also displaced, leaving a central area of clear — but not eosinophilic — cytoplasm (Plates 1.5 and 1.6). The cell body is not shrunken; if anything, it is expanded, with flattening of axonal and dendritic hillocks. A somewhat similar appearance is often seen in the cerebral cortex in Pick's disease (see pp. 278–9). In some cases of motor neuron disease, scattered large round 'ghost' cells, staining very palely and devoid of nuclei, may be seen in the anterior horns of the cord. Their origin is in doubt. Another type of change, which has been attributed, like central chromatolysis, to efforts at axonal regeneration, is the formation of 'torpedoes' (Fig. 3.8) on the axons of cerebellar Purkinje cells. Since Purkinje cells are susceptible to a wide variety of malign influences, including old age, they are commonly depleted, and their earlier position is marked in silver impregnations by the empty processes of basket cells (Fig. 3.9).

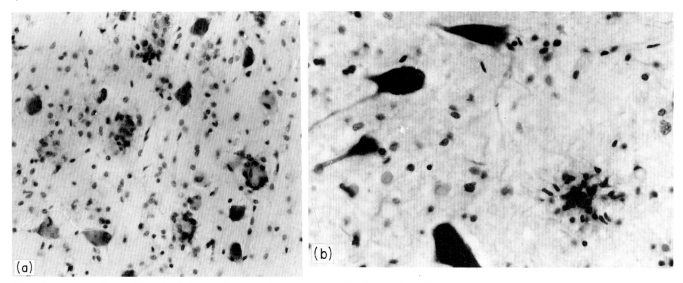

Fig. 3.6. Neuronophagia: (a) in the thalamus of a 4-month-old baby suffering from perinatal hypoxia. Dead thalamic neurons are being devoured by macrophages. Nissl, ×400; (b) in the anterior horn of the spinal cord in a case of multiple system atrophy (p.241). All that remains of a defunct motor cell is a cluster of macrophages. Nissl, ×470.

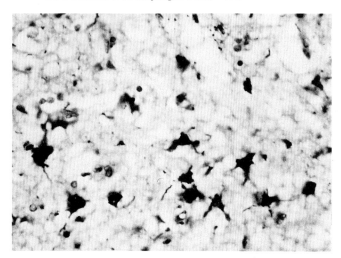

Fig. 3.7. Ferrugination. In an area of old infarction, the bodies of dead neurons in the cerebral cortex, instead of undergoing phagocytosis, have been mummified and impregnated with iron and calcium salts. In an H&E preparation they appear densely basophilic. H&E, ×350. (The resemblance to silver-impregnated neurofibrillary tangles (Fig. 3.10) is fortuitous.)

Changes in neuronal cytoplasm which, in the absence of any knowledge of their causes, are classed as 'degenerative', include Alzheimer's neurofibrillary tangles (Fig. 3.10) and the inclusion bodies, first described by Lewy, characteristic of paralysis agitans (see pp.240–41; Plate 1.4). *Neurofibrillary tangles* occur, mainly but not exclusively, in pyramidal cells of the cerebral cortex and hippocampus. Their relation to dementia in elderly people, and their association with 'senile' plaques (Fig. 3.11), are discussed on pp. 270–73. The histochemistry and ultra-structure of *Lewy bodies* in paralysis agitans, and of the *Lafora bodies* associated with the far

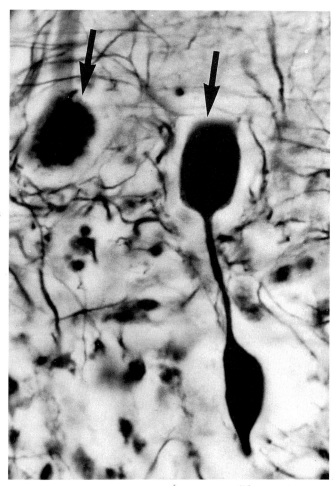

Fig. 3.8. Cerebellar Purkinje cells (arrowed) in a case of multiple system atrophy (p.241). The axon of one cell is expanded by a so-called 'torpedo' — a sign that the distal part of the axon is damaged. Holmes silver, ×1400.

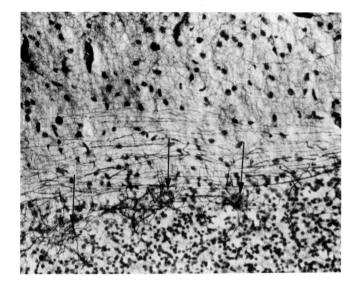

Fig. 3.9. Cerebellar cortex from which Purkinje cells have been lost. The pial surface lies just above the top edge of the edge of the picture. The molecular layer occupies the upper two-thirds and the granule-cell layer the lower third. Between them, the axons of basket cells run parallel to the surface. These terminate in the 'baskets' which normally envelop the bodies of the Purkinje cells. Here, the Purkinje cells have died, leaving empty baskets (arrowed). Holmes silver, ×160.

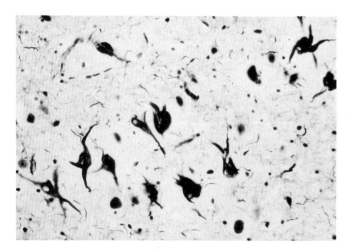

Fig. 3.10. Neurofibrillary tangles in the subiculum (Fig. 2.31) in a case of progressive supranuclear palsy (p.248). von Braunmühl silver impregnation, ×270.

rarer condition of myoclonus epilepsy, have so far revealed nothing to suggest a connection with virus infections. It is otherwise with the eosinophilic cytoplasmic inclusions of rabies, herpes simplex encephalitis and subacute sclerosing panencephalitis. These are described and discussed in Chapter 10.

Striking changes are seen, mainly in the larger cells of the central and peripheral nervous system, in the *lipidoses*. These are for the most part familial disorders, with autosomal recessive inheritance, in which deficiency of an enzyme results in abnormal accumulations of a normal or abnormal lipid

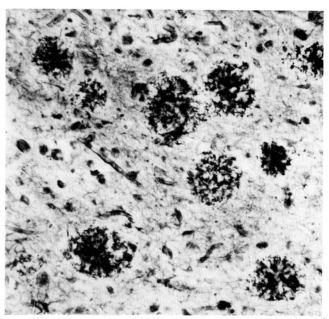

Fig. 3.11. 'Senile' plaques in the cortex of a patient with Alzheimer's disease (p.270). von Braunmühl, ×300.

substance in the cytoplasm of nerve cells (Fig. 19.2). The histological appearances tend to be similar in different types of lipidosis. These conditions are discussed in Chapter 19.

Neuroglia

Neuroglial cells — astrocytes, oligodendrocytes and ependymal cells — originate, like central neurons, from the embryonic neural tube, the common ancestral cell being the spongioblast. The secretory epithelium of the choroid plexus consists of modified ependymal cells.

Astrocytes

Astrocytes are distributed throughout the central (but not the peripheral) nervous system. They have two (perhaps three) known functions (others which have been ascribed to them have not yet been generally accepted). The first of these is based mainly on electron-microscopical studies, which show that while nerve cells have no direct contact with capillary blood vessels, the processes of astrocytes make intimate contact both with nerve cell bodies and with capillaries. It is inferred that certain astrocytes perform the duties of wet-nurses to neurons. The second function is that of reacting to various kinds of local damage — cell death, axonal degeneration, demyelination, etc. — by proliferating, enlarging and putting out long processes which in due course become glial fibres, forming a glial scar (Figs 3.12–3.15). The term *gliosis* is commonly (and confusingly) used to denote both hypertrophy and hyperplasia of astrocytes on the one hand, and glial scarring on the other. We think

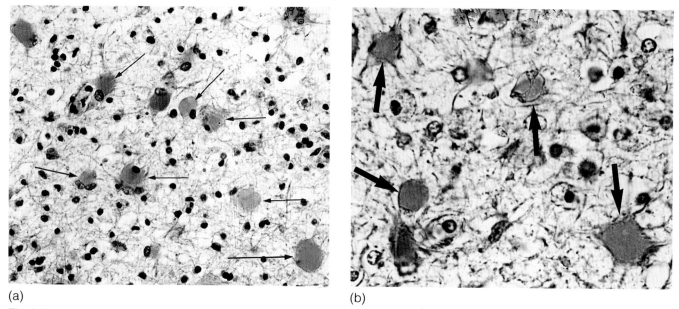

(a)   (b)

Fig. 3.12. Reactive astrocytes (arrowed) in an active plaque of MS. (a) H&E; (b) phosphotungstic acid/haematoxylin. Both ×450.

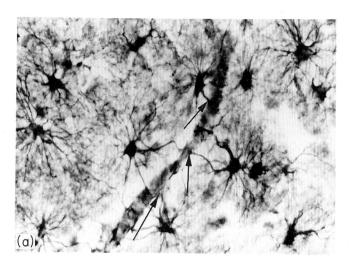

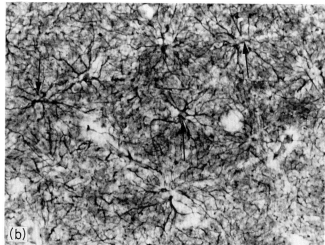

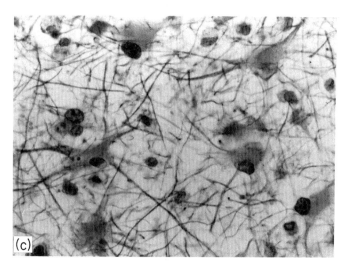

Fig. 3.13. Reactive astrocytes. (a) In the cerebral cortex in a case of Creutzfeldt−Jakob disease. Astrocytes are increased in numbers and in size. Some of the thicker cell processes can be seen terminating in 'end-feet' (arrowed) on the walls of a small blood vessel. Cajal's gold sublimate, ×180. (b) So-called protoplasmic astrocytes in the neighbourhood of a malignant tumour. The cell bodies are smaller than those of the fibrillary astrocytes shown in Fig. 3.13a; the processes are more numerous and more finely divided. In some places (arrowed) glial fibrils can be seen running through the cytoplasm from one process into another. Cajal's gold sublimate, ×180. (c) In a plaque of acute MS. The cells are pleomorphic, and in some instances multinucleate. In biopsy specimens of lesions of this kind there is a temptation to rush into a diagnosis of astrocytoma. Holzer, ×420.

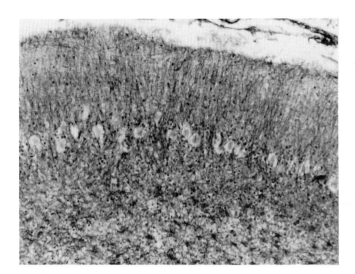

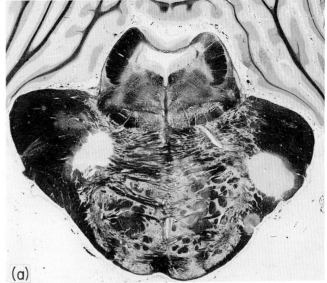

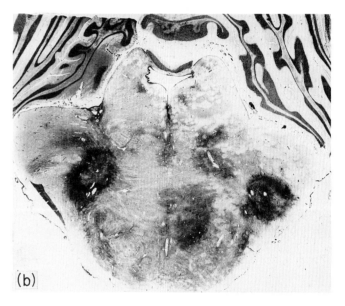

Fig. 3.14. Gliosis of the cerebellar cortex in a case of Creutzfeldt—Jakob disease. There has been a massive loss of neurons in the granular layer (lower half of picture), and almost all the cells seen in this area are reactive astrocytes. Above this, there are Purkinje cells in normal numbers. The molecular layer (above) is crammed with the fibrillar processes of astrocytes (the so-called Bergmann glia) situated in the Purkinje cell layer. The glial fibrils lie parallel with each other (so-called 'isomorphous gliosis') because they are replacing the axons of dead granule cells, which themselves lie at right angles to the surface. Holzer, ×60.

Fig. 3.15. Gliosis in chronic plaques of MS in the pons. Note that the plaques, though roughly symmetrical, are not related to particular neuro-anatomical structures, (a) Myelin stain. (b) Holzer stain, showing so-called 'shadow plaques' (see p.231).

the term is best reserved for the latter. The third function plausibly ascribed to these cells is the maintenance of the *blood—brain barrier* by means of their 'end-feet', which surround the walls of small vessels (Fig. 3.13a) and the similar terminal expansions applied to the pial and ependymal linings of the brain.

In conventional cell stains, and even in metallic impregnations, normal resting astrocytes are unimpressive. The cytoplasm is scanty and the cell outline indistinct. The nucleus is ellipsoid rather than globular, and smaller than that of most nerve cells, rather pale, with a stippling of chromatin. In a reactive astrocyte, the cytoplasm enlarges and becomes more eosinophilic, and the nucleus is displaced to the side (Fig. 3.12). Binucleate forms are not uncommon, and should not be regarded as evidence of neoplasia. In a Holzer preparation (see p.58) one can see cell processes extending in all directions; there are fibrils, presumably the precursors of glial fibres, running from one such process through the cytoplasm, ending in another process, and criss-crossing with other similar fibrils. In metallic impregnations, of which Cajal's gold chloride method is the general favourite, less is seen of intracellular details, but more of the cell processes (Fig. 3.13a and b). Some of these processes, thicker than the rest, terminate as 'end-feet' on the walls of capillaries and venules (Fig. 3.13a). Others, on the surface of the brain and cord, end in intimate contact with the pia mater. Astrocytes, with their processes, may also be demonstrated by treatment with an anti-GFAP (glial fibril-lary acidic protein) antiserum or monoclonal antibody (Fig. 3.30; see p.60).

Following Cajal, a distinction is often drawn between 'fibrillary' and 'protoplasmic' astrocytes (Fig. 3.13a and b), and these terms have been applied to the cells in astrocytic tumours. The physiological significance of this distinction is not known. The change referred to as 'clasmatodendrosis' — i.e. fragmentation of astrocytic processes — is seen in metallic impregnations of what are thought to be moribund astrocytes. Of the few recognized pathological cell changes, two were first described in cases of Wilson's disease

(hepatolenticular degeneration; see p.293). The cells referred to as 'Alzheimer glia, type 1' appear to be grossly
enlarged astrocytes, with bizarre polyploid nuclei (Fig. 19.4).
Similar cells are seen, not only in glial tumours, but also in
Richardson's disease (progressive multifocal leucoencephalopathy; see p.150). Alzheimer type-2 glia is more commonly met with, and appears to be pathognomonic of
hyperammonaemia due to liver failure (see p.302). The
cells appear in conventional cell stains as naked nuclei
within almost empty spaces. These nuclei are pale, globular
or lobulated, larger than those of normal astrocytes, with a
diffuse stipple of chromatin, and a conspicuous nucleolus
(Fig. 19.3). They occur mainly in grey matter, in any region
of the brain.

Oligodendrocytes

Apart from vascular endothelium, oligodendrocytes are the
most numerous cells in the CNS. The 'few dendritic processes' which give them their name are difficult to demonstrate by routine methods, but their nuclei are easily seen.
These are smaller than astrocyte nuclei and contain more
chromatin; in size and staining properties they closely resemble the nuclei of small lymphocytes, from which they
are generally distinguished by their location. In the CNS,
lymphocytes tend to occur in perivascular 'cuffs' (Fig. 3.16),
where they are a sign of an inflammatory process, whereas
oligodendrocytes lie free, or in long or short chains, in
association with myelinated axons (Fig. 3.17). Similar cells
are sometimes seen in unusually large numbers, closely
associated with large nerve cells in the cerebral cortex (Fig.
3.18). The significance of this appearance (so-called *satellitosis*) is not known.

Oligodendrocytes are credited with the function of laying
down, and perhaps of maintaining, myelin sheaths around

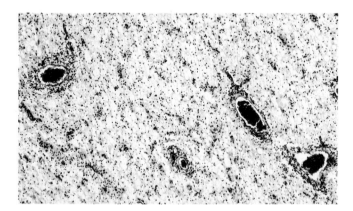

Fig. 3.16. Lymphocytic 'cuffing' of small vessels in cerebral white
matter in a case of subacute sclerosing panencephalitis. This reaction,
often associated with proliferation of microglia, is the most
characteristic feature of inflammatory disorders of the CNS. It is also
commonly seen in vascular and neoplastic disorders, and in
demyelinating diseases such as MS. H&E.

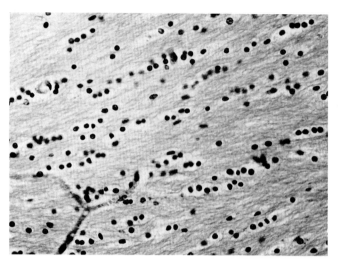

Fig. 3.17. Normal cerebral white matter, showing interfascicular
oligodendrocytes, many of them lying in short chains. H&E, ×250.

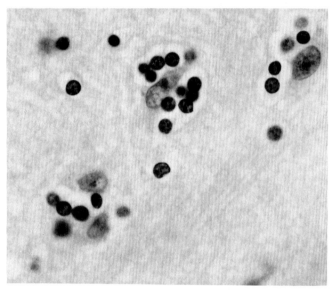

Fig. 3.18. Satellitosis. Nuclei, presumably of oligodendrocytes,
clustered around pyramidal cells in temporal cortex, ×450. (Specimen
from a case of temporal lobe epilepsy.)

axons in the CNS — the role performed by Schwann cells in
the peripheral nervous system. In examining the proximal
parts of cranial and spinal nerve roots, one sees a somewhat
untidy looking transition zone where the two cell types
meet, a millimetre or so from the surface of the cord or
brain stem (Fig. 3.27). In some myelin stains, one can also
see a difference of colour between the central and peripheral
myelin. (In cases with long-standing damage to the posterior
columns, regeneration of sensory nerve fibres may occur,
and the cord is re-invaded by regenerated axons, accompanied
by Schwann cells and invested by myelin of peripheral type
and by collagen-forming fibroblasts, as in Fig. 3.32.) In
demyelinating conditions, and in wallerian degeneration of
myelinated tracts, oligodendrocytes are generally believed

Plate 1

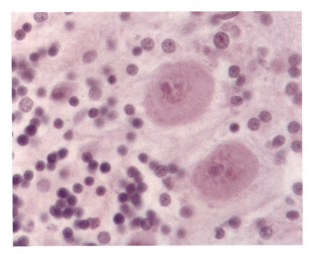

1.1. Cerebellar cortex, with two healthy looking Purkinje cells. The cytoplasm is finely granular and lilac coloured. The nuclei are globular, with flecks of chromatin and well-defined nuclei. H&E, ×800.

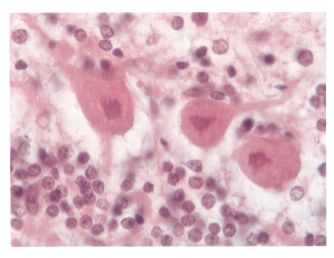

1.2. Purkinje cells from a patient dying after a few hours of hypoxaemia. The cytoplasm is glassy and eosinophilic ('homogenizing change'), and the nuclei are shrunken, deformed, and uniformly basophilic. H&E, ×800.

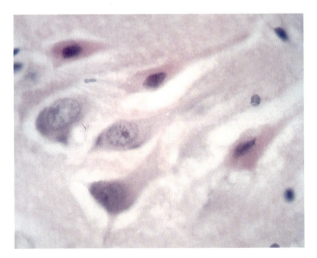

1.3. Hypoxic changes in the pyramidal cell layer of the hippocampus. Three cells in the lower left area appear healthy, whereas three others, in the upper right area, show homogenizing change, with shrinkage, eosinophilic cytoplasm and deformed basophilic nuclei. H&E, ×850.

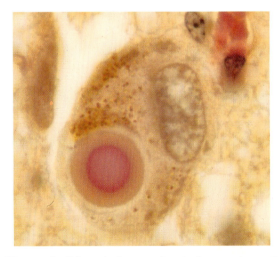

1.4. Pigmented cell from the locus ceruleus in the pons, in a patient with Parkinson's disease. The nucleus is seen on the right; on the left there is a typical laminated Lewy inclusion body. Lendrum's phloxine-tartrazine, ×1600.

Plates 1.5 and 1.6 overleaf

Plate 1 cont.

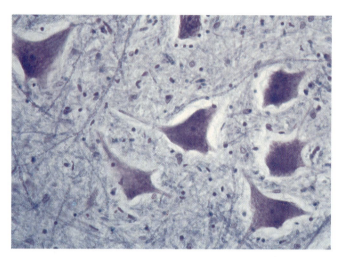

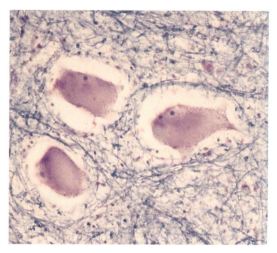

1.5. Normal-looking motor cells from the anterior horn of a spinal cord. The cells are angular (cf. Fig. 3.3), with prominent dendrite hillocks. The cytoplasm is flecked with Nissl substance (tigroid bodies); the nuclei are globular, centrally placed, and contain prominent nucleoli. Klüver−Barrera, ×330.

1.6. Central chromatolysis in three anterior horn cells, the axons of which had been involved in a malignant pelvic tumour. Dendrite hillocks have been reduced, giving the cells a rounded outline. Nissl granules have largely disappeared from the central parts of the cells. The nuclei appear to be flattened against the cell wall, but retain their nucleoli. The appearance is not to be confused with the homogenizing change of hypoxic cells. Klüver−Barrera, ×330.

Plate 2

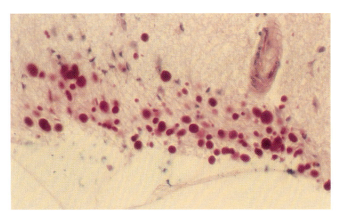

2.1. Accumulation of corpora amylacea in the subpial tissue at the base of the cerebrum. The appearance, though striking, is non-specific. It must not be confused with the picture of cryptococcal meningitis. PAS, ×250.

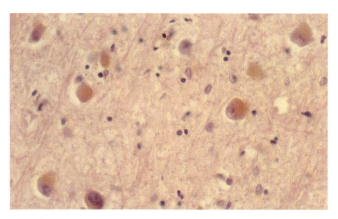

2.2. Lipofuscin in thalamic nerve cells. Buff-coloured lipid may occupy over half the volume of the cell. As with corpora amylacea, the appearance is non-specific, becoming more prominent with increasing age. H&E, ×420.

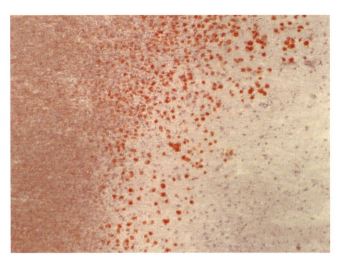

2.3. Lipid phagocytes at the active margin of a plaque of MS. On the left, the fat stain has coloured myelin a pale red; on the right, there is a chronic plaque, from which the myelin breakdown products have been removed by phagocytes and discharged into the bloodstream. Oil red O, ×25.

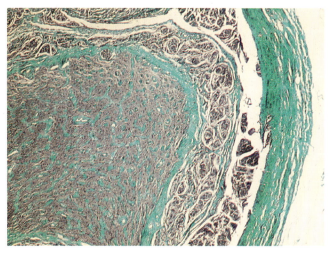

2.4. Meningioma compressing an optic nerve. On the far right of the picture, the dura of the optic foramen is stained green. Proceeding from right to left there follows: a layer of meningioma in the subdural space; the arachnoid (green); meningioma in the subarachnoid space; the pial covering of the optic nerve and finally the nerve itself. The latter is largely demyelinated, but still contains some red-staining myelin sheaths. The fibrous septa within the nerve are stained green. Gomori trichrome, ×25.

Plates 2.5 and 2.6 overleaf

Plate 2 cont.

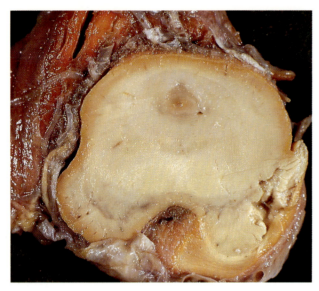

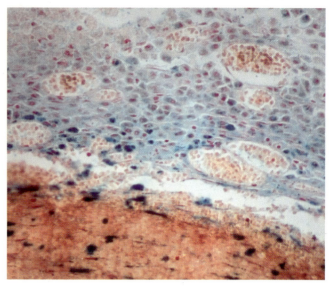

2.5. Superficial haemosiderosis. The patient, a youth aged 21, had undergone a right hemidecortication for intractable epilepsy and behaviour disorder 11 years previously, with good results. Subsequent dribbling intracranial haemorrhage had resulted in superficial haemosiderosis, with obstruction of the CSF pathways. The picture shows brown staining of the surface of the midbrain to a depth of a millimetre or more, and of the tissue surrounding the aqueduct, which has been finally occluded by granular ependymitis. The upper surface of the cerebellum (top of picture) shows a rich dark brown. The right cerebral peduncle (left of picture) is atrophic. The left peduncle has suffered a post mortem tear.

2.6. Transverse section through a chronic subdural membrane, stained for iron. The membrane (upper part of picture) contains numerous deposits of haemosiderin, mostly contained in phagocytes. There is a fibrous stroma, containing scattered thin-walled sinusoid vessels. These vessels are probably the source of the intermittent bleeding which maintains the haematoma. The dark-brown material in the lower part of the picture is altered blood. Perls' stain, ×160.

to die and disappear; it has, however, been suggested that they may sometimes be transformed into astrocytes. Both astrocytes and oligodendrocytes may disappear, along with some nerve cells, in cases of *metachromatic (sulphatide) leucodystrophy* (see p.296).

A peculiar change is seen within the lesions of Richardson's disease (see p.150). Cells thought to be oligodendrocytes acquire large, densely basophilic, nuclei, sometimes with a crescent of pale-staining cytoplasm (Fig. 10.31).

Ependyma

Ependyma, which forms a ciliated one-cell-thick lining to the ventricular system, including the aqueduct and foramina of Luschka, is capable of regenerating to cover local defects in early life (Fig. 3.20), but in later life is unable or unwilling to do so. When, for any reason, the ventricles enlarge, gaps in the ependyma are patched with glial fibres formed by astrocytes, which flatten themselves on the surface.

Where parts of the neural tube or cerebral vesicles close up (as they normally do in the central canal of the cord, at the tips of the posterior horns of the lateral ventricles, and elsewhere) the ependymal cells do not disappear, but lose their epithelium-like arrangement and form clusters or rosettes of rather nondescript cells resembling resting astrocytes (Fig. 3.19), surrounded by glial fibrils. Apart from tumour formation (see pp.181−4), recognized pathological changes in ependyma are few. They include hypertrophy of scattered cells in cases of cytomegalic virus infection (see p.328). In the relatively common condition of 'granular ependymitis', which is often attributable to abnormalities in the ventricular CSF, subependymal astrocytes proliferate, burst through the ependyma, and form a dense mat of glial fibres covering the ependymal cells (Figs 3.20 and 3.21). When this happens in the lining of a ventricle, no harm is done; but if it occurs in a narrow passage such as the aqueduct, it may lead to occlusion, causing obstructive hydrocephalus (see pp.121−3; Fig. 8.4).

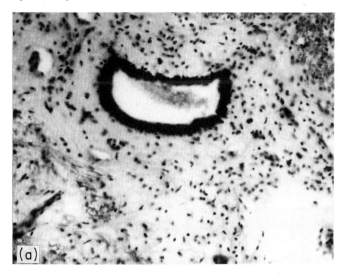
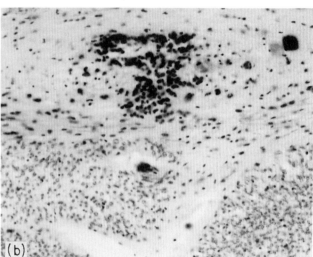

Fig. 3.19. Central canal of the spinal cord. In (a) there is a persistent canal, with ependymal lining. If it were larger, it would constitute a hydromyelic cavity (see p.127). H&E, ×150. In (b) the canal is obliterated, and its position marked by a cluster of nondescript glial cells. This is the more usual appearance. H&E, ×85.

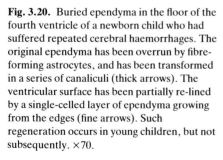

Fig. 3.20. Buried ependyma in the floor of the fourth ventricle of a newborn child who had suffered repeated cerebral haemorrhages. The original ependyma has been overrun by fibre-forming astrocytes, and has been transformed in a series of canaliculi (thick arrows). The ventricular surface has been partially re-lined by a single-celled layer of ependyma growing from the edges (fine arrows). Such regeneration occurs in young children, but not subsequently. ×70.

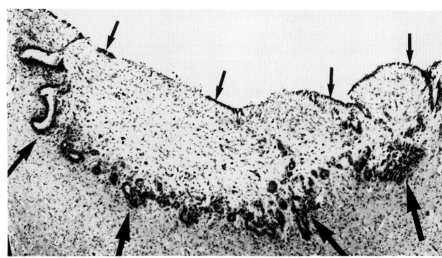

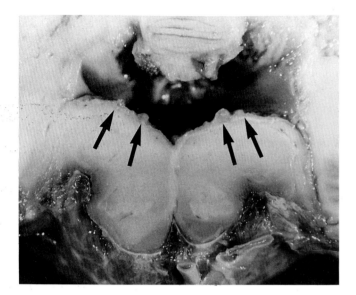

Fig. 3.21. Florid granular ependymitis (arrowed) in the fourth ventricle of a youth who had undergone a right cerebral hemidecortication for intractable epilepsy with severe behaviour disturbances. There was persistent dribbling haemorrhage from the operation site, resulting in superficial haemosiderosis of both pial and ependymal surfaces, and in widespread ependymitis. The picture shows discoloration of the exposed surfaces and atrophy of the right pyramid. Compare with Plate 2.5.

Choroid plexus

Choroid plexus consists of much-divided fronds of highly vascular connective tissue covered with a single-celled layer of cuboidal epithelium (Fig. 3.22). The plexus of the lateral ventricles is formed, in the embryo, by invagination of pia mater through a thinned-out stretch of cortex into the ventricular cavity. The pia carries with it branches of the choroidal arteries, which divide to form capillaries, which in turn join up to form the draining veins. The ependymal cells lining the ventricles are transformed into the secretory epithelium of the choroid plexus. In the lateral ventricles, this invagination occurs along the horseshoe-shaped choroid fissure; similar invaginations occur from the tela choroidea of the third and fourth ventricles. With increasing age, calcium salts are deposited in the choroid plexus, to the point where they are visible in X-rays, and grate on the knife when the brain is being sliced (the *pineal gland* is the other brain structure normally undergoing calcification).

In diagnostic work, choroid plexus commonly attracts attention in smear biopsies (see p.71). Firstly, there is a danger of mistaking a fragment of plexus for a carcinomatous deposit. Secondly, there may be some difficulty in distinguishing between normal plexus and a well-differentiated plexus papilloma. Errors are best avoided by keeping in close communication with the people in the operating theatre.

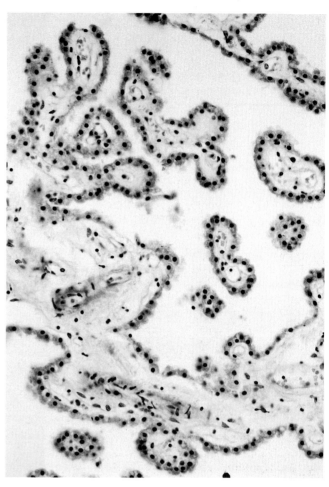

Fig. 3.22. Papillary fronds of choroid plexus in section (H&E, ×240). Compare with the wet-film appearance (Fig. 4.3b).

Microglia

The origins and functions of microglia are still disputed. For many years the general opinion has been that microglial cells are of mesodermal origin, and derived from the monocytes of the blood (also, possibly, from the pericytes of small blood vessels). When brain tissue is damaged, these cells quickly migrate from the bloodstream and begin to clear up the debris. Whether they have a role in the normal physiology of the brain and cord remains undecided. Once inside, they appear to be capable of moving easily through the interstices of the nervous tissue. In time-lapse cinematic studies on neural tissue cultures, phagocytic cells, believed to be microglial, are seen racing through the tissue by means of amoeboid changes of shape, while the neuroglial cells merely perform slow pulsating movements, and nerve cells stay still.

In conventional stains little can be seen of a resting microglial cell apart from a small, dark, irregular nucleus. In the presence of a lesion, a silver impregnation will show

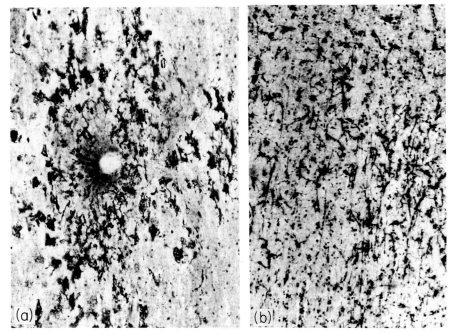

Fig. 3.23. (a) Reactive microglia surrounding a small vessel in a case of acceleration injury to the brain. Weil−Davenport silver impregnation, ×170. Very little would be seen of the reacting cells in a conventional cell stain. (b) 'Rod cells'. Elongated microglial cells in the cerebral cortex from a case of subacute sclerosing panencephalitis. Weil−Davenport, ×170. Rod cells were common in the cerebral cortex in cases of general paralysis of the insane.

active microglia as black silhouettes with bizarre shapes (Fig. 3.23), while cell stains merely show small, nondescript nuclei, as in Fig. 3.6b, where they are engaged in devouring a dead nerve cell. In larger lesions, microglial cells are seen in groups or dense clusters. Later, as they ingest lipids and other substances, they swell and acquire rounded outlines. Their affinity for silver decreases, and they become visible with stains for fat, haemosiderin or bilirubin. Ingested protein, mixed with fat, gives them a foamy appearance in embedded sections, and they become visible in ordinary cell stains (Fig. 3.24). At this stage they are known under a variety of names, including *lipid phagocytes, fat granule cells, Gitter cells,* and *compound granular corpuscles.* Both resting and reactive microglial cells can be demonstrated by means of some of the monoclonal antibodies raised against macrophages (see p.61).

As for other mesodermal elements in the CNS, *fibroblasts* are normally present only in the leptomeninges and around vessels; but when an area of necrosis involves the surface of the brain or cord, fibroblasts from the pia mater readily invade the necrotic tissue, and lay down collagen fibres, which may be mingled with astrocytic fibrils. *Blood vessels* of the CNS differ from those elsewhere in the body in several ways. The major arteries, when healthy, are relatively thin-walled, and possess only one elastic coat. Capillaries and venules are surrounded by the processes of glial cells, which are thought to contribute to the structural basis of the blood−brain barrier. There are no lymphatics in the CNS.

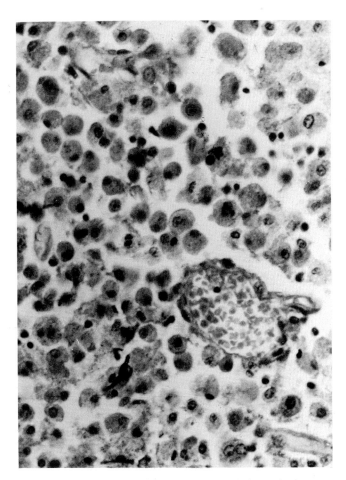

Fig. 3.24. Lipid phagocytes (Gitter cells, compound granular corpuscles) in a recent cerebral infarct. The cells originate as small microglial phagocytes. In frozen sections they show up brilliantly with fat stains. In the course of years they deposit their contents into the lumina of small blood vessels, and disappear. H&E, ×220.

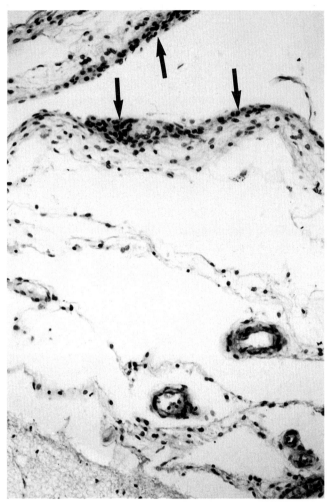

Meninges

These comprise the dura mater (pachymeninx), arachnoid mater and pia mater (leptomeninges). In normal usage, the word 'mater' is omitted. The differences in layout between the cranial and spinal meninges have been described in the previous chapter (p.29). In the cranial cavity, the *dura* consists of two layers, of which the outer layer constitutes the inner periosteum of the skull. Both layers are composed of dense collagenous tissue, poor in blood vessels. The *arachnoid* consists of a thin, but more or less impermeable, layer of connective tissue, patchily covered on its outer surface with *cap cells* (Fig. 3.25). In places, most conspicuously at the vertex of the brain, these cap cells form dense masses (*Pacchionian bodies* or *arachnoid granulations*) which burrow through the inner layer of dura, and project into the venous sinuses enclosed between the two dural layers (Fig. 3.26). It is at these points that CSF is reabsorbed into the bloodstream. Arachnoid cap cells are the characteristic cells of origin of most *meningiomas*. In these, the burrowing tendency of normal cap cells is reproduced; consequently, invasion of the dura is a normal feature of the most benign meningiomas (see p.202).

The *pia* consists, like the arachnoid, of a thin, more or less waterproof, layer of connective tissue, supporting large and small blood vessels. It invests not only the entire CNS, including the buried surfaces of cerebral convolutions, and the Virchow-Robin spaces around penetrating blood vessels, but also the intradural parts of the cranial and spinal nerve roots.

Fig. 3.25. Clusters of 'cap cells' (arrowed) on the outer surface of the arachnoid near the vertex. These are the main cells of origin of the Pacchionian bodies (see Fig. 3.26) which effect the drainage of CSF, and of most meningiomas. The remaining cells composing the arachnoid and pia are nearly all fibroblasts. H&E, ×120.

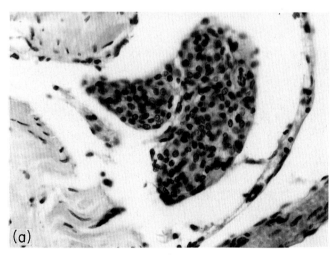
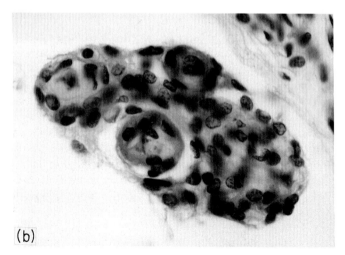

Fig. 3.26. Arachnoid granulations (Pacchionian bodies). (a) An accumulation of arachnoid cap cells projecting into a venous channel in the meninges at the vertex of the brain. H&E, ×180. (b) Another such body, at higher magnification, including a cellular whorl reminiscent of meningioma. H&E, ×250.

Peripheral nerves

The *peripheral nervous system* consists of: the spinal and cranial nerves (other than the olfactory and optic nerves, which in fact are brain tracts); the receptor cells of the special senses in the nasal mucosa, retina, mouth, inner ear and labyrinth; motor, sensory and autonomic nerves distal to the points (about 1 mm from the neuraxis) where neuroglia ends and Schwann cells begin (Fig. 3.27); and sensory and autonomic ganglia. For practical purposes, the *end-organs* on which the nerve fibres terminate are treated as parts of the peripheral nervous system. On the receptor side, these include the corpuscles of Pacini and Meissner; on the effector side, the *motor end-plates* of striated muscle. *Muscle spindles* contain both receptor and motor elements. Unlike the CNS, peripheral nerve contains connective tissue elements and lymphatics.

The *pathological changes* encountered in peripheral nerve are discussed in Chapter 22. They include simple *loss of axons*, which may be caused by proximal trauma, or by vascular lesions, such as occur in polyarteritis nodosa and in diabetes mellitus, or by poisoning, or by inflammation, as in the Guillain−Barre syndrome or in herpes zoster, or as a result of neuronal atrophy, as in motor neuron disease. In order to make even a rough assessment of the severity of axonal loss, accurately-cut transverse sections of the nerve must be examined, with stains for axons and for myelin.

A common, but not very specific, change in peripheral nerve fibres is *segmental demyelination*. This can be observed in accurately-cut thin longitudinal sections. It is more elegantly displayed in teased preparations prepared from fixed nerve (p.86; Fig. 22.4). Here, myelin is lost throughout one or more internodes (segments of myelin extending from one node of Ranvier to the next). Normally, the defect is made good by new Schwann cells; but in the finished job, there will commonly be *two* short internodes, each with its Schwann cell, replacing the original long (0.2−1.0 mm) internode. It should be noted that demyelination of three-dimensional blocks of tissue, such as occurs in the CNS in MS, does not occur in peripheral nerve. Segmental demyelination affects individual nerve fibres without directly affecting their neighbours.

In at least one variety of demyelinating neuropathy, there are successive waves of destruction and restoration of myelin. Each time that this occurs, Schwann cells proliferate and tend to envelop their predecessors. The final picture is of nerve fibres wrapped in multiple layers of Schwann cytoplasm (Fig. 22.9). This phenomenon is commonly known as *onion-bulb* formation, but the pattern is really more that of a rosebud, with imbricated petals, than that of an onion-bulb.

When a peripheral nerve fibre is severed, the part distal to the nerve cell body undergoes *wallerian degeneration*. The axon breaks up into small fragments, which can be stained with silver methods for a few days, after which they

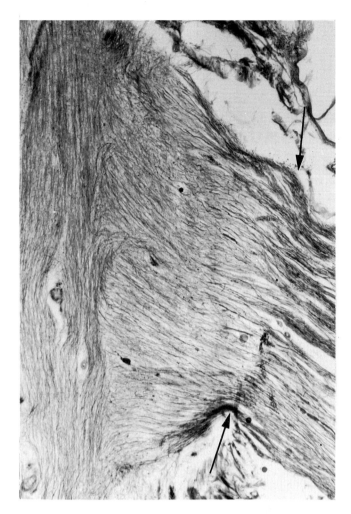

Fig. 3.27. Longitudinal section of spinal cord at the point of entry of a posterior rootlet. Arrows indicate the point where myelin of central type, formed by oligodendrocytes, takes over from the peripheral-type myelin formed by Schwann cells. The nerve fibres can be seen entering the most lateral part of the posterior white column, and bifurcating into ascending and descending branches. Holmes, ×77.

are removed by macrophages. If the fibre is myelinated, the myelin sheath likewise breaks up into droplets, which are reduced to simpler lipids before being phagocytosed. The Schwann cells remain. Meanwhile the central stump degenerates for a few millimetres back; a 'digestive chamber' is formed, in which the axon forms a bulbous expansion, from which a leash of fine axoplasmic filaments emerges. These filaments grow outwards along tissue planes. One of these filaments, if it is lucky, finds the empty connective tissue sheath of the original fibre. The lucky filament continues to grow, and acquires a myelin sheath; the rest are discouraged and disappear. The process is beautifully described and illustrated by Ramón y Cajal (1928).

There appears to be some sort of homoeostatic mechanism, acting in such a way that an under-innervated part of the body induces sprouting in neighbouring nerve fibres until an acceptable density of innervation is established, after which sprouting either ceases or is replaced by a dynamic equilibrium of sprouting and dying-back. This happens on both the sensory and the motor side. Following an attack of poliomyelitis, or in the course of motor neuron disease, surviving motor fibres emit extra terminal sprouts, which induce the formation of new motor end-plates on denervated muscle fibres. In silver impregnations, regenerating fibres can be recognized by their fine calibre, and by periodic fusiform swellings.

By convention, *skeletal muscle* is regarded as part of the neuropathologist's practice. The histology, fine structure, histochemistry and pathology of muscle are discussed in Chapter 23, and techniques of muscle biopsy are dealt with on pp.86–7.

Of the cellular components of the nervous system, nerve cells rarely, Schwann cells and arachnoid cap cells commonly, and neuroglial cells only too often, give rise to *tumours*. The subject is discussed in Chapters 12 and 13.

Staining methods

Some of the most used neuropathological staining methods, and the main indications for their use, are listed below. The list is not, of course, exhaustive. Details of various methods not commonly used in general pathology, or not easily found in technical manuals, are given in Appendix A (p.388).

Nerve cells

For staining nerve cell bodies one or other of the *Nissl* methods is used. These show up nuclei, nucleoli and Nissl substance, and very little else. There is none of the background staining seen in general tissue stains such as haematoxylin and eosin. This makes it possible to estimate neuronal populations in thick (25 μm or more) sections (Figs 3.1, 3.6 and 3.36).

Myelin

For staining myelin, there is a choice between one of the traditional *haematoxylin* stains (Kultschitzky–Pal, Weil, Loyez, etc.) in which myelin appears dark slaty-blue (Figs 2.26, 2.27, etc.) and one of the more recent inventions, such as *Luxol fast blue*. An advantage of the latter is that it can be combined with other stains, in particular, with a Nissl stain, to give a combined picture of nerve cells and myelinated tracts (Plate 1.6). This combination (the *Klüver–Barrera* stain) is very useful in identifying small groups of cells in, for instance, the thalamus and brain stem.

The main use of these stains, not surprisingly, is in locating the places where myelin has been lost. At this point it is worth mentioning that the word *demyelination* is used, in the current literature, in two different senses. As we use

the term, in common with most British authors, it means stripping an axon of its myelin sheath. This happens in the CNS in MS, and in the peripheral nervous system mainly in the form of segmental demyelination. Many American authors, on the other hand, use the term as a synonym for myelin loss, from whatever cause. Those who follow this usage often distinguish between *primary demyelination* (i.e. demyelination in our sense) and *secondary demyelination*, which results from damage to, or disappearance of, myelinated axons. In this usage it is not the axon but the tissue, or the stained section, that is demyelinated. Incomplete or partial loss of myelin is characteristically seen in areas of oedema in the brain or cord, and in the 'shadow plaques' of MS, which are described on p.231.

Both haematoxylin and Luxol fast blue can be used for staining myelin in peripheral nerve, but both these stains are also taken up by connective tissue. In examining samples of peripheral nerve, myelin can be clearly distinguished from connective tissue by the *Gomori trichrome* method, which stains connective tissue blue or green, and myelin red (Plate 2.4).

Glial fibres

Using Nissl and myelin preparations, experience and an alert eye are needed in order to detect local loss of cells or of myelin. On the other hand, a stain for glial fibres will give *positive* evidence of established lesions, by directing attention to areas of fibrous gliosis — for example, small 'shadow plaques' in cases of MS (Figs 3.14 and 3.15). For this, the classical method is the *Holzer* technique. In well-fixed tissue, and in the hands of a good technician, the results of this can be a delight to the eye. Unfortunately, these two conditions do not always prevail. A further drawback is that the method is messy, and involves the use of aniline, the vapour of which is apt to cause headaches, even when the staining is carried out in a fume cupboard. An alternative for showing astrocytes and glial fibres is phosphotungstic acid/haematoxylin (PTAH). This, again, requires well-fixed tissue and an experienced technician. It is useful for differentiating between astrocytes and small nerve cells, the former appearing dark purplish-blue, whereas the latter have a lighter, reddish, tinge. A disadvantage of the method is that it stains myelin as well as glial fibres.

All the above methods are applicable, often with crisper definition than in paraffin sections, to celloidin sections. The disadvantages of celloidin have been mentioned above (p.38).

Axons

For the staining of axons, both central and peripheral, silver impregnations are used. Varieties of these include the Holmes, Palmgren, Bodian and Romanes techniques. We favour the *Holmes* and *Palmgren* methods (see Figs 3.2, 3.3, 3.8, 3.27 and 3.32). Some such method is often needed for distinguishing between demyelination, in which the axons are spared, and degenerative conditions, in which they are not. Silver impregnations can be combined with myelin stains, as in Plate 4.1.

Other stains for paraffin sections

For showing up the 'senile' plaques and neurofibrillary tangles, characteristic of Alzheimer's disease, in paraffin sections, we use a technique devised by Cross (1982) (see p.391). This is a modification of the Palmgren method. An alternative is the von Braunmühl method, which is used on frozen sections (Figs 3.10 and 3.11; see p.391). For intracellular inclusions, such as occur in Parkinson's disease, and in certain viral encephalitides, *haematoxylin and eosin* (H&E) is a useful stain. It is also good for showing acute hypoxic changes in nerve cells, as well as in the examination of tumours, and in differentiating between different types of inflammatory cell. (Most general pathologists, when confronted with a selection of stains, will look first at the H&E. Nothing we say will affect this ingrained habit, but we should like to combat the widespread delusion that a 5 or 10 µm section of CNS tissue, stained with H&E, will provide all the important information on the pathology of the specimen.)

Other methods, in common use in general histopathology, include the *periodic-acid-Schiff* (PAS) reaction, which is useful for demonstrating the yeast in cryptococcal meningitis, and for showing normal and abnormal capillary vessels (Fig. 19.7). It can also be used for detecting 'senile' plaques, and for the stored material in various metabolic storage diseases (see Chapter 19).

Congo Red shows up amyloid in cerebral vessels and in the neurofibrillary tangles and 'senile' plaques of Alzheimer's disease (Plate 7.1). An alternative is a *thioflavine* stain, followed by fluorescence microscopy. An *elastin* stain is used for distinguishing between arteries and the 'arterialized' veins of arteriovenous fistulae, and a *reticulin* stain for mesodermal tumours, or for the sarcomatous elements in certain malignant gliomas (Figs 12.15, 12.36 and 12.40). *Perls'* stain for iron compounds is often useful in showing up small deposits of haemosiderin consequent upon haemorrhage, and 'ferruginated' nerve cells (Fig. 3.7; Plate 2.6).

Fat stains

Since fats are dissolved away in the embedding processes, *frozen sections* are required for the demonstration of fat in the tissues. Of the several stains available we prefer *Oil red O*. The breakdown of myelin gives rise to fatty end-products, which are eventually removed by macrophages and discharged into the bloodstream. In a recent plaque of MS, which is still soft and not toughened by glial fibres, one finds great numbers of lipid phagocytes, whereas an old sclerotic plaque is devoid of fat, except when active extension is taking place at its edges. Staining for fat thus gives valuable information on the chronicity and state of activity of plaques, and of other lesions in which myelin is broken down (Plate 2.3).

Uses of osmic acid

Osmium tetroxide (osmic acid), though it is very expensive and emits toxic fumes, is much used in neuropathology, largely because of its long-established use in neuro-anatomical investigations. It is used as a myelin stain on teased preparations of peripheral nerve fibres (Fig. 22.4). It is also used in the *Marchi* techniques, in which degenerating myelin is stained black, while normal myelin is left unstained (Fig 3.28 and 3.29). As a rule, the Marchi stain becomes positive before the fat stain; for reasons not well understood, frozen sections stained by this method do not always give the same result as when the whole block is stained before cutting.

Metallic impregnations for glia

Staining of *astrocytes* by *Cajal's gold sublimate* method is popular, partly because it is reliable and relatively easy to

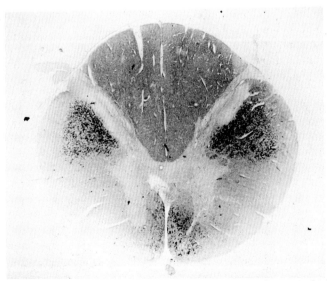

Fig. 3.28. Marchi staining of degenerate pyramidal tracts in a case of motor neuron disease (amyotrophic lateral sclerosis). Note that the tracts on the right of the picture are larger than on the left; but the sum of fibres in the right crossed and left uncrossed tracts is about the same as that of the left crossed and right uncrossed tracts. Asymmetrical decussation of the pyramids is very common. Sometimes the uncrossed tract is totally lacking on one side of the cord. In such cases, one can readily detect a difference in bulk between the anterior white columns by naked-eye inspection of transverse sections. ×8.

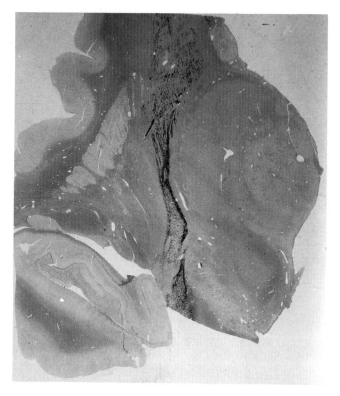

Fig. 3.29. Marchi staining of a degenerate pyramidal tract, cut in a coronal plane, in motor neuron disease. The tract lies well back in the posterior limb of the internal capsule.

carry out, and partly because it gives aesthetic pleasure. Again, for reasons not well understood, the picture is often somewhat different from that seen in Holzer or PTAH preparations on paraffin sections (compare Figs 3.13a and b with Figs 3.13c, 3.14 and 3.15).

Various methods of staining *microglia* in paraffin sections have been published, but none of these has given consistent results in our laboratory. On frozen sections, the *Weil–Davenport* method works consistently well in recently-fixed material; but after a few months' storage in formalin it tends to produce a dust of black precipitate, almost confined to grey matter. The method stains all stages in the development of microglial cells up to the stage of rounded lipid-containing phagocytes (Gitter cells: compound granular corpuscles) (Fig. 3.23). The method can be combined with staining for fat. Some Weil–Davenport preparations show up reactive astrocytes; some even display the processes of oligodendroglial cells, which are otherwise very difficult to impregnate.

For the staining of peripheral nerve fibres and ganglion cell bodies, we use *Schofield's* modification of the Bielschowsky silver technique. This is highly reliable, and very useful in examining the innervation of muscle, both in biopsies and in post mortem material (Figs 22.3, 23.6, 23.7 and 23.38). In some centres, *intravital methylene blue* staining is preferred for muscle biopsies (Harriman 1984). The

position of motor end-plates can also be demonstrated by a histochemical technique (see Fig. 4.39).

The *Golgi* technique, though it has contributed enormously to cellular morphology, is rarely used in diagnostic work.

Electron microscopy

The role of electron microscopy (EM) in diagnostic neuropathology varies from centre to centre, depending on the availability of apparatus and trained staff, and on the interests and expertise of the users. For some purposes, however, EM is really necessary for diagnosis. Nerve and muscle biopsies, and brain biopsies, apart from simple questions of tumour identification, come into this category. The methods are discussed in Chapter 4. For post mortem material, EM is unlikely to be rewarding when the delay between death and post mortem is more than a few hours, with the exception of cases of suspected virus infection. Viruses retain their form more or less intact for many hours after death, and survive formalin fixation. Thus it is often worth while using EM on affected tissues in cases of encephalitis, or as a last resort in otherwise baffling conditions. Even if EM is not carried out, resin-embedded tissue is valuable for the preparation of 1 μm sections — particularly for thin transverse sections of nerve from cases of peripheral neuropathy.

Immunohistological identification of cellular components of the CNS

In recent years increasing use has been made of antibodies to cellular antigens in the identification of cell types in the nervous system. Although the ordinary staining properties of different types of cells are distinct enough for many purposes, the use of antibodies to cell-related antigens is adding further refinement to the identification of cells in the nervous system. It is also adding considerably to knowledge of nervous system development, since immature cells that have not attained full morphological maturity may nevertheless express identifying antigens on the cell surface or in the cytoplasm. The use of antibodies to neurotransmitters, or to enzymes employed in their synthesis, provides a basis for subclassifying neurons, and revealing the extraordinary complexity of their interactions. Although many of these applications of immunohistology are at present beyond the requirements of the diagnostic neuropathologist, it is likely that their use will increase understanding of many nervous system diseases, and that they will eventually find a use in diagnosis. For the present, probably the most widely used antibodies in routine diagnostic use are those directed against glial fibrillary acidic protein (GFAP), which identify normal, reactive and neoplastic astrocytes (Fig. 3.30). Oligodendrocytes react with antibodies to galactocerebroside and with the monoclonal antibody, anti-Leu 7, which detects

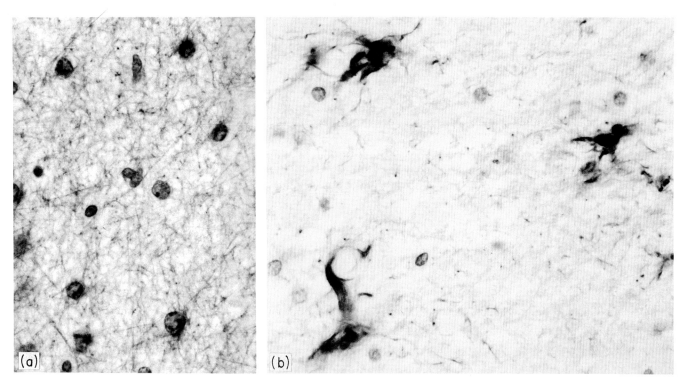

Fig. 3.30. Immunohistochemical staining of astrocytes. (a) Resting. (b) Reactive. GFAP method, ×420.

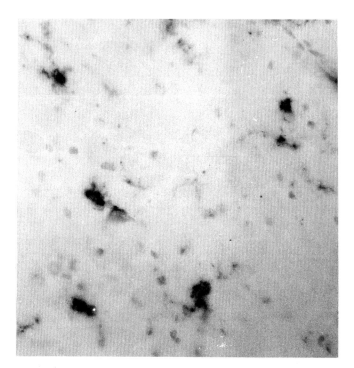

Fig. 3.31. Immunohistochemical staining of microglial cells. EBM11 method, ×420.

myelin-associated glycoprotein, some neural crest-derived cells, and natural 'killer' cells of haemopoietic origin. Neurons can be identified by use of neurofilament antibodies and of antibodies to neuron-specific enolase. There are some macrophage monoclonal antibodies that react with microglial cells (e.g. EBM11) (Fig. 3.31). The use to which some of these and other antibodies can be put in tumour diagnosis is discussed in Chapter 4.

Warnings

Teachers of histopathology are familiar with the tendency of students to turn to the high powers of the microscope before they have scanned the specimen by the low power, and with the need to combat this tendency. The principle that one should survey the wood before examining the trees applies to the exploration of the nervous tissue even more than to the examination of the lungs or liver. Apart from sharply localized lesions, one sample of a liver will look much like another, whereas sections of the lower brain stem may yield quite different information from that derived from the upper brain stem or cervical cord. What is more, the most important bits of information will usually be revealed by the use of the naked eye, hand lens, or dissecting microscope.

In this, as in other activities, it is of some importance to avoid wasting one's time in vain pursuits. In biopsy work, for instance, there is no profit in trying to decide on the exact nature of cells which have been crushed by forceps or frizzled by diathermy. It is therefore important to learn, as soon as possible, to recognize features in histological preparations which are of no pathological significance, or which are actually misleading. Such features are of two main kinds: (i) genuine, but non-specific, tissue changes, and (ii) so-called artefacts. Some of these are listed below.

Non-specific changes in central nervous tissue

By 'non-specific' we mean merely that we do not know what the changes signify, and do not associate them with any well-recognized disease. Some of them may one day turn out to be of great diagnostic importance. It is worth remembering that the great T.H. Huxley spoke of the pituitary gland as a vestigial structure of no physiological importance.

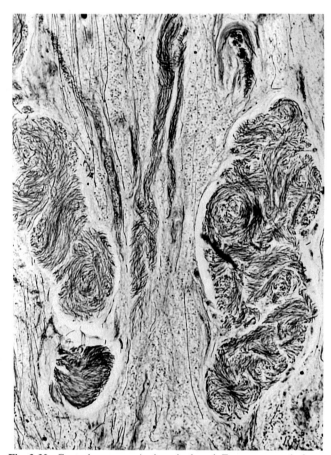

Fig. 3.32. Central neuromas in the spinal cord. Fourteen years before death the patient had suffered a very severe acute polyneuritis, with very slow and incomplete recovery. Although there was little, if any, loss of sensory ganglion cells, there was severe loss of their central processes. Regeneration from sensory ganglia resulted in invasion of the cord by regenerated axons, accompanied by Schwann cells. Within the cord, these fibres formed neuromas, i.e. dense tangles of myelinated axons. In this longitudinal section, stained with silver, surviving CNS tracts contain fine, straight axons, whereas the regenerated fibres are coarse and darkly stained. Holmes silver, ×85.

'Aberrant' nerve fibres

Disputes continue concerning the capacity for sprouting and regeneration of nerve fibres within the CNS, but there is no doubt about the sprouting ability of peripheral nerve fibres. These include the axons of motor neurons, and the central processes of sensory ganglion cells. If for any reason a small or large chunk of spinal cord dies, the necrotic tissue is liable to be invaded by nerve fibres, with Schwann cells in attendance, derived from either anterior or (more commonly) posterior spinal nerve roots. The invading fibres acquire sheaths of myelin of peripheral type (Fig. 11.11). Lacking any orientating influence, they do not form parallel bundles, but get twisted into dense tangles, resembling the neuromas arising from the cut ends of peripheral nerves (Fig. 3.32). The same process may occur on a small scale, and it is not at all uncommon to see tiny neuromas in the substance of the cord or brain stem, with no evidence as to the original lesion.

Calcification

Calcified pineal glands and choroid plexus are normal in later life, and may be visible in straight X-rays of the head. Massive calcification in brain tissue ('brain stones') has been mentioned earlier (p.20). Minor degrees of calcification, unassociated with symptoms, or with any recognized disease, are commonly met with in stained sections. They occur for the most part in elderly people, and are commonest in the lentiform nucleus. They occur either as rows of tiny calcospherites along the course of capillary vessels, or as tubular deposits in the medial wall of larger vessels (Fig. 19.23). They stain positively for iron as well as for calcium.

Corpora amylacea

These are globular basophilic bodies, $10-50\,\mu m$ in diameter, most commonly seen in the subpial tissue of the brain and cord in elderly subjects (Plate 2.1). Favourite locations are the lips of the lateral fissures and the white columns of the spinal cord. They stain positively with PAS and iodine. They are currently believed to develop within astrocyte processes, and to indicate some form of neural decay. They must not be confused with yeasts, such as *Cryptococcus*.

Lipofuscin

This yellowish fatty material accumulates in the cytoplasm of nerve cells with advancing age. It is seen in many sites, but is often most abundant in the large neurons of the thalamus (Plate 2.2).

Subependymal and subpial astrocytes

These normally form sheets of fibroglia, which grow denser with age. Here, too, the change is not regarded as pathological until it is deemed to be excessive. How much is too much is a question individual neuropathologists must decide for themselves, on the basis of their experience. Truly pathological causes include acute and chronic meningitis, and subarachnoid blood from burst aneurysms, head trauma, etc.; and subpial and subependymal gliosis is said to result from repeated epileptic fits.

Myelin pallor

One of the most familiar problems in the histopathology of the CNS lies in deciding whether failure of the myelin in a particular area to take up the stain is due to disease, or to non-specific causes, or to an artefact. 'True' myelin pallor can be caused by oedema (see Chapter 11), demyelination (see Chapter 14), leucodystrophy (see Chapter 19) or by wallerian tract degeneration. Most of the lesions of MS are easily recognized as such, but 'shadow plaques' often give rise to doubts. Doubts of this kind can often be disposed of by the use of a Holzer or similar stain, which reveals a glial reaction to the lesion.

In the spinal cords of elderly people there is sometimes a marginal rim, a millimetre or so wide, of poorly staining, or even absent, myelin. This is often combined with fibrous thickening of the pia mater and subpial gliosis. The cause is generally uncertain. It is important not to mistake this appearance for specific tract degeneration — in particular, of the dorsal and ventral spinocerebellar tracts.

Artefactual causes of myelin pallor are discussed below (p.65).

'Slight cell loss'

This phrase is only too familiar from published neuropathological reports. It may occasionally be taken on trust, but more often it represents an attempt by the author to hedge his bets. He is unsure of his observations; he does not want to be thought to have been neglectful, or to have failed to examine the relevant part; also, he does not wish to commit himself to a positive statement that the tissue is diseased. In a few places, such as the Purkinje layer of the cerebellum, a mild degree of cell loss may actually be detectable without recourse to cell counting. Elsewhere, it is usually exceedingly difficult. Admitting that even we may not be free of sin, we strongly deplore the tendency to report on 'slight cell loss'. Honesty, we maintain, is still the best policy.

A common observation in longitudinal sections of peripheral *nerves* is a more or less regular pattern of waves, as in Fig. 3.33. This is merely the expression of the nerve's elasticity. If the specimen is fixed under moderate longi-

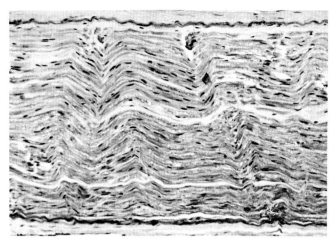

Fig. 3.33. The wavy pattern commonly seen in longitudinal sections of peripheral nerve may be partly due to differential shrinkage of the connective tissue during fixation. ×150.

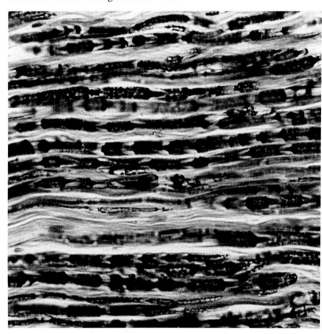

Fig. 3.34. Schmidt-Lantermann clefts. These are very commonly seen in longitudinal sections of myelinated peripheral nerve fibres. Their origin is still disputed. Combined Palmgren and Crystal Scarlet stain. ×440.

tudinal tension, the waves are not seen. Another common appearance is the apparent disruption of myelin sheaths by a series of so-called Schmidt–Lanterman clefts (Fig. 3.34). There has been some dispute as to whether these clefts are natural or artefactual, or a bit of each. At any rate, they do not have a pathological significance. They are discussed by Thomas, Landon & King (1984).

Sections of *muscle* taken from near a tendinous insertion may show features which would be regarded as pathological if they occurred in the belly of the muscle. These include increased perimysial collagen, splitting of muscle fibres, and internal nuclei (see Chapter 23).

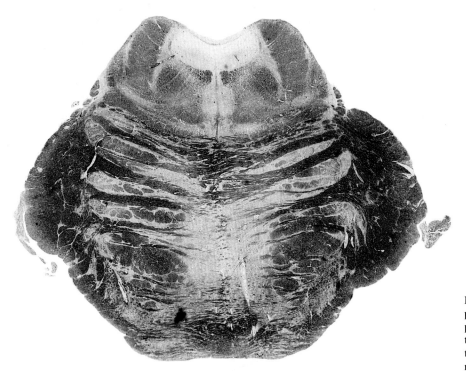

Fig. 3.35. Myelin pallor in the centre of the pons, in the absence of disease, may be due to poor fixation. When the brain is suspended in the formalin bucket from the basilar artery, the pons lies close to the surface of the fluid, resulting in poor penetration of fixative.

Artefacts

In archaeology, the word 'artefact' means an object thought to be the product of human artifice: a stone wall, for instance, or a potsherd, or a flint showing signs of pressure-flaking. In histology, the word means an unintended by-product of a technical procedure, or merely the result of bad technique. Artefacts of these kinds occur at all stages in the processing of pathological material. Tissues decompose if the cadaver is not adequately chilled. If the delay between death and fixation of tissues is excessive, bacteria which entered the bloodstream in the agonal phase may escape into the tissues and proliferate there. When the organisms are of a gas-forming persuasion, this results in the 'Swiss cheese' artefacts illustrated in Fig. 2.18. More commonly, the organisms are non-gas-forming anaerobes. Their presence in the fixed brain tissue is signalled by the appearance of tiny red rings around venules on the cut surfaces. This can be confirmed by Gram stains.

Inadequate or delayed fixation

The effect of inadequate, or delayed, fixation of oedematous brain tissue has already been described (pp.7–8). Apart from oedema, access of formalin may be delayed mechanically — for instance, if the brain is improperly suspended, and parts of the surface are resting on the bottom of the bucket. Hydrostatic pressure may also play a part in fixation.

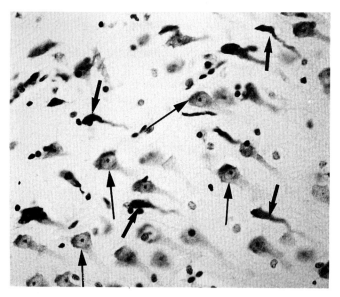

Fig. 3.36. 'Dark cells'. In biopsies of cerebral cortex, the pyramidal cells of layers 3 and 5 appear in stained sections as plump, rounded shapes, with globular nuclei and prominent nucleoli (slender arrows), as compared with the isosceles triangles seen in post mortem material. Near the margins of the specimen, one commonly sees shrunken, dark-staining neurons, often with dark, corkscrew-like apical dendrites (thick arrows). This is a mechanical artefact, without pathological significance. Nissl, ×200.

When the brain is slung from the basilar artery, the part nearest the surface of the fluid, where the hydrostatic pressure is lowest, is the pons. It is not unusual to find that the centre of the pons stains poorly for myelin, as in Fig. 3.35. It is important not to mistake this artefact for the genuine pathological condition of central pontine myelinolysis (p.305).

An artefact most commonly seen in sections from biopsy specimens of cerebral cortex is the so-called 'dark cell'. Near the edge of the specimen one sees shrunken, deformed pyramidal cells, sometimes with prominent, cork-screw-like apical dendrites (Fig. 3.36). It is now generally agreed that this is an effect of mechanical trauma, presumably causing escape of cytoplasm from a previously turgid cell (Duchen 1984).

An artefact which we have encountered in brains removed and fixed in departments other than ours is a widespread deposition of haematoxyphil material in a narrow band deep to the pia covering the cerebral cortex (Fig. 3.37). We, are unable to account for it.

In biopsy material, the commonest artefacts are either mechanical or thermal. A good surgeon is more concerned with the patient's interests than with the pathologist's; he will therefore tend to include damaged tissues in the specimen pot rather than leave them inside the patient. If the specimen is a piece of peripheral nerve, he will make it as short as possible, and apply the jaws of the forceps to the specimen rather than to the remaining cut ends. Thus the pathologist learns to confine his attention to the middle of the specimen. Figure 3.38 shows some artefacts caused by the application of forceps; Fig. 3.39 shows the effects of diathermy on sensitive tissues.

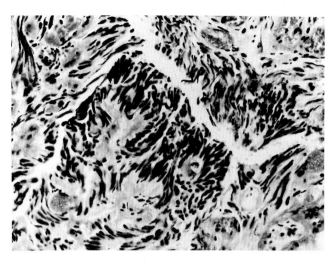

Fig. 3.38. Firm application of the forceps to biopsied tissues often gives rise to bizarre deformations of the affected structures. On occasion, these may mimic pathological changes. ×200.

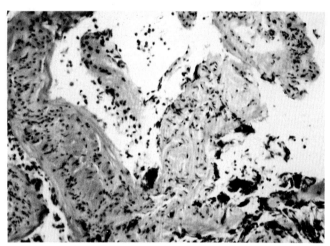

Fig. 3.39. Weird patterns may also be seen in tissues which have been subjected to diathermy. Artefacts from this cause can usually be recognized in an H&E section by a disagreeable purplish discoloration. ×90.

Muscle preparations

Artefacts in histological preparations of muscle include zones of contraction affecting segments of muscle fibres, which then appear abnormally eosinophilic and homogeneous (Fig. 4.37). In frozen sections, ice crystals may leave empty spaces in the centres of fibres.

Artefacts in general constitute a nuisance and, on occasion, a serious trap for the unwary. It is important to recognize them and, as far as possible, avoid their creation. In biopsy work, this may involve a little frank discussion with the surgeons.

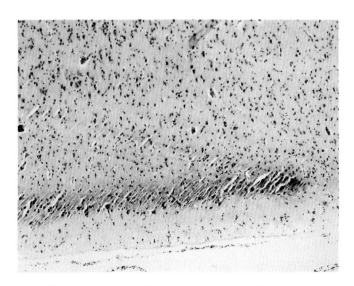

Fig. 3.37. A narrow band of haematoxyphil staining close to, and parallel with, the pial surface, is known locally as the St Elsewhere's artefact. H&E, ×50.

Further reading

Cajal S. Ramón y 1928. *Degeneration and Regeneration in the Nervous System*. Oxford University Press, Oxford.

Cross RB. 1982. Demonstration of neurofibrillary tangles in paraffin sections — a quick and simple method using a modification of Palmgren's method. *Med Lab Sci* **39**, 67–9.

Duchen LW. 1984. General pathology of neurons and neuroglia. In Adams JH, Corsellis JAN, Duchen LW (Eds) *Greenfield's Neuropathology*, 4th edn. Edward Arnold, London, Chapter 1.

Harriman DGF. 1984. Diseases of muscle. In Adams JH, Corsellis JAN, Duchen LW (Eds) *Greenfield's Neuropathology*, 4th edn. Edward Arnold, London, Chapter 21.

Thomas PK, Landon DN, King RHM. 1984. Diseases of the peripheral nerves. In Adams JH, Corsellis JAN, Duchen LW (Eds) *Greenfield's Neuropathology*, 4th edn. Edward Arnold, London, Chapter 18.

Chapter 4
Biopsies

General considerations

Neuropathologists are expected to tackle the interpretation of biopsy specimens from the CNS and its surroundings, peripheral nerves and muscles. They may also be faced with smears, i.e. wet-film preparations from the operating theatre, from tumours, or from brain tissue, for instant diagnosis, and with CSF for cytology.

Clinicians show a proper reluctance to resort to biopsy for the diagnosis of diseases of the CNS. Muscle and nerve biopsies are taken more frequently now than in the past, but brain biopsies are becoming less frequent as new, non-invasive methods of diagnosis are developed. When a brain biopsy has been decided on, it is very important to obtain as much useful information from it as one possibly can. For this, good communication between clinician and pathologist is essential. In practical terms, the pathologist should attend ward rounds, and be readily available for discussion of cases. He should take the trouble to inform himself about findings at operation, and be prepared to demonstrate his own material to clinicians. The clinician, in turn, should be urged to: provide adequate clinical information along with specimens; give due notice to the laboratory about planned operations which may result in biopsy; and learn what kinds of question the pathologist can be expected to answer, and which are beyond his scope. The risk of a missed diagnosis and of an unprofitable or unnecessary operation is greatly lessened if both parties adhere to these guidelines.

When specimens arrive in the laboratory, what is done with them will depend on the nature of the specimen and the likely diagnosis (Fig. 4.1). In order to cover all eventualities it is often best to take a sample to freeze in liquid nitrogen, another for EM following fixation in glutaral-dehyde, and to fix the rest in formalin. This allocation does not allow for microbiological culture, however, and if this is thought necessary, fresh samples in dry, sterile bottles should be sent rapidly to the microbiological laboratory.

Biopsies of tumours

Tumour diagnosis is one of the main tasks of neuropathologists. In biopsy work, a fairly confident early diagnosis can be made in about nine cases out of ten. Among the rest, there is the occasional totally baffling case. Between these extremes, partial or imprecise reports may be helpful to the surgeon. The first question often to be answered is 'is this tumour?'. If the answer is 'no', it is usually possible to describe the tissue as (i) normal brain, (ii) reactive brain, (iii) necrotic debris, or (iv) inflammatory tissue. If the surgeon is convinced, on other grounds, that he is dealing with a tumour (or an abscess), a report of any of these four may help him to decide on his next step. For instance, if the radiology shows a brain tumour, the finding of necrotic debris in a smear makes it almost certain that the tumour is malignant. If the immediate answer is 'yes, this is tumour, but I am not sure what type of tumour', such an answer will usually suffice until further investigations have been carried out, or outside opinions sought.

An important ingredient in good understanding between surgeon and pathologist is that both parties should be fully aware of the common diagnostic pitfalls. For instance, if the pathologist reports on a small biopsy specimen as 'low-grade astrocytoma', the surgeon should be aware that the sample may come from the periphery of a highly malignant glioma; and the pathologist has to remember that not all expanding lesions of the brain are neoplasms, and that it is

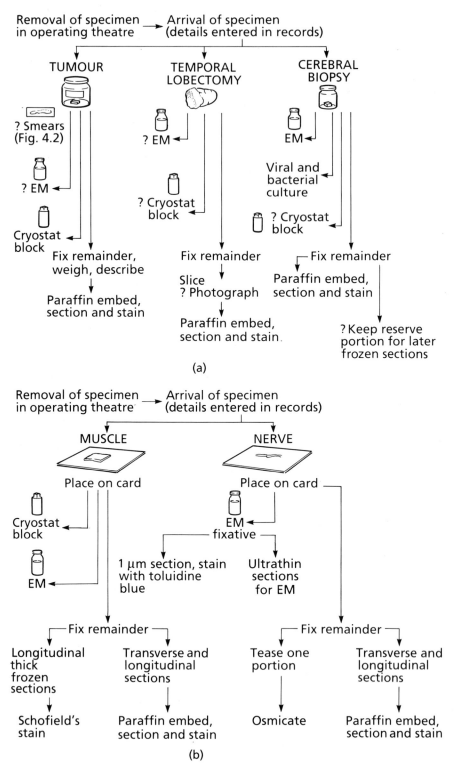

Fig. 4.1. Recommended procedures to adopt when dealing with tumour, temporal lobectomy, and cerebral biopsy specimens (a), or with muscle and nerve biopsies (b).

often difficult to distinguish between reactive and neoplastic astrocytes. In any case of doubt he should confine himself to writing an honest report on what he has actually observed, rather than extrapolate from this to what he thinks he *might* have seen if the surgeon had provided more material.

In dealing with the difficult cases the use of antibodies to relatively cell-specific antigens may be of value (see below). An important practical point arises from the fact that some of these antibodies need to be applied to cryostat sections, necessitating the use of fresh frozen tissue. As one does not know in advance which tumours are going to give rise to diagnostic difficulty, it is advisable to arrange for the rapid transport from the operating theatre to the laboratory of all tissue in an unfixed state, in a screw-topped container to prevent drying out. The pathologist can then decide how best to divide the tissue available for routine histology, cryostat sectioning and smears for rapid diagnosis. EM may also provide diagnostically useful information, and a sample can be appropriately fixed for this purpose if suf-ficient tissue is available. After the main specimen has been fixed, it is described, weighed and embedded, entire or in representative blocks, in paraffin wax.

Choice of stains to perform on paraffin sections will vary according to the supposed nature of the tumour, but H&E is used together with a PTAH stain for presumed gliomas and a Van Gieson stain for meningeal tumours and schwannomas. The PAS stain is helpful for showing mucinous material in carcinomas, choroid plexus tumours, myxopapillary ependymomas and chordomas, and stains for reticulin are helpful in the examination of meningeal tumours and lymphomas. Pituitary tumours require a combined PAS and Orange G or similar stain. Less commonly used but helpful at times are pigment stains for melanin and iron, and nerve fibre stains. Melanin may be present in a number of tumours including meningioma, nerve sheath tumour, ependymoma, medulloblastoma and choroid plexus tumour, as well as melanoma. The use of immunohistological techniques in tumour diagnosis is discussed on p.79, and the histological diagnosis of tumours in Chapters 12 and 13.

Smears in tumour diagnosis (Table 4.1)

For urgent tumour diagnosis there is a choice between smears and frozen sections, or a combination of these. This to some extent depends on personal preference and experience, but with some tumours the choice is largely dictated by their texture. Very soft tumours are best smeared, but with tough tumours frozen sections are to be preferred, though touch preparations, made by dabbing a portion of tough tumour firmly against a glass slide, may contain useful diagnostic features, such as whorl formations from a meningioma. Frozen sections and smears are often complementary. Frozen sections provide valuable information about the architecture of a tumour but less cytological detail

Table 4.1. Questions to answer in smear analysis

If obvious tumour is present:

Is tumour readily identifiable?
If tumour is readily identifiable:
  is it benign-looking?
  is it malignant (necrosis, mitoses)?

If there is doubt about whether tumour is present, consider distinctions between:

fibrillary astrocytoma and gliosis?
glioma and acute MS?
necrotic tumour and brain?
necrotic tumour and pus?
lymphoma and chronic inflammation?
cerebellar tumour and normal/squashed cerebellum?
papilloma and choroid plexus?

If there is no tumour present:

is there normal brain (caution on cerebellar cortex)?
is there reactive brain (swollen astrocytes, etc.)?
is there inflamed brain (cuffed vessels, etc.)?
is there purulent inflammation, or acute infarction?

than smears; blood vessels and their relation to tumour cells are seen clearly in transverse section in frozen sections, while smears provide a good display of considerable lengths of vessels.

Smears are made by placing a small piece of tumour, 2–3 mm across, at one end of a clean glass slide and pressing a second slide firmly across it (Fig. 4.2). Three or four smears can be prepared from different parts of the specimen. They are dried in air, fixed in absolute alcohol for a minute or so and stained with methylene blue (30 seconds) or a similar stain. Excess stain is washed away in tap water (distilled water is not necessary), taking care not to dislodge the smeared tissue. The slide is then dehydrated, cleared and mounted in the usual way (see table below Fig. 4.2). The whole procedure should take less than 10 minutes. Frozen sections are usually stained with H&E.

Many surgeons, faced with the clinical and radiological evidence of a malignant brain tumour, do not engage in open brain surgery. Instead, they approach the site of the tumour with a blunt hollow needle, via a burr-hole, and make smears of the tissue thus obtained. If the tissue proves malignant, no further surgery is undertaken. If the appearances are inconclusive, or if the tumour looks benign, they may proceed to formal surgery. It is particularly on these occasions that the pathologist needs to be circumspect in making a diagnosis, since the smear is all he has to go on. Recently, in some neurosurgical centres, the technique of using multiple CAT-directed or magnetic resonance image-directed biopsies has been evolved. This may result in great difficulties for the pathologist in reaching a firm diagnosis on multiple, very tiny specimens of tissue sent for

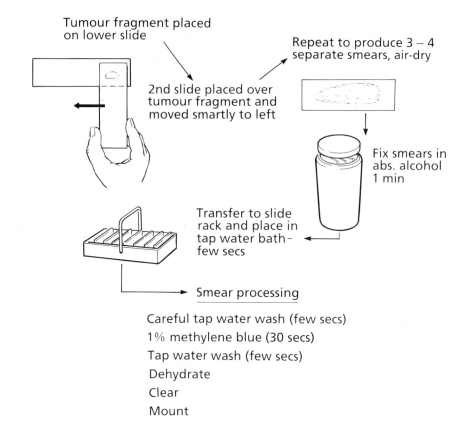

Tumour fragment placed
on lower slide

2nd slide placed over
tumour fragment and
moved smartly to left

Repeat to produce 3 – 4
separate smears, air-dry

Fix smears in
abs. alcohol
1 min

Transfer to slide
rack and place in
tap water bath –
few secs

Smear processing

Careful tap water wash (few secs)

1% methylene blue (30 secs)

Tap water wash (few secs)

Dehydrate

Clear

Mount

Fig. 4.2. Procedure for making smears of
fresh biopsy (or post mortem) tissue.

immediate smears. On other occasions, smears are sent
from the theatre with a request for an immediate opinion,
and are followed by one or more solid specimens, usually in
formalin. In these circumstances it may have to be pointed
out that the smear diagnosis is only provisional. Occasionally,
however, it is a smear which provides the answer, whereas
the stained sections do not.

The following points are offered as guidelines to the
diagnosis of tumours based on their appearance in smears.
Further information of the appearance of CNS tumours in
smears can be found in the monograph by Adams *et al.*
(1981), and the article by Barnard (1981), listed at the end
of this chapter.

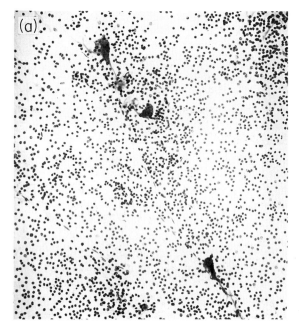

(a)

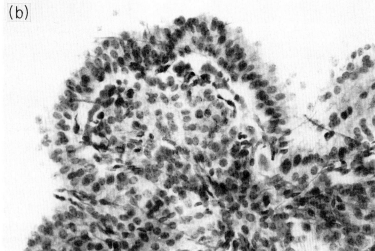

(b)

Fig. 4.3. (a) Smear of normal cerebellar cortex. The small, regular
nuclei are those of granule cells, while the larger, triangular cells are
Purkinje cells. Methylene blue, ×130. (b) Smear of choroid plexus.
Methylene blue, ×150.

Reading a smear (see also Table 4.1)

First of all *check the source of the tissue* (cerebrum, cerebellum, meninges, pituitary fossa, etc.), *assess its overall cellularity* and *decide whether or not it contains tumour.* Bear in mind that 'cellularity' depends on the thickness of the smear, which can be gauged by focusing up and down with the high-power objective. This avoids being deceived into thinking a smear is 'cellular' merely because it is thick. If no tumour is evident at first, search the slides carefully, as the tumour cells may be confined to one corner of one of several slides. If tumour is not present the tissue will consist of normal or 'reactive' brain, or contain some other pathology such as inflammation or infarction, or necrotic, uninter-

pretable debris. The appearance of normal or reactive brain depends on the site. Two normal ingredients of brain are particularly liable to be mistaken for tumour tissue. The first is cerebellar cortex, where the densely packed granule cells may mimic tumour, especially if the cells have been distorted by rough smearing (Fig. 4.3a). Smears of cerebellar cortex, but not tumour, should contain a few large Purkinje cells, and the granule cells should have regular nuclei without mitotic figures. The second is choroid plexus (Fig. 4.3b), which may be mistaken for adenocarcinoma. 'Reactive' brain contains plump, reactive astrocytes and possibly some lipid-filled macrophages, other inflammatory cells and prominent capillaries (Fig. 4.4).

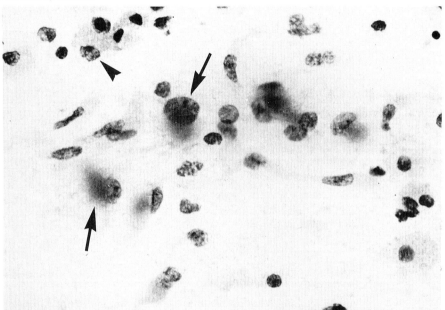

Fig. 4.4. Smear showing reactive cellular constituents in the cerebrum: reactive astrocytes (arrows) and lipid phagocytes (arrow head). Methylene blue, ×240.

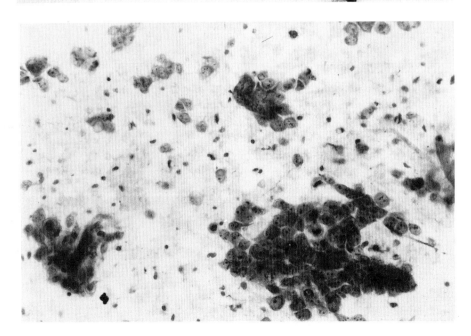

Fig. 4.5. Smear preparation of metastatic carcinoma. The tumour cells are adherent to each other, and therefore form clumps. Methylene blue, ×170.

If tumour is present, examine it at *low power* to gain an idea of the *general arrangement of the cells*. Carcinoma cells tend to form adherent clumps (Fig. 4.5), meningioma cells frequently form whorls (Fig. 4.6), ependymoma and neuroblastoma cells rosettes (Fig. 4.7), and choroid plexus papilloma forms papillary fronds reminiscent of normal choroid plexus (Fig. 4.8). The tumour cells of gliomas, pituitary adenomas and haemangiopericytic meningiomas tend to adhere to vessels and the cells of a lymphoma appear to cuff the vessels, but elsewhere smear quite diffusely (Fig. 4.9). Medulloblastoma cells also tend to smear diffusely. Anaplastic astrocytoma and glioblastoma are noteworthy for the disorderly arrangement of the cells (Fig. 4.10).

Next examine the nature of the tumour cells at *higher power* in more detail. Decide whether most of the tumour cells have well-defined rounded cell boundaries, a feature characteristic of epithelial cells and lymphoid cells. Most gliomas have cells with fine processes. Meningiomas are composed of spindle-shaped cells, some of these also associated with processes. However, in some gliomas and meningiomas cell outlines cannot be clearly discerned at all. Spend some time examining the *cell nuclei*. Always search for *mitotic figures*. They are usually of sinister import, but remember that they can occur in inflammatory cells. They are easy to find in carcinomas, medulloblastomas, lymphomas and malignant meningiomas, and are rare in pituitary

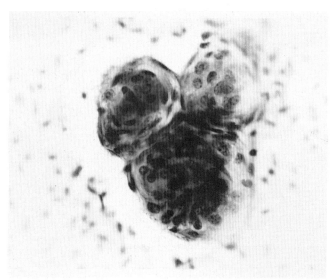

Fig. 4.6. Appearance of whorl formations in a smear preparation from a meningioma. Methylene blue, ×210.

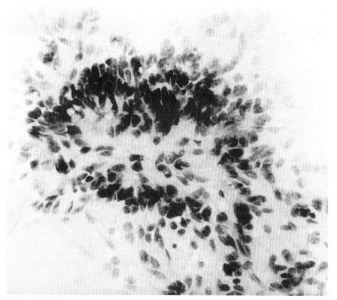

Fig. 4.7. Appearance of an ependymal pseudorosette in a smear preparation. Methylene blue, ×160.

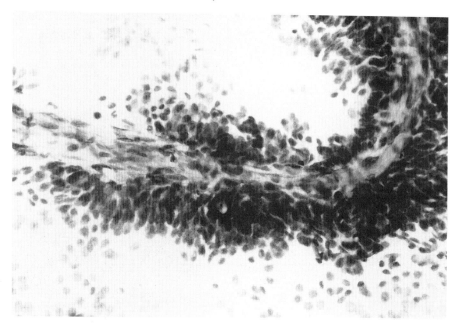

Fig. 4.8. Appearance of a smear preparation from a benign choroid plexus papilloma. Methylene blue, ×170.

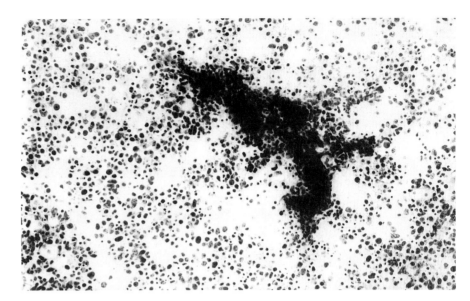

Fig. 4.9. Low-power view of lymphoma tumour cells in a smear preparation. Many tumour cells remain adherent to vessel fragments (centre), while elsewhere they smear diffusely. Methylene blue, ×150.

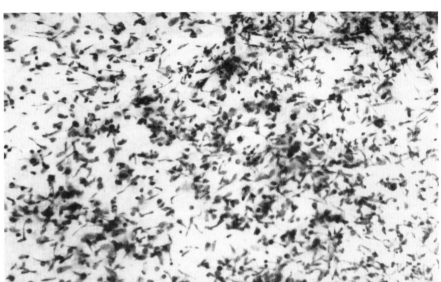

Fig. 4.10. A smear of astrocytoma tumour cells frequently shows a disorderly arrangement of cells. Methylene blue, ×180.

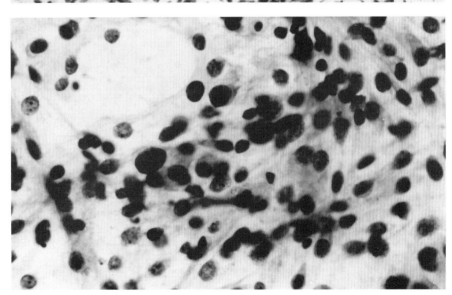

Figs 4.11–4.18. Nuclear morphology in methylene blue-stained smear preparations (×400):

Fig. 4.11. Malignant astrocytoma.

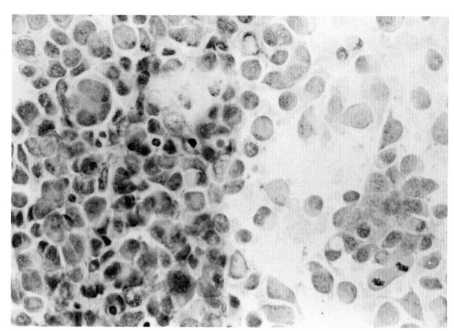

Fig. 4.12. Medulloblastoma.

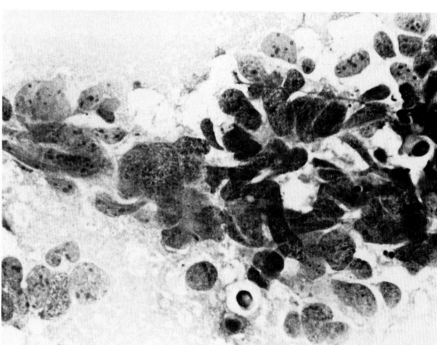

Fig. 4.13. Carcinoma.

adenomas, benign meningiomas, low-grade gliomas, benign nerve sheath tumours and choroid plexus papillomas. Nuclei are pleomorphic in most malignant tumours (gliomas, medullobastomas, carcinomas, lymphomas and malignant choroid plexus tumours) (Figs 4.11–4.16), and in some examples of benign tumours (cerebellar astrocytomas, some schwannomas, meningiomas, subependymal tumours in tuberous sclerosis and pituitary adenomas). Pleomorphic astrocytic nuclei are also found in progressive multifocal leucoencephalopathy (p.150) and acute MS (p.232). Nuclei are usually regular, showing only slight variations in size, in low-grade astrocytomas, oligodendrogliomas and most pituitary adenomas (Figs 4.17 and 4.18). Even the slight variation in size of astrocyte nuclei in low-grade astrocytomas (Fig. 4.17) is a useful feature which distinguishes them from most forms of reactive astrocytosis. Nucleoli are prominent in ependymomas, some carcinomas, melanomas, pituitary adenomas, and some meningiomas and lymphomas (Figs 4.13–4.15), but are usually inconspicuous in other cerebral tumours. Glycogen-containing vacuoles in nuclei are a prominent feature of some meningiomas.

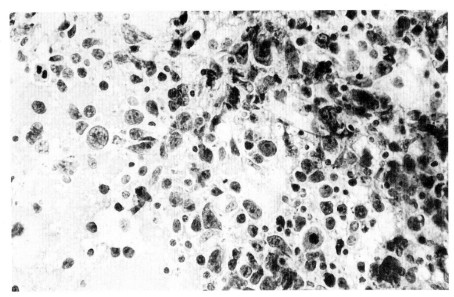

Fig. 4.14. Lymphoma.

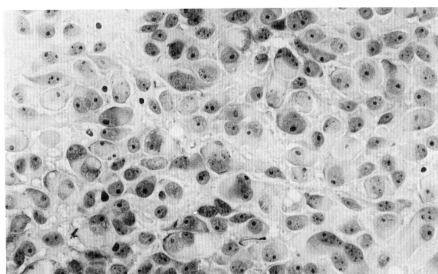

Fig. 4.15. Metastatic melanoma.

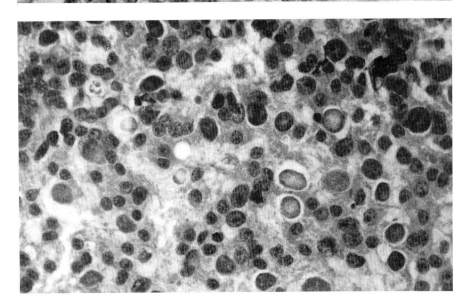

Fig. 4.16. Myeloma (poorly differentiated).

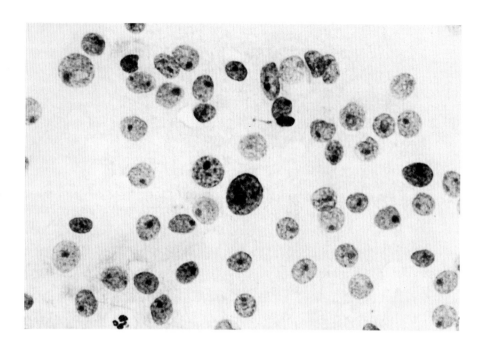

Fig. 4.17. Low-grade astrocytoma (note variation in nuclear size).

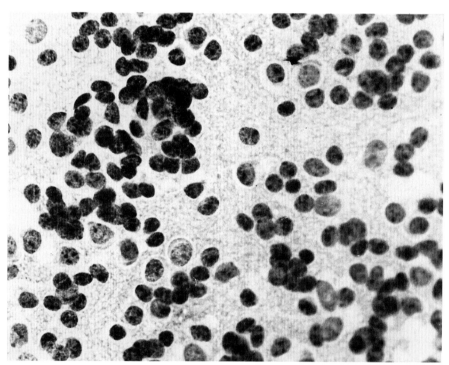

Fig. 4.18. Pituitary adenoma.

Various *miscellaneous features* may be present, providing useful clues to the nature of the tumour as indicated:

1 Normal, or nearly normal, brain occurring in close juxtaposition with clumps of frankly malignant cells — carcinoma.

2 Extracellular, finely fibrillar, metachromatic material (staining pink with aniline blue dyes) — gliomas, especially ependymomas (Plate 3.1); other metachromatic material — chondrosarcoma or chordoma (Plate 3.2).

3 Psammoma bodies — meningioma (benign).

4 Melanin pigment — melanoma or (occasionally) melanocytic meningioma, nerve sheath tumour, ependymoma, medulloblastoma or choroid plexus tumour. (If in doubt whether pigment is melanin or haemosiderin it may be necessary to perform a Perls' stain on another smear.)

5 Many large, multinucleate cells — glioblastoma, osteoclastoma (or osteoclastic reaction), malignant fibrous histiocytoma, carcinoma, reaction to craniopharyngioma or epidermoid/dermoid cyst, inflammatory condition (e.g. tuberculosis).

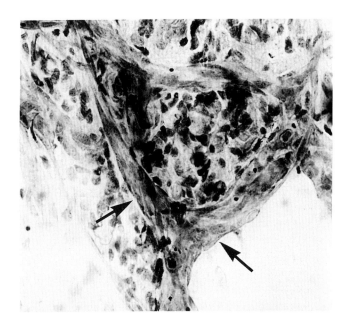

Fig. 4.19. Smear preparation of a malignant glioma, demonstrating hyperplasia of endothelial cells (arrowed). Methylene blue, ×400.

6 Distinct large and small cell populations — germinoma, lymphocytic reaction in a carcinoma, some lymphomas.

7 Keratin — craniopharyngioma, squamous cell carcinoma, epidermoid/dermoid cysts.

8 Frank tumour necrosis — malignant tumour.

9 Endothelial hyperplasia — malignant glioma (Fig. 4.19), cerebellar astrocytoma; rarely, bronchial oat cell carcinoma.

10 Calcium deposits — oligodendroglioma, astrocytoma, pituitary adenoma, meningioma.

11 Numerous mast cells — cerebellar haemangioblastoma.

12 Plasma cells — myeloma (especially if abnormal forms present; Figs 4.16 and 4.20), plasma cell reaction to tumour, infection, etc.

13 Haemosiderin — meningioma, malignant glioma, cerebellar astrocytoma, angioma, schwannoma, cerebellar haemangioblastoma; also, tissue around aneurysms and arteriovenous malformations, and in infarcts.

14 Intense inflammatory cuffing of vessels accompanied by features of 'reactive' brain — encephalitis (Fig. 4.21); rarely, MS.

Finally, smears frequently contain contaminating material, such as bone dust, and especially glove powder (Fig. 4.22). It is almost impossible to try to identify every item in a smear, and it is time wasting and distracting to try to do so.

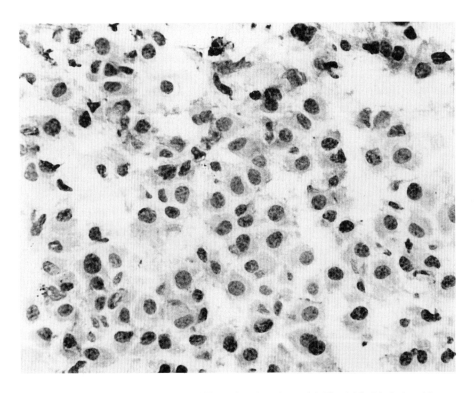

Fig. 4.20. Smear preparation of a well-differentiated myeloma (cf. Fig. 4.16). Methylene blue, ×250.

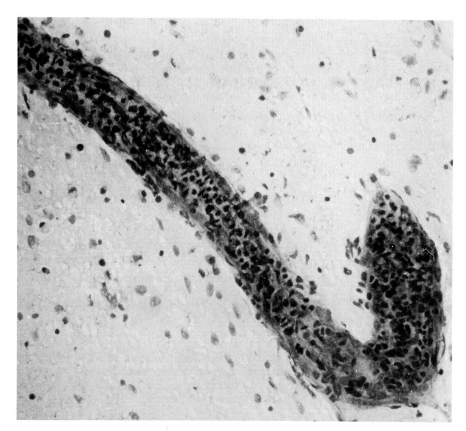

Fig. 4.21. Intense inflammatory cell cuffing of a small blood vessel in a smear preparation from a case of encephalitis. Methylene blue, ×195.

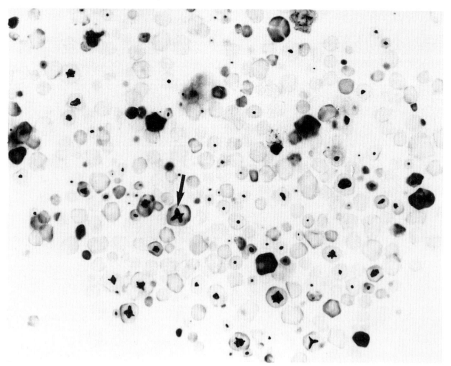

Fig. 4.22. Appearance of glove powder (talc) in a smear preparation. Birefringent particles are visible at the centre of some of them (arrowed). Methylene blue, ×250.

Immunohistological approach to the diagnosis of CNS tumours

Antibodies are now available to a number of antigens which display some degree of specificity for particular lines of cellular differentiation. A number of monoclonal antibodies to common or restricted antigens expressed by neuro-ectodermally derived mature cells and tumours are described by various groups, for example, Carrel *et al.* (1982), Coakham & Brownell (1986). Other antibodies recognize antigens which are common to tumours and fetal neural tissues (Wikstrand *et al.* 1983; Coakham & Brownell 1986). A third group of monoclonal antibodies is directed against antigens shared by CNS and haemopoietic cells (de Tribolet *et al.* 1984; Budka & Majdic 1985). At present there is what seems, to the outsider, a bewildering array of antibodies described by different groups of workers; most of these are not as yet widely available. Individual laboratories have raised antibodies to antigens present in tumour cells, which are suitable for diagnosis, but there is still no generally available 'library' of such antibodies. Such a 'library' would be of great value to neuropathologists, particularly if they could be used on paraffin-embedded tissues, and it is to be expected that something of the sort will soon exist. Meanwhile, a summary of the range of available antibodies is given below. Both polyclonal and monoclonal antibodies to some antigens are now available. Where choice exists, there are practical and theoretical arguments for preferring the use of monoclonal antibodies (Gatter & Mason 1986). Some antibodies require the use of fresh frozen sections (e.g. the anti-macrophage and microglial antibody, EBM11, mentioned below), but most of those described here can be applied to formalin-fixed, paraffin sections. Reactions for some antigens may be improved by pretreatment of paraffin sections with proteolytic enzymes; thus the suppliers' instructions need to be carefully followed. It must be emphasized that antibodies cannot at present be used as tumour-specific reagents, and adjacent sections of a puzzling tumour need to be treated with a panel of antibodies. It is important for each laboratory to become familiar with the appearances obtained in normal tissues and well-differentiated tumours with each antibody before they are tried out on a puzzling tumour.

Immunohistology is most useful in tumour diagnosis in three circumstances: firstly, if the information obtained from an examination of the tumour's architecture and cytology is conflicting, e.g. there may be some features of one type of tumour, and some of another; secondly, if the tissue available is very limited in amount, or too fragmented or distorted to be capable of providing much morphological information; and thirdly, if the tumour is poorly differentiated.

Some of the specificities of widely available antibodies likely to be of use to neuropathologists are summarized below (see also Table 4.2, Bonnin & Rubinstein 1984, Weller 1986 and Perentes & Rubinstein 1987).

Table 4.2. Immunoreactivity of human CNS tumours with a panel of antibodies (prepared in collaboration with Dr C.S. Morris)

	GFAP	EMA	CK	LCA	NF	NK	VIM	S-100	NSE
Astrocytoma	+	−	−	−	−	+	+/−‡	+/−‡	−/+‡
Carcinoma	−	+	+	−	−	+/−	−/+	−/+	−/+
Choroid plexus tumour	+/−	+	+	−	−	+/−	+	+	+
Ependymoma	+	+/−*	+/−	−	−	+	+	−/+	−/+ (focal)
Ganglioneuroma	−	−	−	−	+	−	ND	+	+
Ganglioglioma	+/−	−	−	−	+	−	+/−	+/−	+
Glioblastoma	+	−/+	+/−	−	−	+	+ (focal)	+	+ (focal)
Haemangioblastoma	+/−	−	−	−	−	−	+	−/+ (focal)	+/−
Lymphoma	−	−	−	+	−	−	±	±	−
Medulloblastoma	+/−	−	−	−	+/−	+/−	+ (focal)	+ (focal)	+
Melanoma	−	−	−/+†	−	−	−	+†	+	+ (focal)
Meningioma	−	+/−	+/−	−	−	−	+	+ (focal)	+ (focal)
Myeloma	−	+/−	+/−	+/−	−	−	±	−	−
Neuroblastoma	−	−	−	−	+	+	−	+/−	+
Neurofibroma	−	−	−	−	+/−**	+	+	+	−
Oligodendroglioma	+/−	−	−	−	−	+	−/+	+	+
Schwannoma	−	−	−	−	−	+	+	+	−/±§
Subependymoma	+	−	−	−	−	+/−	+	+	+

GFAP glial fibrillary acidic protein; EMA epithelial membrane antigen; CK cytokeratin; LCA leucocyte common antigen; NF neurofilament; NK natural killer cell/Leu 7; VIM vimentin; NSE neuron-specific enolase; ND not done; +/− usually positive, occasionally negative; −/+ usually negative, occasionally positive.
* positive, in our experience, in benign tumours, and negative in malignant ones.
† may show dual expression of CK and VIM.
‡ dependent on degree of malignancy/anaplasia.
§ NSE may be present in Antoni B areas.
** axons, not tumour cells, are positive.

Antibodies to epithelial cell antigens

Most of these antibodies are directed against cytokeratin or epithelial membrane antigen (EMA). A positive reaction is obtained with carcinomas (Fig. 4.23), normal choroid plexus and choroid plexus tumours. Meningiomas may also give a focally positive reaction with some of these antibodies (Kepes 1986; Theaker *et al.* 1986) (Fig. 4.24). Myeloma and some lymphomas may give a focally positive reaction for EMA, and rarely for cytokeratin. Most gliomas usually give negative reactions with these antibodies, but the focal expression of cytokeratin antigens has been described in some glioblastomas, and benign, but not malignant, ependymomas show some reactivity for EMA (Fig. 4.25).

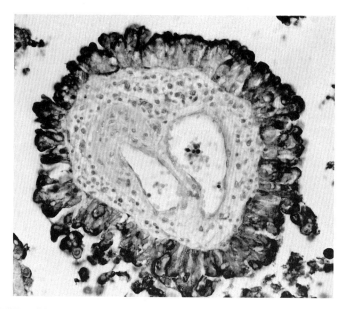

Fig. 4.23 (*right*). Positive reaction for epithelial membrane antigen (EMA) on cells of a metastatic carcinoma. Immunoperoxidase with haematoxylin counterstain, ×250.

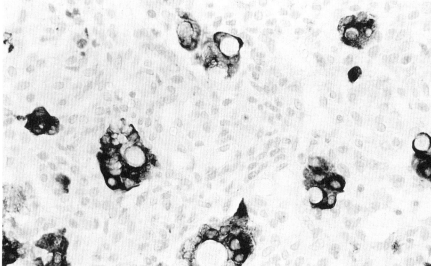

Fig. 4.24. Focal positive reaction for cytokeratin in cells surrounding hyaline bodies (unstained) in a meningioma. Immunoperoxidase with haematoxylin counterstain, ×350. (Courtesy of Dr J. Theaker.)

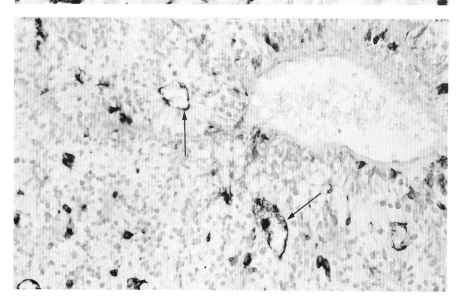

Fig. 4.25. Positive reaction for EMA at the margins of the central lumen of rosettes (arrowed), and in scattered tumour cells in a benign ependymoma. Immunoperoxidase with haematoxylin counterstain, ×100.

Antibodies to vimentin

Vimentin filaments are present in mesenchymal cells and also in glial cells. Gliomas, meningiomas, melanomas, schwannomas, lymphomas and sarcomas give a positive reaction for vimentin. Some carcinomas may also do so. In some studies, though not in all, there has been an inverse relation between the perceived degree of differentiation of astrocytomas and the intensity of reaction for vimentin.

Antibodies to glial fibrillary acidic protein (GFAP)

GFAP is a major cytoplasmic protein which is present in normal and reactive astrocytes. It is also present in gliomas with astrocytic differentiation, and in some cells in glioblastomas, subependymomas and ependymomas (Figs 4.26–4.28). Mixed gliomas containing both oligodendrocytes and astrocytes may show a positive reaction in both cell types (Fig. 4.29). Carcinomas, lymphomas, meningiomas, nerve sheath tumours and neuroblastomas do not react for GFAP. Haemangioblastomas, medulloblastomas and choroid plexus papillomas may contain a few positively reacting cells. Most cells in subependymal giant-cell tumours associated with tuberous sclerosis do not react for GFAP, but do react for neuron-specific enolase.

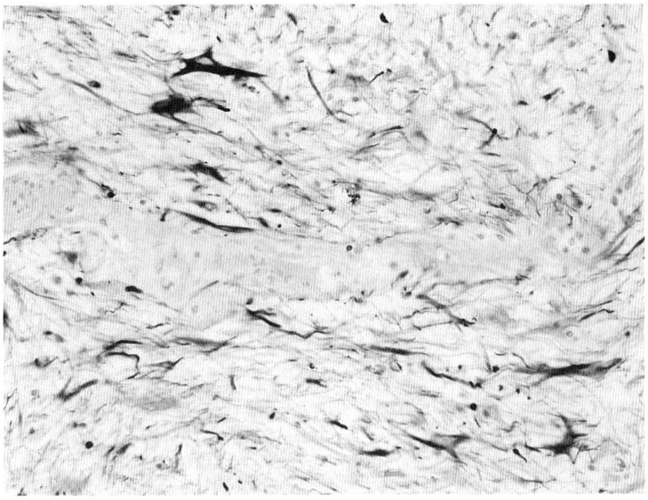

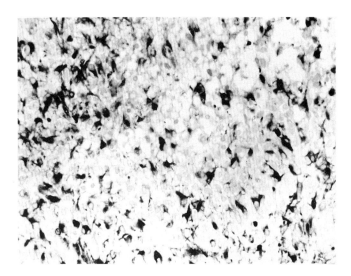

Fig. 4.26. Low-grade, pilocytic astrocytoma, showing positive reaction for GFAP in the processes and some of the cell bodies of the tumour cells. Immunoperoxidase with haematoxylin counterstain, ×250.

Fig. 4.27. Malignant astrocytoma, partly gemistocytic in type, showing a strong reaction for GFAP in the cytoplasm of many, but not all, tumour cells. Immunoperoxidase with haematoxylin counterstain, ×205.

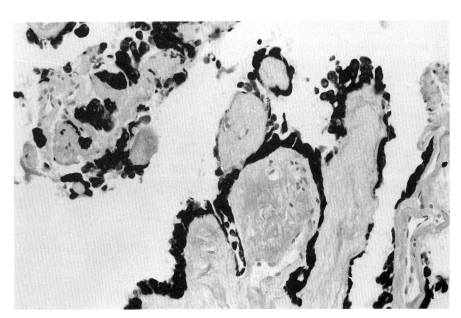

Fig. 4.28. Strong reaction for GFAP in the epithelial cells of a myxopapillary ependymoma. Immunoperoxidase with haematoxylin counterstain, ×250.

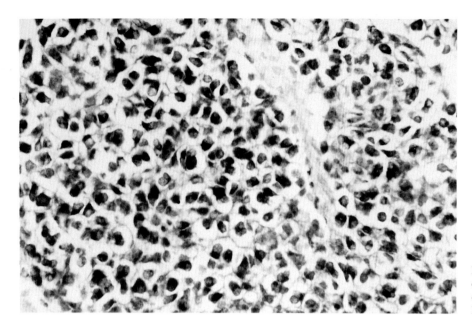

Fig. 4.29. Strong reaction for GFAP in the cell cytoplasm in a malignant oligodendroglioma. Immunoperoxidase with haematoxylin counterstain, ×400.

Antibodies to S-100 protein

S-100 protein is present in glial cells and cells derived from neural crest. It also occurs in small amounts in other cell types, which restricts its value for tumour diagnosis. The following tumours react, at least in some parts of the tumour, with S-100 antibodies; gliomas, benign nerve sheath tumours, melanomas, granular cell myoblastomas, choroid plexus papillomas, some carcinomas and lymphomas. Malignant nerve sheath tumours are not invariably reactive.

Antibodies to neuron-specific enolase

Neuron-specific (γγ) enolase is found in neurons in the CNS and neuro-endocrine cells in other parts of the body. A strong positive reaction with this antibody is obtained with neuroblastomas, melanomas, APUDomas (carcinoids) and oat-cell carcinomas. Subependymal giant-cell tumours in subjects with tuberous sclerosis also react for this antigen. These antibodies are not helpful in distinguishing between different types of 'primitive' tumour, such as neuroblastoma and medulloblastoma, as some reaction tends to be present in all such tumours.

Antibodies to neurofilaments

In general, these antibodies react with neurons, or parts of neurons, such as the axons or dendrites. Tumours giving a positive reaction include neuroblastomas, ganglioneuromas, neurons in gangliocytomas, phaeochromocytomas and some medulloblastomas. Monoclonal neurofilament antibodies are directed against the 68 kd component protein or against one of the two larger molecular weight components. The antibody to the 68 kd component is the one of greatest diagnostic use, since its antigen is the one most regularly found in these tumours.

Antibodies to carbonic anhydrase C

Choroid plexus and its tumours react positively for this antigen.

Antibodies to leucocyte common antigen

All leucocytes react with these antibodies. Lymphomas give a positive reaction, as do most myelomas. Carcinomas, meningiomas and gliomas do not react. Lymphomas identified with these antibodies can be further classified using antibodies specific for T- and B-lymphocytes. Myelomas and B-cell lymphomas can be further classified using antibodies to κ and λ light chains and immunoglobulin heavy chains.

Antibody Leu 7 to human natural killer (NK) cells

This antibody reacts with human NK cells and also with most schwannomas, some neurofibromas, tumours of the APUD series, neuroblastomas and malignant nerve sheath tumours. Most glial tumours, including oligodendrogliomas, and some medulloblastomas, also react with this antibody. Its antigen is thought to be myelin-associated glycoprotein. The pattern of staining produced frequently outlines the cell membranes.

Antibodies to pituitary hormones

These can be used to identify the hormones present in pituitary adenomas (p.211).

Antibodies to macrophages

α-1-anti-chymotrypsin is an antigen which can be used as a relatively specific cell marker for macrophages in the CNS in paraffin sections. Some recently introduced monoclonal antibodies, e.g. EBM11 (Esiri & McGee 1986), 10.1 (Hogg *et al.* 1985) and certain other macrophage antibodies (Franklin *et al.* 1986) react both with macrophages and with normal microglia in cryostat sections. Macrophages, among other leucocytes, also react for leucocyte common antigen, and for class 2 major histocompatibility complex (MHC) antigens.

Other CNS biopsies

The use of biopsy in the diagnosis of non-neoplastic disorders of the CNS is limited to a few metabolic disorders, suspected viral encephalitis and other inflammatory conditions, and the investigation of dementia. Other conditions that may be found, though previously unsuspected, include acute MS, leucodystrophies and neuronal storage disorders. The extent to which use is made of biopsies for diagnosis of these conditions varies from one centre to another according to whether, in the clinicians' opinion, their diagnostic value outweighs any risk. In addition to diagnostic biopsies, there are opportunities to study surgical specimens when temporal lobes are partially resected or a hemispherectomy is performed for the relief of intractable epilepsy. These specimens and their management are discussed in Chapter 18.

Biopsies from cases of *suspected viral encephalitis* should be divided to provide samples for viral and bacterial culture, and, if indicated, animal inoculation studies, a sample for EM and a sample for routine light microscopy (Fig. 4.1a). By light microscopy the sections are scrutinized for changes described in Chapter 10. Snap-frozen tissue for cryostat sec-

tions may also be taken, but, as many microbial antigens are now known to survive formalin fixation, they can be searched for more safely in paraffin sections. Smears can be made and treated with an anti-herpes simplex virus antibody, using the immunoperoxidase technique, if herpes simplex encephalitis is suspected (Fig. 4.30). If the results are negative the results of culture will have to be awaited. Success in detecting microbial antigens depends crucially on having a high-titre, specific antiserum or monoclonal antibody available. Positive and negative control sections or smears should be processed alongside the case under investigation whenever possible.

Cerebral biopsies from cases of *dementia* should be divided perpendicularly to the cortical surface, and one sample frozen for biochemical enzyme assay, another sample fixed in glutaraldehyde for EM, and the remainder fixed in formalin for light microscopy (Fig. 4.1a). After fixation, part of the latter sample is embedded in paraffin wax and sections cut and stained with H&E, Nissl, Congo Red or another amyloid stain, a myelin stain and a modified Palmgren (see Appendix 1) or similar stain for neurofibrillary tangles. Most cases may be expected to show features of Alzheimer's disease (p.270). From such cases a cortical biopsy can be expected to contain several neurofibrillary tangles (Figs 3.9 and 17.7) and some amyloid deposition in leptomeningeal and cortical blood vessel walls (Plate 7.1) and in the cores of plaques. Plaques also may be visible in paraffin sections, but are better displayed in von Braunmühl-stained frozen sections (Fig. 3.10), which can be prepared from the remaining portion of fixed tissue, after the paraffin sections have excluded the diagnosis of Creutzfeldt−Jakob disease. (For precautions to take if this diagnosis is suspected see p. 266.) Some authorities regard the presence of argyrophilic plaques alone as an acceptable criterion for the diagnosis of Alzheimer's disease within certain age limits (at least 10

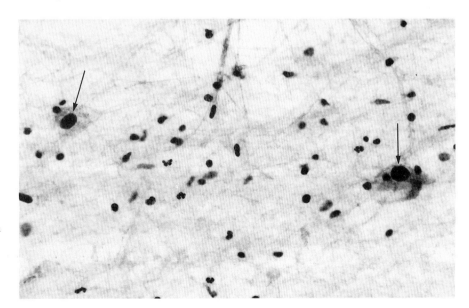

Fig. 4.30. Smear from a cerebral biopsy from a case of suspected herpes simplex encephalitis. A positive reaction in the nuclei of two neurons (arrowed) was obtained with a rabbit antiserum to herpes simplex type 1 virus. Normal rabbit serum gave a negative reaction on a second smear. Immunoperoxidase with haematoxylin counterstain, ×220.

plaques per ×200 field at 66−75 years and at least 15 plaques per ×200 field over 75 years (Khatchachurian 1985).

Brain biopsies performed for *suspected metabolic disease* should contain white matter as well as cortex. The specimen should be divided to provide a snap-frozen sample for biochemical investigation (by prior arrangement with local, or if necessary distant, biochemists), another snap-frozen sample for cryostat sectioning, a third sample for EM and the remainder fixed and processed for light microscopy. Stains for myelin, axons, neurons (Nissl), stored PAS-positive material, and reactive glial cells (PTAH) may be performed on paraffin sections and stains for neutral fat, metachromatic granules and acid phosphatase on cryostat sections. The changes that may be present are described in Chapter 18. The fine structure of any abnormal stored material can be examined by EM.

Cytology of CSF

Investigations on CSF frequently need to be made in a number of different laboratories. Cytological investigation may be the responsibility of the neuropathologist. For this purpose a sample of freshly removed CSF is required and this should be centrifuged as soon as possible at 1150 r/min for 10 minutes onto gelatin coated slides in a cytospin centrifuge. The cytospin preparations obtained are stained with H&E and the May−Grünwald−Giemsa stain (Figs 4.31−4.34).

Immunohistological staining is often useful when trying to identify the nature of tumour cells in CSF and should enable cells to be classified into one of three groups: carcinoma, neuro-ectodermal tumour or lymphoma (Coakham & Brownell 1986).

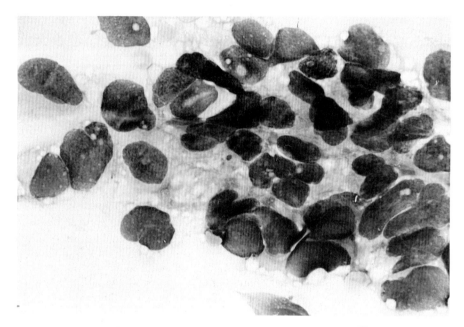

Figs 4.31−4.34. Examples of cytospin preparations of CSF, stained with the May−Grünwald−Giemsa method. (Courtesy of Dr V. Crucioli.)

Fig. 4.31. High-grade glioma, ×700.

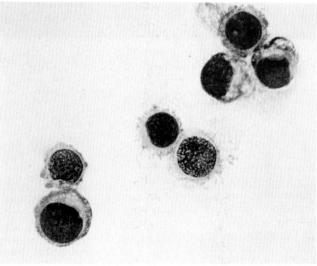

Fig. 4.32. Adenocarcinoma, ×700.

Plate 3

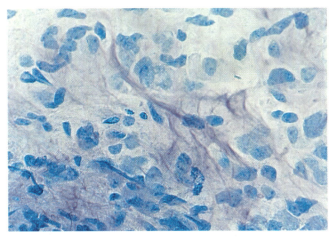

3.1. Smear preparation of a malignant glioma illustrating the appearance of characteristic metachromatic, extracellular fibrillary material (purple). Methylene blue, ×400.

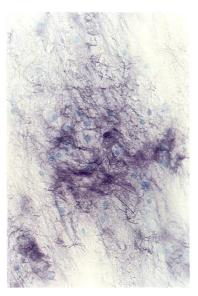

3.2. Abundant, wispy, extracellular, metachromatic strands and scanty, ill-defined cells in a smear preparation of a chordoma. Methylene blue, ×200.

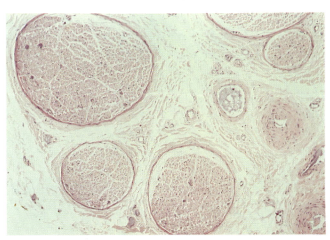

3.3. Low-power view of a transverse section of a normal sural nerve. Note the rounded outline of the nerve fascicles, bounded by the perineurium, with small arteries, arterioles and veins and epineurial connective tissue. H&E, ×40.

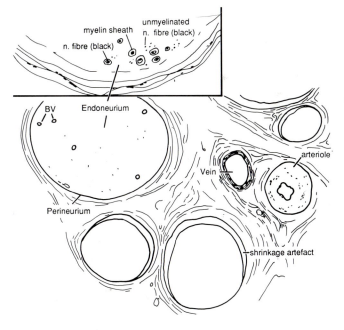

3.4. Drawing to demonstrate the principal features of Plate 3.3. Inset above shows higher power appearances corresponding to those seen in Plates 4.1 and 4.4.

Plate 4

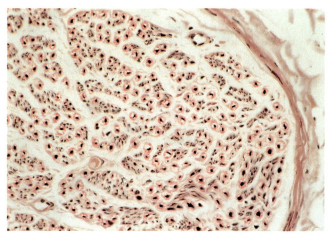

4.1. Combined nerve fibre (black) and myelin (pink) stain on a transverse section of a normal sural nerve. Palmgren/Brilliant crystal scarlet stain (see Appendix 1), ×250.

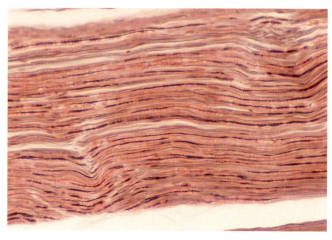

4.2. Longitudinal section of a normal sural nerve stained as in Plate 4.1. ×250.

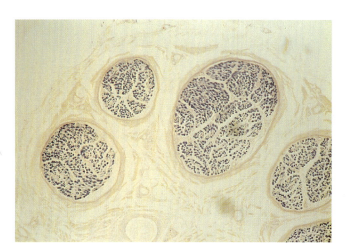

4.3. Transverse section of a normal sural nerve stained for myelin using Page's stain, ×35.

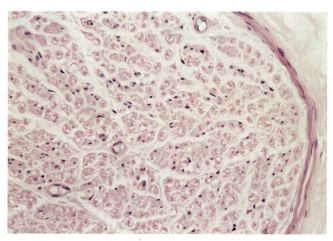

4.4. Close-up view of one of the fascicles shown in Plate 3.3. Blood vessels and Schwann cell nuclei can be seen; myelin sheaths appear pale and vacuolated where fatty constituents have been dissolved out during processing. H&E, ×320.

Plate 5 Normal muscle histochemistry on transverse cryostat sections:

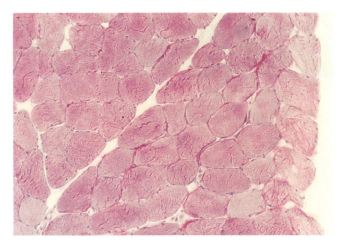

5.1. PAS (glycogen) (type 1 fibres pale), ×200.

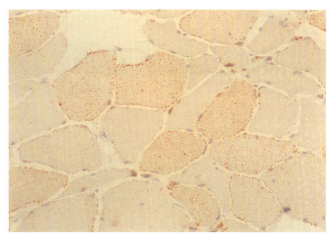

5.2. Oil red O (fat) (more numerous droplets in type 1 fibres), ×260.

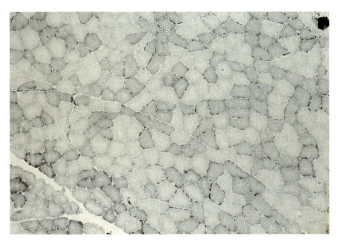

5.3. Succinic dehydrogenase (type 1 fibres dark), ×100.

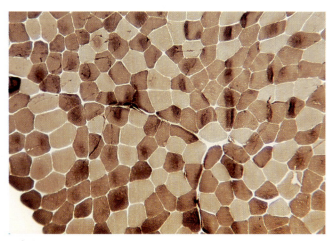

5.4. ATPase (pH 9.4) (type 1 fibres pale), ×100.

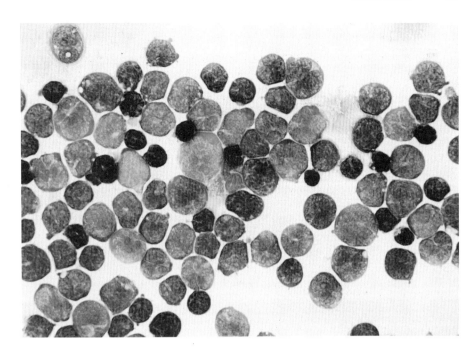

Fig. 4.33. Lymphoma (centroblastic, centrocytic type), ×700.

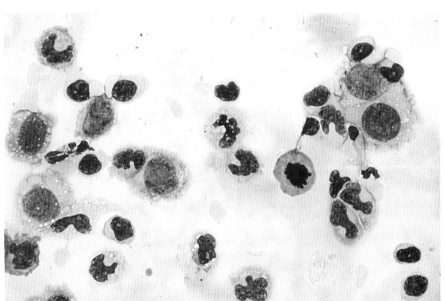

Fig. 4.34. Germinoma (leucocytes and tumour cells, including one in mitosis), ×560.

Nerve biopsies (for staining techniques see Appendix 1)

Examination of a nerve biopsy can provide a definitive diagnosis in only a relatively small number of diseases: amyloidosis, leprosy, neuropathy due to vasculitis, sarcoidosis or paraproteinaemia. In other cases it may help by narrowing the range of possible diagnoses to be considered by the clinician. The choice of nerve to biopsy is important. As it should leave no motor deficit or important sensory deficit, and at the same time be readily accessible to the surgeon, the choice often falls on the sural nerve. Artefactual changes are easily produced in peripheral nerves and for

this reason the biopsy specimen needs to be removed gently. It should measure 1.5–3.0 cm in length. The tips of the cut ends are discarded as they are likely to have been compressed by forceps during removal. A small portion is rapidly immersed in glutaraldehyde fixative for resin embedding and EM. Occasionally it is necessary to take an additional portion to snap-freeze for cryostat sectioning, for example if immunofluorescence or metachromatic stains are to be used. The remainder is placed on a card to which it will adhere after a few minutes, before being dropped into fixative. After fixation the nerve is divided to provide carefully orientated transverse and longitudinal sections after paraffin embedding, and a separate portion is reserved for teasing and osmicating. Several 1 µm sections are prepared from the resin-embedded material for light microscopy after staining with toluidine blue (Fig. 4.1b), and ultrathin sections for microscopy prepared from selected blocks. Paraffin sections are stained with H&E, van Gieson, myelin and axon stains. Useful techniques are those that combine myelin and axon stains in the same section, such as Palmgren's stain combined with Page's myelin stain, or brilliant crystal scarlet (Plate 4.1; Appendix 1). The sections are examined for qualitative changes indicative of disease (Chapter 22) and can also be submitted to simple quantitative analysis (p.332). The appearances of a normal sural nerve processed in some of the ways described are shown in Plates 3.3 and 3.4, Plate 4 and Figs 4.35 and 4.36. It should be borne in mind that nerve pathology can quite frequently be detected in skin or conjunctival biopsies, in which case resort to a nerve biopsy may not be necessary.

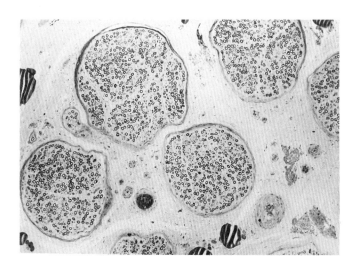

Fig. 4.35. Transverse 1 µm section of resin-embedded normal sural nerve. Individual myelinated nerve fibres can be easily seen, their sheaths appearing as dark rings. Toluidine blue, ×40.

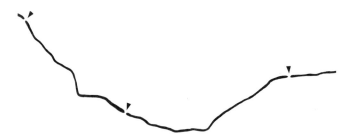

Fig. 4.36. Osmicated and teased preparation of a fibre from a normal sural nerve. Individual internodes are visible between the nodes of Ranvier (arrow heads). ×90.

Muscle biopsies

Muscle biopsy can provide important diagnostic information about primary muscle diseases described in Chapter 23 and about some systemic disorders such as polyarteritis nodosa or sarcoidosis, or some of the metabolic diseases described in Chapter 19. It can also provide confirmation of a denervating process affecting motor neurons. Muscle has considerable regenerative power, and there is a greater choice of sites for biopsy than there is for nerve biopsy. The site for biopsy must be carefully chosen, however. Severely wasted muscles should be avoided, as the end results of either primary muscle or neurogenic wasting diseases are often indistinguishable. On the other hand, a muscle that is barely affected by disease may show only minimal and non-specific changes. Muscles that have been recently subjected to electromyography should also be avoided as they are liable to show confusing artefacts due to trauma. If possible the muscle biopsied should be one familiar to pathologists and therefore one for which information on normal fibre diameters is available. Whenever possible the biopsy should be taken from near the mid-point of the muscle in order to include some motor end-plates. Certainly the samples removed should avoid the tendinous insertions, since features such as nemaline rods and central nuclei, usually interpreted as pathological, may occur at these sites in normal muscle. Muscle biopsies should measure 2−3 cm in the long axis of the fibres and 1.0−1.5 cm in the other dimensions. Some experts like the muscle to be clamped *in situ* before removal to prevent it from undergoing contraction after removal. This certainly makes for finer preservation of ultrastructure, but it is unlikely that any features of diagnostic importance will be missed if this is omitted. After removal the muscle specimen should be placed on card and a small portion removed for glutaraldehyde fixation and EM (Appendix A). (The specimen should be handled gently, as artefacts due to hypercontraction are easily produced by rough handling (Fig. 4.37).) Then a transverse slice is removed from one end to be snap-frozen in cooled isopentane in liquid nitrogen for cryostat sectioning. A further sample may be needed for biochemistry, and this also should be snap-frozen. Occasionally special biochemical studies may be indicated, for example for investigation of malignant hyperpyrexia or mitochondrial myopathies, and arrangements for these should be made with a biochemist before the biopsy is taken. The remainder of the sample is allowed to adhere to the card for a few minutes before being immersed in formalin. After fixation portions are processed for paraffin embedding, and sections, transverse and longitudinal to the direction of the fibres, are stained with H&E and van Gieson stains. If a disease causing patchy pathology (such as myositis or arteritis) is suspected, sections at several levels through the embedded block should be examined if the initial sections show no pathology. The final remaining

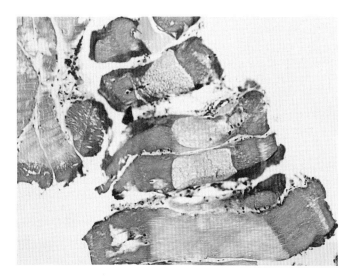

Fig. 4.37. Hypercontraction artefact in a muscle biopsy. This change should not be mistaken for hyaline necrosis. H&E, ×90.

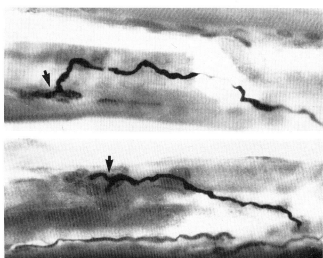

Fig. 4.38. Appearance of normal motor end-plates (arrowed) in Schofield's silver stain of muscle. ×360.

sample in formalin is cut into longitudinal sections and stained with Schofield's silver method or an alternative (intravitam methylene blue) to show nerve fibres and motor end-plates (Fig. 4.38).

Histochemical stains on cryostat sections have an important diagnostic role. Sections should be cut transversely, and sequential sections stained with H&E, and modified trichrome stains. Choice of routine histochemical reactions is to some extent a matter of personal preference. The use of marker enzyme reactions involved in major energy-producing pathways enables a clear distinction to be drawn between the different fibre types (p.344). As a routine we perform the PAS reaction for glycogen, oil red O for fat, the succinic dehydrogenase reaction as an example of a mitochondrial enzyme, and the myosin ATPase reaction at pH 9.4 to provide good fibre-type distinction (Plate 5). In selected cases this last reaction may also need to be carried out at pH 4.6 and pH 6.3, and occasionally it is helpful to perform the acid phosphatase and phosphorylase reactions, the latter two particularly if glycogen storage disease is suspected, or if excess glycogen is found with the PAS stain. The non-specific esterase reaction is useful for identifying motor end-plates in frozen sections (Fig. 4.39). Histochemical methods for demonstrating acetyl cholinesterase activity also locate motor end-plates. Details of the performance and interpretation of these reactions can be found in Dubowitz (1985). A point that is not always realized is that even in a frozen section glycogen is liable to leach out during processing, a pitfall that can be avoided by first dipping the section in celloidin. In examining these reactions, and the routinely stained sections, attention is paid to the presence of pathological features and to quantitative abnormalities in the muscle (Chapter 23).

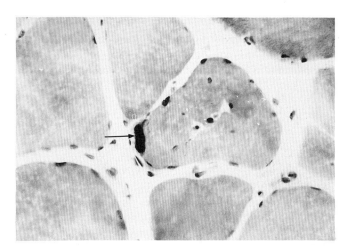

Fig. 4.39. Cryostat transverse section of muscle, showing strong reaction for non-specific esterase (arrowed) (red reaction product) at the site of a motor end-plate. ×360.

Rectal biopsies

Full-thickness rectal biopsies are occasionally referred to a neuropathologist for assessment of the autonomic ganglion cell population. Certain metabolic diseases can be diagnosed, or at least suspected, from the appearances of these cells and of nearby mucosal macrophages, as described in Chapter 19. In Hirschsprung's disease it is necessary for the surgeon carrying out a resection of the abnormal segment of bowel to be satisfied that there is a normal complement of ganglion cells in the ends of the bowel which are to be anastomosed. This requires that frozen sections be examined from the clearly identified upper and lower resected margins and checked for the presence of ganglion cells. A histochemical reaction for acetylcholinesterase may be helpful for this purpose (Patrick *et al.* 1980).

Further reading

Adams JH, Graham DI, Doyle D. 1981. *Brain Biopsy: the Smear Technique for Neurosurgical Biopsies*. Chapman and Hall, London.

Barnard RO. 1981. Smear preparations in the diagnosis of malignant lesions of the central nervous system. In Coss LG, Coleman DV (Eds) *Advances in Clinical Cytology*. Butterworths, London, pp. 254–69.

Bonnin JM, Rubinstein LJ. 1984. Immunohistochemistry of central nervous system tumours. Its contribution to neurosurgical diagnosis. *J Neurosurg* **60**, 1121–33.

Budka H, Majdic O. 1985. Shared antigenic determinants between human hemopoietic cells and nervous tissues and tumours. *Acta Neuropathol (Berl)* **67**, 58–66.

Carrel S, de Tribolet N, Mach, JP. 1982. Expression of neuroectodermal antigens common to melanomas, gliomas and neuroblastomas. 1. Identification of monoclonal anti-melanoma and anti-glioma antibodies. *Acta Neuropathol (Berl)* **57**, 158–64.

Coakham HB, Brownell B. 1986. Monoclonal antibodies in the diagnosis of cerebral tumours and cerebrospinal fluid neoplasia. In Cavanagh JB (Ed.) *Recent Advances in Neuropathology 3*. Churchill Livingstone, Edinburgh, pp. 25–53.

de Tribolet N, Carrel S, Mach JP. 1984. Brain tumour-associated antigens. In Rosenblum ML, Wilson CB (Eds) *Progress in Experimental Tumour Research*. Karger, Basel.

Dubowitz V. 1985. *Muscle Biopsy, a Practical Approach*, 2nd edn. Baillière Tindall, London.

Esiri MM, McGee JO'D. 1986. Monoclonal antibody to macrophages labels macrophages and microglial cells in human brain. *J Clin Pathol* **39**, 615–21.

Franklin WA, Pulford K, Brunangelo F *et al.* 1986. Immunohistological analysis of human mononuclear phagocytes and dendritic cells using monoclonal antibodies. *Lab Invest* **54**, 322–36.

Gatter KC, Mason DY. 1986. The use of monoclonal antibodies in the histopathologic diagnosis of human malignancy. In Fer MF, Greco FA, Oldham RK (Eds) *Poorly Differentiated Neoplasms and Tumours of Unknown Origin*. Grune and Stratton, New York, pp. 399–429.

Hogg N, Takac, L, Palmer BG, Selvendran Y, Allen C. 1985. The p150, 95 molecule is a marker of human mononuclear phagocytes: comparison with expression of class II molecules. *Eur J Immun* **16**, 240–8.

Kepes JJ. 1986. The histopathology of meningiomas. A reflection of origins and expected behaviour? *J Neuropath Exp Neurol* **45**, 95–107.

Khatchachurian ZS. 1985. Diagnosis of Alzheimer's disease (Conference Report). *Arch Neurol* **42**, 1097–104.

Patrick WJA, Besley GTN, Smith II. 1980. Histochemical diagnosis of Hirschprung's disease and a comparison of the histochemical and biochemical activity of acetylcholinesterase in rectal mucosal biopsies. *J Clin Pathol* **33**, 336–43.

Perentes E, Rubinstein LJ. 1987. Recent applications of immunoperoxidase histochemistry in human neurooncology. An update. *Arch Pathol Lab Med* **111**, 796–812.

Theaker JM, Gatter KC, Esiri MM. Fleming KA. 1986. Epithelial membrane antigen and cytokeratin expression by meningiomas: an immunohistological study. *J Clin Pathol* **39**, 435–39.

Weller RO. 1985. The immunopathology of brain tumours. In Bleehen NM (Ed.) *Tumours of the Brain*. Springer, Berlin, pp. 19–33.

Wikstrand CJ, Bourdon MA, Pegram CN, Bigner DD. 1983. Human foetal brain antigen expression common to tumours of neuroectodermal origin. *J Neuroimmunol* **3**, 43–62.

Chapter 5
Injuries to the Head and Spinal Column

Types of head injury

In Britain, and in many other parts of the world, the commonest causes of head injury are road traffic accidents and falls. Elsewhere, it may be otherwise. In Papua New Guinea, for instance, the commonest such injury is said to be due to the falling of a coconut from a great height. Apart from accidents, the common causes include gunshot wounds (self-inflicted or otherwise), sport, and deliberate mayhem, such as occurs in boxing. In the Oxford records there is a single case of a javelin wound in the brain. The Oxford neurosurgeon Joe Pennybacker, in a list of personally handled cases of head injury sustained in the course of sport, after many instances of trauma from boxing, cricket,

football and equitation, concluded with a single entry under the heading 'chess'. The patient, while waiting for his opponent to move, had tilted his chair too far backwards and cracked his skull.

Causes and effects

Figure 5.1 is a much simplified diagram of the ways in which the brain may be affected following an injury. Much of it is self-explanatory; but it is worth drawing attention to some important features. The first is that when death is due to intracranial disaster, the *immediate* cause usually lies in the *brain stem*. As an illustration of this point, we can quote a case in the Oxford file of a man who directed a revolver

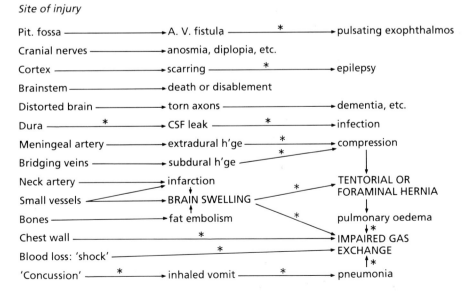

Fig. 5.1. Oversimplified diagram, showing some of the immediate and delayed effects of injury on the brain. Arrows indicate causal sequences. Asterisks show points at which medical or surgical intervention may be helpful. Capital letters indicate major immediate threats to life.

89

bullet through both temporal lobes, destroying the thalamus on the way. He remained alive, in a decerebrate state, for five days, after which he died from tentorial herniation due to cerebral sepsis and swelling. The diagram makes clear the number of different paths leading to death from either tentorial or foraminal herniation.

Brain and chest

The second important feature is the close relationship between the brain and the *respiratory system*, and the complexity of their interactions. In the first place, it is common knowledge among neurosurgeons and their anaesthetists that defective ventilation of the patient on the operating table will cause his brain to darken and swell. Chest injuries, pulmonary oedema and pneumonia are among the common causes of impaired gas exchange. A concussed person is liable to vomit, and the inhalation of vomitus may lead to a pneumonia which threatens life. In the second place, experience in the post mortem room points to a close association between pulmonary oedema and foraminal, rather than tentorial, herniation; and it is believed by some that pressure on the lower medulla may provoke pulmonary oedema by way of vagal irritation. If this is so, we are faced with the possibility of a vicious quadrilateral of (i) impaired gas exchange → (ii) brain swelling → (iii) foraminal herniation → (iv) pulmonary oedema → (i) impaired gas exchange ...

Haemorrhages and contusions

A third feature of the diagram is the number of different ways in which *intracranial bleeding* may give rise to a fatal herniation. Two of these — acute epidural and subdural haemorrhages — are dealt with on p.97. Less familiar, at textbook level at least, are the haemorrhages, often large and disruptive, which occur at sites of cerebral and cerebellar

contusion. This may be partly due to inconsistency in the use of the word '*contusion*'. As we use it, it means merely abrasion of the brain surface, with tearing of pial and arachnoid membranes and of superficial blood vessels. If the torn vessels are large or medium-sized veins, a contusion will give rise to a subdural haematoma. If they consist of small arteries, capillaries and venules, they are likely to go into protective spasm, and bleeding is arrested by spasm and clotting, possibly assisted by arterial hypotension due to 'shock'. Renewed bleeding at a later stage may be due to a rise in blood pressure, or to other causes. This *delayed haemorrhage* may be massive and disruptive, ploughing into tissue already suffering from ischaemic damage, giving rise to large subdural haematomas, and resulting in fatal herniation. The entire lesion, as displayed at post mortem, is commonly referred to as a 'contusion', whereas we think that a distinction should be drawn between the original contusion and the subsequent *contusional haemorrhage*. Our evidence for this view comes from the histological examination of a series of nine fatal head injuries, with survivals of up to 13 days. In those with more than 3 days' survival, there were cellular reactions, inflammatory and glial, datable to the time of injury. No such reactions were seen in relation to the major haemorrhages, which appeared to be terminal. The impression that the original lesions had been more or less trivial was reinforced by the fact that most of the patients had talked coherently at some time after the injury.

Coup−contrecoup lesions

A further feature of these nine cases was that all of them had had a fall on the back of the head, and sustained a linear fracture of the occipital bone on the side of impact. Underlying this fracture was a contusion of the undersurface of the cerebellum; and a further contusion was present in the surface of the *opposite* frontal lobe (Figs 5.2

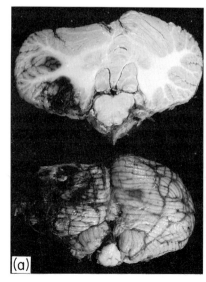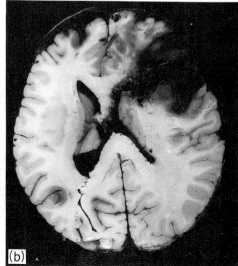

Fig. 5.2. Contusional haemorrhages. Woman aged 57, concussed for 20 min following a fall on the back of the head, causing a linear fracture of the left occipital bone. Fully conscious for 3 hours, then lapsed into coma. Acute subdural haematoma evacuated through a burr-hole, without improvement. Died 54 hours after injury. Post mortem findings of foraminal herniation: contusions of left cerebellar hemisphere and right frontal lobes, both giving rise to haemorrhages into the brain substance and subdural space. (a) Cerebellum, surface and slice. (b) Horizontal slice, showing massive haemorrhage into right frontal lobe, extending to the lateral ventricle. The right hemisphere is swollen, with subfalcine herniation and flattening of convolutions.

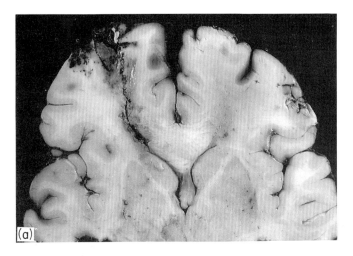

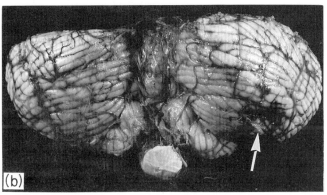

Fig. 5.3. Cerebral oedema associated with contusional haemorrhage. Man aged 70, concussed for half an hour following a fall on the back of the head, causing a linear fracture of the right occipital bone. Fully conscious for 24 hours, then lapsed into coma. Left subdural haematoma removed; no improvement. Died 13 days after the injury. Post mortem findings: transtentorial hernia, due to intracerebral haemorrhages, mainly in the left frontal lobe, with surrounding oedema. (a) Horizontal slice, showing haemorrhagic slit extending from left frontal pole to the anterior horn of the lateral ventricle. The surrounding tissue is oedematous, and the lateral ventricles are compressed. (b) Trivial contusion on undersurface of cerebellum (arrowed). There is no foraminal hernia.

and 5.3). In every case a massive haemorrhage had occurred from one or other of these contusions; in one case, from both. All nine cases were examples of the classical *coup–contrecoup* pattern of damage, described in detail by Courville in 1942.

Post mortem examination

In a case of head injury one is concerned with two main questions: (i) the mechanism of the injury, and (ii) the cause of death. These two are often related, as when the head injury is combined with a neck injury causing crushing of the cervical cord. Points of importance for the forensic aspects of the case are, first, the form and distribution of superficial bruises, scratches and lacerations, and second,

the site and form of bony injuries to the skull, face, spinal column and elsewhere. Instructions on the examination of injured bodies (including the estimation of alcohol levels in the blood) and on the interpretation of one's findings are given in textbooks of forensic pathology. As to the immediate cause of death, this is to be found, in most cases, in the brain stem. In the most severe cases of acceleration injury of the brain, with instant death, one may find a tear running half-way through the midbrain, which is tethered within the posterior cranial fossa, and cannot withstand an extreme swirling movement of the cerebral hemispheres. In cases where death was not instantaneous, the cause is likely to be a tentorial or foraminal hernia, due to haemorrhage, or brain swelling, or a combination of these. If no hernia is present, it is well to look elsewhere for the cause of death: in the cervical cord, for instance, or in the chest.

If the case has no clinical antecedents, as often occurs with fatal road traffic accidents, it is justifiable to dissect and slice the brain fresh, and discard it after looking for significant lesions, such as contusions, tears and haemorrhages. If the victim of the accident was the driver of a crashed vehicle, and shows no evidence of a blow on the head, but is found to have suffered a cerebral haemorrhage, it should be borne in mind that the haemorrhage may have caused the accident. If the patient has survived a few days or even hours in hospital, there is likely to be some clinical interest in the case. The surgeon concerned may wish to be present at the post mortem; and if his interest is still unsatisfied the brain should be fixed, uncut, for later dissection.

Types of traumatic lesions in the brain

Lesions which may come to light in slices of the fixed brain include *'ball' haemorrhages*, a centimetre or less in diameter, commonly in the white matter underlying the cerebral cortex (Fig. 5.4). These are attributable to uprooting of small penetrating vessels by superficial *shearing strains*. If the vessel is an arteriole, there may be an area of softening in the territory formerly supplied by the vessel. Somewhat larger areas of softening may be present in cases with extensive subarachnoid bleeding, with a few days' survival. These are attributable to *vasospasm* (see p.100).

Fat embolism

If there are focal softenings, or areas of brain swelling, and especially if chest lesions have been found, blocks should be taken from sensitive areas — hippocampus, thalamus and cerebellum — in order to look for evidence of generalized hypoxia. Scattered petechial haemorrhages in the central white matter, most conspicuous in the corpus callosum, are characteristic of *fat embolism* (Fig. 5.5). In such cases, frozen sections may show fat globules in small vessels in the cerebral cortex, though not in the affected white matter.

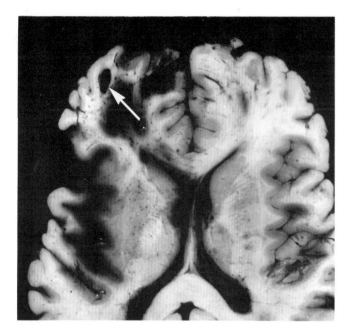

Fig. 5.4. 'Ball' haemorrhage (arrowed) associated with a contusion of the left frontal pole. There is subarachnoid blood in the left lateral fissure.

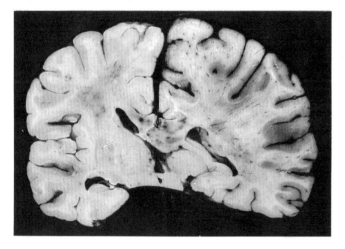

Fig. 5.5. Cerebral fat embolism in a man aged 21, 4 days after a severe chest injury. There was acute infarction, due to thrombosis, in the right internal carotid territory. The cerebral white matter shows numerous petechial haemorrhages, most prominently in the corpus callosum. (Courtesy of Dr Betty Brownell.)

This, along with the demonstration of similar globules in lung capillaries, is regarded as sufficient evidence of cerebral fat embolism.

Acceleration injuries and concussion

Other lesions, characteristic of cases in which the brain has undergone a sudden *acceleration* relative to the dura mater and skull, are large or small tears, with brown discoloration, on one side or other of the corpus callosum, and in a superior

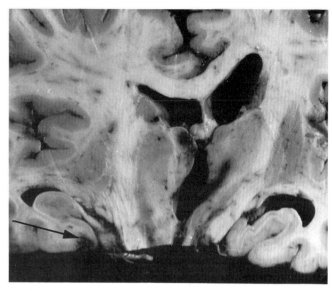

(a)

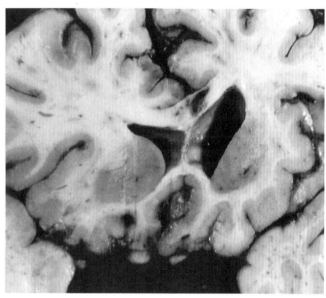

(b)

Fig. 5.6. Acceleration injuries. Haemorrhagic tears: (a), (b) and (c — *facing page*) in corpus callosum; (d — *facing page*) in superior cerebellar peduncles. Arrows show bruising from the edge of the tentorium.

cerebellar peduncle at the level of the upper pons (Fig. 5.6d). The former are attributable to a side-to-side swirling movement of the cerebral hemispheres, which has been checked by the falx cerebri, causing lateral tension in the corpus callosum. The latter are caused by a similar swirling movement, causing tension at the upper end of the brain stem. When such lesions are visible to the naked eye, sections from the area will reveal numerous other lesions, of microscopic dimensions, and without haemorrhage. These are readily demonstrable in paraffin sections from the presence

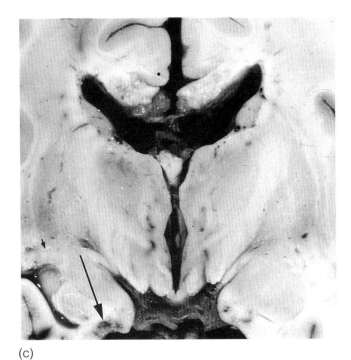

(c)

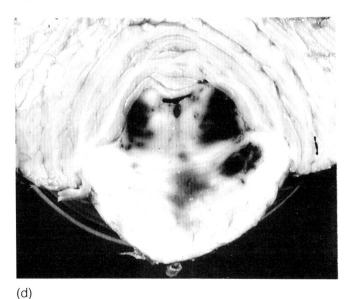

(d)

Fig. 5.6. (*continued*)

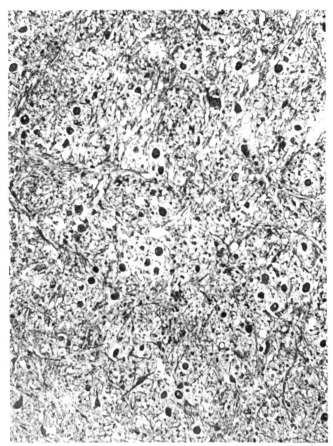

Fig. 5.7. 'Retraction balls'. Blobs of axoplasm, stained by the Palmgren method, in the midbrain of a man of 49 dying a few days after an acceleration injury. ×210.

of so-called *retraction bulbs*, i.e. blobs of axoplasm extruded from the ends of torn axons (Fig. 5.7). They are best seen in metallic axon stains, but are visible in ordinary cell stains such as H&E. In cases with 2 or more days' survival, frozen sections stained by the Weil–Davenport method will show numerous small clusters of active microglial cells (Fig. 5.8). These clusters are common, and may be found anywhere in the brain, in cases of acceleration injury. They have repeatedly been observed in cases of 'concussion', i.e. short-lived loss of consciousness following a blow on the head, without subsequent neurological deficits, in which death was due to causes outside the head. These lesions cannot of course be held responsible either for the concussion itself or for subsequent headaches. Concussion is a transient state, whereas torn axons remain torn. The headaches, if they occur, are more naturally attributed to the thin films of subdural and subarachnoid blood which are commonly seen on the surface of the brain after the mildest of head injuries. It is possible that multiple scattered lesions may account for some of the cerebral atrophy observed in the brains of professional boxers. These, however, often show lesions of a quite different type: a large cavity (cavum septi) separating the two leaves of the septum lucidum (cf. Fig. 16.10), and neurofibrillary tangles in nerve cells in the substantia nigra and medial temporal cortex.

Vigil coma

Some cases of severe head injury, having been nursed through the critical acute phase, may linger on for a matter of years in a state sometimes called 'vigil coma'. The

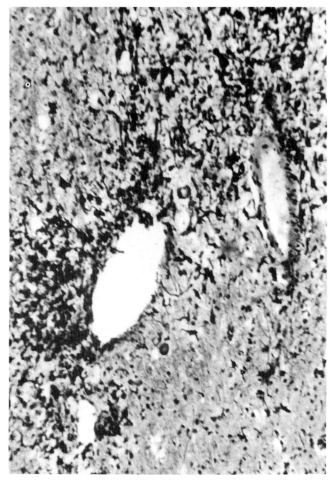

Fig. 5.8. Same case as in Fig. 5.7. Active microglia around vessels in the corpus callosum, stained by the Weil–Davenport method, ×210.

patients have alternate periods of sleep and wakefulness; during the latter they follow moving objects with their eyes, but do not speak, obey commands, or execute purposive movements. Strich (1956), in a series of such cases, demonstrated gross atrophy of the cerebral white matter, with degeneration of corticofugal pathways and of certain fibre tracts in the brain stem, but no major destructive lesion involving cortex, basal ganglia or hindbrain. She attributed these changes to widespread tears in the white matter, caused by accelerations within the skull. In other cases of protracted vigil coma following injury, there may be post mortem evidence of severe cerebral hypoxia at the time of injury, in the form of cell loss and fibrous gliosis in the hippocampus and other areas of cerebral cortex, thalamus, putamen, and cerebellum, where Purkinje cells have largely disappeared. Such cases may also show the shrivelled remains of old infarcts.

Other lesions

Other lesions attributable to acceleration include avulsion of olfactory bulbs (the lesion held responsible for post-traumatic anosmia), tearing of the pituitary stalk, tearing of cranial nerves (in particular the 3rd and 6th), and cortical contusions due to shearing stresses. Impact on the sharp edge of a dural fold may produce visible bruises in the cingulate gyrus, on the under-surface of the parahippocampal gyrus, and on the lateral surface of a cerebral peduncle. Cortical lesions are held responsible for most cases of *post-traumatic epilepsy*; but in a long-standing case of this condition it may be difficult to distinguish the original lesion from similar lesions acquired in the course of epileptic fits.

Brain stem haemorrhages

Haemorrhages in the upper brain stem due to acceleration need to be distinguished from those due to distortion in the course of a tentorial herniation. This may not always be easy if a hernia is in fact present. Points of distinction are that the former are generally quickly fatal, and are asymmetrical, being most severe on one side of the tectum, involving the superior cerebellar peduncle (Fig. 2.13), whereas haemorrhages due to herniation tend to be symmetrical, and most severe in the midline (Fig. 2.12). In either case, the medulla is very rarely involved.

Missile wounds

Immediately-fatal missile wounds are rarely of more than forensic interest. On the other hand, non-fatal missile wounds of the cerebral hemispheres, with several years' survival, can be of great interest to students of 'higher' brain functions — speech, for instance, or music — in cases with good neurological and psychological follow-up. The lesions are non-progressive, and usually uncomplicated by vascular disease; and the patients are not, as a rule, ill. When such a case presents itself in the post mortem room, the pathologist should show it due respect, i.e. should not cut it before fixation, or leave it sitting on a tray. After fixation, the brain should be carefully and systematically sliced, and the slices photographed. If the pathologist is not prepared to conduct a careful anatomical study himself, he should, ideally, get in touch with someone who is so prepared.

Spinal injuries

At first sight, the spinal cord appears to be very well protected from mechanical injuries. On the other hand, the structure providing this protection may itself participate in causing damage to the cord. This happens both as a result of 'natural' disease processes such as cervical spondylosis and rheumàtoid arthritis, and from trauma to the vertebral column causing a sudden narrowing of the spinal canal, with acute compression of the cord (Fig. 5.9). The circumstances under which this happens vary somewhat according to whether the injury is accidental or intentional.

Fracture-dislocation

The common accidents causing paraplegia and tetraplegia are falls (including dives into shallow water) and traffic accidents, resulting in *fracture-dislocation* between two adjacent vertebrae. The frequency of different types of intentional cord injury depends on local cultural differences. In some cultures, stab wounds in the back are common. In

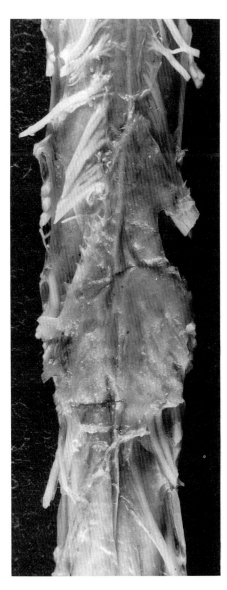

Fig. 5.9. Anterior aspect of the lower cervical and upper thoracic cord from a man of 29 who 10 years earlier had dived into shallow water and suffered a fracture dislocation, with a complete crush at cord level C6. There is a pad of scar tissue overlying the cord at this level.

some parts of southern Africa, we are told, the insertion of a spoke from a bicycle wheel into the spinal canal is practised. In Britain, after the practice of simple suspension by the neck was discontinued, judicial killings were for many years carried out by means of a sudden drop, arrested by a noose around the subject's neck. Textbooks of pathology are for some reason rather reticent about the mechanisms involved. According to one account, there is separation of upper cervical vertebrae, causing stretching and rupture of the cord and lower brain stem; according to another, there is a fracture-dislocation, in the course of which the odontoid peg is driven into the lower medulla. In either case, the effect will be an immediate tetraplegia. Loss of consciousness, and death, will presumably ensue after an interval, being due either to asphyxia from paralysis of respiratory movements or to interruption of blood supply to the brain, or both.

It is easy to miss a *neck injury* at post mortem. In any case of blunt head injury followed by death, the cervical spine should be manipulated; if it shows unnatural mobility, or local bruising, and if circumstances permit, the upper part of the vertebral column should be removed, replaced with a length of baton wood, X-rayed, and fixed entire for later dissection. In one common form of fracture-dislocation the displaced vertebra quickly returns to its normal position, and the X-ray may show very little unless the picture is taken with the vertebrae in their abnormal, twisted, relationship.

The usual mechanism of cord transection in a case of fracture-dislocation is a scissor-like action between the pedicle and lamina of one vertebra and the body of its neighbour. Sections taken from the point of maximum constriction of the cord, stained for axis cylinders, will show whether the transection was complete or partial. For a week or so following an injury, the silver stain will show retraction-bulbs at points where axons have been severed. With a long-standing lesion, the question can be answered by looking for degeneration in ascending and descending tracts in axon and myelin stains on sections taken a few centimetres above and below the lesion (Fig. 5.10).

Arterial lesions

In the dissection of the specimen, the foramina transversaria should be explored, and the *vertebral arteries* examined at all levels from the sixth to the first cervical vertebrae. If both vertebral arteries are torn or occluded, or if one is rudimentary, as is often the case, and the other is occluded, death may be attributable to ischaemia of the brain stem. A few years ago, an unusual case of fatal neck trauma was examined in Oxford. The patient, a previously healthy young man, presented with coma and respiratory failure. There was no bony injury, but the first two centimetres of one vertebral artery were thrombosed; and there were fresh

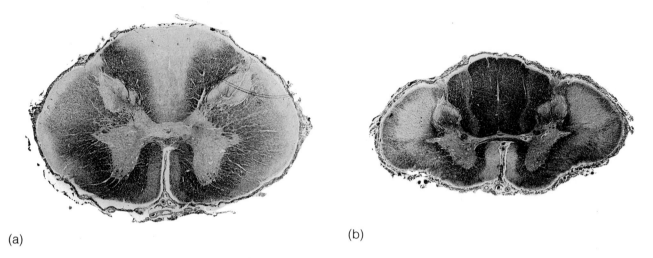

(a)　　　　　　　　　　　　　　　　　　(b)

Fig. 5.10. Same case as in Fig. 5.9. Myelin-stained sections of cord at upper cervical (a) and mid-thoracic (b) levels. In (a) there is wallerian degeneration of the gracile funiculi and spinocerebellar tracts, and marginal myelin pallor, attributable partly to degeneration of short ascending fibres. There is also some pallor of the crossed and uncrossed corticospinal tracts, probably attributable to retrograde degeneration. In (b) the crossed and uncrossed corticospinal tracts are wholly degenerate, and there is pallor in the anterolateral columns, presumably due to damage to other descending fibres.

infarcts, due to emboli, in the brain stem and cerebellum. On enquiry, it emerged that the young man had been practising yoga, spending hours at a time upside down, resting on the back of his head and neck.

A rare complication of non-penetrating injury to the soft tissues of the neck is damage to the intimal coat of a carotid artery. This may lead to thrombosis and later to occlusion and/or embolism. Post-traumatic hemiplegia calls for a careful examination of the opposite common and internal carotids at post mortem.

Further reading

Adams JH. 1984. Head injury. In Adams JH, Corsellis JAN, Duchen LW (Eds) *Greenfield's Neuropathology*, 4th edn. Edward Arnold, London, Chapter 3.

Courville CB. 1942. Coup–contrecoup mechanism of cranio-cerebral injuries: some observations. *Arch Surg* **45**, 19–43.

Crompton R. 1985. *Closed Head Injury: its Pathology and Legal Medicine*. Edward Arnold, London.

Strich SJ. 1956. Diffuse degeneration of the cerebral white matter in severe dementia following head injury. *J Neurol Neurosurg Psychiat* **19**, 163–185.

Chapter 6
Intracranial Haemorrhage

Questions facing the pathologist who finds a collection of blood within the cranial cavity include the following: What was the source of the blood? How had it spread? When did it occur? What caused the bleeding? Is there evidence of previous episodes of bleeding? Was the haemorrhage sufficient to cause death, whether directly or indirectly?

Epidural blood

Epidural blood — that is, blood lying between the skull and the dura mater — can be attributed with near certainty to trauma. The classical epidural haematoma arises from a branch of a middle meningeal artery which has been punctured by a splinter of bone, driven inwards by the impact of a blunt object such as the toe-cap of a boot. The bone most commonly involved is the thinnest part of the vault, namely the squamous temporal, which is traversed by the middle meningeal artery and its branches. The dura underlying the vault is less adherent than at the base, and can be stripped away from the bone by blood at systolic pressure. Puncture of a basal artery (for instance, of an internal carotid by a fracture of the sphenoid bone) will result in subdural, rather than epidural, bleeding; or, on occasion, in a carotico-cavernous fistula. This lesion must be looked for in cases with the clinical finding of pulsating exophthalmos.

Subdural blood

Subdural blood, lying between the dura and arachnoid membranes, may arise from various causes, mostly involving a tear at some point in the arachnoid. The commonest of these are traumatic tearing of bridging veins, ruptured aneurysms, and extensions from deeper sources, such as traumatic or spontaneous cerebral or cerebellar haemorrhages. The bridging veins transmit blood from the surface of the brain to the venous sinuses in the dura mater. This occurs at many points, above and below the tentorium; but whereas the brain stem and cerebellum are fairly tightly packed into the subtentorial space, and are thus not liable to undergo much displacement in the course of an acceleration injury, the bridging veins of the cerebral hemispheres are liable to damage from overstretching. Such tearing occurs when there is excessive deformation of the skull during birth (see Chapter 21); otherwise it is almost always a result of sudden acceleration of the head.

The subdural compartment, like the pleural cavities, is normally a *potential* space, with free, lubricated gliding between the apposed surfaces. How much gliding occurs when the head is given an accelerating blow has been vividly demonstrated, through a transparent 'skull', in experimental animals. The greatest movements of the brain relative to the dura and skull take place at the vertex, where large bridging veins leave the arachnoid to run into the superior longitudinal sinus. These will tolerate anteroposterior displacements of small extent — that is, of a centimetre or so; with larger displacements they are liable to be torn, releasing blood into the subdural and subarachnoid compartments.

Chronic subdural haematoma

Occasionally, a subdural haematoma of venous origin may quickly become big enough to cause a fatal cerebral compression. More commonly, the bleeding ceases, and the clot is gradually resorbed, leaving a delicate membrane stained with blood pigments. Such residua are commonly observed months or years after brain surgery. An alternative outcome

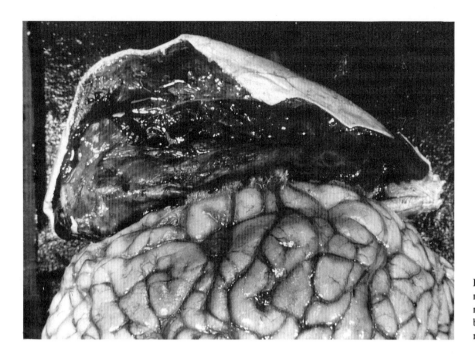

Fig. 6.1. Chronic subdural haematoma, in a man of 70. One year earlier he had suffered a minor blow to the head. The source of bleeding appeared to be a torn bridging vein running into the superior sagittal sinus.

is the formation of a chronic subdural haematoma (Figs 6.1 and 11.1). This consists of a mass of altered blood, part solid and part fluid, enclosed in a fibrous membrane, which is formed from connective tissue elements in both dura and arachnoid. The membrane is thicker on its inner aspect, and is adherent to the arachnoid in one or more places. Histological examination of the membrane usually reveals a laminated structure, with alternate layers of connective tissue and blood residues, indicating that the bleeding has been episodic (Plate 2.6). In places the tissue is highly vascular, and contains many thin-walled sinusoid vessels which are probably the source of the repeated haemorrhages. Chronic subdural haematomas are typically found either in young children suffering from some form of brain damage, or in old people with more or less atrophic brains, as in Fig. 11.1. Why this should be so is not altogether clear. It may be that resorption of the original haematoma is hindered if the brain tends to shrink away from its membranes.

Subarachnoid blood

This is readily distinguished from subdural blood by the fact that it cannot be simply wiped off the surface of the brain. When the arachnoid is torn, as commonly happens in cases of head injury, or when an aneurysm ruptures outwards, subdural and subarachnoid blood are found together. The commonest sources of subarachnoid blood are traumatic contusions, ruptured aneurysms, and haemorrhages into the brain substance, either above or below the tentorium. The latter may reach the subarachnoid space either by direct eruption at the surface of the brain or by irruption at some point into the ventricular system, reaching the sub-

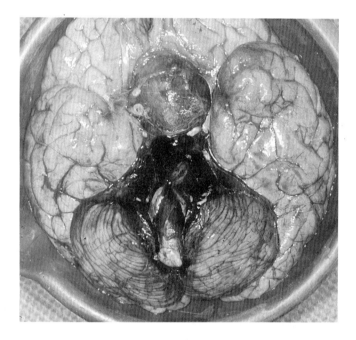

Fig. 6.2. Blood in the basal cisterns. A large aneurysm, seen in the upper part of the picture, had ruptured into the anterior horn of a lateral ventricle, and the whole ventricular system had filled with blood. The blood at the base had escaped from the fourth ventricle via the foramina of Luschka. (Courtesy of Dr Betty Brownell.)

arachnoid space by way of the fourth ventricle and the foramina of Luschka and Magendie, where blood may be seen emerging (Fig. 6.2) even before the brain is dissected.

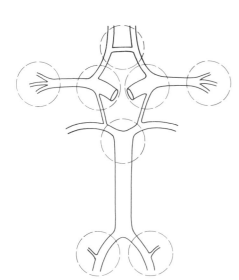

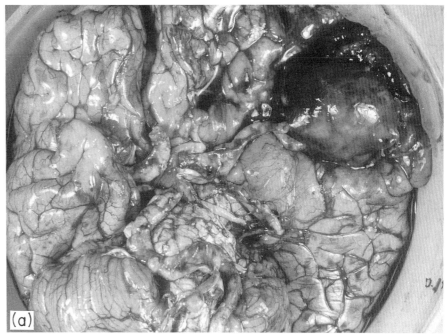

Fig. 6.3. Diagram of the basal arteries, including the circle of Willis. The commonest sites for aneurysm formation are ringed. Of these the commonest are the neighbourhood of the anterior communicating artery (top of diagram) and the middle cerebral arteries.

Fig. 6.4. Giant aneurysm of left middle cerebral artery, Man, aged 58. (a — *above*) Base of brain. (b — *below*) Aneurysm cut open. The mass consists almost entirely of organized thrombus, with very little liquid blood. The basal arteries, including the one carrying the aneurysm, are irregularly dilated and calcified.

Aneurysms

When the suspected source of subarachnoid blood is a ruptured aneurysm, it is advisable to look for the aneurysm before the brain is fixed. Formalin transforms a clot, with the consistency of red-currant jelly, which can be easily cleared away by superficial dissection in the post mortem room, to a hard, crumbly mass, which disrupts the brain tissue when it is sliced, and may make it very difficult to distinguish a thin-walled aneurysm from its surroundings. To start with, the likeliest situation of the aneurysm may be guessed at, after observing where the blood is most abundant. After cutting through the arachnoid at this point, the clot may be cleared away piecemeal by blunt dissection until the aneurysm, and its point of rupture, have been identified. Even when angiography has already demonstrated an aneurysm, it is best to identify the source of bleeding in this way. Aneurysms are often multiple, and the offending lesion is not necessarily the one most obvious in the angiogram. In any case, it is worth locating the actual point of rupture, if only for the interest of the clinicians concerned with the case. Figure 6.3 gives an indication of the most usual sites for the formation of aneurysms. In general, they form at points of bifurcation of cerebral arteries. There is as yet no general agreement as to their causes. Some examples are shown in Figs 6.4–6.7.

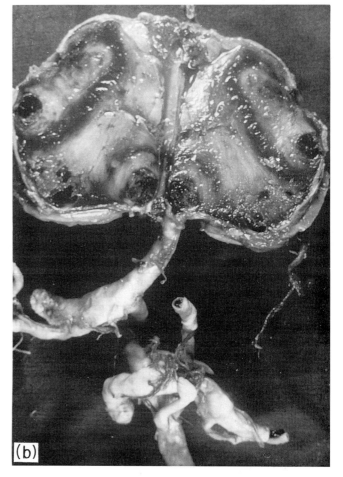

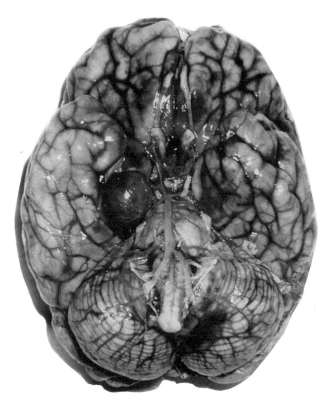

Fig. 6.5. Aneurysm of the posterior cerebral artery in a 15-year-old (an unusual finding at this age).

Apart from subarachnoid haemorrhage, ruptured aneurysms are a major cause of *intracerebral bleeding*. When the point of rupture faces the surface of the brain, blood at arterial pressure is pumped directly into brain tissue. This is particularly likely to happen when the aneurysm is embraced on two sides by cerebral cortex, as is the case with aneurysms of the anterior communicating and middle cerebral arteries. In the former, blood may even irrupt into the anterior horn of a lateral ventricle; in the latter, into the inferior horn. Reports on long series of cases of fatal intracerebral haemorrhage have indicated that in about a fifth of the cases the cause of the haemorrhage was a ruptured aneurysm (Greenhall 1977).

Complications

Subarachnoid bleeding, whatever its source, may give rise to two complications, both of clinical significance: *ventricular dilatation* and *arterial spasm*. The former has been ascribed to impaired absorption of CSF in the arachnoid granulations, leading to back-pressure and raised intracranial tension (see Fig. 8.1). It is usually transient in non-fatal cases. The latter is a well-recognized feature in angiograms following subarachnoid haemorrhage. It can be severe and prolonged enough to cause areas — often multiple, often small — of cerebral infarction. These are commonly, but not exclusively, areas supplied by branches of the main artery bearing the ruptured aneurysm. Various histological changes may be seen in vessels which have undergone spasm. The most conspicuous of these changes, in cases with survival of a month or more, is a reduction of the lumen, due to proliferation of the tunica intima (Fig. 6.8). In the histological examination of fatal cases it is worth looking for areas of infarction, and for evidence of earlier bleeds, in the form of haemosiderin deposits in the meninges. In cases of ruptured aneurysm, histological sections of the aneurysm itself will show the transition from the wall of the artery, which possesses an elastic lamina, and that of the aneurysm, which does not.

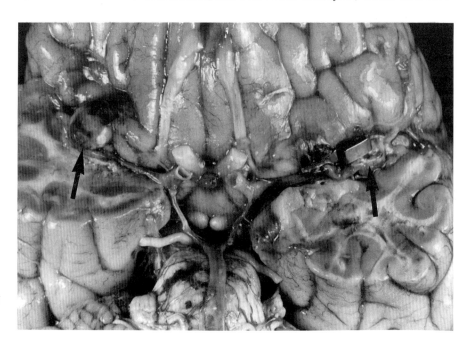

Fig. 6.6. Bilateral middle cerebral artery aneurysms (arrowed) in a 49-year-old man. A clip had been applied to the one on the right of the picture. The temporal poles have been cut away.

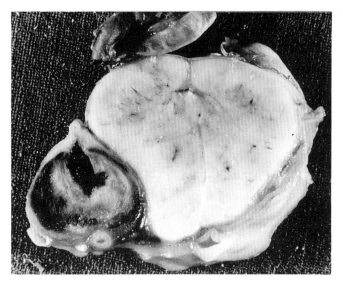

Fig. 6.7. Transverse section of vertebral artery aneurysm indenting the lower medulla. Male, aged 57.

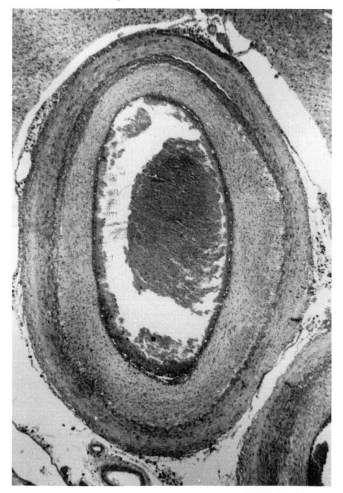

Fig. 6.8. Intimal thickening in a pericallosal artery, three months after a subarachnoid haemorrhage. Angiograms at that time showed severe and widespread arterial spasm. Note that the other coats of the artery are perfectly healthy. There is no surrounding haemorrhage or exudate. H&E, ×35.

Intracerebral bleeding

When the source of bleeding lies inside the brain, it is often wise, before fixation, to extract as much of the clot as can conveniently be dislodged without disrupting the brain. This makes it easier to slice the brain after fixation. If the size of the clot is of interest, it can be weighed on its own. (Of course, if the only purpose of the post mortem is to satisfy a coroner as to the cause of death, it is an economy to slice the brain on the spot). After slicing, the following should be looked for: vascular malformations, tumours, aneurysms lurking in secluded places, and traces of earlier haemorrhages. Abnormally dilated veins should be looked for, as these may be the only evidence of an *arteriovenous malformation* which has destroyed itself in an explosive rupture. Most vascular malformations, however, are immediately recognizable from their strange tangles of vessels surrounded by haemosiderin deposits (Figs 16.15 and 16.16), and often from their gritty resistance to the knife. The different types of malformation — telangiectases, cavernous angiomas, arteriovenous fistulae and the rest — are well described by Russell & Rubinstein (1977). Venous angiomas are not uncommonly the origin of 'spontaneous' haemorrhage in the region of the cerebellar vermis.

In what follows we discuss intracerebral haemorrhage in adult brains. Those occurring around the time of birth are discussed in Chapter 21.

'Spontaneous' cerebral haemorrhage

The commonest site of 'spontaneous' intracerebral haemorrhage is the *lentiform nucleus* (Fig. 6.9). A relevant factor here may be the normal disposition of the branches of the lateral striate (lenticulostriate) group of arteries (Fig. 6.10). These, after reaching and supplying the putamen, make a right-angled turn inward and upward to supply the caudate nucleus. It has been suggested that the intravascular stresses at the bend may result in (i) the formation of microaneurysms (the so-called Charcot–Bouchard aneurysms) and (ii) actual rupture of the vessel. There is as yet no generally accepted view on the frequency and distribution of micro-aneurysms, and on the causal connections between micro-aneurysms, spontaneous bleeding and arterial hypertension. The subject is discussed, with admirable restraint, by McCormick & Schochet (1976).

In the brains of patients who have in the past made a good recovery from a hemiplegic stroke, it is not unusual to see a well-defined cavity, containing tarry fluid, in one putamen (Fig. 7.1). In such cases it is reasonable to suppose that the patient's hemiplegia was caused by oedema surrounding the haematoma and involving the posterior limb of the internal capsule, and that recovery was related to the subsidence of the oedema.

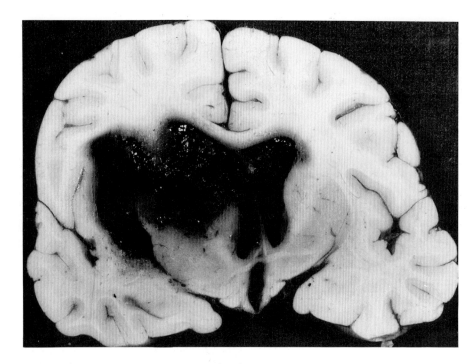

Fig. 6.9. Acute haemorrhage into the lentiform nucleus, erupting into the ventricular system, in a 60-year-old woman.

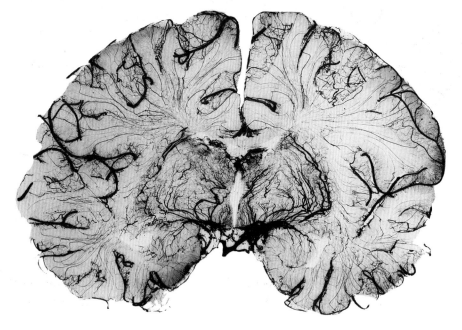

Fig. 6.10. X-ray photograph of a centimetre-thick coronal slice at level A1, following post mortem injection of a radio-opaque fluid into the aorta. Note in particular the nearly right-angled upward bend of the lateral striate group of arteries as they pass through the putamen on their way to the caudate nucleus. (Preparation by Dr Michael Dunnill.)

Thalamus, brain stem, cerebellum

Apart from the lentiform nucleus, the commoner sites of spontaneous haemorrhage include the *thalamus* (Fig. 6.11), the vermis of the *cerebellum* (Fig. 6.12), and the *pons* (Fig. 2.14). Haemorrhages within the spinal canal are rare; the relatively common arteriovenous fistulae, or 'angiomas' of the cord, usually present with infarction and paraplegia rather than with subarachnoid or intramedullary haemorrhage (see p.31). Haemorrhages in the pons may originate

in at least three ways, which may be rather difficult to distinguish. Firstly, there are 'spontaneous' haemorrhages, generally fatal, sometimes producing a dramatic onset of hyperthermia. Some of these may arise from vascular anomalies, which are destroyed in the course of the haemorrhage. Secondly, they may be the direct result of trauma. A characteristic traumatic lesion is a tear, with consequent haemorrhage, in one or other superior cerebellar peduncle (Fig. 2.13). The third, and almost certainly the commonest, cause of bleeding in the pons is distortion of the upper brain

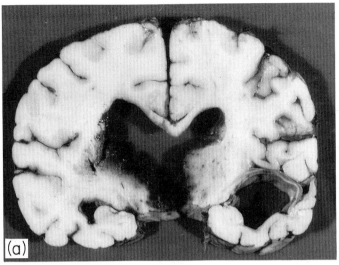
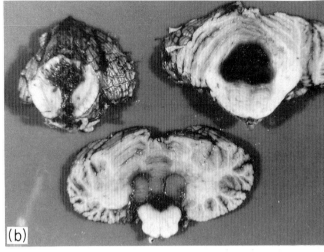

Fig. 6.11. Repeated cerebral haemorrhages in a hypertensive woman, dying aged 61. (a) 6½-year-old encapsulated haematoma in right temporal lobe and fresh haemorrhage in left thalamus erupting into lateral and third ventricles; (b) extension of this into the tegmentum and fourth ventricle.

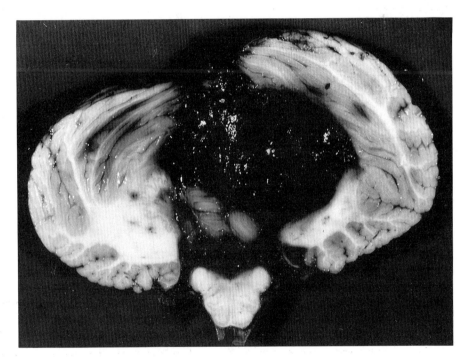

Fig. 6.12. Cerebellar haemorrhage in a woman aged 64, under treatment with an anti-coagulant for deep leg vein thrombosis.

stem, with rupture of its intrinsic vessels, in the course of transtentorial herniation (Fig. 2.12). In a case of head injury the second and third causes may be combined.

Phlebothrombosis

Among the more dramatic types of cerebral haemorrhage are those due to *thrombosis of major collecting veins* or dural venous sinuses (Fig. 6.13). The patterns of bleeding are characteristic of the vessels involved; for instance, thrombosis of an internal cerebral vein causes bleeding in the thalamus and basal ganglia on the same side, while if the great vein of Galen is affected, these lesions are bilateral. At the vertex, thrombosis of a major bridging vein causes haemorrhage in the parasagittal cortex and white matter, and with thrombosis of the superior sagittal sinus the lesions are bilateral. When such thromboses occur, there is almost always an underlying systemic disorder, or a nutritional defect. They are particularly associated with marasmus in children.

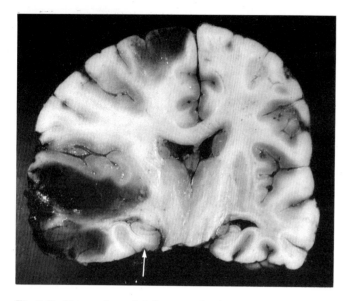

Fig. 6.13. Haemorrhages in left temporal and superior frontal areas, due to cortical venous thrombosis, in a woman aged 40. Note the intense swelling of the left hemisphere, causing a shift to the right and tentorial herniation. There is an indentation of the left parahippocampal gyrus from pressure on the edge of the tentorium (arrowed).

Blood disorders

Massive or *multiple intracerebral haemorrhages* may be found in a variety of blood disorders, including *haemophilia*. They occur in various types of *leukaemia*, especially the more acute forms. *Thrombocytopenia*, however caused, predisposes to haemorrhage. In addition, cerebral haemorrhage is a well-recognized hazard of the therapeutic use of *anticoagulants*.

Vascular diseases

Diseases of blood vessels giving rise to brain haemorrhages include various types of cerebral *amyloid (congophilic) angiopathy* (for details, see Tomlinson & Corsellis 1984). In one of these, a rare familial form first reported from Iceland, fatal apoplectic strokes occur in previously healthy middle-aged subjects. In another familial form, severe changes in cerebral arteries, giving rise to infarcts and/or haemorrhages throughout the central nervous system, are coupled with peculiar 'plaque' formations resembling, but not identical with, the 'plaques' associated with either Alzheimer's disease or the Gerstmann–Sträussler syndrome (pp.270–73 and p.276). A sporadic form of cerebral amyloid angiopathy unassociated with systemic amyloidosis is said to account for up to 20% of 'strokes' due to cerebral haemorrhage in elderly subjects (Fig. 6.14). As in Alzheimer's disease, the affected vessels are situated in the cerebral cortex and overlying leptomeninges. Other features of Alzheimer's disease may be present in these cases, but in most of them dementia is not mentioned in the clinical notes. It is probable that if Congo Red staining were carried out routinely in cases of fatal cerebral haemorrhage, many more cases of these conditions would be found.

Causes of minor haemorrhages

Minor haemorrhages, not giving rise to massive clots, arise from a wide variety of causes, of which the commonest is probably a minor head injury. After a fatal traffic accident, without serious impact on the head, it is common to find flecks of fresh blood on both surfaces of the arachnoid. These are presumably due to tearing of capillary and other small vessels by shearing stresses between the brain and the

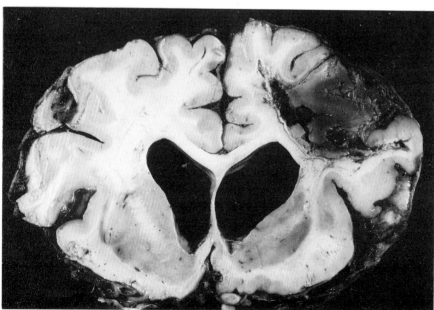

Fig. 6.14. Four-month-old haematoma, partly encapsulated, in the right frontal lobe of a demented woman aged 81 with cerebral congophilic angiopathy. There is severe cerebral atrophy, with dilated ventricles.

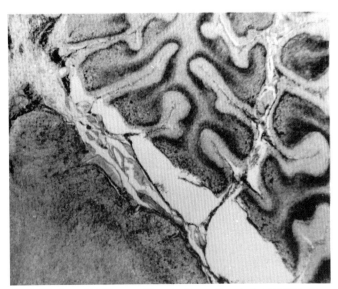

Fig. 6.15. Superficial haemosiderosis. Case of hemispherectomy, at aged 8 years, for infantile hemiplegia with intractable epilepsy. Good result for 3 years, followed by deterioration and death at age 15, due to persistent intracranial bleeding. Note the erosion of the exposed surface of the cerebellum. Nissl, ×40.

dura. (Incidentally, they may be contributory causes of post-concussion headaches.) Similar shearing stresses, affecting rather larger penetrating vessels, may give rise to 'ball' haemorrhages in or just below the cerebral cortex (Fig. 5.4).

Diffuse *petechial haemorrhages*, or brain purpura, may likewise be due to a variety of conditions, which include thrombocytopenia, fat embolism (Fig. 5.5) and acute encephalitis (Fig. 10.37). With these, the danger to life comes from swelling of the affected brain tissue, which may give rise to fatal herniation. Finally, brain tumours of many kinds may bleed. The typical mottled or speckled appearance of the cut surface of a malignant glioma is largely due to small haemorrhages within the tumour.

Superficial haemosiderosis

A common effect of repeated, or dribbling, releases of blood into a ventricle or into the subarachnoid space is a diffuse yellow−brown staining of the exposed ependymal and pial surfaces of the brain and spinal cord (Plate 2.5). This state of superficial haemosiderosis (sometimes mislabelled haemochromatosis) is for the most part well tolerated by the affected nervous tissue. The exception is the cerebellar cortex, which in its exposed parts shows erosion of the molecular layer and loss of Purkinje cells (Fig. 6.15).

Dating of lesions

When the diagnosis in a case of intracranial haemorrhage is obvious to the naked eye, histological examination of the affected tissue may be no more than a ritual gesture. In cases which have survived a fatal haemorrhage by a day or more, or in which there is evidence of repeated haemorrhages, it may be desirable to make an estimate of the age of a lesion. This can be done, approximately at least, by looking for inflammatory tissue reactions and the breakdown products of blood in paraffin sections stained with H&E or Perls' stain for iron, and for microglial and astrocytic reactions in frozen sections with silver impregnations and fat stains.

Further reading

Greenhall RCD. 1977. *Pathological findings in acute cerebrovascular disease and their clinical implications*. D.M. thesis, University of Oxford.

McCormick WF, Schochet SS. 1976. *Atlas of Cerebrovascular Disease*. WB Saunders, Philadelphia.

Russell DS, Rubinstein LJ. 1977. *Pathology of Tumours of the Nervous System*. 4th edn. Edward Arnold, London.

Tomlinson, BE, Corsellis, JAN. 1984. Ageing and the dementias. In Adams JH, Corsellis JAN, Duchen LW (Eds) *Greenfield's Neuropathology*. 4th edn. Edward Arnold, London, Chapter 20.

Chapter 7
Infarction, Hypoxia, Cerebral Vascular Disease

Definitions

Infarction, as the word is applied to the CNS, is an imprecise term. This is because of differences in vulnerability between different cellular elements of the CNS to oxygen deprivation. For example, a hypoxic episode lasting long enough to kill off the Purkinje cells of the cerebellum may leave the neighbouring granule cells intact. An episode which kills all the nerve cells may leave the neuroglia (astrocytes and oligodendrocytes) alive; and when nerve cells and neuroglia are fatally damaged, microglial phagocytes and vascular endothelium survive. In common usage, the terms 'infarct' and 'softening' are generally interchangeable, and denote the state when mesodermal cells — microglia (which later become lipid phagocytes), fibroblasts and endothelial cells — are the sole survivors. Some causes of softening other than infarction are shown in Table 7.1.

Occasionally one finds a recent lesion in which all degrees of hypoxic damage are represented. In the centre is a patch of coagulative necrosis, from which the blood supply has been totally and permanently cut off. There are no living cells, but one can discern the ghostly outlines of dead nerve cells, and of myelin sheaths, which still take up a small amount of myelin stain. Outside this is a zone of softening, consisting purely of lipid phagocytes and small blood vessels. Beyond this is a zone containing swollen-bodied fibre-forming astrocytes, as well as microglial phagocytes mopping up the debris of axoplasm and myelin arising from wallerian degeneration of nerve fibres. The same elements are present in the outer zone, with the addition of a few surviving nerve cells. The signs of wallerian degeneration may stretch far beyond this point.

Sequelae of infarction

The after-effects of cerebral infarction differ according to the age of the patient. In adults the infarcted area at first swells and softens. From then on the central region of total necrosis begins to shrink, as it is invaded at its edges by new capillaries and phagocytes, which gradually remove the debris. The final state is a soft sponge-like substance, traversed by strands of glial and collagenous fibres. Outside this the tissue also shrinks, largely as a result of wallerian degeneration of interrupted axons. Myelin debris is phagocytosed, and there is a moderate astrocytic reaction. Infarcted cerebral cortex is reduced to a thickness of 2–3 mm, of which the outer millimetre consists of a relatively tough membrane, supplied by capillaries, and strengthened by fibroblasts derived from the pia mater.

In infants, including those who have suffered brain damage at birth, the pattern is different. Owing, no doubt, to pressure from the growth of the rest of the brain, the infarcted tissue is not converted into a spongy mass, but is condensed into a solid glial scar of almost woody hardness. Where cerebral cortex is involved, there is a tendency to spare the crowns of the gyri, which continue to grow, with more or less normal myelination and maturation of nerve cells. If the brain is examined at operation or post mortem some years later, the convolutions may look fairly normal from the outside; but, on section, the gyri appear as mushroom-like excrescences on the surfaces of a gliotic mass, from which the cortex in the depths of the sulci has been removed (Fig. 16.14). This condition, referred to as *ulegyria*, is characteristic of the tissue removed in cases of infantile hemiplegia with intractable epilepsy (see pp.261 and 325).

Table 7.1. Patterns of softening in the CNS

Site	Common causes
Putamen, insula, lips of lateral fissure (as in Fig. 7.16)	Occlusion of MCA, with patent anastomotic channels from ACA and PCA
Entire MCA territory (as in Fig. 7.1)	Occlusion of ICA or MCA, with inadequate anastomotic channels
Inferior temporal and calcarine cortex (as in Figs 7.18 and 7.20)	Atheroma, occludng PCA branches
	Pinching of PCA branches in course of transtentorial herniation (p.9)
Laminar, of cerebral cortex (as in Figs 7.4 and 7.5)	Hypoxaemia Hypoglycaemia (p.303)
Arterial border zones (as in Fig. 7.19)	Heart failure: prolonged arterial hypotension
Temporal lobe, insula and cingulate gyrus (as in Fig. 10.1)	Herpes simplex encephalitis (p.144)
Globus pallidus, bilateral (as in Fig. 20.1)	Carbon monoxide poisoning (p.310)
Patches in cerebral hemispheres as in:	
Fig. 7.10	Embolism from heart or atheromatous plaque in ICA
Fig. 7.3	Vasospasm following subarachnoid haemorrhage
Figs 7.21 and 7.22	Small-vessel disease
Fig. 19.19	Ammonaemic encephalopathy
Fig. 11.6	Acute MS
Fig. 9.3	Heubner's arteritis
Mamillary bodies	Wernicke's encephalopathy (p.316)
Multiple, pinhead-sized, mainly subcortical (as in Fig. 10.26)	Progressive multifocal encephalopathy (p.150)
Centre of pons (as in Fig. 19.26)	Central pontine myelinolysis (p.305)
Symmetrical patches in brain stem (as in Fig. 19.6)	Leigh's encephalopathy (p.294)
Dorsolateral area of lower medulla (as in Fig. 7.11)	Occlusion of VA or PICA
Spinal cord (total transverse or anterior two-thirds)	Occlusion of radicular artery by trauma or aortic atheroma Ant. spinal artery thrombosis Oedema (e.g. in acute MS)
Spinal cord, scattered foci	Nitrogen embolism (p.118)
Posterior and lateral columns (as in Fig. 20.12)	Subacute combined degeneration (p.318)
Anterior grey horns (as in Fig. 10.18)	Poliomyelitis (p.147)

ACA anterior cerebral artery; MCA middle cerebral artery; PCA posterior cerebral artery; ICA internal carotid artery; PICA post inferior cerebellar artery; VA vertebral artery.

'Pathoclisis'

Selective vulnerability of different types of nerve cell (sometimes dignified with the term 'pathoclisis') is an undisputed fact. In some cases, the difference may depend on the metabolic habits of the cells concerned; in others, on their state of activity at the critical moment. This suggests itself when one sees 'hypoxic' cells randomly mixed with normal-looking cells of the same type, as in Plate 1.3. There are also regional differences, which may be due to differences in the local blood supply. For instance, cortex in the depth of a cerebral sulcus is often more vulnerable than at the crowns of neighbouring gyri, as in Fig. 7.3; and at the edge of an infarct the lesion tends to extend further into layers 2 and 3 than into layers 1 and 4. In some cases of generalized cerebral hypoxia (or hypoglycaemia; see Fig. 7.5) one finds widespread *laminar necrosis* of the cerebral cortex, most marked in layers 2 and 3 (Fig. 7.4). The greater vulnerability of sector H1 (the Sommer sector; see Figs 2.31 and 7.6) of the hippocampus can perhaps be explained on the basis of its vascular supply; but other possibilities have been suggested, and the question remains unanswered.

'Stroke'

In cases of 'stroke' due to cerebral infarction (see Figs 7.1–7.6) the immediate danger to life comes, not from the loss of vital centres in the brain, but from *swelling* of the infarcted tissue, attributable to sudden breakdown of the blood–brain barrier (Fig. 7.1). Death in the acute phase of a stroke, either ischaemic or haemorrhagic, is nearly always due to tentorial herniation, with compression and distortion of the upper brain stem (see p.9). The infarcted tissue is either pale, as in Fig. 7.1, or more or less haemorrhagic, as in Fig. 7.2. The reason for this difference is not always clear; but in some cases haemorrhage may ensue when arterial pressure is re-applied to softened tissue — for example, when an embolus impacted in an artery is lysed or broken up.

The 'respirator brain'

Advances in techniques of intensive care have resulted in a new pathological entity — the so-called 'respirator brain'. After 20 minutes or so of cardiac arrest, the whole brain is dead; but the heart can be restarted, and artificial respiration will keep the rest of the body alive. When the brain comes to be examined, it is discoloured, dark and rather soft. Histologically, it shows universal coagulative necrosis, with recognizable anatomical features, but no living cells. Today, as the clinical diagnosis of brain death is made with more confidence, the respirator brain is less frequently seen.

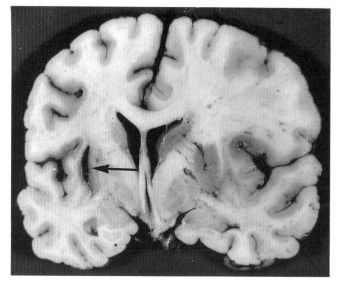

Fig. 7.1. Two-day-old infarction, due to embolism, in the territory of the right middle cerebral artery in a hypertensive women aged 61. The tears in the right corpus striatum are artefacts, probably caused during removal of the brain, due to softening of the territory of the lateral striate artery territory, while the medial striate territory, supplied by the anterior cerebral artery, remains firm. The infarcted tissue is pale and swollen, with a midline shift to the left, diencephalic downthrust (cf. Fig. 2.8), grooving of the right parahippocampal gyrus and subfalcine herniation of the right cingulate gyrus. In addition there is an old, slit-like haemorrhagic cavity in the left putamen (arrowed).

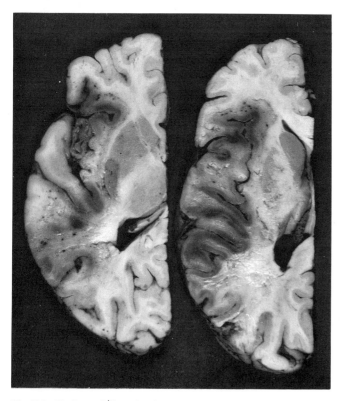

Fig. 7.2. Horizontal slices showing haemorrhagic infarction of the territory of an occluded left middle cerebral artery in an 84-year-old hypertensive woman. Right hemiplegia 4 weeks before death.

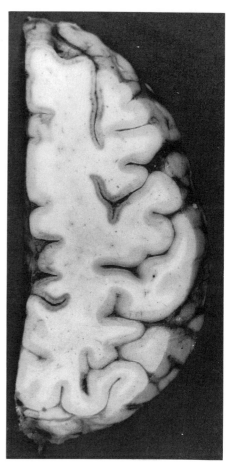

Fig. 7.3. Acute infarction in the territory of the right anterior cerebral artery, affecting the depths of sulci more than the crowns of the gyri. Man aged 47, with severe vasospasm following rupture of an aneurysm of the anterior communicating artery.

Causes of hypoxia

A great many factors, several of which may act in conjunction or additively, may be operative in producing local or generalized hypoxia in the brain.

Affecting oxygenation of blood

1 Lack of oxygen in inhaled air (e.g. self-asphyxiation by a child playing with a plastic bag).
2 Paralysis of, or mechanical interference with, breathing movements (e.g. motor neuron disease, pulmonary collapse).
3 Impaired gas exchange (e.g. in pneumonia, pulmonary oedema, emphysema).
4 Blocked airway (e.g. tumour, inhaled foreign body, oedema of glottis).

Affecting oxygen-carrying power of blood

1 Anaemia, chronic or acute, from blood loss.
2 Carbon monoxide poisoning.

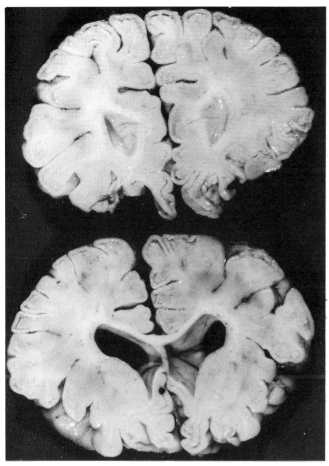

Fig. 7.4. Widespread laminar necrosis of cerebral cortex in a man aged 63, who suffered a postoperative cardiac arrest. Resuscitated, but remained in deep coma, on artificial ventilation, for 6 weeks.

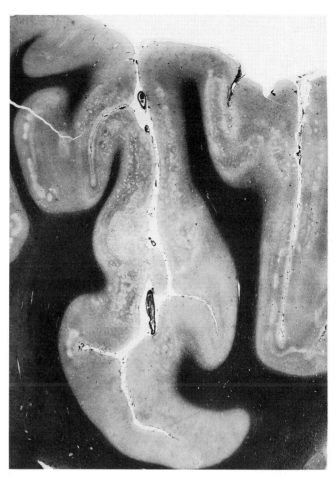

Fig. 7.5. Cortical necrosis, most severe in the depths of sulci, 3 days after an overdose of insulin.

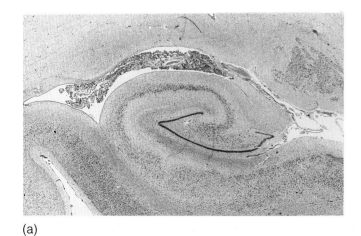

(a)

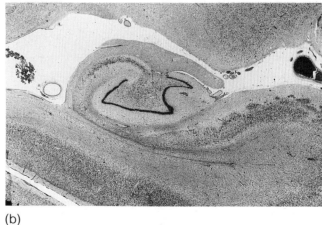

(b)

Fig. 7.6. Photographs of left hippocampus, in coronal section, at level P2; Nissl, ×5. (a) Normal. (b) Severe cell loss and shrinkage in the Sommer sector (H1; see Fig. 2.31), following repeated cardiac arrests, in a man aged 50.

Affecting circulation of blood to head

1 Arterial hypotension (e.g. in shock or heart failure).
2 Partial or total occlusion of arterial lumina (e.g. coarctation of common carotid, atherosclerosis and other arteriopathies, thrombosis, embolism).
3 Vasospasm (especially after subarachnoid haemorrhage).
4 Venous occlusion, with back-pressure.

Affecting oxygen uptake by CNS tissues

1 Increased demand for oxygen ('consumptive hypoxia'). It is believed by some that this is a major cause of cell loss in the hippocampus and cerebellar cortex following protracted epileptic fits.
2 Hypoglycaemia (e.g. insulin overdose, islet-cell tumour).
3 Toxic or metabolic disorders (e.g. hyperammonaemia, avitaminosis (vit B_1)).

Although any of these factors may affect the severity and distribution of a cerebral infarct, the major causes of infarction are those causing blockage of arterial lumina — namely atheroma, thrombosis and embolism, and combinations of these. All three are included, along with spontaneous or hypertensive haemorrhage, under the commonly used heading of 'cerebrovascular disease'.

Infarction due to atheroma

The commonest and most easily identified site at which the arterial supply of the brain is compromised is the bulbous lower end of the internal carotid artery. Atheroma is rarely seen in the common carotid, which runs straight from its origin upwards. At its bifurcation, the blood flow becomes turbulent; and atheromatous narrowing of the origins of the internal and external carotids is exceedingly common in

later life (Fig. 7.7). From time to time one is astonished to find that both internal carotids are more or less occluded, although the cerebral hemispheres show no significant softenings. In such cases it is supposed that the cutting-off of the cerebral arterial supply has been gradual, allowing time for expansion of alternative routes, including the vertebral/basilar system, and certain anastomotic pathways from the external carotids. Part of the explanation may lie in the observation that there is a rough inverse relationship between the degree of atheromatous narrowing of the internal carotids and the severity of atheroma of the anterior part of the circle of Willis. This suggests that high arterial pressure is conducive to atheroma, and that narrowing of the internal carotids in the neck protects the cerebral arteries.

The process of compensating for narrowing of this or that artery may take place from a very early age. Gross, presumably congenital, inequalities of size between the two internal carotids, and even more commonly between the two vertebral arteries, are not unusual in young subjects, and are matched by compensatory asymmetries in the circle of Willis, which in any case has a very variable pattern.

Sites of atheroma

Selection of sites for the development of atheroma in arteries supplying the brain may depend on factors other than turbulence and blood pressure. Atheroma is rarely seen in those parts of the internal carotid and vertebral arteries which are encased in bony canals. This suggests that atheroma may be encouraged by the artery's freedom to wriggle with each pulse wave.

Atheroma of the arteries at the base of the brain is very common in elderly subjects — at least, in over-fed populations. Any vessel may be affected; but severe narrowings, which can be held responsible for infarcts, are most commonly seen around the bifurcation of an internal carotid, in

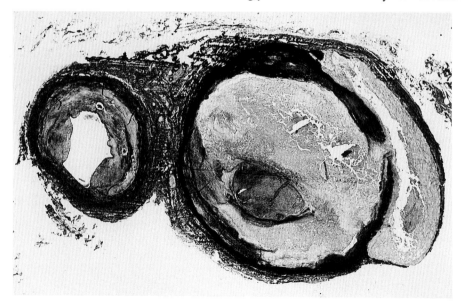

Fig. 7.7. Transverse section through the left internal and external carotid arteries close to their origin, from a man aged 60 with a recent right-sided hemiplegic stroke. The internal carotid (right side of picture) is totally occluded by atheroma and thrombus — the external carotid partially so.

the more proximal parts of the middle and posterior cerebral arteries, and in the basilar and vertebral arteries (Fig. 7.8). Histological changes in these vessels are much the same as those seen in small- and medium-sized arteries elsewhere in the body (Fig. 7.12). Less commonly, arteries of the vertebral/basilar system are not narrowed but elongated, tortuous, expanded, and irregularly calcified (Fig. 7.9). These changes are reminiscent of the disease of the abdominal aorta that commonly gives rise to aortic aneuryms. It is by no means clear whether these two forms of atherosclerosis belong to the same spectrum of disease.

'Cerebral thrombosis'

In clinical parlance, the term 'cerebral thrombosis' is used freely in cases of non-haemorrhagic infarction of parts of the brain, whether the cause of the infarct is thrombosis, atheroma or embolism, or a combination of these. In practice, it is often not possible to be sure of the cause, even after a careful post mortem examination and histological examination of suspect vessels. For instance, one may find an atheromatous narrowing near the origin of a middle cerebral artery, with the residual lumen blocked by thrombus, and be unable to decide whether the thrombus had formed locally, or been lodged as an embolus from the heart or from the carotid sinus. Clotting may, of course, occur over a large extent of the artery *distal* to an occlusion.

Embolism

Embolization of the brain commonly occurs from one of two sites: the heart and a carotid sinus. On the left side of the heart thrombus may form and become loosely attached to the endocardium overlying a myocardial infarct. It may also form, in a fibrillating heart, in the left atrium. Small emboli may also arise from vegetations, infected or otherwise, on the mitral or aortic valves. In bacterial endocarditis, these may give rise to mycotic aneurysms, most commonly at some point in the course of a middle cerebral artery (p.136). Emboli from the carotid sinus may be either dislodged chunks of atheromatous debris, or fragments of thrombus overlying a raw area of the intima. In either case, the embolus is likely to be impacted, according to its size and friability, at the bifurcation of the internal carotid artery, or at some point in the course of the middle cerebral artery. Sometimes (presumably when the embolus is very friable) a shower of small emboli may lodge in the lumina of penetrating arterioles, giving rise to multiple softenings in the cerebral white matter and basal ganglia. In the acute phase, these softenings, with their sharply defined edges, may suggest a diagnosis of MS, and have been called 'fool's plaques' (Fig. 7.10).

Cerebral emboli originating in the lungs appear to be uncommon, apart from fat emboli in cases with broken

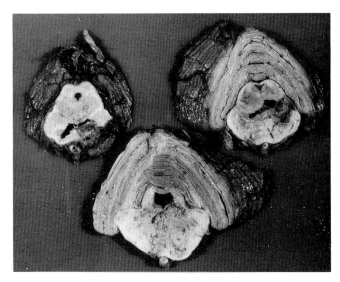

Fig. 7.8. Multiple brain stem infarcts, due to atheroma of the basilar artery, in a hypertensive 83-year-old woman.

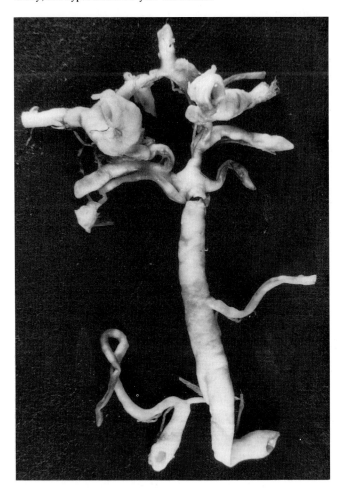

Fig. 7.9. Calcification of basal arteries. The pattern of arteries is highly asymmetrical (for instance, the basilar is supplied almost entirely by one vertebral), and there are several fusiform aneurysms. Being brittle, the basilar artery has snapped at its upper end during dissection.

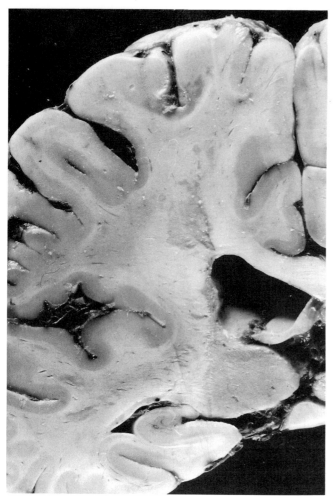

Fig. 7.10. 'Fool's plaques'. These are well-defined grey areas of infarction, superficially resembling plaques of MS, in the central white matter. 92-year-old man, with 3 weeks' history of confusion and right hemiparesis. At post mortem the heart was enlarged and scarred, with fragments of thrombus in the left ventricle. The lesions in the brain are attributable to a shower of small emboli from this source.

bones, and metastases from malignant tumours and septic foci. Very rarely, phlebothrombosis in a systemic vein gives rise to a 'paradoxical' embolism via a patent foramen ovale. An initial pulmonary embolism may increase the pressure on the right side of the heart, and so divert a second embolus into the left atrium (Gleysteen & Silver 1970). We have encountered one such case.

Embolization in the territory of the vertebral arteries appears to be rare. Infarcts in the brain stem and cerebellum are usually readily accounted for by atheroma of a vertebral artery, occluding the origin of one or more of its branches. This is the usual finding in the condition known to clinicians as the lateral medullary syndrome (see p.375), which is due to occlusion at its origin of a posterior inferior cerebellar artery (PICA) (Figs 7.11 and 25.2). We have encountered only one case of embolization (other than malignant) in the

hindbrain. This was in a case of (presumably traumatic) thrombosis at the origin of a vertebral artery. The case is briefly described on pp.95–6.

Arterial spasm

Arterial spasm, lasting long enough to cause infarction, is a well-documented complication of massive subarachnoid bleeding, whether from trauma or from rupture of an aneurysm. It is discussed above (p.100). In this connection, it is worth remembering that a direct neurosurgical approach to an aneurysm entails the risk of trauma, and subsequent thrombosis, in the artery bearing the aneurysm, giving rise to a large and, on occasion, disastrous infarct.

Patterns of infarction

There are certain commonly occurring patterns of cerebral infarction, which can be fairly satisfactorily accounted for on the basis of the normal distribution of cerebral arteries and points of anastomosis between them. Figures 7.12–7.15 show the normal distribution of the brain arteries. Points worth noting are:

1 There are anastomoses between the terminal branches of the anterior, middle and posterior cerebral arteries on the surface of the brain, but not in the interior. The penetrating arteries, including those supplying the thalamus and basal ganglia, are end-arteries, with clearly defined territories.

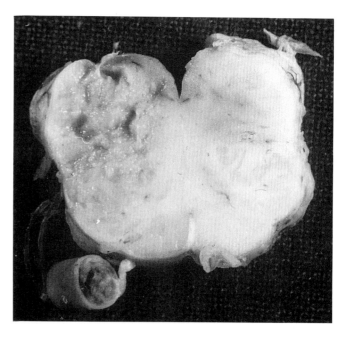

Fig. 7.11. Lateral medullary infarction, due to thrombosis of the left vertebral artery (lower left), occluding the origin of the posterior inferior cerebellar artery, in a 62-year-old woman.

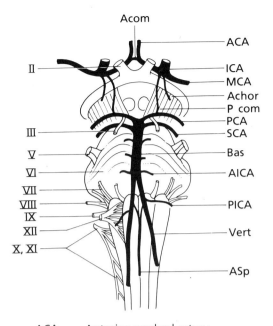

ACA	Anterior cerebral artery
Acho	Ant. choroidal artery
A com	Ant. communicating artery
AICA	Ant. inf. cerebellar artery
ASp	Ant. spinal artery
Bas	Basilar artery
ICA	Internal carotid artery
MCA	Middle cerebral artery
PCA	Posterior cerebral artery
P com	Post. communicating artery
PICA	Post. inferior cerebellar artery
SCA	Superior cerebellar artery
Vert	Vertebral artery

Fig. 7.12. The basal arteries of the brain. The circle of Willis comprises the proximal parts of the anterior and posterior cerebral arteries, and the anterior and posterior communicating arteries.

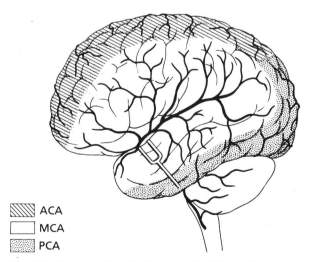

Fig. 7.13. The superficial distribution of the left middle cerebral artery.

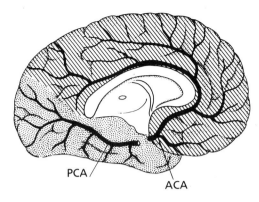

Fig. 7.14. The distribution of the anterior and posterior cerebral arteries on the medial surface of the right cerebral hemisphere.

2 The anterior communicating artery usually has a fair-sized calibre. If the first part of, say, the right anterior cerebral artery is clipped in the course of surgery, the left anterior cerebral artery will usually take over the supply of its territory via the anterior communicating artery.

3 There is a reciprocal relationship in the size of the posterior communicating artery and the first part of the posterior cerebral artery on the same side. When the former is large and the latter small, the posterior cerebral territory is supplied mainly by the internal carotid artery, and the basilar artery is smaller than usual. There is a similar reciprocal relation in the sizes of the left and right vertebral arteries.

4 The blood supply of the cerebellum is variable. Usually the superior cerebellar artery supplies the rostral third, the anterior inferior cerebellar artery (AICA) is small, and the PICA supplies about two-thirds of the cerebellar hemisphere. Quite often, however, the AICA is large, and the PICA correspondingly small, on one or both sides.

Figure 7.16 shows the effect of occlusion of a middle cerebral artery (MCA) when the anterior (ACA) and posterior (PCA) cerebral arteries are fully patent. The central part of the MCA territory — part of the lentiform nucleus, insula, and opercula of the lateral fissure — are softened, while the border zones are kept alive by the ACA and PCA via surface anastomoses.

In Fig. 7.1 the entire MCA territory is infarcted. This is usually the result of an occlusion, by embolism, of the upper end of the internal carotid artery. The ACA territory is supplied, via the anterior communicating artery, from the opposite ACA. The territory of the lateral striate arteries, which arise from the MCA in the lateral fissure, is softened; that of the medial striate, coming from the recurrent branch of the ACA, is firm, with a clear line of demarcation. Figure 7.17 shows the effect of acute internal carotid occlusion when take-over by the ACA is not achieved. Figure 7.18 shows a long-standing infarct in the territory of the PCA.

Arterial blood pressure falls continuously between the aorta and the capillary bed. In the cerebral arteries, the

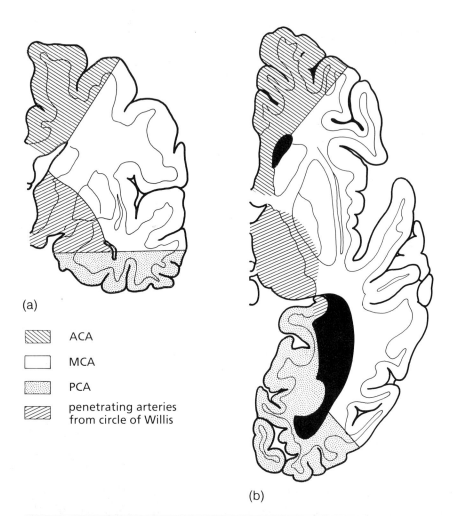

(a)

⬚ (hatched)	ACA
☐ (white)	MCA
▦ (stippled)	PCA
⬚ (hatched)	penetrating arteries from circle of Willis

(b)

Fig. 7.15. The territories of the anterior, middle and posterior cerebral arteries (a) in a coronal slice at level A1, and (b) in a horizontal slice at mid-thalamic level.

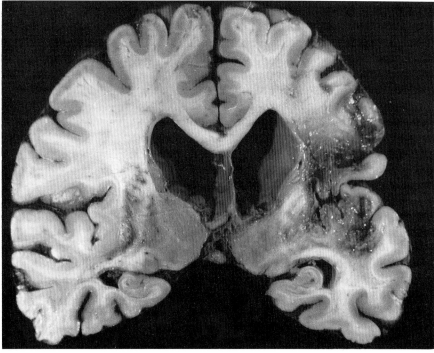

Fig. 7.16. Infarct of 6 months' standing, due to an embolus originating in the right carotid sinus, affecting the right insula and inferior frontal gyrus, in a 59-year-old diabetic man.

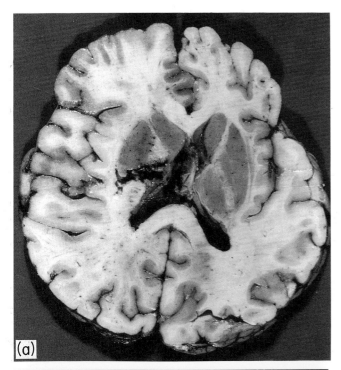

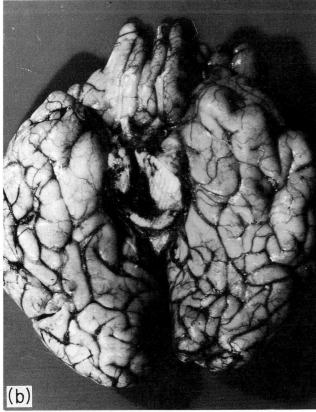

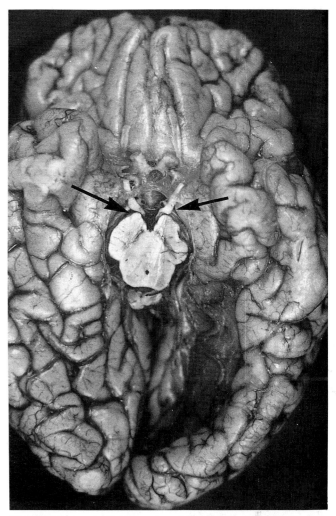

Fig. 7.18. Long-standing infarction of the territory supplied by a branch of the left posterior cerebral artery. The artery itself can be seen winding around the lateral surface of the midbrain. (In passing, note the close relationship between the posterior cerebral arteries and the oculomotor nerves (arrowed). In the presence of a diencephalic downthrust, the nerve is kinked by the artery, giving rise to the important clinical sign of the fixed dilated pupil.)

Fig. 7.17. Acute infarction of the territories of the left anterior and middle cerebral arteries, due to thrombotic occlusion of the left common and internal carotid arteries, in a 57-year-old woman. (a) Horizontal slice, showing swelling, with subfalcine herniation, of the anterior two-thirds of the left hemisphere. (b) The cause of death was haemorrhagic disruption of the upper brain stem, caused by transtentorial herniation.

pressure is at its lowest at the termination of their branches, i.e. at the points where they form anastomoses with the terminations of neighbouring arteries. This supplies a very plausible explanation of the common association of border-zone infarcts (Fig. 7.19) with severe or protracted heart failure. Similar border-zone infarcts may be seen in the same cases at the junction of the territories of the superior and inferior cerebellar arteries.

Cerebral infarcts may result from *pinching* of arteries, rather than from occlusion of their lumina. This can be caused by distortion, as from a tumour; but the most familiar instance is in cases of unilateral cerebral swelling or compression, with tentorial herniation. On the side opposite the swelling, the backward-directed branches of the PCA are squeezed against the free edge of the tentorium. This

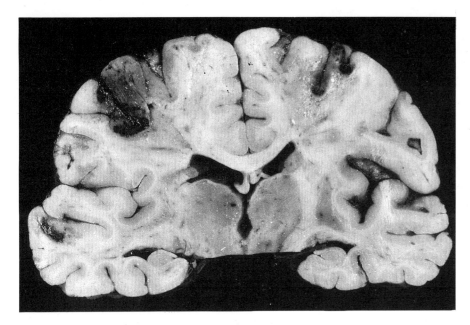

Fig. 7.19. Border-zone ('watershed') infarcts, in a 47-year-old woman with aortic valve disease leading to heart failure. Confusion and coma for one month before death. There is haemorrhagic softening in the border zones of the middle and anterior cerebral arteries on both sides, and of the middle and posterior cerebral arteries on the left side. There were similar softenings in the border-zones of the superior and inferior cerebellar arteries on both sides.

interrupts the supply to the under-surface of the temporal and occipital lobes, and of the calcarine cortex. If the patient survives (a rare occurrence) he is left with a homonymous hemianopia. The infarct itself is almost always haemorrhagic (Fig. 7.20). Even more dramatic haemorrhage occurs in infarcts due to venous occlusion (Fig. 6.13). These are discussed on p.103. Infarcts due to traumatic tearing of vessels are discussed on pp.95–6.

Lacunes

On slicing the brain of an elderly person, one commonly sees multiple small rarefactions (so-called *lacunar state*) in the thalamus and basal ganglia — most conspicuously in the lentiform nucleus (Fig. 7.21). On close inspection, small vessels can usually be seen at the centres of these lacunes (Fig. 7.22). They are regarded by some as mini-infarcts, but their causes are still uncertain. They are associated with atheroma of the small arteries at the base. Clinically, they are suspected of playing a part in senile tremor and other Parkinson-like disturbances. Much more rarely, one finds multiple softenings and rarefactions in the cerebral white matter, associated with hyaline, thickened arterioles. The patients are usually elderly, hypertensive, and more or less demented. The condition is sometimes referred to as *Binswanger's disease* (p.276), although it is not very clear what Dr Binswanger originally described.

'Strokes' and hypertension

Whereas the association of cerebral haemorrhage with chronically raised blood pressure seems to be well established, the part played by hypertension in cerebral infarction is not yet clear. A causal link between raised blood pressure

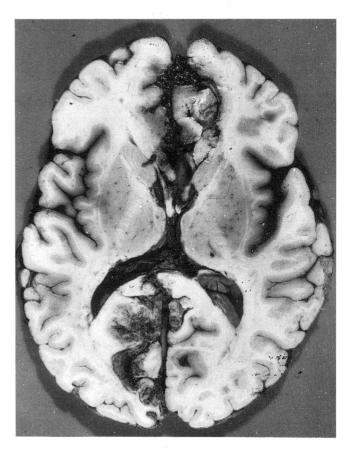

Fig. 7.20. Acute haemorrhagic infarction of part of the territory of the left posterior cerebral artery. Man, aged 53, with rupture of an aneurysm of the anterior communicating artery.

and atheroma may well exist, but there are objections to most of the simple theories of the nature of such a link. The arteriolar changes seen in Binswanger's disease are common in other parts of the body in chronic hypertensives; but whereas hypertension is common, Binswanger's disease is rare.

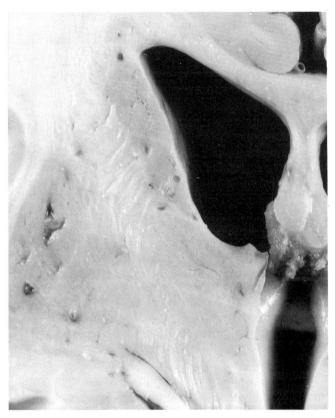

Fig. 7.21. Rarefactions ('lacunes') in the corpus striatum. Man, aged 65, with long-standing hypertension (heart weight, 500g) and 18 months' progressive dementia.

Hypertensive encephalopathy

This, in contrast, is a rare, fulminating, usually fatal condition associated with *sudden* elevation of the blood pressure, such as may occur in malignant hypertension and toxaemia of pregnancy. In the brain, the characteristic finding is of fibrinoid necrosis of small vessels, with petechial haemorrhages, and a variable amount of oedema of white matter.

An enlarged heart is regarded as good evidence of chronic hypertension. It is therefore prudent to record the weight of the heart at post mortem in all cases suspected of cerebral circulatory disorder.

Infarcts in the spinal cord

These are not very common, and when they occur the causes are generally different from those of infarcts in the brain. The main artery is the anterior spinal, which is continuous from its origin from the two vertebral arteries to the conus medullaris, and is fed by two or three major radicular arteries. If any of these feeding arteries is occluded, some part of the cord is likely to be infarcted.

Common causes of occlusion

1 *Compression of the nerve root* carrying a major radicular artery as it passes through an intervertebral foramen. The compressing agent is usually a tumour, benign or malignant. Benign offenders include schwannomas and meningiomas; malignant ones include carcinomas (especially Pancoast's tumour of the lung), myelomas, lymphomas and neuroblastomas. As causes of paraplegia, these are probably at least as common as tumours inside the spinal canal.

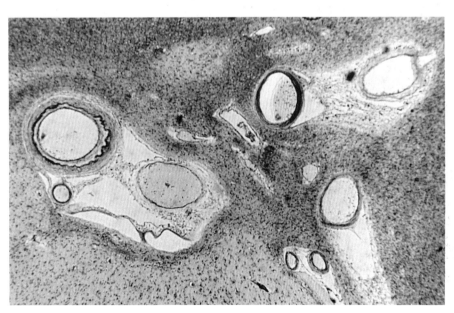

Fig. 7.22. Rarefactions related to small vessels in the corpus striatum of a hypertensive woman aged 85, suffering from general debility and mental confusion. H&E, ×35.

2 *Occlusion of a radicular artery* at its origin from an atheromatous aorta, causing a reduction in perfusion pressure.

3 *Trauma*. This includes unfortunate cases where surgery at the back of the abdomen (for instance, in the course of a lumbar sympathectomy) results in damage to a relevant nerve root and artery.

4 *Nitrogen embolism*. In divers, too rapid decompression may result in release of bubbles of nitrogen into the bloodstream, giving rise to decompression sickness (caisson disease, the 'bends'). In fatal cases, fresh softenings may be found, especially in the white columns of the thoracic cord. With longer survival, upward and downward tract degeneration occurs.

5 *Spinal 'angioma'*. An uncommon condition, known at various times as 'subacute necrotizing myelitis', 'angiodysgenetic necrotizing myelopathy', 'Foix−Alajouanine disease' and 'angiomatosis of the spinal cord', is now generally regarded as the result of a fistulous communication between the arterial supply and the venous drainage of the lower part of the spinal cord. How the fistula arises is not known. The disease presents, in adult life, as a progressive motor and sensory paraplegia. Exposure from behind shows the lower half of the cord covered with what looks like a tangled mass of dilated veins (Fig. 2.22), but careful dissection shows that this mass is composed of a single, extremely tortuous, thick-walled vein. Similar, but much smaller, tortuous veins may be seen running along the roots of the cauda equina. Under the microscope, the affected veins are seen to be 'arterialized', with thick, fibrous walls, devoid of the smooth muscle fibres and elastic laminae characteristic of arteries — a change liable to occur wherever veins are subjected to near-arterial pressures. Their lumina are more capacious than those of normal superficial veins. The small intrinsic vessels of the cord, on the contrary, have thick, hyaline walls, and the lumina are either diminished or abolished. The cord tissue itself shows a mixture of infarction, gliosis and wallerian degeneration, often with a few surviving nerve cells in the central parts. Thrombosis may be seen in both extrinsic and intrinsic vessels.

Arterial disease

Diseases of arteries, other than atheroma, causing ischaemic lesions in the CNS, include temporal (giant-celled) arteritis, polyarteritis nodosa, and endarteritis obliterans (Heubner's arteritis). The first of these, when it occurs in the brain, spinal cord or meninges, does not differ histologically from the same disease in other parts of the body. The second is more often encountered by neuropathologists in the shape of temporal artery biopsies than in post mortem material. Briefly, it is a granulomatous panarteritis characterized by giant cells of Langhans type. It is very rarely seen in intracranial vessels.

Endarteritis obliterans

Endarteritis obliterans is a condition associated with meningitis, especially with *chronic* meningitis — syphilitic, tuberculous or fungal (see Chapter 9, pp.131−4). It affects small- and medium-sized superficial arteries which lie bathed in purulent or granulomatous exudate (Fig. 7.23). The characteristic histological feature is that although the medial coat and elastica are well preserved, the intimal coat is thickened — sometimes to the point of complete occlusion of the lumen — by new-formed connective tissue. Why this should happen is a mystery, but there may well be a common causal link between this intimal thickening and that seen following subarachnoid haemorrhage (see p.100). Infarcts due to endarteritis may be extensive, and may involve important areas of central grey matter. They, along with the effects of obstructive hydrocephalus (see p.121), take the blame for poor results following successful treatment of the infection in cases of tuberculous meningitis.

Congophilic angiopathy, mentioned above (p.104) as a cause of intracerebral bleeding, may also be complicated by thrombosis of diseased vessels, with consequent infarction (Fig. 7.24) (see Griffiths *et al.* 1982).

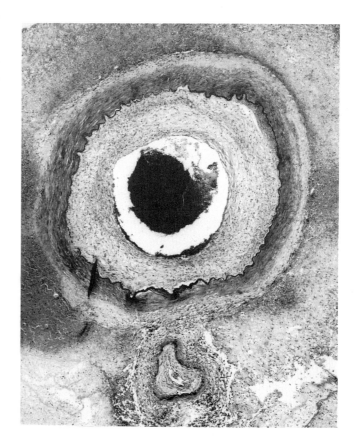

Fig. 7.23. Endarteritis obliterans (Heubner's arteritis). Woman aged 36, with a 4-week history of tuberculous meningitis, ×35.

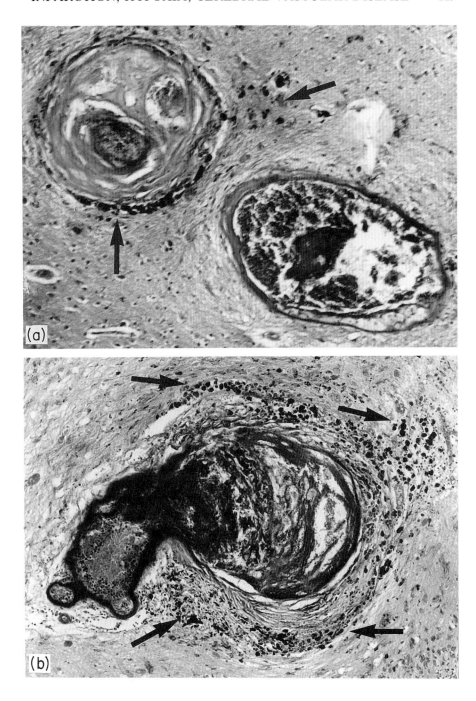

Fig. 7.24. Familial congophilic angiopathy. Case 1 of Griffiths *et al.* (1982). (a) Vessels in cerebral cortex, one containing fluid blood, the other half-occluded by thrombus. (b) Vessel in cerebellum, occluded by organized thrombus, with leakage into surroundings. Accumulations of siderin phagocytes are indicated by arrows. PAS, ×75.

Effects of blood disorders

In general, any blood disease in which spontaneous intra-vascular clotting occurs is liable to produce infarction — anaemic if it affects arteries or arterioles, more or less haemorrhagic if it occurs in veins or venules. In *thrombotic thrombocytopenic purpura* both blood and small blood vessels are affected. (For the pathology of this condition, see Brierley and Graham 1984, pp.186–7.)

Recommendations

In conclusion, we would make the following recommendations for the post mortem examination in a case of clinically diagnosed cerebrovascular disease.

1   In the post mortem room, examine the heart carefully; in particular, weigh it, as this may provide the best evidence for chronic arterial hypertension. Take, and preferably fix for later dissection, as much as is accessible of the common and internal carotid arteries. If the cord is involved in the

disease, and if circumstances permit, take and fix the vertebral column, with the abdominal aorta attached.

2   At post mortem and in the subsequent cut-up, check the patency of the carotid and vertebral arteries in the neck. Examine the circle of Willis, observe its anatomical pattern, and note points of narrowing by atheroma or thrombus. If infarcts are found, compare their outlines with those of arterial territories.

3   Take blocks for histology, not only from areas of obvious disease but from areas (e.g. hippocampus and cerebellum) known to be vulnerable to hypoxia. Take sections of selected arteries and look for changes not only of atheroma, but also of other arteriopathies.

4   When infarcts are found, aim at giving a plausible account of their causation.

Further reading

Brierley JB, Graham DI. 1984. Hypoxia and vascular disorders of the central nervous system. In Adams JH, Corsellis JAN, Duchen LW (Eds) *Greenfield's Neuropathology*, 4th edn. Edward Arnold, London.

Chester EM, Agamanolis DP, Banker BQ, Victor M. 1978. Hypertensive encephalopathy: a clinicopathologic study of 20 cases. *Neurology* **28**, 928–39.

Gleysteen JJ, Silver D. 1970. Paradoxical arterial embolism: collective review. *Am Surg* **36**, 47–54.

Griffiths RA, Mortimer TF, Oppenheimer DR, Spalding MK. 1982. Congophilic angiopathy of the brain. *J Neurol Neurosurg Psychiat*, **45**, 396–408.

Chapter 8
Hydrocephalus, Cysts and Syrinxes

Hydrocephalus

Hydrocephalus (in the vernacular, water on the brain) in practice means enlarged cerebral ventricles. The term 'external hydrocephalus', which denoted enlargement of the cerebral subarachnoid spaces, has dropped out of use, as it is no more than an aspect of cerebral atrophy. The terms 'communicating' and 'non-communicating' hydrocephalus are still used. They denote the presence or absence of communication, via the apertures of the fourth ventricle, between the ventricular system and the subarachnoid space. Mention has already been made (pp.26–7) of naked-eye changes in cases of hydrocephalus, and of some of the causes of ventricular enlargement.

The most important of these causes (important because it may threaten life) is interference with the circulation of CSF, leading to back-pressure. A short account of the CSF pathways is given below, with particular mention of the points where such interference may occur, and which therefore need attention when examining a hydrocephalic brain. Obstruction at several points may occur, as in cases of congenital hydrocephalus due to the Chiari type 2 malformation, which is discussed on pp.252–4.

CSF pathways: points of obstruction

The main source of CSF is the choroid plexus of the lateral ventricles, with contributions from the plexuses of the third and fourth ventricles. Resorption of fluid occurs, on a small scale, at many points on the cerebral and spinal arachnoid; but the main site of resorption is in the arachnoid granulations (Pacchionian bodies; see Fig. 3.26) associated with the superior longitudinal sinus and bridging veins on the vertex of the brain. When production of CSF outruns absorption, pressure builds up in the lateral ventricles, which expand in consequence.

The only recognized cause of CSF over-production is a functioning *papilloma of the choroid plexus* (p.190), which may arise within any of the four ventricles, producing a symmetrical hydrocephalus, most marked in the lateral ventricles. Defective absorption of CSF, thought to be due to blood corpuscles choking the arachnoid granulations, is a common effect of subarachnoid haemorrhage — usually, but not always, transient (Fig. 8.1).

Between the choroid plexus and the arachnoid granulations there are various points where the flow of CSF may be obstructed, of which the first are the *interventricular foramina* (of Monro). A rare benign (but potentially fatal) lesion, which may obstruct one or both foramina, often transitorily, is the so-called *colloid cyst of the third ventricle*. This invariably arises in the roof of the ventricle, close to the foramina, where it dangles from a short stalk (Fig. 8.2). When the brain is sliced, it may become detached. It should be looked for in cases with a history of recurrent severe headache, especially if the onset and cessation are sudden. The third ventricle itself may be blocked by tumour — in particular, by *ependymomas*, *craniopharyngiomas*, and *teratoid tumours* (including germinomas) in the pineal region (see pp.181, 209, 220–21).

A more frequent site of obstruction is the *aqueduct*. Kinking of the aqueduct is probably the main reason for the association of hydrocephalus with posterior fossa tumours (see Fig. 8.3). Surgical removal of the tumour often suffices to relieve the hydrocephalus. Compression of the aqueduct occurs with expanding pontine gliomas and with pineal tumours. Actual blockage of the lumen may occur acutely,

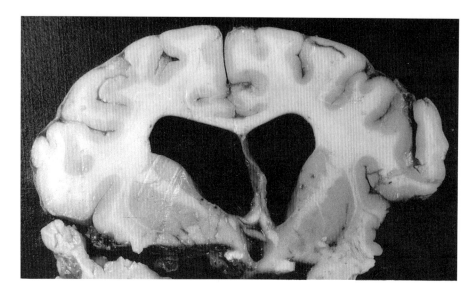

Fig. 8.1. Hydrocephalus following repeated subarachnoid bleeding from an aneurysm of the right posterior communicating artery, in a woman aged 77. Note flattening of the convolutions, indicating that the hydrocephalus is due to obstruction rather than to cerebral atrophy.

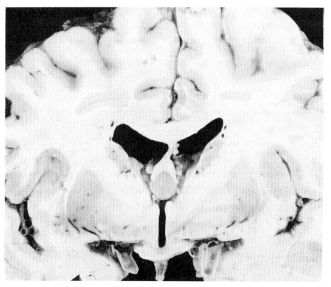

Fig. 8.2. Colloid cyst of third ventricle. Incidental finding in a 55-year-old man. Note proximity to interventricular foramina. (Courtesy of Dr T.H. Moss.)

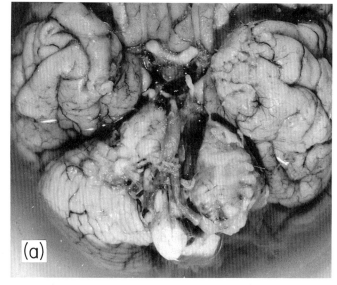

(a)

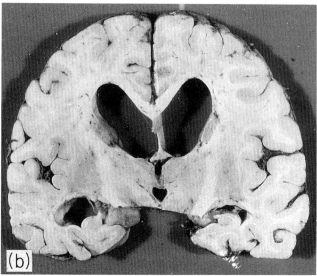

(b)

Fig. 8.3 (*right*). (a) Undersurface of the brain in a woman of 82 with a recurrent tumour (schwannoma) of the left acoustic nerve. Much of the left cerebellar hemisphere was removed at the time of operation, about 10 years earlier. (b) Obstructive hydrocephalus resulting from distortion of the brain stem.

from intraventricular haemorrhage, or gradually, as a result of progressive granular ependymitis (see p.53), in the condition generally known as *aqueduct stenosis* (Fig. 8.4). There are also cases of congenital atresia, or 'forking' of the aqueduct (Russell 1949; see Fig. 8.5). In all these conditions, the lateral and third ventricles are dilated, but not the fourth; and there is an associated flattening of the cerebral convolutions.

Narrowing or obliteration of the lateral and median apertures of the fourth ventricle (foramina of Luschka and Magendie) is almost always due to fibrosis following a subacute or chronic (or inadequately treated) meningitis (Fig. 8.6). In such cases the fourth ventricle shares in the general dilatation. A chronic meningitis — in particular, tuberculous meningitis — may also result in dense fibrous adhesions between the edge of the tentorial opening and the surface of the midbrain, blocking the subarachnoid pathway

of the so-called *cisterna ambiens*. Finally, there is a danger that the flattening of the cerebral convolutions, caused by raised intraventricular pressure, may interfere with the passage of fluid through the cerebral sulci on its way to the arachnoid granulations, creating a vicious circle. Blockage of the intercellular channels in the granulations by blood cells is mentioned above (p.100).

The patency or otherwise of the interventricular foramina and aqueduct is easily observed in brain slices. The lateral apertures are likewise easily displayed, if they have not already been exposed. They are recognizable by their glossy ependymal lining. The median aperture may be hard to distinguish because of post mortem tearing of the delicate velum overlying the lower end of the fourth ventricle. For similar reasons the patency of the cisterna ambiens may be hard to determine if the brain has been removed from the skull in the customary fashion.

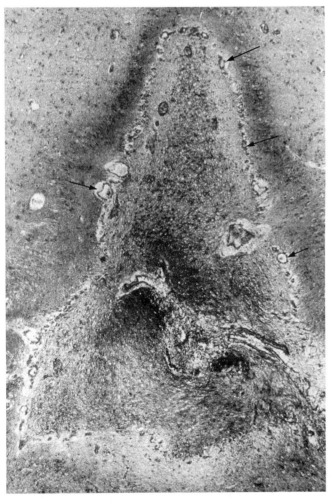

Fig. 8.4. Proliferation of neuroglia, with new vessel formation, in the aqueduct of a patient with tuberculous meningitis. The aqueduct is totally blocked. The remains of the ependyma can be seen in the form of tiny canaliculi (arrowed) around the edge of the blockage. The stimulus to glial proliferation was probably haemorrhage from repeated needling of the lateral ventricles. PTAH, ×40.

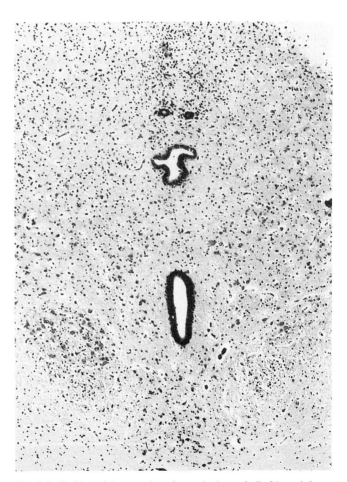

Fig. 8.5. Forking of the aqueduct, from a hydrocephalic 24-week fetus. H&E, ×100.

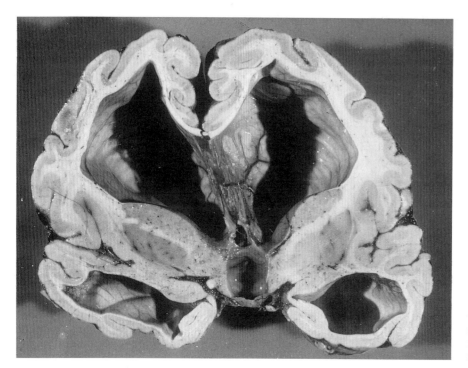

Fig. 8.6. Severe obstructive hydrocephalus in a 20-year-old man, treated in childhood for tuberculous meningitis. The site of obstruction was the cisterna ambiens (i.e. the subarachnoid space surrounding the midbrain). Note the preferential loss of white matter, as against grey.

Non-obstructive causes of ventricular enlargement

The pathology of so-called *'normal-pressure hydrocephalus'* is still in dispute. It seems that in some such cases the intracranial pressure is not consistently normal, but is raised during certain periods of the day or night. Also, there has often been an alleviation of symptoms, and a decrease in ventricular size, following a shunting procedure. In any case coming to post mortem, a meticulous search for possible obstructive lesions should be carried out. For a recent review, see Anderson (1986).

The term *'otitic hydrocephalus'*, referring to a condition of raised intracranial pressure, with papilloedema, associated with otitis media, has become obsolete since the demonstration by air ventriculography that in such cases the ventricles are not enlarged but reduced in size. The increased pressure is attributed to brain swelling consequent upon phlebothrombosis of the lateral sinus and its tributaries.

Enlargement of the lateral ventricles, without signs of raised intraventricular pressure, may be due to *loss of brain tissue*, from a variety of causes. One of these is perinatal cerebral hypoxia or ischaemia, which produces characteristic lesions in the central cerebral white matter on one or both sides (see pp. 324–5). Not uncommonly, the brains of lifelong mental defectives, or of sufferers from so-called cerebral palsy, show a deficiency of cerebral white matter on one side or both, compensated by a lateral and upward extension of the body of the lateral ventricle (Fig. 8.7). These extensions tend to have a roughly square outline, unlike the rounded shape of ventricles subjected to raised internal

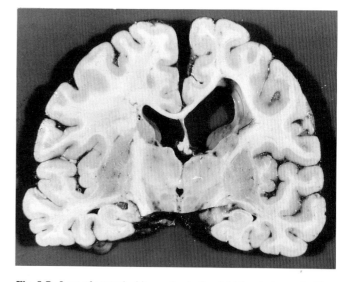

Fig. 8.7. Loss of central white matter in the right hemisphere of a 76-year-old mental defective, with spastic left hemiplegia from infancy. The lesion, which may occur on one side or both, is a characteristic result of perinatal circulatory disturbance.

pressure. In general, loss of cerebral tissue is reflected in a visible thinning of the corpus callosum (Fig. 8.8).

Infarcted brain tissue, having been swollen in the acute phase, thereafter shrinks as the necrotic material is removed by macrophages. *Old infarcts* are probably the commonest cause of local compensatory dilatation of the ventricles. Other common causes include *demyelination*. Myelin constitutes more of the brain's bulk than do nerve cells, glial

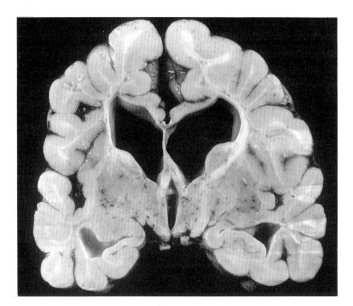

Fig. 8.8. Loss of cerebral white matter on both sides, in a 13-year-old girl whose mother suffered from toxaemia in pregnancy. The child was retarded, quadriplegic and epileptic. Note the virtual disappearance of the corpus callosum; also the relative sparing of the crowns of the gyri, as compared with the sulci (*ulegyria*; see p.325 and Fig. 16.14).

cells and their processes. In some cases of severe MS, much of the cerebral myelin is destroyed, and the ventricles may be conspicuously enlarged (Fig. 14.9). In *Huntington's chorea* the caudate nuclei lose their neurons and shrivel, causing symmetrical compensatory dilatation of the anterior horns of the ventricles (Fig. 8.9). The same may occur in *Pick's disease*, with the additional feature of dilatation of the

inferior horns, due to atrophy of the temporal cortex and white matter (Fig. 8.10). Similar dilatation of the fourth ventricle is seen in cases of 'system' degenerations of the brain stem and/or cerebellum (Fig. 8.11). Unilateral enlargement of a temporal horn may be seen in cases of temporal lobe epilepsy (see Chapter 18).

Intracranial cysts

Intracranial cysts are of various kinds. Cystic cavities in the centra ovalia, alongside the lateral ventricles, are generally the end-result of perinatal circulatory disturbances (see pp.323–4). They are commonly referred to as *porencephalic cysts* (Fig. 21.8). Among the commoner causes of cysts in the brain are *tumours*, in particular those of the astrocytic series, ranging from the benign cerebellar astrocytoma of childhood to the more malignant types of glioma in the cerebral hemispheres of adults (Fig. 11.5; see pp.176 and 164). Cysts of large and life-threatening size are associated with haemangioblastomas of the cerebellum (p.195). In these, progressive enlargement of the cyst is often responsible for the patient's symptoms, which can be relieved temporarily by drawing off the contained fluid.

A rarer cause of intracerebral cysts is *sequestration* of some part of a lateral ventricle — in particular, of a temporal horn, with inclusion of a frond of the choroid plexus. This may give rise to the clinical features of an expanding lesion, whereas loculation of the tip of an occipital horn, containing no choroid plexus, does not cause symptoms.

Not uncommonly one finds, on slicing a brain, that the septum lucidum is split, with a fluid-filled cavity between

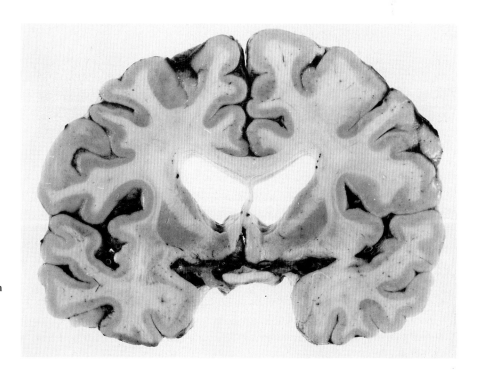

Fig. 8.9. Coronal slice at level A1 from a man aged 52 with Huntington's chorea. The ventricles are large because of atrophy of the corpus striatum. There is no obvious wasting of cortex or white matter, and the corpus callosum is of normal bulk.

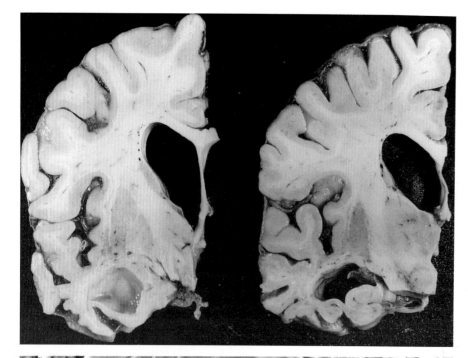

Fig. 8.10. Coronal slices, at levels A1 and P1, from the left hemisphere of a man aged 67 with Pick's disease. In this individual there was atrophy of the caudate nucleus. The main visible abnormality is an extreme atrophy of the temporal cortex and white matter, with compensatory dilatation of the inferior horn of the ventricle.

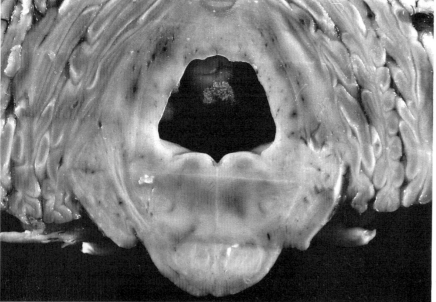

Fig. 8.11. Enlarged fourth ventricle in a woman aged 76 with pontocerebellar atrophy.

the two leaves (Fig. 16.10a). The cavity, referred to as a *cavum septi*, is said to be relatively common in professional boxers. It is lined with neuroglial fibres, whereas loculated ventricles are at least partially lined by ependyma.

Arachnoid cysts

These consist of clear fluid enclosed between reduplicated layers of arachnoid membrane. They may cause symptoms by pressure on underlying structures, or appear as incidental post mortem findings. They are commonly called 'congenital', but are very rarely found in the brains of newborn babies;

their origin is obscure. They are found in various sites above and below the tentorium, but are commonest within a lateral fissure, lying between the frontal and temporal lobes (Fig. 8.12). Fortunately, they are seldom encountered within the spinal dura, where their expansion might result in an irreversible paraplegia. The subject is reviewed by Shaw & Alvord (1977).

Subdural fluid collections (other than haematomas) overlying the brain have been attributed either to valvular traumatic tears in the arachnoid, with leakage of CSF, or to imbibition of fluid by chronic haematomas. Both types are referred to as *subdural hygromas*.

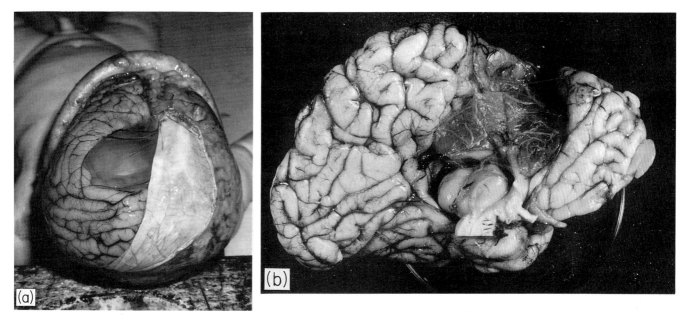

Fig. 8.12. Large left frontoparietal arachnoid cyst in a 10-week-old infant with multiple malformations. Cot death. (a) View from above, before removal of the brain. (b) Medial view of left hemisphere, after fixation. There is no corpus callosum.

Hydromyelia and syringomyelia

From childhood onward the 'central canal' of the spinal cord is for the most part not a canal at all, but a rather irregular column of ependymal cells, Among these there may be short stretches of an ependyma-lined tubule, less than 1 mm in diameter, and of no known clinical or pathological significance. Where the contained fluid comes from is not known. A longer stretch, of greater calibre, wholly or partially lined with ependyma, is dignified by the term *hydromyelia*. A longitudinal cavity in the cord, unconnected with the central canal, having no ependymal lining, is referred to as a '*syrinx*', and the condition is called *syringo-* *myelia* (Fig. 8.13). Occasionally one may find a syrinx as well as a patent canal in a single transverse section. In such cases, upward and downward exploration may reveal a communication between the two cavities. One is then tempted to suppose that fluid secreted into a hydromyelic canal has erupted into the cord substance, and proceeded to track upward and downward along fibre tracts. More often, no such communication is found. What is more, repeated efforts to trace a connection between the syrinx and the fourth ventricle have failed; and the problem of the origin of the fluid remains unsolved. Lasting fame awaits the solver.

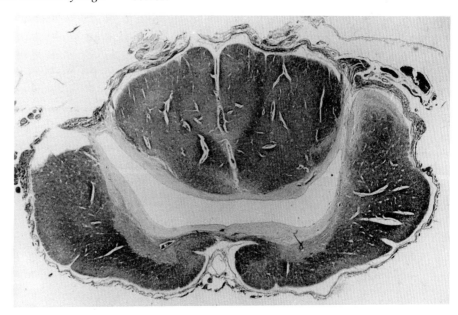

Fig. 8.13. Syringomyelia. The patient, a 60-year-old woman, had an obstructive hydrocephalus due to a vascular hamartoma in the fourth ventricle, and a syrinx extending from the second to the fifth cervical segment. There was also an exaggerated lordosis of the cervical spine.

Pathology

Before interference, a spinal syrinx is an extended longitudinal cyst, blowing out the cord to about double its normal cross-sectional area. The lower cervical and upper thoracic segments are the most commonly affected. After interference by surgeon or pathologist, the cord collapses; being tethered at the sides by the denticulate ligaments, it undergoes anteroposterior flattening. The wall of the cavity consists of glial fibres, sometimes reinforced with collagen fibres. The thickness of the wall is thought to correspond to the age of the lesion. Examination of transverse sections shows that the cavity grows mainly at the expense of grey matter; the white columns are also reduced in area, but here, as in other instances of the effects of pressure, the reduction appears to be largely due to demyelination, with relative preservation of axis cylinders. The amount of destruction of grey matter can be roughly assessed from the degree of fibre loss in anterior roots at the affected levels; loss of pyramidal tract fibres at levels below the syrinx is some indication of the severity of damage to the spinal white matter. Damage to the white commissure, which is believed to be responsible for dissociated sensory loss, with defective painful and thermal sensation over a few segments, is hard to assess histologically.

The *routine examination* of a syringomyelic cord should include an attempt to account for the patient's recorded disabilities in terms of damage to the grey matter of the cord and interruption of fibre tracts. It must also include a careful search for *associated lesions*, particularly in the form of *tumours* or evidences of past *trauma*. Intrinsic tumours with associated cysts, which may track up and down the cord, including ependymomas and haemangioblastomas, may sometimes be the actual source of the cyst fluid; but there is also an unexplained association of syringomyelia with extrinsic spinal tumours such as meningioma and schwannoma, and even with tumours in the posterior fossa. In some cases of spinal trauma, a syrinx appears, usually above the level of the lesion, and slowly enlarges. A wide variety of *congenital deformities* of the skull, vertebral column and neuraxis have been associated with syringomyelia; the mechanisms involved are generally as obscure as in cases of 'primary' or 'idiopathic' syringomyelia. One of the more plausible theories envisages a valvular opening at the point of entry of a posterior nerve root into a syrinx which has extended into the posterior grey horn, with inward leakage of subarachnoid fluid caused, perhaps, by lengthening, shortening and twisting movements of the cord. For reviews of the subject see Netsky (1953), Gardner (1973), Barnett, Foster & Hudgson (1973), and Larroche (1984).

Syringobulbia

The term syringobulbia seems to imply that a similar pathological process occurs in the lower brain stem, but this is not necessarily the case. Commonly the lesions in question are not enclosed cysts, but slits, extending from the floor of the fourth ventricle into the substance of the medulla oblongata (Fig. 8.14). The lesions may be on one side or both. Whether or not they communicate with the ventricle, it seems that they do not present as expanding lesions, but produce disturbances by destruction of nerve cells and interruption of fibre tracts. Their cause is unknown. There are several reported cases in which syringobulbia and syringomyelia coexisted, but we know of none in which there was a demonstrable continuity between the two lesions. Even so, it is advisable in such cases to make a very careful

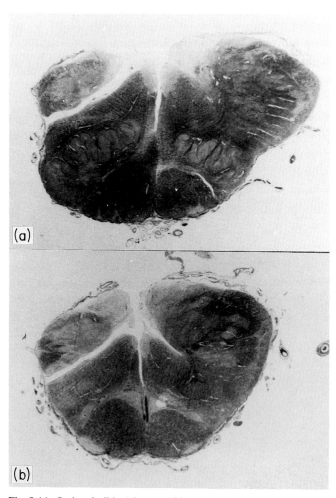

Fig. 8.14. Syringobulbia. Man aged 22, with bony deformity of upper cervical spine, associated with Chiari type 1 malformation, syringobulbia and cervical syringomyelia. Presented with 3-month history of paraesthesiae. (a) Upper medulla. (b) Lower medulla. The patient's left side is on the left side of the pictures. Myelin stain. The main cavity extends from the fourth ventricle to the pial surface on the left.

search, at microscopic level, for evidence of such continuity; in any and every case of syringomyelia a hunt should be made for possible communications between the syrinx and the subarachnoid space. The classical work on syringobulbia by Jonesco-Sisesti (1932), is now available in English translation.

Further reading

Anderson M. 1986. Normal pressure hydrocephalus. *Br Med J* **293**, 837–8.

Barnett HJM, Foster JB, Hudgson P (Eds). 1973. *Syringomyelia*. WB Saunders, Philadelphia.

Gardner WJ. 1973. *The Dysraphic States*. Excerpta Medica Foundation, Amsterdam.

Jonesco-Sisesti N. 1932. *Syringobulbia: a contribution to the pathophysiology of the brainstem*. Translated by RT Ross, 1986. Praeger, New York.

Larroche J-C. 1984. Malformations of the nervous system. In Adams JH, Corsellis JAN, Duchen LW (Eds) *Greenfield's Neuropathology*, 4th edn. Edward Arnold, London, Chapter 10.

Netsky MG. 1953. Syringomyelia: a clinicopathological study. *Arch Neurol Psychiat* **70**, 741–75.

Russell DS. 1949. *Observations on the pathology of hydrocephalus*. Medical Research Council Report Series no 265. HMSO, London.

Shaw CM, Alvord EC. 1977. 'Congenital' and arachnoid cysts and their differential diagnosis. In Vinken PJ, Bruyn GW (Eds) *Handbook of Clinical Neurology*. North-Holland, Amsterdam, **31**, 75–135.

Chapter 9
Pyogenic Infections and Granulomas

When faced with the neuropathological examination of a case of possible CNS infection the main aims are to establish (i) the *cause* of the infection (Table 9.1), (ii) the *route* by which the nervous system was reached by the organism, and (iii) the *effects* the infection has had on the nervous system itself. This may be a relatively straightforward task, for example in a case of classical acute leptomeningitis due to pneumococcal infection with associated pneumonia and bacteraemia. On the other hand, in another case infection may not have been considered in the differential diagnosis, the naked-eye appearances at post mortem examination may be unremarkable, and the organism may be a relatively uncommon one. The pathologist needs to be particularly alert for infection when examining material from patients who, for one reason or another, may be suspected of being immunodeficient.

Routes of infection

Bacteria reach the nervous system and its membranous coverings either via the bloodstream or by spread from a nearby focus of infection. Blood-borne spread of bacteria to the nervous system may occur from a focus of established infection elsewhere (e.g. osteomyelitis, septic arthritis, endocarditis, bronchiectasis, skin sepsis). Common local sources of infection are the paranasal air sinuses, middle ears and bones of the skull and spine. Infection arising in a middle ear may spread backward and laterally into mastoid air cells, upward into the ipsilateral temporal lobe or backward into the ipsilateral cerebellar hemisphere, and in a frontal sinus may easily reach the adjacent frontal lobe. It is remarkable how readily bones of the skull may be eroded by pus under raised pressure. Infection may also

gain direct access to the CNS in patients with malformations, such as a meningomyelocele, a skull fracture, particularly at the base of the skull, or with a shunt inserted in a ventricle. Acute meningitis, cerebral abscess, epidural abscess or subdural empyema may all develop from local spread of infection. The virulence of the invading organism, the effectiveness of the host defences, and the speed of commencing appropriate antibiotic therapy all influence the outcome. Highly virulent pneumococci, on reaching the brain, are liable to cause a focal purulent encephalitis rather than an abscess because there is no time available for capsule formation to take place to contain the infection. Many organisms can multiply rapidly in the CSF, which provides an excellent culture medium, relatively removed from immune defences. Organisms in the subdural space are difficult to eradicate because of the low vascularity of the dura, and the poor penetration of antibiotics unless these are instilled directly. Organisms of relatively low virulence, such as cryptococci and other fungi, and toxoplasmosis, are generally encountered in immunosuppressed, very young, or elderly and debilitated patients, and may evoke little in the way of an inflammatory response.

Consequences of infection

There are important secondary effects of infections in and around the nervous system that may complicate the picture. They include oedema, acute, possibly fatal, vascular events such as sagittal sinus thrombosis with venous infarction, cerebral arterial infarction due to arteritis, and hydrocephalus.

Several important practical considerations follow from the foregoing comments:

1 As far as possible, an *aseptic technique* should be adopted

when performing a post mortem examination on cases suspected of having an infective aetiology, at least until specimens have been taken for microbiological investigation.

Table 9.1. Organisms causing meningitis and/or granulomas in and around the brain (commoner organisms are indicated in bold)

Bacteria
Actinomyces (Gram + branching filaments)
Bacillus anthracis (Gram + rods)
Borrelia burgdorfii (spirochaetes)
Brucella species (Gram − cocco-bacilli)
Coliforms (Gram − rods)
Haemophilus influenzae (Gram − rods)
Klebsiella species (Gram − rods)
Listeria monocytogenes (Gram + rods)
Meningococcus (Gram − cocci in pairs)
Mycobacteria tuberculosis (Gram +, acid-fast rods)*
Other mycobacteria (Gram +, acid-fast rods)*†
Nocardia species (Gram + branching filaments)
Pneumococcus (Gram + cocci in pairs)
Proteus species (Gram − rods)
Pseudomonas (Gram − rods)
Serratia species (Gram − rods)†
Staphylococci (Gram + cocci)
Streptococci (Gram + cocci in chains)
Treponema pallidum (spirochaetes)*

Fungi
Aspergillus (septate hyphae)*†
Blastomyces (yeast)*
Candida albicans (yeast)*†
Cladosporidium (septate hyphae)*
Coccidiomyces (yeast)*
Cryptococcus (yeast)*†
Histoplasma (yeast)*
Zygomycetes (mucor) (non-septate hyphae)*
  (especially in diabetics)

Protozoa and metazoa
Amoebae* (some)†
Cysticercus (with cysts)*
Echinococcus and other tapeworms (with cysts)*
Micronemiasis
Onchocerca
Paragonimus
Schistosoma*
  S. japonicum mainly in the brain
  S. haematobium and *mansoni* mainly in the spinal cord
Strongyloides
Toxocara
Toxoplasma*† (and infants)
Trichinella

Viruses
Enteroviruses
Herpes simplex type 2 virus
HTLV1 (see p.157)
HIV † (see p.153)
Lymphocytic choriomeningitis virus
Paramyxoviruses (especially mumps)

* may be associated with granulomas.
† opportunistic infections.

These should be sent to the laboratory with sufficient information to ensure that appropriate media are used for culture. Additional samples of CSF and serum may be stored deep-frozen in case they are needed for estimation of microbial antibody titres at a later stage.

2 Observations need to be made regarding the *source of infection*. In cases of bacterial infection the frontal air sinuses and middle ears must be carefully entered and inspected, and swabs taken from them for culture. A track leading from the sinus to the meninges may be identifiable. Sources of infection need also to be sought elsewhere in the body (e.g. lungs, pleural and peritoneal cavities, heart valves, joint spaces, bones). Skull bones need to be inspected for fractures, particularly at the base following head injury.

3 A careful search needs to be made for evidence of systemic diseases that are associated with immunodeficiency, such as Hodgkin's disease or other lymphoma, sarcoidosis or acquired immune deficiency sydrome (AIDS). It should be remembered that previous splenectomy predisposes to pneumococcal infection.

Leptomeningitis

Acute meningitis

In classical cases this diagnosis is easily made. There is a purulent exudate readily visible in the subarachnoid space (Fig. 9.1). This may be more marked over the vertex or at the base. The brain itself often appears congested and swollen, and occasionally these features, together with the presence of a few petechial haemorrhages, may be all there is to note on naked-eye examination (Fig. 9.2). Death in such fulminating cases can result directly from the cerebral swelling and associated brain stem compression.

Small penetrating vessels at the surface of the cortex and brain stem are surrounded by acute inflammatory cells which occupy the superficial perivascular spaces. Acute hypoxic (homogenizing) changes (p.46) may be seen in cortical and hippocampal neurons. The subarachnoid space and leptomeninges contain a neutrophil polymorph infiltrate. Fibrin strands are also frequently seen. Organisms may be demonstrated with appropriate stains, unless treatment with antibiotics during life has largely eradicated them. Outside the CNS there may be adrenal or skin haemorrhages, and evidence of more widespread intravascular coagulation.

Chronic meningitis

When the inflammatory process in the subarachnoid space continues for more than a week or two, secondary effects on the brain are liable to develop. One of these is hydrocephalus, caused by interruption of the normal CSF circulation by fibrin and, later, granular ependymitis at the aqueduct, gliosis or fibrosis around the outlet foramina of

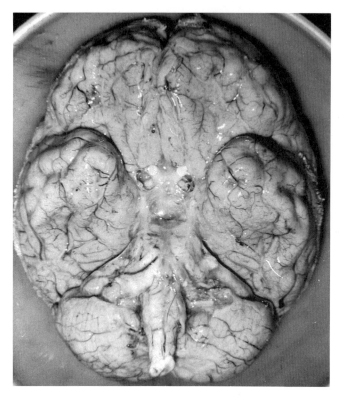

Fig. 9.1. Base of the brain from a case of acute meningitis. There is a thin film of pus obscuring the under-surface of the brain.

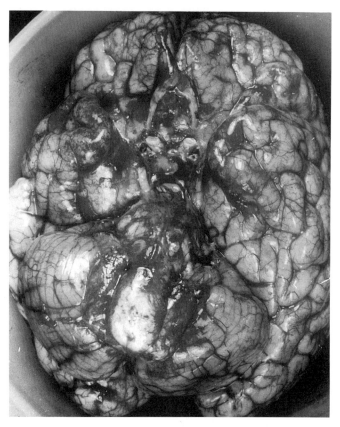

Fig. 9.2. Base of the brain from a case of fulminating pneumococcal meningitis. Petechial subarachnoid haemorrhages and severe brain swelling with foraminal herniation are evident. Frank pus formation has not occurred, though microscopy showed a neutrophil polymorph infiltrate throughout the subarachnoid space.

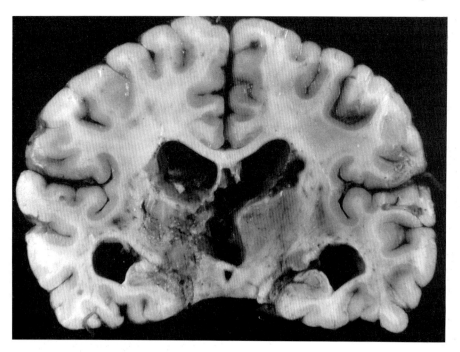

Fig. 9.3. Coronal slice across the cerebrum from a patient with a 6-week history of tuberculous meningitis. There is infarction of the left thalamus, left hippocampus and right caudate nucleus (haemorrhagic) due to arteritis. Hydrocephalus is also present. Note also inflammatory exudate in hippocampal fissures.

the fourth ventricle, and fibrosis in the subarachnoid space. The degree of hydrocephalus may be quite gross (Fig. 8.6). A second important complication is the development of multiple cerebral infarcts (Fig. 9.3), due to narrowing of, and thrombosis in, arteries affected by endarteritis obliterans (p.118; Fig. 7.23). This consists of intimal proliferation, and inflammation of all layers of the arterial wall, but particularly of the adventitia. The hydrocephalus and infarcts are readily visible to the naked eye, as is the collagenous thickening of the leptomeninges, chiefly at the base (Figs 9.4 and 9.5). The endarteritis requires microscopy to be appreciated. With infection due to organisms producing chronic meningitis, there are also likely to be microscopic granulomas. These contain lymphocytes, macrophages, plasma cells, epithelioid cells and multinucleate giant cells (Fig. 9.6). Some organisms produce more diffuse, mononuclear inflammation. Cerebral infarction is particularly common in fungal infections, when it may be due to invasion of artery walls by hyphal growth, followed by local thrombosis (Fig. 9.7). The organisms themselves can be identified with appropriate stains (Gram for bacteria, Ziehl–Neelsen for *Mycobacteria*, PAS and methenamine silver stains for fungi, Giemsa for protozoa, Levaditi for spirochaetes).

Cranial and spinal nerve roots are often inflamed and damaged in chronic meningitis (Fig. 9.8). Dorsal spinal root involvement is particularly characteristic of tertiary syphilis, and gives rise to *tabes dorsalis*. Cases of tabes are still seen, and the characteristic finding in the spinal cord is of patchy secondary degeneration of posterior column nerve fibres (Fig. 2.24b). Residual inflammation in treated cases is either sparse or absent.

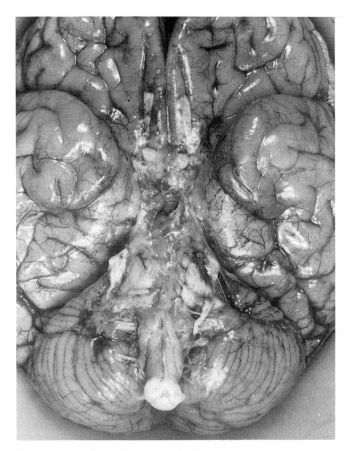

Fig. 9.4. Base of brain from a case of tuberculous meningitis. Anatomical features and the basilar artery are largely obscured by an opaque, gelatinous exudate in the subarachnoid space.

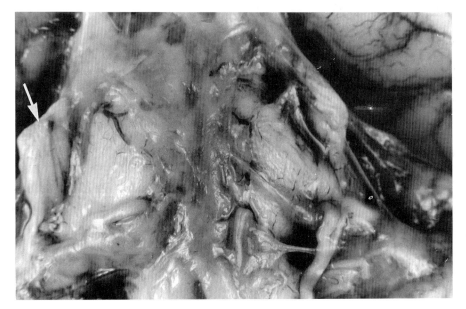

Fig. 9.5. Close-up view of the ventral surface of the pons from a case of tuberculous meningitis (same case as in Fig. 9.4). An arrow marks the stump of the right trigeminal nerve at the lateral border of the pons.

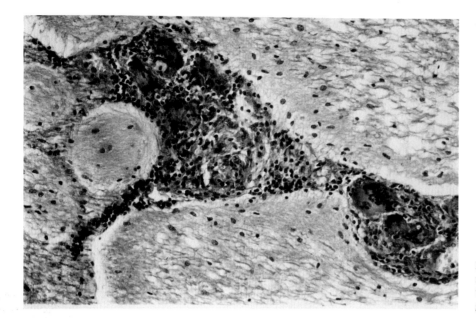

Fig. 9.6. Subarachnoid granulomas in chronic meningitis due to sarcoidosis. Inflammation takes the form of coalescing, non-caseating granulomas. H&E, ×200.

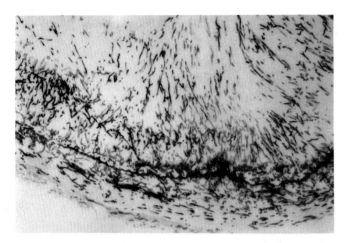

Fig. 9.7. Transverse section of a segment of artery wall from a case with arteritis due to aspergillus infection. Hyphal structures, many of them radially orientated, are shown with the methenamine silver stain. ×70. (Slide courtesy of Dr P. Gallagher.)

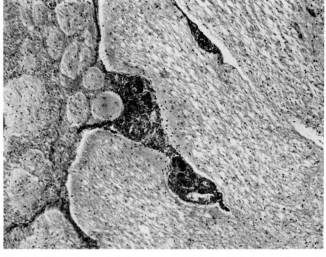

Fig. 9.8. Chronic meningitis due to sarcoidosis with inflammation and fibrosis around cranial nerve roots (left) at the base of the brain. H&E, ×60.

A granular *ependymitis* is almost invariably present in cases of chronic meningitis, since the inflammatory process reaches all the regions lying close to the CSF. The foci of granulomatous inflammation and gliosis form small nodules on ependymal surfaces (Fig. 9.9). Initially these contain inflammatory cells and reactive astrocytes (Fig. 9.10). Later on, the inflammatory cells disappear, leaving a small gliotic nodule. These nodules are caused not only by previous inflammation, but also by a variety of irritants, including blood or high-protein exudates reaching the CSF.

Chronic spinal arachnoiditis

Occasionally symptoms and signs of spinal root compression are found to be due to an *adhesive arachnoiditis* in which collagenous thickening and chronic inflammatory cell infiltration of the arachnoid occur (Fig. 9.11). In some subjects this develops after injection of radiological contrast medium, particularly Myodil, into the subarachnoid space. Sequestered remains of such material may be evident lying free or in macrophages if the opportunity arises to examine the arachnoid membrane microscopically. In other cases there is no obvious predisposing cause. Organisms are not usually identifiable.

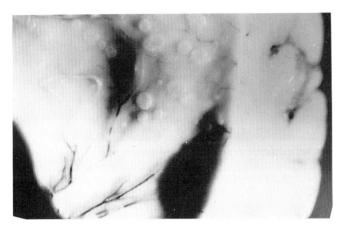

Fig. 9.9. View of the lateral ventricular surface from a case of tabes dorsalis in which there was, in addition to spinal root damage, a marked ventriculitis. Granulomatous nodules project above the normal ependyma-lined surface.

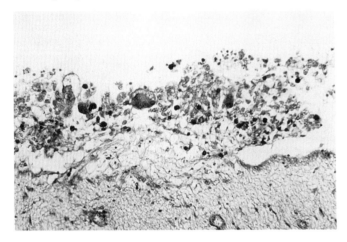

Fig. 9.10. Low-power view of a section through an ependymal granulation such as those seen in Fig. 9.9. The ependyma is disrupted and inflammatory and glial cells contribute to the cellular nodule projecting into the ventricular cavity above. H&E, ×120.

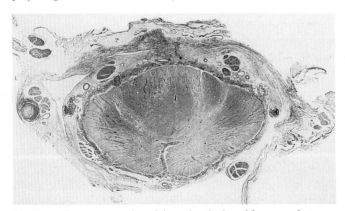

Fig. 9.11. Transverse section of thoracic spinal cord from a patient who suffered from chronic MS, and who had had a spinal myelogram 30 years before she died. There is a focal, densely fibrotic arachnoiditis enveloping the cord and roots at this level. An old, demyelinated plaque is present in the right anterolateral region of the cord. H&VG, ×8.

Subdural empyema

Pus in the subdural space usually spreads from a focus of local osteomyelitis or paranasal sinus infection. There may also be associated acute meningitis. In contrast to the subarachnoid pus present in acute meningitis, pus in the subdural space is easily wiped from the surface of the brain (Fig. 9.12). It may spread diffusely or loculate in pockets, for example alongside the falx. There is a relatively high incidence of venous sinus thrombosis associated with subdural empyema. This in turn may give rise to haemorrhagic cerebral infarction (see p.103).

Epidural abscess

This occurs around the spinal dura, and is usually caused by local spread of pyogenic infection, expecially with *Staphylococcus aureus*, from neighbouring vertebrae. Pus is liable to collect in a number of communicating pockets. Many neutrophils accumulate initially, later to be replaced by granulation tissue. Such abscesses are commonest in the thoracic region, and may extend over several segments of the spinal

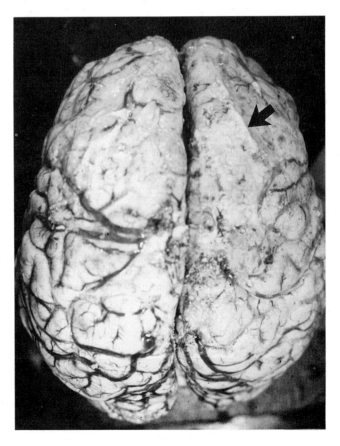

Fig. 9.12. View of the cerebral hemispheres from above in a case of acute subdural empyema. Pus forms a layer that is easily wiped from the surface of the arachnoid (arrowed).

cord. Thrombosis of spinal vessels may complicate the picture. Epidural granuloma formation is a not infrequent complication of tuberculosis of the spine.

Brain abscess

Abscesses may occur anywhere in the brain, but are particularly common in white matter. Those with a local cause have particular sites of predilection, as mentioned above. They may also be multiple, especially when the organisms are blood-borne. Initially they consist of a small focus of liquefaction necrosis, or purulent encephalitis. As this expands the centre fills with pus and a wall is formed, composed of glial fibrils and a little collagen. This wall is relatively fragile and, if the abscess is situated near the ependymal surface, may be insufficient to prevent it from rupturing into the ventricle. Almost invariably a striking degree of oedema is found surrounding a brain abscess (Fig. 9.13). The herniation to which this gives rise is often the immediate cause of death. Sections for microscopy should be taken from the abscess wall, which may be laminated, and the surrounding brain. Degenerate white blood cells, fibrin and organisms are found to occupy the abscess cavity; glial and collagen fibres, reactive astrocytes, inflammatory cells and a few fibroblasts form the capsule, and oedema and congested vessels, with swollen endothelial cells, are found in the surrounding brain. Bacteria are the organisms usually responsible for a brain abscess, but other organisms can be involved, and should be considered, particularly if bacterial cultures are negative. Bacterial abscesses often contain a mixed flora which includes anaerobic organisms. Clues to other organisms may be available; for example, free-living amoebae occasionally give rise to brain abscesses and, since

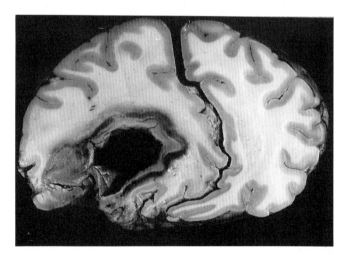

Fig. 9.13. Coronal slice through a left frontal lobe abscess. Pus at the centre had been dislodged during slicing. The dark rim separating the abscess cavity from the surrounding brain corresponds to a zone of hyperaemic blood vessels. There is surrounding oedema and marked shift of midline structures to the right.

they gain entry to the brain along the olfactory route, usually produce haemorrhagic necrosis of the olfactory bulbs, a feature not seen in cases of bacterial abscess. Some other protozoa and fungi, listed as causes of granulomas in Table 9.1, may also cause abscesses if the extent of the damage is sufficient to produce liquefaction necrosis of the brain.

Purulent encephalitis associated with subacute bacterial endocarditis

Septic emboli arising from infected heart valves occasionally give rise to solitary or multiple brain abscesses. If of sufficient size, they may also block an artery and cause cerebral infarction, which is liable to become infected by extension from the septic embolus. The presence of numerous neutrophil polymorphs in and around the edge of an infarct should raise the suspicion of this diagnosis, and a Gram stain should be performed to look for organisms. Another possible consequence of a septic embolus lodging in a cerebral artery is the development of a *mycotic aneurysm* caused by local infection and weakening of the arterial wall. This in turn may rupture, causing haemorrhage into the brain or subarachnoid space. Organisms released into the subarachnoid space may give rise to meningitis.

Granulomas

Granulomatous inflammation in the brain produces lesions which can vary in size from microscopic nodules to gross space-occupying masses. The latter form ill-defined regions of granular, yellowish, partly calcified necrosis (Fig. 9.14) They can occur anywhere, in grey or white matter, and abutting on the ventricular or pial surfaces. There is usually an associated chronic meningitis. Oedema is not usually as conspicuous as around an abscess. Microscopy should be undertaken on the granuloma itself and on neighbouring regions of the brain and meninges. The main lesions generally consist of diffusely arranged or clustered mononuclear inflammatory cells, including epithelioid cells, lymphocytes, plasma cells and frequently multinucleate giant cells. Sometimes there are well-defined granulomas (Fig. 9.15), and there may be foci of necrosis. Organisms responsible for granulomas in the CNS are varied (see Table 9.1) and attempts to identify them should rely both on culture and on appropriate stains. Remnants of parasites are responsible for some cases. Occasionally the organisms may not be evident in sections of the lesion, but serological evidence of the pathogen may be obtainable. Some organisms are confined to particular geographical locations. Information about diseases caused by such organisms can be found in Scaravilli (1984), or Brown & Voge (1982). Granulomas in immunosuppressed patients are due to a slightly different range of organisms from those with intact immunity (Table 9.1), and may be associated with impairment of antibody

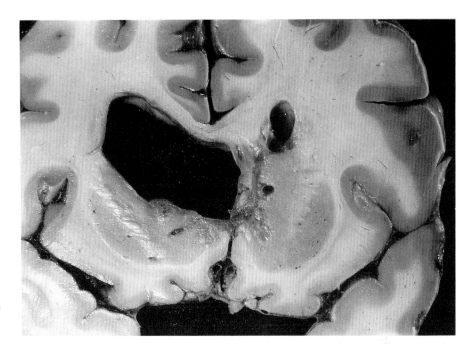

Fig. 9.14. Coronal slice across the frontal lobes from a case of sarcoidosis. There is ventricular dilatation and granular scarring in the septum and paraventricular parts of the caudate nuclei.

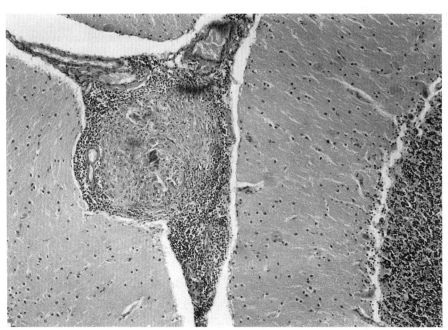

Fig. 9.15. Sarcoid granuloma with a multinucleate giant cell at its centre, in the subarachnoid space overlying the cerebellum. H&E, ×120.

production. A search for extracranial granulomas should be undertaken in any case examined post mortem.

Sarcoidosis is a rare cause of granulomatous disease of the brain and leptomeninges (Figs 9.8 and 9.14—9.16). The granulomas produced are histologically indistinguishable from those caused by identifiable pathogens, apart from the absence of organisms. The diagnosis of sarcoidosis of the CNS is one that can only be made after other causes of granulomas have been excluded, and it is supported if there was a positive Kveim test obtained during life, and if

lesions are found at characteristic sites elsewhere in the body. Some cases, however, appear to have lesions confined to the CNS and its wrappings.

Histiocytosis X

In this condition, now generally considered as a single entity, but formerly recognized as three related conditions — eosinophilic granuloma, Hand—Schüller—Christian disease, and Letterer—Siwe disease — focal granulomatous inflam-

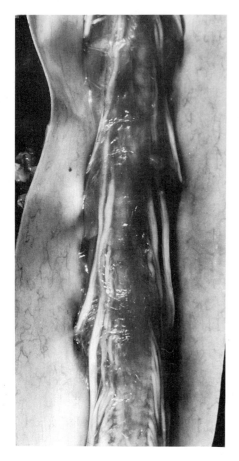

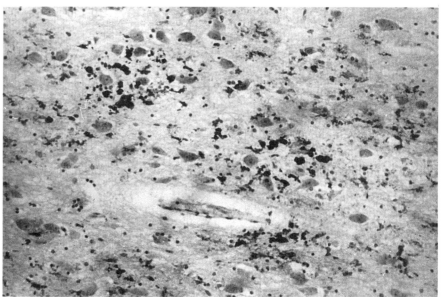

Fig. 9.16 (*left*). Posterior surface of the spinal cord and leptomeninges from a case of sarcoidosis. The leptomeninges are diffusely thickened, and have a slightly gelatinous appearance. There is also some accumulation of blood pigments, probably as the result of repeated lumbar puncture.

Fig. 9.17 (*above*). Granular, PAS-positive material in macrophages and microglia in the hypothalamus from a case of Whipple's disease. PAS stain, ×360.

mation develops at various sites, usually within the bones of the skull, the pituitary gland, meninges or brain (particularly the hypothalamus). The spinal cord and cauda equina are also occasionally involved. Inflammatory cells found in the lesions include epithelioid cells, foamy histiocytes, multinucleate cells, lymphocytes, plasma cells and interdigitating reticulum cells. Eosinophil leucocytes are abundant in *eosinophilic granuloma*, which is the most benign form of histiocytosis X.

Lymphomatoid granulomatosis

This is an unusual condition which occasionally affects the brain, and causes focal inflammatory lesions containing mononuclear inflammatory cells and obliterative changes in small blood vessels.

Whipple's disease

Whipple's disease is another rare disorder that may affect the brain and cause severe neurological abnormalities. In such cases there are deposits in the brain of macrophages laden with PAS-positive granular material (Fig. 9.17), identifiable ultrastructurally as bacteria. The organism responsible is a corynebacterium.

Further reading

Brown WJ, Voge M. 1982. *Neuropathology of Parasitic Infections.* Oxford University Press, Oxford.

Harriman DGF. 1984. Bacterial infections of the central nervous system. In Adams JH, Corsellis JAN, Duchen LW (Eds) *Greenfield's Neuropathology*, 4th edn. Edward Arnold, London, pp. 236−59.

Scaravilli F. 1984. Parasitic and fungal infections of the nervous system. In Adams JH, Corsellis JAN, Duchen LW (Eds) *Greenfield's Neuropathology*, 4th edn. Edward Arnold, London, pp. 304−37.

Chapter 10
Encephalitis and Myelitis

In this chapter we discuss various diseases that cause inflammation of the brain. In many of these conditions the inflammatory process also involves the meninges so that the condition produced is a meningoencephalitis. If the white matter is preferentially involved, the term leucoencephalitis is used, while polioencephalitis denotes inflammation predominantly affecting the grey matter. Inflammation of the spinal cord is referred to as myelitis, and of the brain and spinal cord as encephalomyelitis.

Table 10.1. Organisms causing human encephalitis and meningoencephalitis

Viruses
Herpes simplex
Herpes zoster
Cytomegalovirus (in immunocompromised subjects or fetus)
Herpes B virus (after monkey bite — very rare)
Enteroviruses (e.g. polio)
Adenoviruses (rare)
Paramyxoviruses (e.g. SSPE and immunosuppressive measles encephalitis)
Rabies
Lymphocytic choriomeningitis virus
JC papovavirus (in immunocompromised subjects) (PML)
Arthropod-borne viruses
Rubella (fetus and newborn)
Human immunodeficiency virus (HIV) (AIDS)

Rickettsiae
Typhus or typhus-like fevers
Q fever

Parasites
Plasmodium
Toxoplasma (in newborn and immunocompromised)
Trypanosomes

The tempo of encephalitic diseases varies from acute, even fulminating, causing death within a few days, to indolent and progressive over months or years. Acute forms present with combinations of headache, signs of raised intracranial pressure, particularly drowsiness or coma, epilepsy, and variable focal neurological signs. Subacute encephalitis clinically tends to combine features of epilepsy and progressive focal neurological signs of widespread CNS disease. Most cases of encephalitis are either infective or allergic in origin; of the infective agents involved, viruses form the most important group in western countries (Table 10.1). Occasionally the possibility of infection may not have been considered clinically, and such cases can only be resolved satisfactorily if the pathologist is alert to this possible aetiology and takes appropriate specimens for microbiology and microscopy. Even if infection has been considered likely by the clinicians concerned, it is frequently not possible to confirm the diagnosis until a post mortem examination is performed. Opportunistic viral infections such as cytomegalovirus and JC papovavirus need to be considered, mainly in adults who have been immunosuppressed; likewise with measles encephalitis in immunosuppressed children.

Viral encephalitis

In contrast to bacteria and fungi, viruses depend for replication on the presence of suitable host cells. Aseptic meningitis due to viral infection is well recognized and relatively common, but generally self-limiting, so that pathologists are seldom required to investigate such cases. The commonest identified cause of viral meningitis is mumps. Viral encephalitis and myelitis, due to infection of cells of the brain and spinal cord, tend to produce more serious disease, though the extent of the damage produced is extremely variable. The range of viruses pathogenic to the nervous system is extensive. Some gain entry to the brain via the bloodstream (e.g. arboviruses), whereas others take a neural route to the CNS after initial replication in extraneural tissues and uptake into peripheral nerves (e.g. rabies).

Post mortem examination in cases of suspected viral encephalitis

At post mortem examination an aseptic technique should be adopted, and specimens should be taken for microbiology and EM before fixing the brain and spinal cord in formalin. In cases of suspected Creutzfeldt—Jakob disease, which is associated with the presence of a transmissible agent (which does not, however, cause an encephalitis) special precautions are needed, and these are described on p.266.

Close liaison with clinical colleagues and microbiologists is important to ensure that specimens for culture and EM are taken from the most appropriate sites, preferably from CNS tissues that appear inflamed but not frankly necrotic. Throat swabs and samples of faeces should be sent for viral culture as well as samples from the CNS and CSF. CSF and serum samples should also be collected for estimation of viral antibody titres. A rise in the serum antibody titre to a particular virus is not by itself sufficient evidence to implicate that virus as the cause of encephalitis. However, by comparing antibody titres in CSF with those in serum it is possible to find out if intrathecal synthesis of antibody to a specific virus has taken place. If it has, this is good evidence for the presence of the virus within the CNS, even when attempts to culture the virus are unsuccessful. In viral encephalitis there is usually also evidence of oligoclonal immunoglobulin in the CSF, but this is a less specific indicator of an infective aetiology than finding evidence of intrathecal viral antibody, as oligoclonal immunoglobulin is also produced in some conditions not known to have viral aetiology, such as MS.

Macroscopic examination of the CNS and choice of blocks for microscopy

On naked-eye inspection of the brain from a case of viral encephalitis there may be little abnormality of note. If the illness was acute, there is likely to be some generalized swelling and congestion, possibly with a few petechial hae-morrhages on the pial surface. The meninges may be slightly cloudy. Herpes simplex encephalitis is exceptional in that there are usually extensive and severe macroscopic abnor-malities, with, in the acute phase, swelling, haemorrhage and softening centred on one or both temporal lobes (Fig. 10.1). If the patient survives until months or years later there is destruction and collapse of the same regions (Fig. 10.2). In chronic forms of encephalitis there is likely to be some degree of cerebral atrophy, granular discoloration of the white matter, and fibrous thickening of the leptomeninges (Fig. 10.3). Secondary effects of encephalitis, such as venous thrombosis and infarction, uncal herniation with infarction in posterior cerebral artery territory, or effects of prolonged and repeated epileptic fits, may be present and must not be allowed to divert attention from the underlying disease.

Biopsy specimens from cases of suspected encephalitis

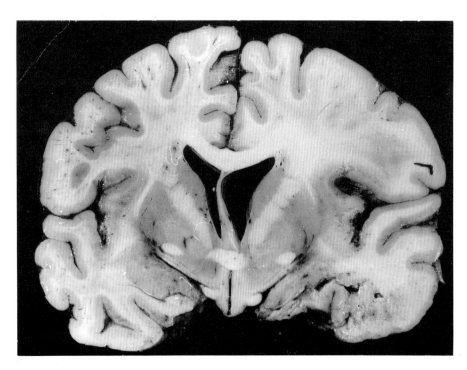

Fig. 10.1. Coronal slice through the temporal and frontal lobes of the brain from a case of acute herpes simplex encephalitis. There is softening and necrosis of medial and inferior parts of the temporal lobes, more extensive on the right. The insula is also affected on both sides. The right cerebral hemisphere is swollen, causing a shift of midline structures to the left, and a downthrust of diencephalic structures. The slight dilatation of the right lateral ventricle has resulted from compression of the third ventricle and foramen of Munro.

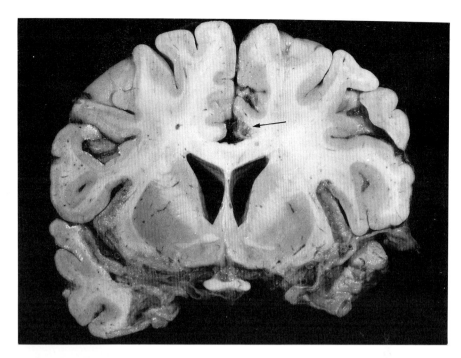

Fig. 10.2. Coronal slice through the temporal and frontal lobes of the brain from a patient dying 8 weeks from onset of herpes simplex encephalitis. At this stage oedema has subsided, and there is collapse of the affected parts, in this case the whole of the temporal lobe and insula on the right, and medial and superior aspects of the temporal lobe and the insula on the left. Note also necrosis of the right cingulate gyrus (arrowed).

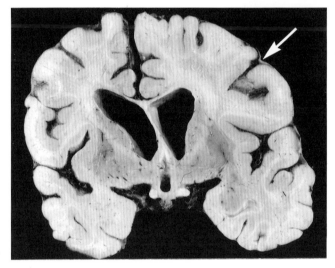

Fig. 10.3. Coronal slice through the frontal and temporal lobes of the brain from a case of subacute sclerosing panencephalitis (SSPE) in which the disease lasted 7½ years. Note marked, generalized atrophy with ventricular enlargement, grey discoloration of cerebral white matter, severe narrowing of the corpus callosum and leptomeningeal thickening (arrowed).

should be divided under aseptic conditions to provide samples for microbiology, EM and histology, as described in Chapter 4 (p.83).

When preparing blocks for microscopy from post mortem cases, samples should be taken from areas which appear normal as well as from those that are obviously abnormal, and from transition zones in between. Samples from each major cerebral lobe, hippocampus, basal ganglia, thalamus and several levels of the brain stem and cerebellum should

be taken, and whenever possible samples should also be examined from cervical, thoracic and lumbar levels of the spinal cord and from dorsal root ganglia. This wide sampling of the CNS is necessary because, although the *type* of damage caused by viral infections tends to be stereotyped, the location and distribution of the damage is often characteristic of particular viruses. Further information can be gained from a search for inclusion bodies, though these are rarely pathognomonic in isolation. The most reliable evidence about the cause of encephalitis comes from culture of a specific organism, and from the use of immunohistological studies used to detect the presence of specific viral antigens. Immunoenzyme techniques can demonstrate a variety of viral antigens if high-titre specific antisera or monoclonal antibodies are applied to sections of formalin-fixed, paraffin-embedded tissues (Figs 10.4 and 10.12). In acute viral encephalitis the chance of detecting viral antigens is much greater at the start of the illness, and they are likely to be detectable for no more than a few weeks at most, and often for only a few days. Methods for the detection of viral-specific nucleic acid sequences are now coming into use for diagnosis. The *in situ hybridization* technique can be used not only on frozen but also on paraffin sections (Burns *et al*. 1986). However, as viral nucleic acid sequences have been detected in several studies in material from normal brains, the use of these highly sensitive probes for diagnosis of active viral infection of the nervous system needs further study before it is adopted routinely. It should be remembered that the mere presence of viral nucleic acid in a cell is not evidence of active, pathogenic infection, particularly in the case of viruses that are known to be able to establish latent infections in the nervous system. Demonstration of viral

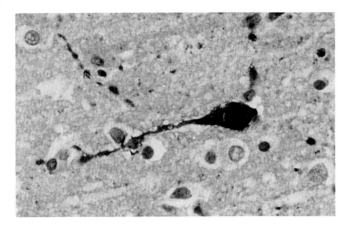

Fig. 10.4. Measles virus antigen demonstrated in neuron nucleus, cytoplasm and processes by application of a rabbit antiserum to measles virus to a paraffin section of cerebral cortex from a case of SSPE. Peroxidase reaction with weak haematoxylin counterstain, ×570.

protein antigens or culture of virus remain, in our opinion, the most reliable tools for diagnosing most forms of viral encephalitis.

Pathological features common to most forms of viral encephalitis

Cell death or alterations

Most viruses causing encephalitis produce lysis of host cells, though the extent of this is variable, and the cell types affected differ. In most instances neurons are killed, an event which attracts to the site a group of phagocytic cells

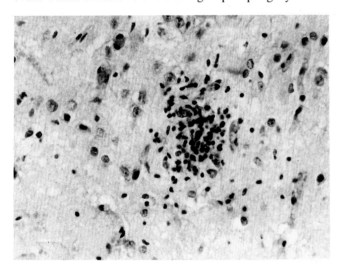

Fig. 10.5. Focus of neuronophagia in the cerebral cortex from a patient with a renal transplant, on immunosuppressive therapy. The clinical history did not suggest any neurological disease, but post mortem examination of the brain showed scattered foci such as this in the cerebrum and cerebellum, one of which was associated with a typical CMV inclusion body in a neuron (Fig. 10.8). H&E, ×180.

whose role is to ingest the debris. This process is called neuronophagia (Fig. 3.13). Neuronophagic cell clusters should be carefully searched for in grey matter. They are most conspicuous when considerable numbers of large neurons are killed more or less simultaneously, as occurs, for example, in acute poliomyelitis. When cell death is less selective, involving not only neurons but also glial cells, frank tissue necrosis is seen, as in acute herpes simplex encephalitis. Cell death may also occur on a relatively small scale and over an extended period of time, as in subacute sclerosing panencephalitis (SSPE), or in the glial nodule encephalitis which occurs in some immunosuppressed patients (Fig. 10.5). In these cases neuronophagia may be found only after prolonged searching.

Cell structure may be altered without cell lysis in some forms of encephalitis. Examples of such change are the development of neurofibrillary tangles in some neurons in SSPE, and of bizarre changes in astrocyte nuclei in progressive multifocal leucoencephalopathy (PML) (Fig. 3.21).

Inclusion bodies

These are also alterations of cell structure which occur in a number of viral infections. They usually contain virus-coded material. Most characteristic are Negri bodies, cytoplasmic inclusions found in neurons in rabies. They consist of one or several hyaline eosinophilic bodies lying close to the nucleus (Fig. 10.6). Round or oval, intranuclear, eosinophilic inclusion bodies, larger than nucleoli, and usually surrounded by a halo of clear nucleoplasm, are found in neurons and oligodendrocyte nuclei in SSPE and 'immunosuppressive' measles encephalitis (Cowdry type A inclusions) (Fig. 10.7). They are also sometimes present in neurons in herpes simplex encephalitis. Large intranuclear inclusion bodies are seen in the brain in adult and congenital CMV infection (Figs 10.8 and 21.14; see p.328). Basophilic, enlarged oligodendrocyte nuclei are present in PML (Fig. 10.31).

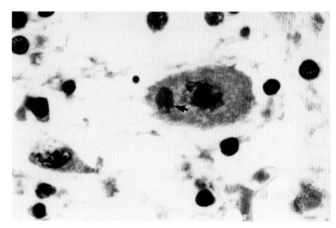

Fig. 10.6. Negri body (arrowed) in the cytoplasm of a cerebellar Purkinje cell from a case of rabies. H&E, ×760.

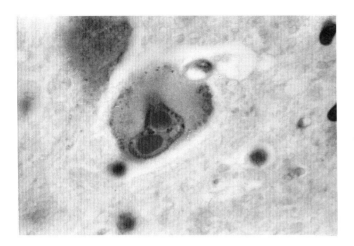

Fig. 10.7. Intranuclear eosinophilic inclusion bodies surrounded by a pale halo in cortical neurons from a case of immunosuppressive measles encephalitis. H&E, ×650.

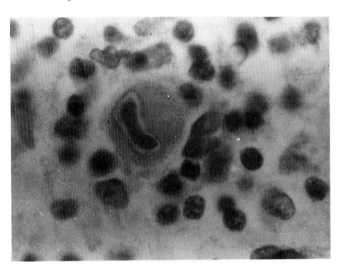

Fig. 10.8. Intranuclear inclusion body in a neuron in the dentate nucleus of the cerebellum from a patient with a renal transplant (same patient as in Fig. 10.5). H&E, ×740.

Inflammation

Inflammatory cell infiltration, oedema and congestion occur in the brain in all forms of acute viral encephalitis. Initially the infiltrating cells are neutrophil polymorphs, but these are replaced within two or three days by mononuclear inflammatory cells. Some petechial or larger haemorrhages are also common, particularly in herpes simplex encephalitis. After 10–15 days plasma cells become prominent in addition to lymphocytes and macrophages. These inflammatory cells form dense cuffs of cells in perivascular spaces and also extend into neighbouring brain parenchyma (Figs 3.16 and 10.9). The leptomeninges also contain some inflammatory cells (Fig. 10.10). Inflammation persists for months or even years after an episode of acute encephalitis, though in

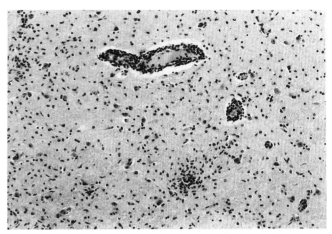

Fig. 10.9. Encephalitic focus in the thalamus from an 8-year-old child with a 2-week history of acute meningoencephalitis associated with serological evidence of Coxsackie infection. There is perivascular cuffing with mononuclear inflammatory cells, and parenchymal microglial and lymphocytic infiltrates. H&E, ×160.

diminishing amount. In persistent infection, such as in SSPE, the cuffing continues to be prominent. In immunosuppressed patients it is reduced or absent even in the presence of abundant viral antigen.

Glial reaction

Microglial cells show an increase in size and number in viral encephalitis (Fig. 3.23b). The microglial reaction is greatest at sites of maximum damage, but also occurs in a much more widespread distribution. Astrocytes also show reactive change in and around sites of damage, and later on produce dense glial scars. Focal accentuation of astrocytic and microglial reactions, termed glial nodules, are particularly characteristic of viral encephalitis.

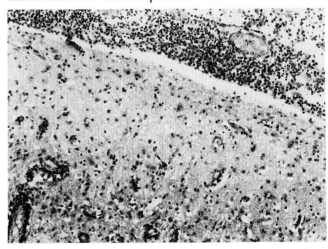

Fig. 10.10. Cortex and leptomeninges (top right) from a case of acute herpes simplex encephalitis. There is an intense mononuclear inflammatory cell infiltrate in the leptomeninges as well as in the cortex. H&E, ×140.

Histological features of specific forms of viral encephalitis

Some of the types and locations of lesions characteristic of specific viral infections are given below (see also Fig. 10.11). For further details see Booss & Esiri (1986).

Herpes simplex encephalitis (type 1) (Figs 4.30, 10.1, 10.2, 10.10, 10.12 and 10.13)

Sites of most severe damage: both temporal lobes, one usually being more affected than the other; under-surfaces of frontal lobes, insula, cingulate gyrus, amygdala, hippocampus. Very rarely there is a primary brain stem encephalitis.

For neonatal infection with the type 2 virus see p.329.

Histological features: intense perivascular and parenchymal inflammation, oedema and necrosis, particularly in the cerebral cortex, maximal in the first few weeks, diminishing gradually over succeeding months; inflammation also in leptomeninges and subcortical white matter; inclusion bodies may be present in neuron nuclei in the first week or two; viral antigen is demonstrable in neuron and glial cytoplasm and nuclei in the first few weeks; herpes virions are detectable by EM in the first few weeks.

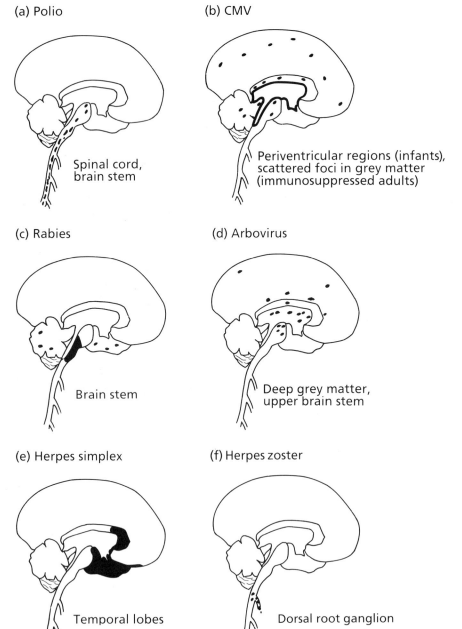

(a) Polio — Spinal cord, brain stem

(b) CMV — Periventricular regions (infants), scattered foci in grey matter (immunosuppressed adults)

(c) Rabies — Brain stem

(d) Arbovirus — Deep grey matter, upper brain stem

(e) Herpes simplex — Temporal lobes

(f) Herpes zoster — Dorsal root ganglion

Fig. 10.11. Variations in topographical sites of maximal damage to the nervous system in different viral infections.

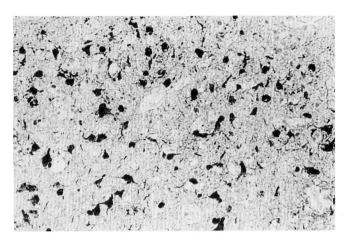

Fig. 10.12. Demonstration of herpes simplex (type 1) virus antigen in cerebral cortex in acute herpes simplex encephalitis using the immunoperoxidase technique. There is infection of many neurons and glial cells. Haematoxylin counterstain, ×105.

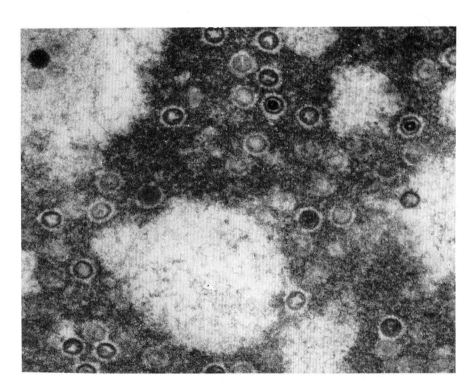

Fig. 10.13. Intranuclear particles of herpes virions in acute herpes simplex encephalitis. Uranyl acetate and lead citrate, ×57660.

Herpes zoster (Figs 10.14–10.16; see also p.339)

Sites of most severe damage: spinal or cranial sensory ganglia and nerve related to dermatome of skin eruption; spinal cord or brain stem at the same level shows milder changes; occasionally associated thrombosis in nearby major cerebral artery.

Histological features: acute, intense inflammation, congestion and sometimes haemorrhage in one or more ganglia initially, with degeneration of sensory neurons; wallerian degeneration and inflammation in segmental nerve; milder inflammation in CNS at the same segmental level and in adjacent ganglia; viral antigen and herpes virions demonstrable in ganglion and nerve in the first few days only; granulomatous arteritis or thrombosis in the major cerebral artery ipsilateral to the site of cranial zoster occasionally occurs a little later, and in these cases herpes virions or viral antigen may be demonstrable in cells of the media of the vessel wall. In immunosuppressed patients varicella zoster virus occasionally causes a multifocal, generally periventricular, demyelinating disease with inclusions in oligodendrocyte nuclei.

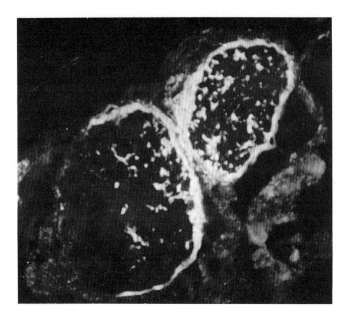

Fig. 10.14. Demonstration of Varicella zoster virus antigen by immunofluorescence using a rabbit antiserum on a frozen section of frontal nerve from a case of acute ophthalmic zoster. ×60.

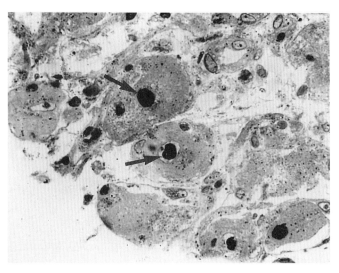

Fig. 10.15. Semi-thin, resin-embedded section from the trigeminal ganglion from a case of acute ophthalmic zoster. Intranuclear inclusion bodies are present in some neurons (examples arrowed). Toluidine blue, ×280.

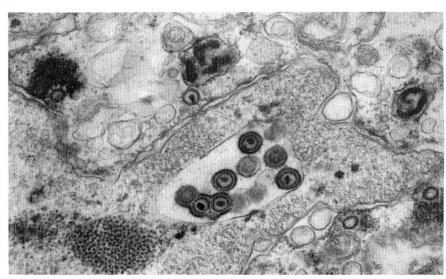

Fig. 10.16. Varicella zoster virions in trigeminal neurons from the case illustrated in Figs 10.14 and 10.15. Uranyl acetate and lead citrate, ×43 800.

Cytomegalovirus (CMV) (Figs 10.5, 10.8 and 21.13–15; see also p.328)

Sites of most severe damage: in congenital infection see p.328; in immunosuppressed adults, patchy foci scattered throughout grey matter of the brain.

Histological features: in congenital infection see p.328; in adults, foci of neuronophagia; intranuclear inclusion bodies occasionally identifiable; virus detectable with antisera using immunoperoxidase technique.

Herpes B virus (very rare)

Sites of most severe damage: spinal cord or brain stem segment related to the site of a monkey bite.

Histological features: intense inflammation and necrosis with petechial haemorrhages and neuronophagia; inclusion bodies in neurons and oligodendrocytes.

Epstein–Barr (EB) virus

In rare, fatal cases the brain usually shows generalized oedema, with no more than an occasional, sparse perivascular inflammatory cell infiltrate.

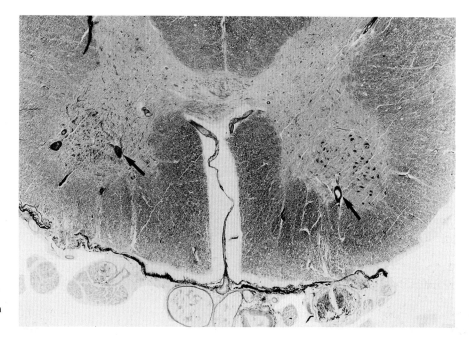

Fig. 10.17. Low-power view of cervical cord section from a case of acute poliomyelitis. Note intense perivascular cuffing in both anterior grey horns (arrowed) and destruction of motor neurons on the left. LBCV, ×14.

Rabies (Fig. 10.6)

Sites of most severe damage: brain stem, especially grey matter of the pons and medulla; also hypothalamus, and in spinal paralytic form, spinal cord and dorsal root ganglia; milder changes in thalamus, basal ganglia, hippocampus, cerebral cortex and cerebellum.

Histological features: intense congestion with petechial haemorrhage, moderate inflammation, neuronophagia, little astrocytic reaction; Negri inclusion bodies, most easily found in large neurons, especially pyramidal cells of the hippocampus, and Purkinje cells of the cerebellum (but not invariably present). Viral antigen detectable in formalin-fixed material with widespread distribution; also present in peripheral nerves and salivary glands, etc. Virus particles visible by EM in Negri bodies and elsewhere in neurons.

Poliomyelitis (Figs 2.25c, 10.17 and 10.18)

Sites of most severe damage: anterior horns, with spread into adjacent grey and white matter of the spinal cord, maximal at segmental levels worst affected clinically; brain stem grey matter, especially the reticular formation, is also usually affected in severe cases, with milder changes in hypothalamus, precentral motor cortex and dentate nuclei of the cerebellum.

Histological features: congestion and intense inflammation with neuronophagia in the first few weeks, gradually diminishing over the next few months. Years later there is loss of anterior horn cells, residual gliosis, wasting of anterior nerve roots and profound atrophy of groups of muscle fibres in affected muscles. Identical lesions rarely occur with other enterovirus infections.

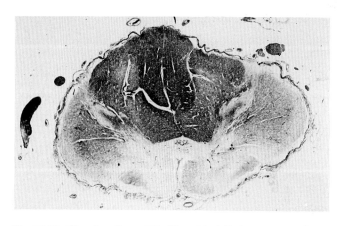

Fig. 10.18. Chronic poliomyelitis. The subject died many years after the acute illness. This low-power view of the cervical cord shows shrinkage of the anterior grey horns and pallor of anterolateral white matter. Myelin stain.

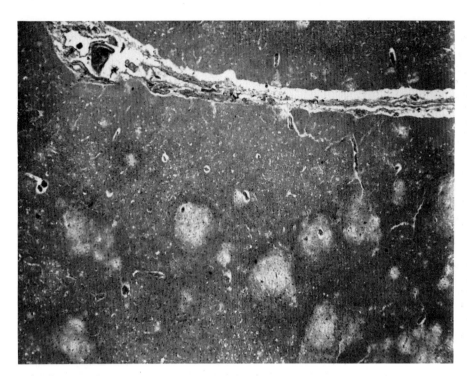

Fig. 10.19. Japanese B encephalitis. Low-power view of the late-stage appearance showing the cerebral cortex surrounding a sulcus, with numerous, acellular, necrotic foci scattered in the cortex. H&E, ×38. (Slide courtesy of Prof. R. Iizuka.)

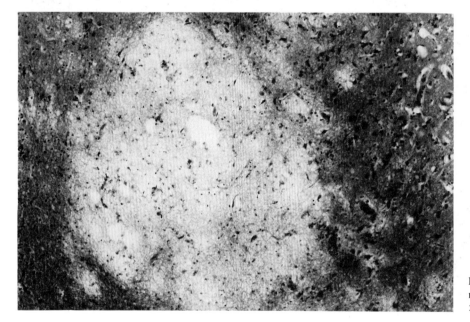

Fig. 10.20. Higher power view of one of the necrotic foci illustrated in Fig. 10.19. H&E, ×250.

Arbovirus (arthropod-borne virus) (Figs 10.19 and 10.20)

Sites of most severe damage: grey matter of the basal ganglia, thalamus and hypothalamus; also upper brain stem, cerebral cortex and cerebellum; occasionally cervical spinal cord.

Histological features: congestion, inflammation and neuronophagia at the acute stage; some acellular foci of necrosis which persist.

Lymphocytic choriomeningitis

Sites of most severe damage: spinal cord, brain stem, cerebral cortex and/or subcortical white matter; meninges always prominently affected.

Histological features: parenchymal necrosis, and intense inflammation of meninges and underlying CNS; viral antigen has been demonstrated in frozen sections.

Plate 6

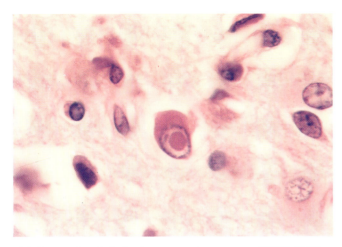

6.1. Intranuclear inclusion in a neuron from a case of SSPE. H&E ×900.

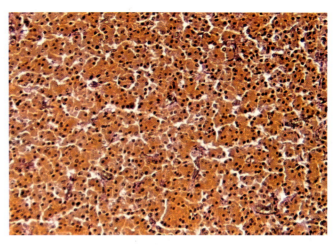

6.2. Intermingled eosinophil and chromophobe cells in a growth-hormone-secreting pituitary adenoma. Orange G/PAS, ×150.

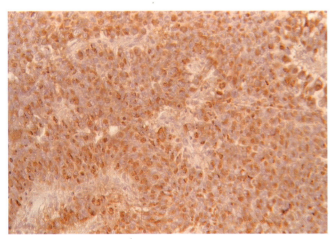

6.3. Prolactin-secreting chromophobe pituitary adenoma. The section has been treated with a prolactin antiserum, and demonstrates reaction product in all the tumour cells (brown). Immunoperoxidase with haematoxylin counterstain, ×100.

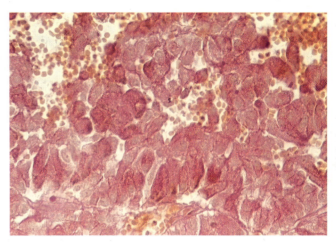

6.4. Basophil tumour cells in an ACTH-secreting pituitary adenoma. Orange G/PAS, ×500.

Plates 6.5 and 6.6 overleaf

Plate 6 cont.

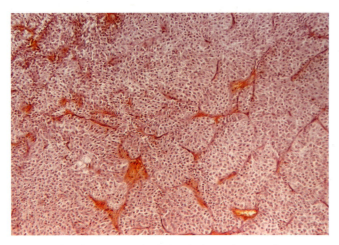

6.5. Non-functioning, chromophobe pituitary adenoma. Orange G/PAS, ×150.

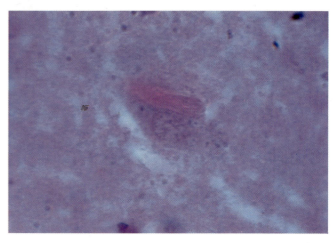

6.6. Hirano body (pink) lying adjacent to a hippocampal pyramidal neuron. H&E, ×800.

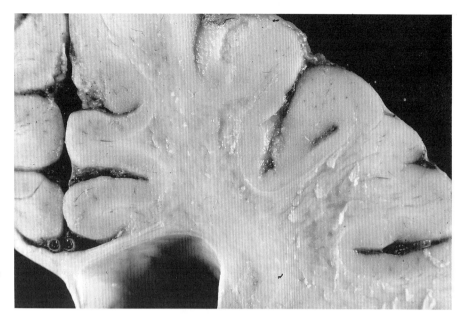

Fig. 10.21. Close-up view of cerebral white matter in a coronal slice through the cerebrum from a case of SSPE with an illness duration of 7 years. Note grey discoloration of the white matter, which has an altered, rubbery texture.

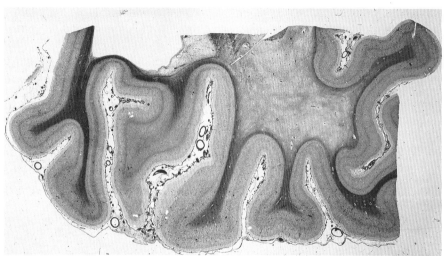

Fig. 10.22. Low-power view of a section of the occipital lobe cortex and white matter from a case of SSPE. There is marked pallor of myelin staining in the white matter. LBCV, ×2.5.

Subacute sclerosing panencephalitis (SSPE) (Figs 10.3, 10.4, 10.21–10.23 and Plate 6.1)

Sites of most severe damage: widespread in cerebral cortex, white matter and brain stem. In some cases grey matter is worst affected, in others white matter.

Histological features: widespread subacute inflammation with many lymphocytes, plasma cells and macrophages, marked astrocytic and microglial reactions, neuronophagia, neuron and oligodendrocyte loss and loss of myelin in white matter; inclusion bodies in oligodendrocyte and neuron nuclei; measles virus antigen demonstrable in formalin-fixed material by immunoperoxidase technique in cells with inclusion bodies and other neurons and oligodendrocytes; paramyxovirus nucleocapsids present in nuclei by EM in cells with inclusion bodies.

Immunosuppressive measles encephalitis (Figs 10.7, 10.24 and 10.25)

Changes are similar to those of SSPE, but there is less myelin damage and astrocytic reaction, and very little inflammation.

Note that both SSPE and 'immunosuppressive' measles encephalitis are rare complications of measles infection. The most frequent CNS complication of measles infection is perivenous encephalomyelitis (p.154).

Progressive rubella encephalitis

Sites of most severe damage: cerebrum, especially cerebral white matter, and cerebellum.

Histological features: widespread subacute inflammation

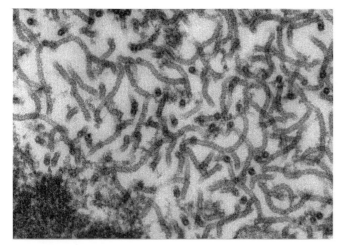

Fig. 10.23. Intranuclear nucleocapsids from the brain of a case of SSPE. Uranyl acetate and lead citrate, ×87 500. (Photograph courtesy of Mrs J. E. Richmond.)

with mononuclear cells, microglial and astrocytic reaction, diffuse myelin loss, cerebellar atrophy with Purkinje and granule cell loss; amorphous basophilic deposits in parenchyma and blood vessel walls, sometimes with calcification. For congenital rubella infection of the brain without progressive features see p.328.

Progressive multifocal leucoencephalopathy (PML: Richardson's disease) (Figs 10.26–10.33)

Sites of most severe damage: multiple foci in cerebrum, especially at junction of cortex and white matter, and in white matter; cerebellar white matter, or brain stem.

Histological features: multiple small rounded foci of demyelination; sometimes larger, irregular areas probably formed by coalescence of smaller ones; these foci lack normal oligodendrocytes but contain reactive astrocytes and variable

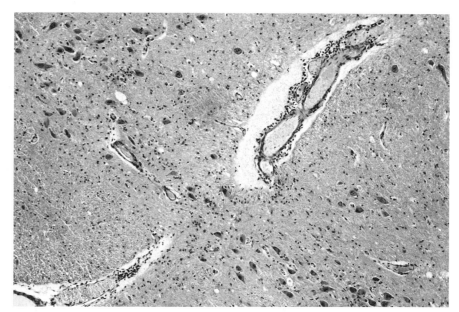

Fig. 10.24. Midbrain section from a case of immunosuppressive measles encephalitis. There is sparse perivascular inflammation and some loss of cells in the substantia nigra, seen traversing the figure from top left to bottom right. H&E, ×120.

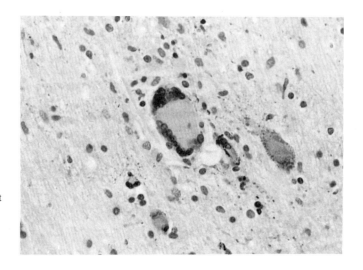

Fig. 10.25. Multinucleate giant cell in the hypothalamus from a case of immunosuppressive measles encephalitis. There is a focal reaction for measles antigen at the periphery of the cell, close to the nuclei. Immunoperoxidase reaction with rabbit antimeasles serum, counterstained with haematoxylin, ×360.

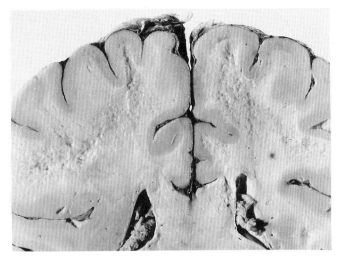

Fig. 10.26. Progressive multifocal leucoencephalopathy (PML). Coronal slice through the cerebrum at the level of the splenium of the corpus callosum, showing multifocal areas of discoloration, necrosis and pitting of the white matter.

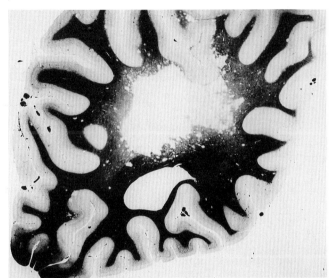

Fig. 10.27. Low-power view of myelin-stained section of the left parieto-occipital region from a case of PML. There is a large, irregular area of confluent demyelination in the white matter. Several small, satellite foci of demyelination are seen just beyond the margin of the large lesion.

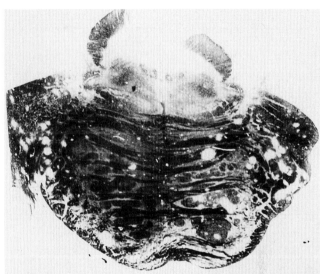

Fig. 10.28. Low-power view of myelin-stained section of the pons from a case of PML showing multiple small foci of demyelination. ×2.

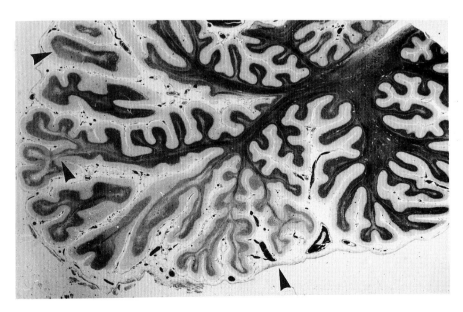

Fig. 10.29. Low-power view of myelin-stained section of the cerebellum from a case of PML. Multiple foci of granule cell loss and myelin pallor are present (arrow heads).

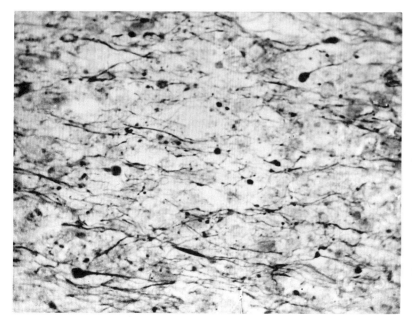

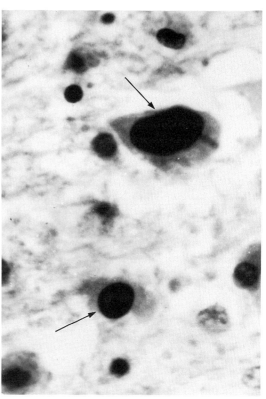

Fig. 10.30 (*above*). Axon stain showing appearances in a demyelinated focus in PML. Many axons survive, but some show fragmentation and end-bulb formation. Holmes stain, ×300.

Fig. 10.31 (*right*). Homogeneous, basophilic inclusions in enlarged oligodendrocyte nuclei in PML (arrowed). H&E, ×900.

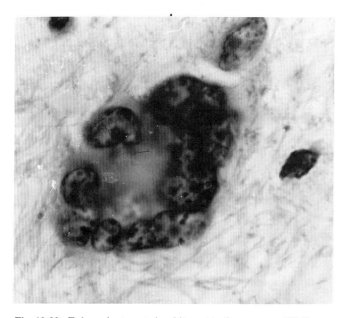

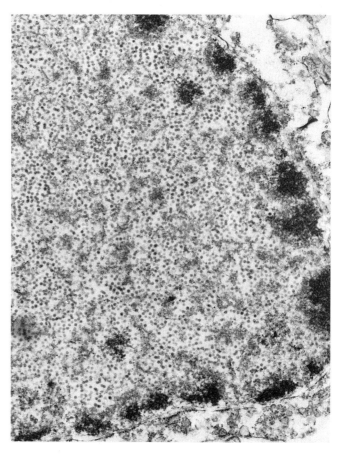

Fig. 10.32. Enlarged astrocyte in white matter from a case of PML. The cell contains several large nuclei. H&E, ×1590.

Fig. 10.33 (*right*). Part of the nucleus from the edge of a demyelinated lesion of PML. The nucleus is packed with papovavirus particles. Uranyl acetate and lead citrate, ×27 000.

numbers of microglial cells and macrophages containing neutral fat; enlarged basophilic oligodendrocyte nuclei are found at the margins of the lesions; astrocytes in the demyelinated foci and elsewhere may contain pleomorphic nuclei and are sometimes multinucleate; demyelinated foci contain surviving axons; foci of granule cell loss occur in the cerebellum; papovavirus antigens may be demonstrable in frozen sections, and papovavirus particles are visible by EM in oligodendrocyte nuclear inclusions.

Human immunodeficiency virus (HIV: acquired immune deficiency syndrome (AIDS)) (Figs 10.34–10.36)

HIV-specific nucleic acid and viral antigens have been demonstrated in the brain in AIDS patients with neurological symptoms. The predominant cell types containing the virus seem to be macrophages, or multinucleated giant cells probably derived from them (Koenig *et al.* 1986; Wiley *et al.* 1986). A diffuse encephalopathy is one of the commonest findings and this has been attributed to the effects of the virus. It is characterized by diffuse loss or focal loss of myelin, particularly in cerebral white matter, with a lesser degree of axonal loss (Navia *et al.* 1986), and in some cases vacuolar change and rarefaction of the tissue. There may also be a myelopathy, particularly of the upper spinal cord, with pallor and vacuolation in the myelin sheaths of the white matter. There is only sparse lymphocytic inflammation, or else an absence of inflammatory cells associated with these lesions, except that multinucleate giant cells may be found in perivascular spaces in affected areas and in basal ganglia. HIV particles have been shown by EM in such

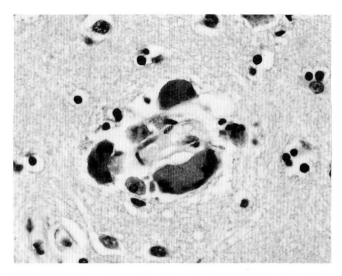

Fig. 10.35. Perivascular multinucleate giant cells in the basal ganglia region from a case of AIDS encephalopathy. In contrast to those illustrated in Fig. 10.33, these cells contain intracytoplasmic pigment. H&E, ×360. (Section courtesy of Dr B. Horten.)

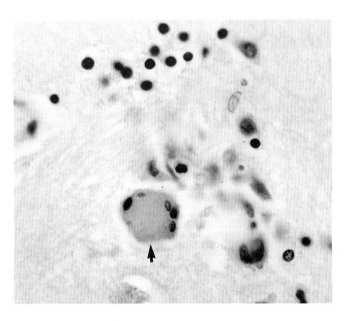

Fig. 10.34. Perivascular multinucleate giant cells (arrowed) in the basal ganglia region from a case of AIDS encephalopathy. H&E, ×340.

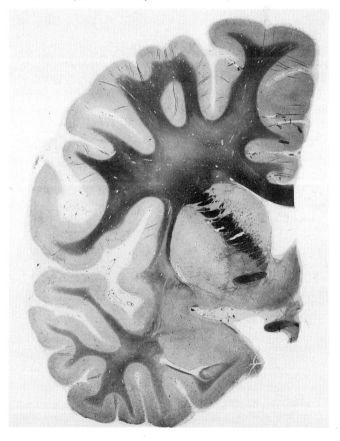

Fig. 10.36. Low-power view of a myelin-stained section showing caudate nucleus, putamen and neighbouring white matter. In contrast to the normal intensity of myelin staining, seen in the corpus callosum and internal capsule, diffuse pallor is seen in the main cerebral white matter.

cells. This encephalopathy is seen in children with AIDS as well as in adults (Epstein *et al.* 1985) (see also p.329). Areas that are most at risk for HIV-associated encephalopathy, and therefore the areas that should be examined to establish the diagnosis, are the central cerebral white matter, amygdala, hippocampus, putamen, and frontal and temporal cortex (de la Monte *et al.* 1987). In addition, AIDS sufferers frequently develop CNS lesions caused by other pathogens, most frequently a glial nodule encephalitis probably due to CMV, though this may be due to the HIV itself in some cases, and PML. Also described is a myelitis associated with the presence in the CNS of herpes simplex type 2. Toxoplasmosis (p.158) and cryptococcal infection (Chapter 9) commonly occur in the brain in AIDS sufferers, but these infections are associated more with focal symptoms and signs of neurological disease than with diffuse encephalopathy or dementia. Peripheral neuropathy with inflammation and demyelination (p.337) or axonal degeneration also occurs quite commonly in AIDS, and CNS lymphoma (p.193) has a higher incidence in AIDS sufferers and other immunodeficient individuals than in the general population.

Allergic encephalitis

Allergic encephalitis was first encountered at the end of the nineteenth century when it was found to be a not uncommon complication of the use of Pasteur's vaccine against rabies. It also occurred in a small proportion of subjects vaccinated against smallpox, and still occurs following certain exanthematous diseases, particularly measles. The condition is thought to be due to an immune attack directed against myelin, and the most severe lesions occur in white matter. It may also occur after non-specific upper respiratory tract and gastrointestinal infections, or occur apparently 'out of the

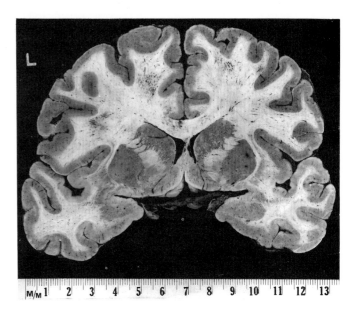

Fig. 10.37. Coronal slice through the heads of the caudate nuclei from a case of acute haemorrhagic leucoencephalitis. Small petechial haemorrhages are present in the cerebral white matter and corpus callosum.

blue'. Two variants of allergic encephalitis are recognized: an acute form, with pathological features which we shall refer to as *perivenous encephalomyelitis* (PVEM), and a hyperacute form known as *acute haemorrhagic leucoencephalitis* (Hurst's disease; AHLE). They are both acute diseases with a clinical history lasting only a matter of days in some fatal cases, and with a slow and often incomplete recovery if the patient survives. There are no confirmatory laboratory tests and the clinical diagnosis is sometimes missed, especially if there is no preceding febrile illness.

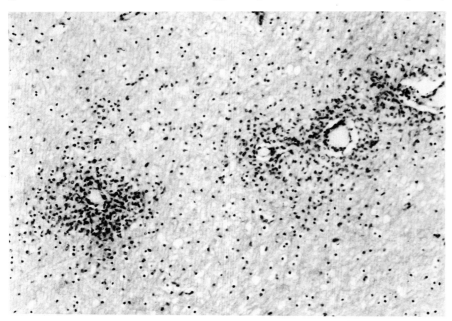

Fig. 10.38. Perivenous inflammatory infiltrate in perivenous encephalitis. Particularly characteristic is the manner in which the inflammatory cells fan out into the neighbouring parenchyma, rather than remaining as dense cuffs, largely confined to the Virchow–Robin spaces. H&E, ×130.

Most cases examined at post mortem die in the acute phase of the disease. In these cases the brain is swollen and congested and there may be a few petechial haemorrhages. Tentorial or foraminal herniation is common. The fixed and sliced brain shows little of note apart from swelling and prominent vascular markings in PVEM. In AHLE there are, in addition, multiple petechial haemorrhages in white matter (Fig. 10.37), and the cerebral swelling is at times asymmetrical, giving rise to shift of midline structures.

The diagnosis can only be confirmed by microscopy. Blocks for this purpose should be taken from congested, swollen areas of cerebral white matter, since these are often the most severely affected parts. The spinal cord should also be examined, since this frequently contains lesions, particularly at the thoracic level. On microscopy the characteristic finding in PVEM is of a dense mononuclear inflammatory infiltrate occupying the perivascular spaces around veins and venules, and spilling over into the immediately adjacent CNS parenchyma. Very acute cases may also show some neutrophils in the infiltrate. The inflammation is most florid in white matter but occurs also in grey matter (Figs 10.38 and 10.39). The inflammatory cells consist of lymphocytes,

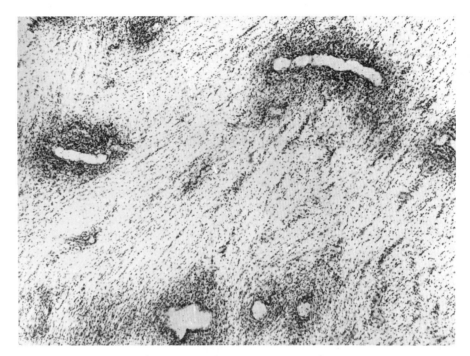

Fig. 10.39. Intense perivenous inflammatory cell cuffing from the cerebrum of a case of perivenous encephalitis. Nissl, ×120.

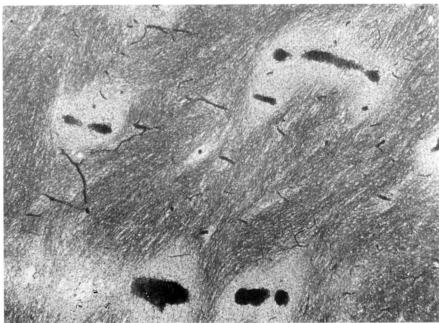

Fig. 10.40. Myelin-stained section adjacent to that shown in Fig. 10.39 demonstrating the perivenous loss of myelin. ×120.

mainly T-cells, macrophages and microglial cells. Accompanying this inflammation there is demyelination in the regions immediately surrounding the inflamed vessels (Fig. 10.40). Some axons may show mild damage, but most are intact (Fig. 10.41). Further away there is pallor of myelin staining which is attributable to oedema. The endothelium of affected veins appears swollen but the vessels are patent. Reactive astrocytes and macrophages containing neutral fat may be seen in and around the demyelinated zones if survival has lasted for at least a week. At a later stage, months or years after the acute episode, there is perivenous rarefaction and some more diffuse myelin loss with fibrillary gliosis, maximal around widened, fibrotic perivascular spaces (Fig. 10.42). Inflammation at this stage has largely resolved.

AHLE is a fulminating disease in which there is widespread necrosis of small vessels, with fibrin deposition in and around their walls. Plasma protein exudation is apparent in the perivascular tissue, which appears pale and necrotic, with fragmentation of both axons and myelin. Some inflammation is also seen and a high proportion of the cells are neutrophils, which infiltrate the vessel walls and perivascular spaces and invade the adjacent sleeves of necrotic parenchyma (Fig. 10.43). Multiple petechial haemorrhages also surround many of the affected vessels (Fig. 10.44). The leptomeninges are congested and moderately inflamed. Some cases of allergic encephalitis show pathological changes intermediate between those of classical PVEM and AHLE, or features of both diseases are found in different parts of the CNS.

The cause of allergic encephalitis is poorly understood, but there is a similar experimental disease which is produced when laboratory animals are immunized with CNS myelin

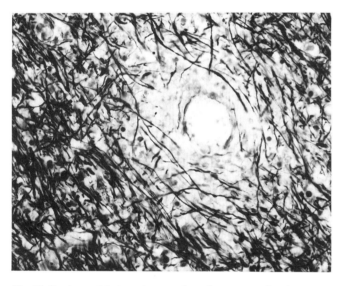

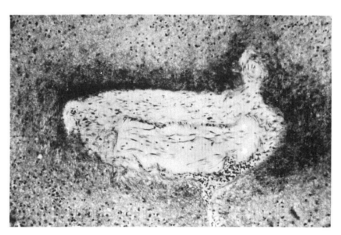

Fig. 10.42. Late effects of perivenous encephalitis. Inflammation has largely subsided, but there is fibrosis in the perivascular space, and intense gliosis in the surrounding neuropil. PTAH, ×120.

Fig. 10.41. Axon stain in perivenous tissue from a case of perivenous encephalitis. Many axons remain intact in the inflamed zone. ×150.

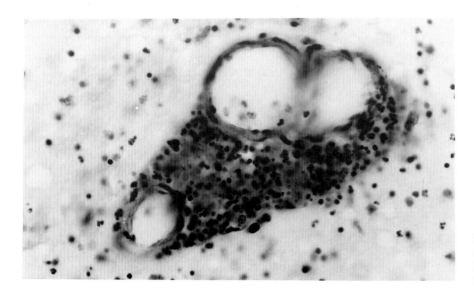

Fig. 10.43. Perivenous inflammatory cell infiltrate in acute haemorrhagic leucoencephalitis. The majority of cells are neutrophil polymorphs. H&E, ×220.

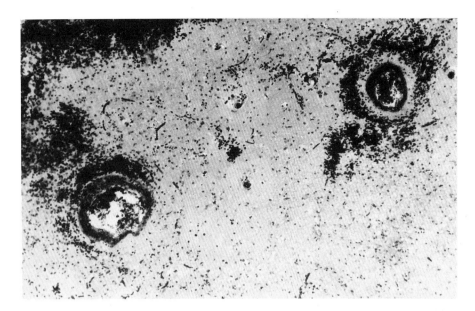

Fig. 10.44. Intense congestion, perivenous and more diffuse haemorrhages in cerebral white matter from a case of acute haemorrhagic leucoencephalitis. PTAH, ×100.

antigens along with adjuvant. Perivenous demyelination and inflammation are produced in the classical form of this experimental disease, which involves injecting Freund's adjuvant with the myelin antigen. A condition closely resembling AHLE is produced if pertussis vaccine is substituted for Freund's adjuvant in the inoculum. The role in the human disease of the preceding viral infections in triggering the allergic reaction is not clear. Viruses are not usually demonstrable in the CNS in these diseases.

While considering varieties of allergic encephalitis it should be mentioned that acute lesions of MS show intense mononuclear inflammation with demyelination (Chapter 14), and therefore closely resemble those of PVEM. The clinical histories of these two diseases are, however, usually different,

and histologically the lesions of acute MS extend further from the vein walls and show more evidence of a glial reaction. This reflects the usually longer duration of disease in MS. However, occasional cases show features of both diseases (Fig. 10.45). Experimental forms of allergic encephalitis resembling MS have now been produced in some laboratory animals.

Tropical spastic paraparesis

There is a form of neuromyelopathy recognized in some tropical countries in which inflammatory changes and degeneration occur in the spinal cord, nerve roots and sensory ganglia. The inflammatory reaction is chiefly

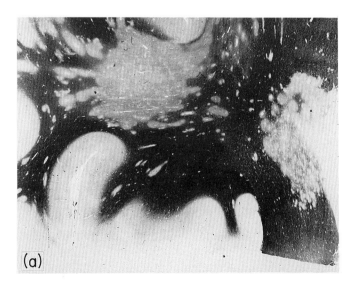

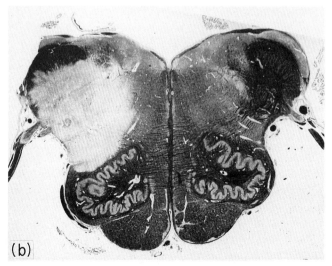

Fig. 10.45. Myelin-stained sections of the cerebrum (a) and medulla (b) from a case of perivenous encephalitis in which, in addition to the characteristic perivenous inflammation and demyelination, seen in (a), there were also more extensive plaques of demyelination resembling those seen in MS (a and b). (a) ×2; (b) ×4.

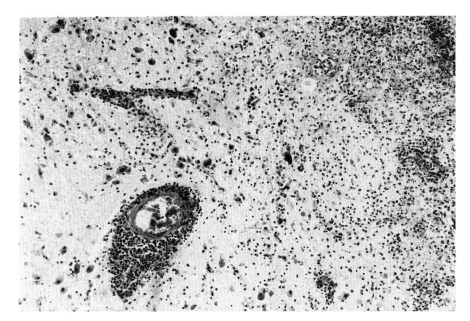

Fig. 10.46. Intense diffuse and perivascular inflammation in cerebral toxoplasmosis. H&E, ×80.

perivascular and includes lymphocytes, plasma cells and macrophages. Similar slight changes may extend upward into the brain. Long-standing cases show little inflammation but prominent leptomeningeal and perivascular fibrosis at the same sites. Neuron loss is seen in the spinal grey matter and sensory ganglia, with axonal loss in lateral and posterior columns of the spinal cord. Evidence of elevated antibody titres to the retrovirus HTLV1 in serum and CSF have recently been described in cases from Jamaica, Colombia and Martinique (Gessain *et al.* 1985; Rogers-Johnson *et al.* 1985). Some clinically similar cases in West Africa, in which, however, the inflammation is lacking, have been ascribed on the basis of epidemiological evidence to chronic cyanide poisoning related to high consumption of cassava (see p.311).

Other forms of encephalitis and myelitis

Purulent encephalitis is discussed in Chapter 9, and parenchymal syphilitic lesions in Chapters 9 and 17.

Rickettsial encephalitis

Rickettsial diseases are acute, systemic infections, caused by bacterium-like organisms, usually transmitted to man by insect vectors. The organisms have a predilection for invading and multiplying in the endothelial cells of small blood vessels. A skin rash usually develops. Neurological involvement results if vessels of the nervous system or leptomeninges are colonized. Lesions consist of a focal vasculitis affecting small blood vessels, sometimes accompanied by small infarcts. The diagnosis is usually made on the basis of serological tests demonstrating a rise in antibody titre to one of the Rickettsiae, coinciding in time with the systemic illness.

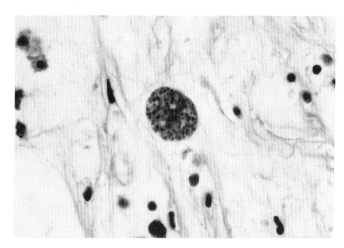

Fig. 10.47. Toxoplasmosis cyst, one of several widely distributed in the lesion illustrated in Fig. 10.46. H&E, ×400.

Parasitic infections

Most parasitic infections of the brain and leptomeninges provoke formation of granulomas (Chapter 9). *Toxoplasmosis* in neonates or immunosuppressed adults may, however, cause an encephalitis reminiscent of viral encephalitis, with inflammation, glial nodules, focal necrosis and late calcification (Fig. 10.46). Toxoplasma cysts can usually be identified in the lesions (Fig. 10.47). In *cerebral trypanosomiasis* (sleeping sickness) there is a diffuse meningoencephalitis with cuffing of vessels by lymphocytes and plasma cells and with some reactive astrocytosis in cerebral white matter. Cerebral and cerebellar white matter, basal ganglia and brain stem tend to be the areas most affected, and the cerebral cortex is relatively spared. Morula cells (plasma

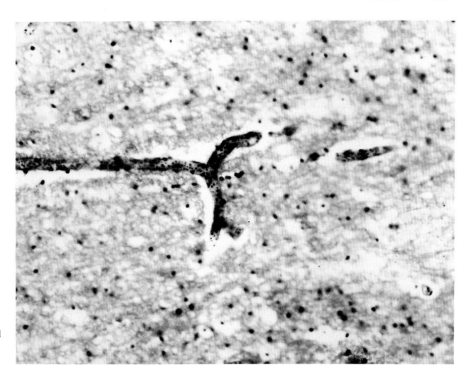

Fig. 10.48. A focus of white matter oedema and rarefaction centred on a small vein packed with parasitized erythrocytes in a case of cerebral malaria. H&E, ×100.

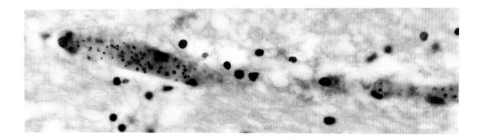

Fig. 10.49. Higher power view of the parasitized erythrocytes shown in Fig. 10.48. H&E, ×380.

cells distended with immunoglobulin) occur in perivascular spaces and in the brain.

Cerebral malaria results chiefly from infection with *Plasmodium falciparum*. The diagnosis is made on the basis of acute neurological disease in a subject whose blood contains malaria parasites. The lesions in the brain in fatal cases are widely distributed and centred on small blood vessels, many of which can be seen to contain large numbers of parasitized red blood cells (Figs 10.48 and 10.49). In addition to the congestion and presumed stasis of blood in capillaries and other small vessels, the vascular endothelium appears swollen, and extravasated red cells and proteinaceous fluid may be seen around them. There is also necrosis of the perivascular brain parenchyma, with focal loss of myelin staining in white matter, and accumulation of reactive microglia and astrocytes in the vicinity. The pathogenesis of cerebral malaria is not fully clarified, but opinion is more in favour of a hypoxic/toxic mechanism than of an immunological one.

Encephalitis of undefined aetiology

Rasmussen's encephalitis

Rare cases of chronic encephalitis, with epilepsy as one of the chief presenting features, were first described by Rasmussen (1978). Almost all those affected have been children. Histopathological studies have been made on surgically removed tissues, including temporal lobectomy and hemispherectomy specimens. They show a subacute or chronic meningoencephalitis affecting chiefly cerebral cortex, but also white matter, with perivascular mononuclear inflammatory cells, microglial nodules and foci of neuronophagia. Inclusion bodies have not been seen, and viral culture and EM studies have failed to reveal viruses or other organisms in the brain. The cause of this disease therefore remains unknown.

Brain tumours

These act similarly, but as a rule more slowly. A slowly-growing tumour such as a meningioma may be accommodated by demyelination of central white matter, which thus loses bulk while keeping most of its axons intact (Fig. 11.2). A fast-growing tumour, on the other hand — a glioblastoma, say, or secondary carcinoma — may enhance its deadly

potential by causing an oedematous reaction in the surrounding brain tissue (Figs 11.3 and 11.4). With some tumours — notably with gliomas of the astrocytic series — space occupation is as much due to the formation of an associated cyst (Fig. 11.5) as it is to expansion of the solid tumour tissue. The tumours most commonly met with are *gliomas*, which are described in the next chapter. The commonest of these, alas, is the fast-growing malignant *glioblastoma*. This occurs mainly in men and women over 50 years of age. Among younger adults, the slower-advancing diffuse *astrocytoma* is commoner. *Lymphomas* are relatively rare, but often highly malignant. Of the extrinsic tumours, the relatively benign meningioma is the most frequent in elderly people: in young people, pituitary adenomas and craniopharyngiomas are relatively common. In some parts

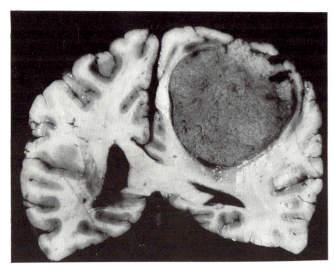

Fig. 11.2. Large meningioma indenting the right parietal lobe in a woman aged 52, with a 9-month history of headaches. Died in operating theatre. Loss of white matter is mainly attributable to demyelination of axons in white matter, owing to compression. The tumour is histologically benign, and non-invasive.

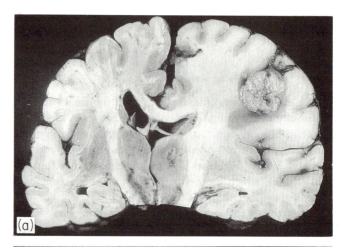

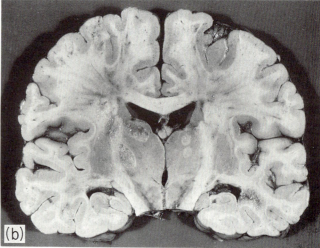

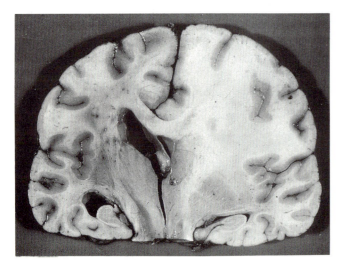

Fig. 11.3. Oedema of the right frontal lobe, associated with a malignant astrocytoma, situated anteriorly to this, in a man aged 30, with a 2-month history of headaches; final state, mute and incontinent. Note the midline shift, subfalcine hernia, flattening of convolutions, and grooving and bruising of the right parahippocampal gyrus. The corpus callosum, here and in Fig. 11.4a, is tilted downward on the right, indicating that swelling is more intense in the upper than in the lower part of the hemisphere.

Fig. 11.4. Metastatic tumours. (a) Bronchial carcinoma. Deposits are seen in the right thalamus and middle frontal convolution. There is severe associated oedema, with midline shift and subfalcine hernia. (b) Carcinoma of the lung. Deposits are widely dispersed in cortex, white matter and thalamus; but there is no apparent oedema or displacement.

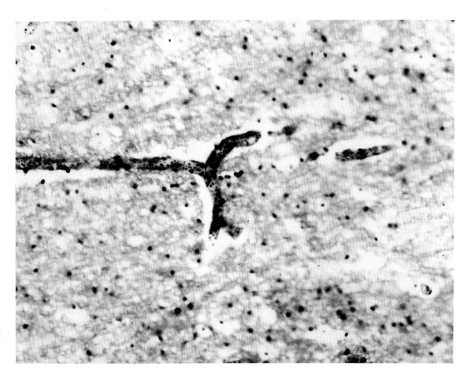

Fig. 10.48. A focus of white matter oedema and rarefaction centred on a small vein packed with parasitized erythrocytes in a case of cerebral malaria. H&E, ×100.

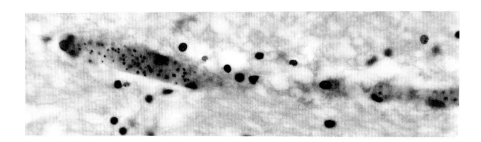

Fig. 10.49. Higher power view of the parasitized erythrocytes shown in Fig. 10.48. H&E, ×380.

cells distended with immunoglobulin) occur in perivascular spaces and in the brain.

Cerebral malaria results chiefly from infection with *Plasmodium falciparum*. The diagnosis is made on the basis of acute neurological disease in a subject whose blood contains malaria parasites. The lesions in the brain in fatal cases are widely distributed and centred on small blood vessels, many of which can be seen to contain large numbers of parasitized red blood cells (Figs 10.48 and 10.49). In addition to the congestion and presumed stasis of blood in capillaries and other small vessels, the vascular endothelium appears swollen, and extravasated red cells and proteinaceous fluid may be seen around them. There is also necrosis of the perivascular brain parenchyma, with focal loss of myelin staining in white matter, and accumulation of reactive microglia and astrocytes in the vicinity. The pathogenesis of cerebral malaria is not fully clarified, but opinion is more in favour of a hypoxic/toxic mechanism than of an immunological one.

Encephalitis of undefined aetiology

Rasmussen's encephalitis

Rare cases of chronic encephalitis, with epilepsy as one of the chief presenting features, were first described by Rasmussen (1978). Almost all those affected have been children. Histopathological studies have been made on surgically removed tissues, including temporal lobectomy and hemispherectomy specimens. They show a subacute or chronic meningoencephalitis affecting chiefly cerebral cortex, but also white matter, with perivascular mononuclear inflammatory cells, microglial nodules and foci of neuronophagia. Inclusion bodies have not been seen, and viral culture and EM studies have failed to reveal viruses or other organisms in the brain. The cause of this disease therefore remains unknown.

Brain tumours

These act similarly, but as a rule more slowly. A slowly-growing tumour such as a meningioma may be accommodated by demyelination of central white matter, which thus loses bulk while keeping most of its axons intact (Fig. 11.2). A fast-growing tumour, on the other hand — a glioblastoma, say, or secondary carcinoma — may enhance its deadly potential by causing an oedematous reaction in the surrounding brain tissue (Figs 11.3 and 11.4). With some tumours — notably with gliomas of the astrocytic series — space occupation is as much due to the formation of an associated cyst (Fig. 11.5) as it is to expansion of the solid tumour tissue. The tumours most commonly met with are *gliomas*, which are described in the next chapter. The commonest of these, alas, is the fast-growing malignant *glioblastoma*. This occurs mainly in men and women over 50 years of age. Among younger adults, the slower-advancing diffuse *astrocytoma* is commoner. *Lymphomas* are relatively rare, but often highly malignant. Of the extrinsic tumours, the relatively benign meningioma is the most frequent in elderly people: in young people, pituitary adenomas and craniopharyngiomas are relatively common. In some parts

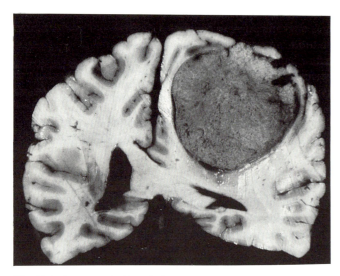

Fig. 11.2. Large meningioma indenting the right parietal lobe in a woman aged 52, with a 9-month history of headaches. Died in operating theatre. Loss of white matter is mainly attributable to demyelination of axons in white matter, owing to compression. The tumour is histologically benign, and non-invasive.

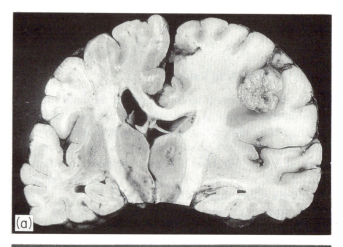

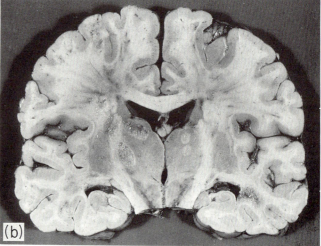

Fig. 11.4. Metastatic tumours. (a) Bronchial carcinoma. Deposits are seen in the right thalamus and middle frontal convolution. There is severe associated oedema, with midline shift and subfalcine hernia. (b) Carcinoma of the lung. Deposits are widely dispersed in cortex, white matter and thalamus; but there is no apparent oedema or displacement.

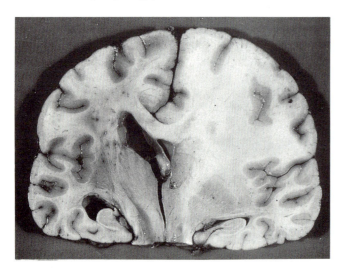

Fig. 11.3. Oedema of the right frontal lobe, associated with a malignant astrocytoma, situated anteriorly to this, in a man aged 30, with a 2-month history of headaches; final state, mute and incontinent. Note the midline shift, subfalcine hernia, flattening of convolutions, and grooving and bruising of the right parahippocampal gyrus. The corpus callosum, here and in Fig. 11.4a, is tilted downward on the right, indicating that swelling is more intense in the upper than in the lower part of the hemisphere.

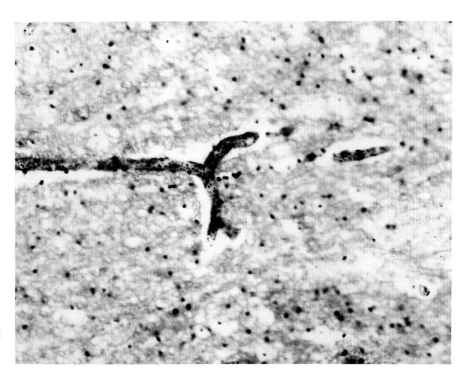

Fig. 10.48. A focus of white matter oedema and rarefaction centred on a small vein packed with parasitized erythrocytes in a case of cerebral malaria. H&E, ×100.

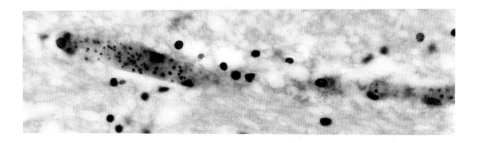

Fig. 10.49. Higher power view of the parasitized erythrocytes shown in Fig. 10.48. H&E, ×380.

cells distended with immunoglobulin) occur in perivascular spaces and in the brain.

Cerebral malaria results chiefly from infection with *Plasmodium falciparum*. The diagnosis is made on the basis of acute neurological disease in a subject whose blood contains malaria parasites. The lesions in the brain in fatal cases are widely distributed and centred on small blood vessels, many of which can be seen to contain large numbers of parasitized red blood cells (Figs 10.48 and 10.49). In addition to the congestion and presumed stasis of blood in capillaries and other small vessels, the vascular endothelium appears swollen, and extravasated red cells and proteinaceous fluid may be seen around them. There is also necrosis of the perivascular brain parenchyma, with focal loss of myelin staining in white matter, and accumulation of reactive microglia and astrocytes in the vicinity. The pathogenesis of cerebral malaria is not fully clarified, but opinion is more in favour of a hypoxic/toxic mechanism than of an immunological one.

Encephalitis of undefined aetiology

Rasmussen's encephalitis

Rare cases of chronic encephalitis, with epilepsy as one of the chief presenting features, were first described by Rasmussen (1978). Almost all those affected have been children. Histopathological studies have been made on surgically removed tissues, including temporal lobectomy and hemispherectomy specimens. They show a subacute or chronic meningoencephalitis affecting chiefly cerebral cortex, but also white matter, with perivascular mononuclear inflammatory cells, microglial nodules and foci of neuronophagia. Inclusion bodies have not been seen, and viral culture and EM studies have failed to reveal viruses or other organisms in the brain. The cause of this disease therefore remains unknown.

Behçet's disease

Behçet's disease is characterized clinically by recurrent ulceration of the mouth and genitalia, and iridocyclitis. In some cases there are also neurological abnormalities, the pathology of which consists of multiple, focal, ill-defined areas of congestion and softening. The commonest sites affected are the brain stem, especially the midbrain, basal ganglia, hypothalamus and internal capsule. These areas should be included among those examined microscopically in this disease. Both grey and white matter are affected, and contain inflammatory, necrotic foci with perivascular lymphocytes, microglial nodules in grey matter, and a more diffuse microglial and astrocytic reaction (Figs 10.50 and 10.51). There is loss of myelin and to a lesser extent of axons and neurons. Vessels show relatively little pathological change. The leptomeninges adjacent to affected parenchyma are mildly inflamed. The cause of the disease is not known.

Occasional cases of encephalitis occur in which *no definite diagnosis* can be made. The inflammation may predominate in grey or white matter, with or without neuronophagia, and in the absence of perivenous demyelination or inclusion bodies. Provided these distinguishing features have been carefully searched for, and microbiological studies have been taken far enough to exclude identifiable causes of encephalitis, the pathologist will have taken the matter as far as can be expected.

Encephalitis associated with carcinoma

Subacute or chronic encephalitis occurs in some patients with carcinoma, particularly oat-cell carcinoma of the bronchus. The primary tumour in such cases is almost invariably small, and metastatic spread is limited to regional lymph nodes. The brain shows little abnormality externally. In slices there may be a suggestion of ill-defined softening and discoloration in grey matter at almost any level of the neuraxis. The regions that merit particular attention in any individual case are those to which the clinical signs and symptoms were referable, and samples for microscopy should be taken from these areas and also from other major subdivisions of the nervous system (cerebral cortex, white matter, basal ganglia, thalamus, several levels of the brain stem and spinal cord and dorsal root ganglia). The areas predominantly affected are grey matter and they show perivascular cuffing with mononuclear inflammatory cells, chiefly lymphocytes, loss of neurons and neuronophagia (Fig. 10.52). Microglia proliferate, and astrocytes are variably reactive. Inflammation and neuron loss do not always go hand in hand. There tends to be a predominant area of damage, for example in the cerebral cortex, where the hippocampus and medial temporal lobe are particularly likely to be involved, or in the basal ganglia, thalamus, brain stem, or spinal cord. Mild inflammation is more widely spread. The sensory ganglia may show loss of neurons with satellite cell proliferation accompanying involvement of the CNS or in isolation. This ganglioradiculitis is accompanied by secondary degeneration of nerve fibres in posterior columns of the spinal cord. Such cases usually show evidence of a sensory neuropathy clinically. Cases with ataxia show one of two rather different lesions in the cerebellum: inflammation and loss of neurons in the dentate nuclei, or severe depletion of Purkinje cells and to a lesser extent of granule cells, without inflammation. Serum or CSF of cases of the latter type have occasionally been shown to contain an antibody which reacts with cerebellar Purkinje cells.

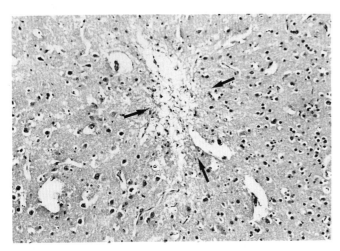

Fig. 10.50. Microscopic focus of rarefaction (arrowed) in the cerebral cortex from a case of Behçet's disease. H&E, ×80.

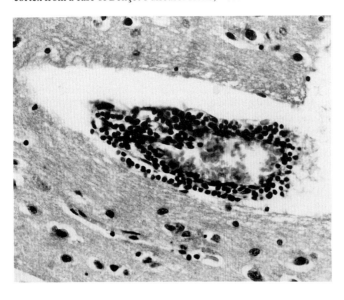

Fig. 10.51. Behçet's disease. Lymphocytic perivascular cuffing in the brain. H&E, ×230.

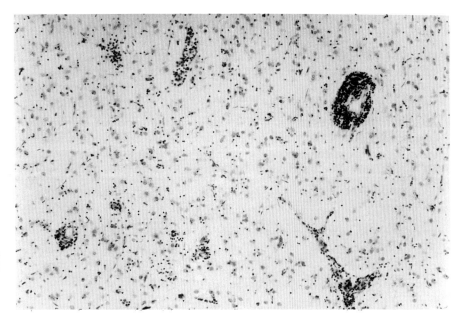

Fig. 10.52. Low-power view of a section of the putamen from a case of encephalitis associated with oat-cell carcinoma of the lung, showing perivascular lymphocytic cuffing and microglial nodules. H&E, ×80.

Encephalitis lethargica

A world-wide epidemic of encephalitis lethargica (von Economo's encephalitis) occurred during, and in the decade after, the First World War. No aetiological agent was identified, but the epidemiology and pathology were consistent with a viral cause. The epidemic overlapped in time with a world-wide outbreak of influenza, and this has led to speculation that a neurovirulent strain of influenza virus may have been involved. Occasional sporadic cases that fit the clinical pattern of the disease have continued to be described, but again no agent has been identified. Fever, somnolence and impaired oculomotor function characterize the acute phase of the disease. In a significant proportion of the survivors parkinsonian symptoms and oculogyric crises occurred. Patients who died in the acute phase of the disease had a polioencephalitis more or less limited to the brain stem, particularly the midbrain and diencephalon, with congestion, inflammation and neuronophagia. The brains of subjects with post-encephalitic parkinsonism showed severe neuron loss and gliosis in the midbrain, particularly the substantia nigra, and some neurofibrillary tangles resembling those seen in Alzheimer's disease, in some remaining neurons.

Further reading

Allergic encephalitis

Leibowitz S, Hughes RAC. 1982. *Immunology of the Nervous System*. Edward Arnold, London.

Wisniewski HM, Lassmann H, Brosnan CF *et al*. 1982. Multiple sclerosis: immunological and experimental aspects. In Matthews WB, Glaser GH (Eds) *Recent Advances in Clinical Neurology* 3. Churchill Livingstone, Edinburgh, pp. 95–124.

Parasitic encephalitis

Brown WJ, Voge M. 1982. *Neuropathology of Parasitic Infections*. Oxford University Press, Oxford.

Scaravilli F. 1984. Parasitic and fungal infections of the nervous system. In Adams JH, Corsellis JAN, Duchen LW (Eds) *Greenfield's Neuropathology*, 4th edn. Edward Arnold, London, pp. 304–37.

Tropical spastic paraparesis

Gessain A, Vernant JC, Maurs L *et al*. 1985. Brain antibodies to human T-lymphotropic virus type 1 in patients with tropical spastic paraparesis. *Lancet* 2, 407–10.

Rogers-Johnson P, Gajdusek DC, Morgan OStC *et al*. 1985. HTLV I and HTLV III antibodies and tropical spastic paraparesis. *Lancet* 2, 1248–9.

Viral encephalitis

Booss J, Esiri MM. 1986. *Viral Encephalitis: Pathology, Diagnosis and Management*. Blackwell Scientific Publications, Oxford.

Brownell B, Tomlinson AH. 1984. Virus diseases of the central nervous system. In Adams JH, Corsellis JAN, Duchen LW (Eds) *Greenfield's Neuropathology*, 4th edn. Edward Arnold, London, pp. 260–303.

Burns J, Redfern DRM, Esiri MM, McGee JO'D. 1986. Human and viral gene detection in routine paraffin embedded tissue by in situ hybridisation with biotinylated probes: viral localisation in herpes encephalitis. *J Clin Pathol* **39**, 1066–73.

de la Monte SM, Ho DD, Schooley RT *et al*. 1987. Subacute encephalomyelitis of AIDS and its relation to HTLV-III infection. *Neurology* **37**, 562–9.

Epstein LG, Sharer LR, Joshi VV *et al.* 1985. Progressive encephalo-pathy in children with acquired immune deficiency syndrome. *Ann Neurol* **17**, 488–96.

Haase AT, Pagano J, Waksman B, Nathanson N. 1983. Detection of viral genes and their products in chronic neurological diseases. *Ann Neurol* **15**, 119–21.

Johnson RT. 1982. *Viral Infections of the Nervous System*. Raven Press, New York.

Johnson RT, McArthur JC. 1987. Myelopathies and retrovirus infections. *Ann Neurol* **21**, 113–16.

Kennedy PGE. 1988. Neurological complications of human immuno-deficiency virus infection. *Postgrad Med J* **64**, 180–7.

Koenig S, Gendelman HE, Orenstein JM *et al.* 1986. Detection of AIDS virus in macrophages in brain tissue of AIDS patients with encephalopathy. *Science* **233**, 1089–93.

Levy RM, Bredesen DE, Rosenblum ML. 1985. Neurological manifes-tations of the acquired immune deficiency syndrome (AIDS): ex-perience at UCSF and review of the literature. *J Neurosurg* **62**, 475–95.

Navia BA, Cho E-S, Petito CK, Price RW. 1986. The AIDS dementia complex. II Neuropathology. *Ann Neurol* **19**, 325–51.

Petito CK, Cho E-S, Lemann W, Navia BA, Price RW. 1986. Neuro-pathology of acquired immune deficiency syndrome (AIDS): an autopsy review. *J Neuropath Exp Neurol* **45**, 635–46.

Wiley CA, Schrier RD, Nelson JA, Lampert PW, Oldstone MB. 1986. Cellular localisation of human immunodeficiency virus infection within the brains of acquired immune deficiency syndrome patients. *Proc Natl Acad Sci USA* **83**, 7089–93.

Other forms of encephalitis

Price TR, Wisseman CL, Woodward TE. 1977. Rickettsial diseases. In Goldensohn ES, Appel SH (Eds) *Scientific Approaches to Clinical Neurology*. Lea and Febiger, Philadelphia, pp. 515–26.

Rasmussen T. 1978. Further observations on the syndrome of chronic encephalitis and epilepsy. *Appl Neurophysiol* **41**, 1–12.

Chapter 11
Space-occupying Lesions

Types of expanding lesion

In the earlier chapters stress is laid on the importance of tentorial and foraminal herniations as causes of death. In this chapter we discuss the various causes of such herniations. Inevitably, there will be some repetition of points made in other chapters. We also discuss some lesions within the spinal canal, which by their expansion cause paraplegia or tetraplegia rather than sudden death.

The effects of expanding lesions depend on several factors, including their position, their size and their rate of expansion. In general, the effects of intracranial expanding lesions differ according to whether they lie above or below the tentorium. Treating the supratentorial lesions first, we have to consider the following:

1 Haematomas, intrinsic or extrinsic.
2 Neoplasms, intrinsic or extrinsic.
3 Abscess.
4 Obstructive hydrocephalus.
5 Cerebral oedema.

Intracranial haemorrhage

Intracranial haemorrhage is discussed in Chapter 6. In general, the effects of a massive supratentorial haemorrhage, whether in the brain substance or outside it, will be: to shift midline structures to the opposite side, producing a sub-falcine hernia (Figs 2.8c and 11.1), with compression and distortion of the lateral ventricles; to force diencephalic structures downward through the tentorial opening (Figs 2.8 and 2.9); to apply lateral compression to the midbrain via the ipsilateral uncus and parahippocampal gyrus (Fig. 2.12); to press the opposite cerebral peduncle against the free edge of the tentorium (Fig. 2.10); and to kink one or both oculomotor nerves where they cross the posterior cerebral arteries. Branches of the opposite posterior cerebral artery may be pinched, causing infarction of occipital cortex, including the striate area (Fig. 7.20).

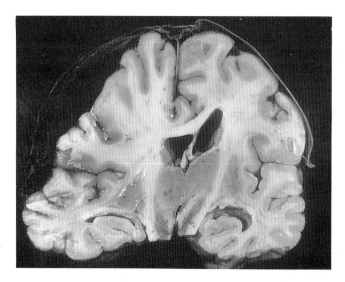

Fig. 11.1. Effects of a large chronic subdural haematoma. The brain has been sliced coronally, with much of the dura, and the underlying haematoma, in place. There has been a remarkable degree of displacement of midline structures to the right, and the left cingulate gyrus has virtually wrapped itself around the free edge of the falx. In contrast, the convolutions are not flattened, and the ventricles appear to be of normal size. Explanation: the brain was already atrophic at the time of injury, and there was ample room for the haematoma to expand without causing a fatal transtentorial hernia.

Brain tumours

These act similarly, but as a rule more slowly. A slowly-growing tumour such as a meningioma may be accommodated by demyelination of central white matter, which thus loses bulk while keeping most of its axons intact (Fig. 11.2). A fast-growing tumour, on the other hand — a glioblastoma, say, or secondary carcinoma — may enhance its deadly potential by causing an oedematous reaction in the surrounding brain tissue (Figs 11.3 and 11.4). With some tumours — notably with gliomas of the astrocytic series — space occupation is as much due to the formation of an associated cyst (Fig. 11.5) as it is to expansion of the solid tumour tissue. The tumours most commonly met with are *gliomas*, which are described in the next chapter. The commonest of these, alas, is the fast-growing malignant *glioblastoma*. This occurs mainly in men and women over 50 years of age. Among younger adults, the slower-advancing diffuse *astrocytoma* is commoner. *Lymphomas* are relatively rare, but often highly malignant. Of the extrinsic tumours, the relatively benign meningioma is the most frequent in elderly people: in young people, pituitary adenomas and craniopharyngiomas are relatively common. In some parts

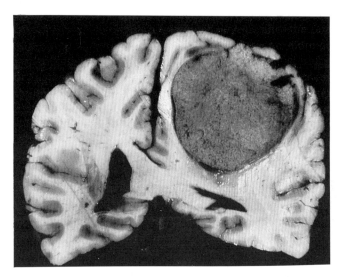

Fig. 11.2. Large meningioma indenting the right parietal lobe in a woman aged 52, with a 9-month history of headaches. Died in operating theatre. Loss of white matter is mainly attributable to demyelination of axons in white matter, owing to compression. The tumour is histologically benign, and non-invasive.

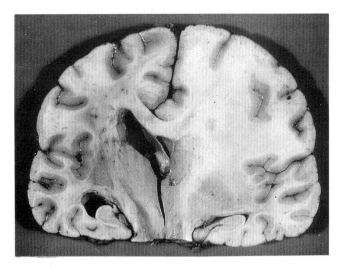

Fig. 11.3. Oedema of the right frontal lobe, associated with a malignant astrocytoma, situated anteriorly to this, in a man aged 30, with a 2-month history of headaches; final state, mute and incontinent. Note the midline shift, subfalcine hernia, flattening of convolutions, and grooving and bruising of the right parahippocampal gyrus. The corpus callosum, here and in Fig. 11.4a, is tilted downward on the right, indicating that swelling is more intense in the upper than in the lower part of the hemisphere.

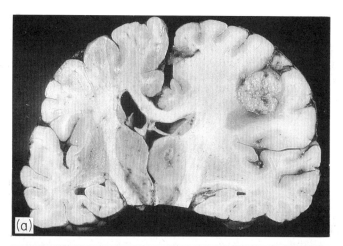

(a)

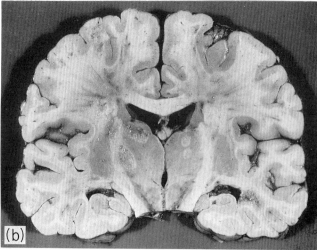

(b)

Fig. 11.4. Metastatic tumours. (a) Bronchial carcinoma. Deposits are seen in the right thalamus and middle frontal convolution. There is severe associated oedema, with midline shift and subfalcine hernia. (b) Carcinoma of the lung. Deposits are widely dispersed in cortex, white matter and thalamus; but there is no apparent oedema or displacement.

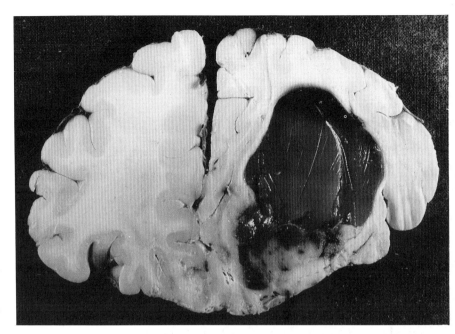

Fig. 11.5. Cyst associated with a relatively small right frontal malignant astrocytoma, in a woman aged 50. Main complaints, headaches and epileptic fits. (The congealed cyst fluid, which would normally be yellow or colourless, is darkened by haemorrhage.)

of the world non-neoplastic tumours such as tuberculomas are all too frequent.

Abscesses (see Chapter 9) may be blood-borne, most commonly from an infected lung, or arise by inward extension from an infected frontal sinus or middle ear (Fig. 9.13).

Obstructive hydrocephalus

Obstructive hydrocephalus may be due to tumours (see p.121). The aqueduct may be partially or totally blocked even by small tumours in the tectum or in the pineal region, or merely by kinking due to other posterior fossa lesions. Here it should be noted that an expanding lesion in the posterior fossa tends to resist a transtentorial downthrust, and herniation, when it occurs, is likely to take place at the foramen magnum. Tentorial herniation is the natural result of acute distension of the lateral ventricles due to aqueduct stenosis or an impacted cyst of the third ventricle.

Cerebral swelling: oedema

Acute cerebral swelling has a variety of causes. The old distinction between *dry swelling*, in which there is extra fluid in blood vessels or within brain cells, and *cerebral oedema*, in which fluid seeps into intercellular spaces, may be theoretically sound, but it is very difficult to apply in individual cases. In practice, it seems that the former, but not the latter, may be reduced by intravenous osmotic agents such as mannitol and urea. It is oedema which constitutes the biggest threat to life in the neurosurgical and acute neurological wards. The patient, for instance, who dies in the acute phase of non-haemorrhagic stroke is killed not by the loss of vital brain tissue, but because of distortion of his upper brain stem by a herniated parahippocampal gyrus propelled downward by swelling of the infarcted tissue (see p.107).

Among the causes of acute dry swelling of the brain the most familiar are *hypoxaemia* and *hypercapnia*. When the brain is exposed at operation, trouble with the airway is quickly betrayed by congestion and darkening of pial vessels and a tendency of brain tissue to rise out of the wound. The process can usually be quickly reversed. Oedema, on the other hand, implies an increase in the water content of the brain, which is less easily controlled. The physiology of the process has been studied intensively in recent years; and at present the prevailing view is that there are two main types of cerebral oedema: the *vasogenic*, which affects white matter more than grey, and the *cytotoxic*, which affects mainly glial cells and neurons. The two may both occur, it seems, in the same brain. For further discussion, see Miller & Adams (1984).

Cerebral oedema occurs in many different conditions. It is one of the main bugbears of surgeons concerned in the management of head injury. In acute infarction, it affects the tissue adjacent to the infarct, and it may be difficult to determine the boundary between the softening due to irreparable loss of blood supply and that due to oedema of the surrounding tissue. Oedema due to toxic and metabolic disturbances is particularly apt to occur in young children, and is the main neuropathological finding in, for instance, Reye's syndrome (p.303). It occurs in the neighbourhood of many tumours, including benign growths such as meningiomas, and malignant ones such as secondary carcinomas (Fig. 11.4). It occurs in association with inflammatory lesions, both focal and diffuse, and in this context it is worth noting that the lesions of acute MS have an inflammatory character, and may give rise to intense swelling (Fig. 11.6).

Both before and after fixation, oedematous brain is un-naturally soft. In slices of fixed brain, the affected white matter is slimy to the touch, and often yellowish in colour. If it is adequately fixed, the tissue, though softer than normal, is still resilient: unfortunately, formalin is slow to penetrate oedematous tissue, and without special pre-cautions (see p.7) the result may be a sour-smelling, almost fluid, substance resembling toothpaste.

In histological preparations the affected areas stain poorly for myelin (Fig. 11.7); it is not always clear to what extent this is due to actual myelin breakdown. If oedema has persisted for more than a day or so, one sees numerous swollen-bodied astrocytes, presumably engaged in the busi-ness of laying down the fibres which form the meshwork of post-oedematous gliosis (Fig. 11.8). (These cells, incidentally, may be very conspicuous in a diagnostic smear preparation; the pathologist has to be cautious in making the diagnosis between reactive astrocytosis and gemistocytic astrocytoma.)

Effects of expanding lesions in the head

In general, the effect of expanding *supratentorial lesions*, including cerebral oedema, is, first, to drive fluid out of the lateral ventricles and subarachnoid spaces, then to thrust the diencephalon downward, and finally to cause trans-tentorial herniation and distortion of the upper brain stem. There are three important exceptions to this rule. Firstly, in young children, whose cranial sutures have not yet closed, the cranial cavity may be expanded by pressure from within, so that transtentorial herniation is avoided. Secondly, if the expanding lesion involves the posterior parts of the hemi-spheres, the whole tentorium will be pressed downwards, in

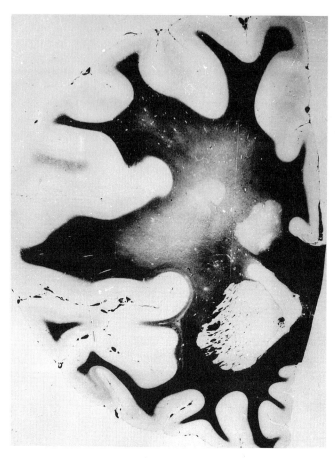

Fig. 11.7. Same case as in Fig. 11.6. A myelin-stained section of the left frontal lobe shows two distinct demyelinated areas in the central white matter. Around the smaller of these is a wide area of oedema, in which myelin is not destroyed, but stains feebly.

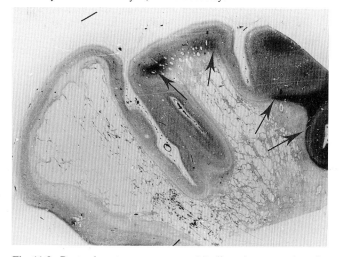

Fig. 11.8. Postoedematous spongy state. Myelin stain on a section of cortex from another case of acute MS, of Schilder type, in a 12-year-old girl dying after an illness lasting 5 months. In this case, and in the one illustrated in Figs 11.6 and 11.7, the clinical diagnosis was of a rapidly-growing tumour. Here, the oedema had subsided by the time of death, leaving a spongy tissue in which, surprisingly, many demyelinated axons remained. In the picture, a few patches of surviving subcortical myelin are seen (arrowed). ×2.2.

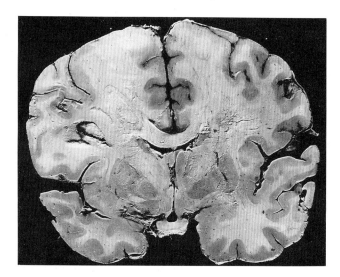

Fig. 11.6. Acute MS, of Balò type, in a 21-year-old woman, with a total history of 5 weeks. The dark lesion in the left hemisphere is a haemorrhagic needle-track. The whole brain is swollen, with flattened convolutions and compressed ventricles.

which case pressure is transferred to the posterior fossa, favouring a foraminal rather than a tentorial herniation. Thirdly, a very slowly expanding lesion — a meningioma, for instance, or hydrocephalus due to a partial or intermittent occlusion of the aqueduct — may result in diffuse demyelination of white matter, i.e. compensatory brain shrinkage.

Expanding lesions in the posterior fossa

These include tumours arising in the base of the skull (chordoma, chondroma, chemodectoma), meningiomas and nerve sheath tumours (especially schwannoma of the eighth cranial nerve) (pp.198–200) and cerebellar abscesses. Intrinsic tumours include *diffuse astrocytoma* of the brain stem (a condition at one time referred to as 'hypertrophy of the pons'), the relatively benign *circumscribed astrocytoma* of the cerebellum (p.176) and the highly malignant *medulloblastoma* of the cerebellum (p.190). The first two of these tend to occur in children or young adults, the third in infants and young children. The commonest cerebellar tumour in elderly people is probably *secondary carcinoma*; middle-aged people are more liable to develop a cerebellar *haemangioblastoma* (p.195). This, in spite of its sinister-sounding name, is usually a benign tumour, completely removable by surgery if caught in time. Although it is a tumour of vasoformative tissue, and so presumably unrelated to the glioma family, it has a close similarity to the benign astrocytoma of the cerebellum, in that it produces symptoms mainly through the formation of an expanding cyst, which is usually much larger than the tumour itself. *Ependymomas*, of various degress of malignancy, arise in the aqueduct, fourth ventricle and lateral aperture (foramen of Luschka), whereas they are relatively rare in the lateral and third ventricles. They are apt to send tongues of tumour out through the foramina into the subarachnoid space (Fig. 12.21). At operation it may be possible to peel these away cleanly, so that the free passage of fluid is re-established; the tumour, however, is usually adherent at some point to a structure which it would be imprudent to disturb. A benign variant, sometimes encountered in routine examination of the medulla, is the *subependymoma*, or subependymal astrocytoma (p.184). This is usually a small nodule, harmlessly tucked into the lower end of the fourth ventricle, and only rarely growing to a size capable of obstructing the lateral apertures.

Lhermitte–Duclos disease

This is a rare but interesting condition, presenting clinically as a posterior fossa tumour. In this the granule cells in a circumscribed area of cerebellar cortex undergo gross hypertrophy. The resulting expansion is increased by myelination of the axons of the granule cells. Purkinje cells, and cerebellar white matter, are squeezed out of existence; what remains is a thick, much-folded blanket of soft pale tissue. The condition is described on p.264.

In general, the effects of expanding lesions in the posterior fossa are threefold, with differences of emphasis in different cases. First, there is the damage to cells and fibre tracts due to infiltration or to pressure. (In cases of diffuse astrocytoma, in which the whole brain stem is infiltrated by hyperplastic or neoplastic astrocytes, it is sometimes astonishing how little interference with function seems to have occurred. In the case of the cerebellum, a great deal of tissue may be lost before clinical ataxia becomes troublesome.) Second, there is in most cases some obstruction of CSF pathways, causing dilatation of the lateral and third ventricles (see p.121). The presence of a small tumour in one cerebellar hemisphere may be enough to produce a kink in the upper brain stem, impeding the flow of fluid through the aqueduct. Children appear to be particularly at risk in this respect: almost any tumour in the posterior fossa of a child is likely to cause raised pressure and papilloedema.

The third effect is to promote *herniation*, which may be either upward or downward (see pp.21–5). In either case, life is threatened. Of the two, downward displacement, with impaction of the lower medulla and cerebellar tonsils in the foramen magnum, is by far the commoner. This may well be because in many cases upward pressure is countered by a downward thrust due to high pressure in the lateral and third ventricles.

The risk of foraminal herniation is enchanced if there is already a congenital prolongation of one or both cerebellar tonsils (Chiari type 1 malformation) or if the capacity of the posterior fossa is reduced by a congenital or acquired deformity of the base of the skull, such as platybasia or Paget's disease.

Expanding lesions in the spinal canal

These may lie in the spinal cord, subarachnoid space, meninges, or extrathecal space, or in the vertebral column. The effects are exerted on the cord, or nerve roots, or both.

Intrinsic neoplasms of the cord

These are mostly *gliomas*, of which the commonest is an ependymoma or subependymoma arising from the central canal (Fig. 11.9). Some of these are well circumscribed, and can even be shelled out by the surgeon through an incision between the posterior white columns. Diffuse astrocytomas are less common, and secondary carcinomas, though they occur, are rare. Ependymomas are also found growing from the *filum terminale*, which normally consists of little more than pia and ependyma. These are usually benign, and can be dissected cleanly away from the surrounding roots of the cauda equina. They are hard to distinguish from schwannomas by the naked eye. *Haemangioblastomas* also

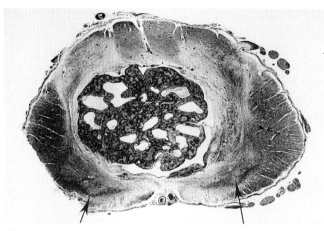

Fig. 11.9. Myelin-stained section from the cervical cord of a woman aged 53 with a two-year history of progressive tetraparesis. The tumour is a cystic ependymoma. The tissue surrounding it shows a mixture of necrosis and oedema. The white columns are reduced in bulk, but still contain axons. The grey matter of the anterior horns (arrowed) is fairly well preserved.

occur in the substance of the cord, but not as commonly as in the cerebellum.

Whereas the brain can expand at the expense of ventricular and subarachnoid spaces, and is finally restricted by the folds of the dura mater, the cord is contained in a relatively inelastic tube of pia mater. It can increase its volume somewhat in the cervical region by becoming more circular and less elliptical in cross-section (Fig. 11.10); beyond this, as the intrapial pressure increases, the circulation of blood is embarrassed, and necrosis may ensue. The other recourse is demyelination of long tracts. It is remarkable how much function can be transmitted through grossly attenuated long tracts in cases with slowly progressive lesions such as

syringomyelia and benign ependymomas. In such cases it seems also that the pia itself may undergo a fair amount of stretching. This is not so in a case of acute inflammatory oedema, such as occurs in the more fulminant forms of MS (Fig. 11.11). In the Dévic type of MS, the cervical and upper thoracic cord, and sometimes the optic nerves, undergo necrosis, apparently as a consequence of ischaemia from pressure. The necrotic tissue is then squeezed upward and downward, like toothpaste from a tube, forming plugs in the structurally weakest part of the cord, at the base of the posterior columns, or even into entering nerve roots (Fig. 11.12).

Subarachnoid tumours

The tumours most commonly occurring in the subarachnoid space are *schwannomas* arising from the sheaths of nerve roots. In von Recklinghausen's disease (Fig. 13.5a) these may be multiple, lying in the subarachnoid or extrathecal space, or appear as 'dumb-bell' tumours on both aspects of the dura. *Meningiomas*, which are usually intrathecal, may also be of dumb-bell form. *Carcinoma* deposits, though rare in the cord substance, are relatively commonly seen as nodules attached to the leptomeninges and nerve roots (Fig. 13.5b). There is also a condition of *meningeal carcinomatosis* in which malignant cells are thickly plastered over the cord and roots, more or less obliterating the subarachnoid space. The appearance and the clinical features somewhat resemble those of a chronic, e.g. tuberculous, meningitis; the condition is sometimes referred to as 'carcinomatous meningitis'. Obliteration of the subarachnoid space by tumour is also seen in some cases of medulloblastoma, with 'seeding' from the cerebellum. Here, the tumour can be seen invading the cord through the pia in many places.

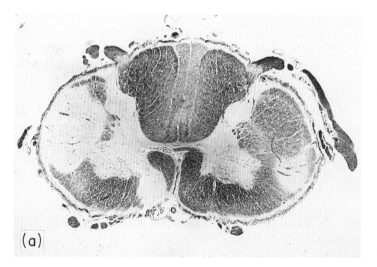
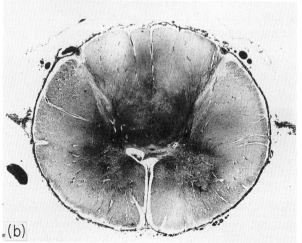

Fig. 11.10. Swelling of the cervical cord in acute MS. (a) Chronic case, showing three well-demarcated plaques. The dimensions and shape of the section are normal. (b) Acute case, showing a combination of demyelination and oedema. The swelling has resulted in a circular cross-section, with a tightly-stretched pia. Myelin stains.

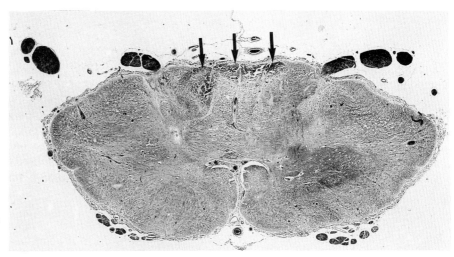

Fig. 11.11. Myelin-stained section from the seventh cervical segment in a woman aged 34 with MS. Four years earlier, there had been an acute attack of neuropticomyelitis, leaving her blind, and paralysed in the right arm and both legs. There was necrosis of the upper thoracic cord, and a postoedematous state of the lower cervical segments. On the right side (left side of the picture) all the nerve cells, and most of the axons, have disappeared. Some cells, and myelinated axons, remain in the left anterior horn. Anterior roots are wasted; posterior roots are intact. There has been invasion of the necrotic posterior columns by myelinated fibres derived from posterior roots (arrowed).

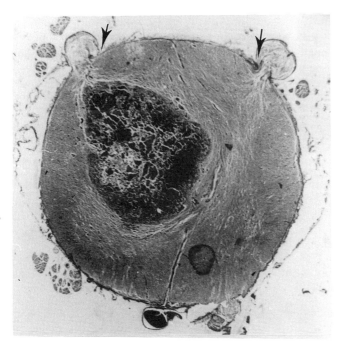

Fig. 11.12. Case of metastatic carcinoma. The lumbar cord is expanded by tumour. The pial sheath is tightly stretched, and cord tissue is herniating through the posterior root entry zones (arrowed).

Extrathecal expanding lesions

These include *tumours* and *abscesses*. Any of these may interfere with cord function by compression. In cases of carcinoma with paraplegia, the results of decompression are often disappointing, because the functional disturbance turns out to be due not to compression but to infarction of the cord. Carcinomatous infiltration of a spinal root carrying a major radicular artery only too often results in irreversible cord ischaemia. (This, of course, is not a reason for withholding operation if there is a remote chance of relieving cord compression.) The commonest of the compressing tumours are *meningiomas* and *schwannomas*, followed by various *lymphomas*, in particular Hodgkins' disease, and *myelomas*. Below the conus medullaris, there is room for small tumours to grow without causing symptoms (Fig. 11.13). Larger ones cause trouble by compressing the roots of the cauda equina, which are capable of some degree of recovery, provided that the major nerves within the pelvis are not eroded by malignancy.

As causes of cord compression, *spinal deformities*, congenital or acquired, are probably commoner than spinal tumours. In the elderly the commonest of these are *prolapsed intervertebral discs* and *cervical spondylosis*. In younger people traumatic *fracture-dislocations* are more frequent. Other lesions of the vertebral column which may cause narrowing of the spinal canal include tuberculous *spinal caries*, *rheumatoid arthritis*, *spondylolisthesis*, *Paget's disease*, and congenital deformities affecting the atlas and axis vertebrae. For a satisfactory post mortem examination of such cases, a careful study of the vertebral column, preferably combined with X-rays of the relevant part, as well as of the cord itself, should be carried out.

In the lumbosacral region, *disc protrusions* may compress nerve roots near their point of entry into intervertebral foramina, and even affect the calibre of the spinal canal. Thoracic disc protrusions tend to be small, limpet-shaped midline excrescences, and seldom cause disability. Protrusions in the cervical region are commoner (no doubt because of the greater mobility in the neck), and more of a threat to life. Not only is the cord itself at risk from anteroposterior compression, but its blood supply may be compromised by pressure on the anterior spinal artery. In *cervical spondylosis*, stripping of anterior and posterior longitudinal ligaments in the vicinity of degenerate discs gives rise to formation of new bone — *osteophytosis*. Anteriorly, this is a comparatively harmless process; posteriorly, the osteophytes encroach on the spinal canal (Fig. 2.20), and thus decrease the margin of safety in the face of sudden movements — especially that of

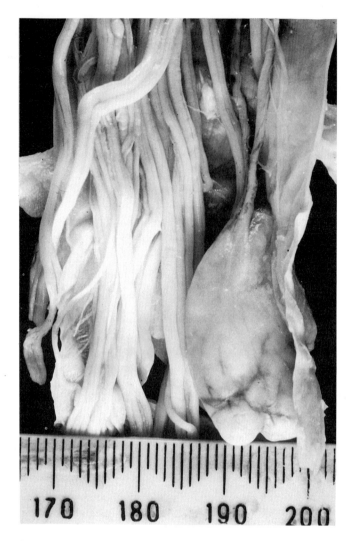

Fig. 11.13. Incidental finding of a schwannoma attached to a sacral rootlet. There is plenty of room in this part of the subarachnoid space. At higher levels a tumour of this size would undoubtedly have caused paraplegia from cord compression.

over-extension of the neck. A further effect of posterior osteophytes is that they form fibrous adhesions with the theca, thus hampering up-and-down movements of the spinal cord, and adding to the risks from sudden movement of the neck. The effects of spinal trauma are discussed on pp.94–5.

The spinal cord may undergo compression by a variety of expanding *cystic lesions*, all of them rare, histologically benign, and for the most part developing from embryonic rests. They include *dermoids* and *epidermoids* (see p.210), *arachnoid cysts*, which occasionally protrude through the dura into the extrathecal space, and *enterogenous cysts*. The latter lie in the cervical or thoracic subarachnoid space in front of the cord, and are lined by a columnar epithelium, usually of gastrointestinal type or, very rarely, of bronchial type. In some cases, they communicate with a similar cystic lesion in the mediastinum.

In examining cases in which myelopathy is thought to have ensued from pressure on the cord, the general rule is to take sections from above and below the lesion, and to look for loss of fibres in the ascending (spinocerebellar and posterior column) and descending (pyramidal) tracts respectively (see Fig. 5.10).

Further reading

Miller J Douglas, Adams J. Hume. 1984. The pathophysiology of raised intracranial pressure. In Adams JM, Corsellis JAN, Duchen LW (Eds) *Greenfield's Neuropathology*, 4th edn. Edward Arnold, London, Chapter 2.

Chapter 12
Tumours Arising in the Brain and Spinal Cord

This chapter and the following one aim to provide an overview of tumours of the nervous system. It is not our intention to deal comprehensively with their natural history, incidence and aetiology. These can be found in reference works on tumours of the nervous system such as those listed at the end of the chapter. What we hope to provide in these two chapters is a guide to the diagnosis of tumours, indicating the signposts that we have found useful along the way. Management of surgical specimens, interpretation of smears, and brief consideration of the role of immunohistological techniques in tumour diagnosis can be found in Chapter 4.

CNS tumour classification

The main requirement regarding surgical specimens is to provide the surgeon with a name for the tumour and some indication of its likely growth potential. This is not as straightforward as it might seem, for the classification of CNS tumours has long been a matter of debate, and small biopsies of gliomas do not always provide a reliable guide to prognosis. In any case, the surgeon, looking for guidance in management and treatment of the case, and for indications of the prognosis, will have other (and often more significant) clues than the histological report: the patient's clinical history, the neurological examination, radiological findings, and so on. If the neuropathologist merely reports on the most malignant features of the material examined, the surgeon should be satisfied. For post mortem diagnosis, on the other hand, the points of interest are not only the histological details of the tumour, but also its effects on the functions of the brain or spinal cord, the correlation of focal brain damage with clinical signs, and the evidence on the tumour's mode of spread and on the way in which it has contributed to the patient's death.

With regard to tumour classification, we have adopted the relatively simple system set out in Table 12.1. This is less elaborate than that proposed by the WHO in 1979, but is sufficient for present purposes. The different tumours are considered below and in Chapter 13 in the order in which they appear in Table 12.1, items 1–6 being contained in this chapter and items 7–14 in Chapter 13. Mention should also be made of the widely used classification and grading of gliomas proposed by Kernohan et al. (1949), which has commended itself to surgeons and others wishing to relate clinical outcome to histological findings in gliomas. This procedure is not without its pitfalls, largely on account of the tendency for some gliomas not only to contain different areas that would fit the criteria for different grades in the Kernohan classification, but also to become progressively less well differentiated with time. Despite these reservations, there is, of course, a need to provide the surgeon with as accurate a definition as possible of the nature of the tumour specimen received, and Kernohan's proposals in this regard have yet to be bettered. A disputable system of tumour classification is a recent proposal to categorize many childhood tumours of the CNS as 'primitive neuroectodermal tumours' (Rorke et al. 1985; Rubinstein 1985). Whether this term may have some use when only a very small biopsy is available is open to debate, if there is sufficient evidence to indicate a more precise diagnosis, such as medulloblastoma, ependymoma or neuroblastoma, it is desirable that this should be stated in any report on a childhood CNS tumour.

Table 12.1. Classification of CNS tumours

1 *Gliomas*
   With predominantly astrocytic differentiation
   With predominantly oligodendroglial differentiation
   With predominantly ependymal differentiation
   Glioblastoma (and gliosarcoma)

2 *Choroid plexus tumours*
   Papilloma
   Carcinoma

3 *Medulloblastoma*

4 *Tumours containing neurons*
   Neuroblastoma
   Gangliocytoma
   Ganglioglioma
   Ganglioneuroma

5 *Primary CNS lymphoma*

6 *Haemangioblastoma*

7 *Nerve sheath tumours*
   Schwannoma
   Neurofibroma
   Malignant nerve sheath tumours

8 *Meningioma (and meningeal sarcoma and melanoma)*

9 *Craniopharyngioma*

10 *Dermoid and epidermoid cysts*

11 *Pituitary adenomas*

12 *Pineal and parapineal tumours*
   Teratoma
   Germinoma
   Pineal parenchymal tumours

13 *Tumours extending to CNS from local source*

14 *Tumours metastatic to the CNS*

Items 7–14 are discussed in Chapter 13.

Post mortem examination of cases of CNS tumour

In examining the CNS in cases with tumours at post mortem, the presence of midline shift, herniations, other consequences of intracranial space occupation (Chapter 11) and other associated CNS disease should be noted. If the tumour caused epilepsy, the brain may show pathological changes associated with this condition (Chapter 18). It is of course important to carry out a careful examination of extracranial viscera looking particularly for sources of metastatic deposits. These include carcinoma, lymphoma, leukaemia and sarcoma. In cases of malignant disease treated with chemotherapy or radiotherapy, and in diseases associated with immunosuppression, one has to look for the effects these may have on the CNS. There may also, rarely, be evidence of: extracranial spread of primary CNS or pituitary tumour to other sites; endocrine effects of pituitary adenomas; and extracranial pathology associated with intracranial or spinal

tumours such as von Recklinghausen's disease (p.198), tuberous sclerosis (p.262) or Lindau's syndrome (p.262).

The spinal cord should be examined along with the brain if there was any clinical suspicion of spinal cord disease or if tumours known to disseminate via CSF pathways have been earlier diagnosed. These include medulloblastoma, choroid plexus tumours, melanoma, ependymoma, and carcinomas, particularly those arising in the breast or stomach.

Macroscopic and microscopic features of intrinsic neuroepithelial tumours

Glial tumours

By definition, gliomas are tumours of neuroglial cells, that is, astrocytes, oligodendrocytes and/or ependymal cells. As all these cells are derived from the cells labelled 'spongioblasts' by embryologists, it is not surprising to find that in many neuroglial tumours there is a mixture of cell types and patterns reminiscent of two or even three of the normal types and patterns. In consequence, it is often difficult to classify a particular tumour as *an* astrocytoma, *an* oligodendroglioma, or *an* ependymoma, whereas there is no such difficulty in speaking of *a* glioma. This point should be borne in mind when reporting on a small sample of tumour from a biopsy. The fact that the fragment of tissue has the appearance of gemistocytic astrocytoma does not exclude the possibility that another part of the tumour may have the features of an oligodendroglioma, or (as is very often the case) that elsewhere in the tumour there are areas of anaplastic malignancy.

A remarkable characteristic — one might almost call it a virtue — of gliomas in general is their reluctance to metastasize, or perhaps the reluctance of other parts of the body to accept glioma metastases. Since there are no lymphatics in the CNS, this channel of spread is unavailable to gliomas; although they are well supplied with veins, reports of glioma metastases in lungs are exceedingly rare. Experimentally explanted tumours, on the other hand, are said to flourish. Even the kind of seeding through the CSF pathways so characteristic of medulloblastomas, which are generally regarded as primitive neural tumours, rarely occurs. Glioblastomas and oligodendrogliomas do indeed reach, and transgress, the pial membrane, and continue to grow for a certain distance in the subarachnoid space, whence they may re-invade the brain. Fragments of malignant glioma may also become detached and adhere to ependymal surfaces, whence they may grow back into the brain. What it is that inhibits their wider spread is not known.

Gliomas composed predominantly of astrocytes

It is unfortunate that one word — astrocytoma — is used to cover at least two very different tumours. The first is diffusely spread through a region of the CNS. It has no clearly defined boundaries (Fig. 12.1) and in most cases is inoperable, simply because its removal would entail an unacceptable loss of functioning nervous tissue (the exception is a glioma of an optic nerve; if it does not involve the chiasma, it can be removed at the expense of the already compromised sight in one eye). This diffuse type of astrocytoma is nevertheless regarded as relatively benign, in that it grows slowly, and is compatible with several years' useful life. In contrast, there are tumours composed of astrocytes, unmixed with nervous tissue, and having well-demarcated margins. Except in a few vital areas in the brain stem, these can be completely removed surgically with good hope that they will not recur. They are most commonly met with in the cerebellum in young people. On the assumption that they are true neoplasms, rather than local glial reactions to some congenital malformation, they constitute the benign end of the spectrum of malignancy in gliomas. They are often separated from the diffuse astrocytomas under the clumsy title of 'benign cerebellar astrocytoma of childhood'. Benign, in fact, they are, provided they are removed; otherwise the child will die from the effects of mounting pressure in the posterior cranial fossa. This pressure is usually due not to the size of the tumour, which remains small, but to the expansion of an associated cyst. In most cases it is this that causes the patient's symptoms.

A real and practical difficulty arises in making the distinction between low-grade astrocytoma and reactive gliosis. In one variety of glioma a region of the brain or spinal cord is expanded — sometimes grotesquely so — by the presence

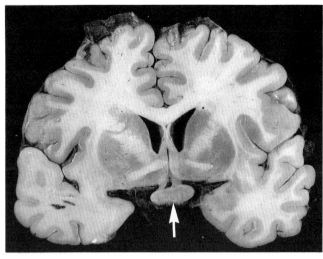

Fig. 12.2. Coronal slice across the frontal and temporal lobes and optic chiasm from a case with diffuse expansion of the optic chiasm by an astrocytoma (arrowed).

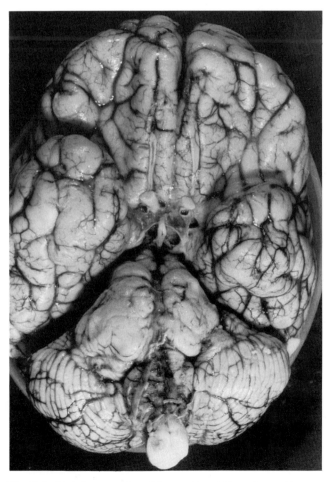

Fig. 12.3. Nodular expansion of the pons by a diffuse glioma. The basilar artery lies in a groove surrounded by the asymmetrically expanded base of the pons.

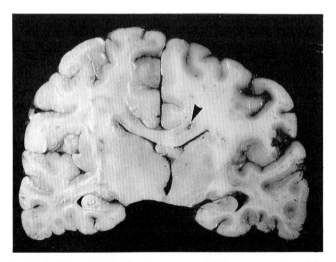

Fig. 12.1. Coronal brain slice from a case of diffuse astrocytoma of the left cerebral hemisphere. The left side of the cerebrum and diencephalon are diffusely enlarged, particularly the thalamus, and midline structures are pushed over to the right. Lateral and third ventricles are compressed. The corpus callosum is infiltrated with tumour on both sides and contains a cyst on the right (arrow head). Notice how the infiltrated structures in the left hemisphere retain their original form as they expand (e.g. hippocampus).

174   CHAPTER 12

of vast numbers of well-differentiated astrocytes lying between and among nerve cells and their processes. This may occur in many parts of the CNS, including the optic nerves and brain stem (Figs 12.2 and 12.3). The clinical findings in such cases show that the nervous elements are functioning more or less normally. The histological appearance, one feels, could as well be designated 'pathological hyperplasia of astrocytes' as 'diffuse astrocytoma' — apart, that is, from the prognostic implication of the latter term, which is that the process will continue relentlessly until the space-occupying aspect of the condition kills the patient, or blinds him, as the case may be.

Gliosis, in the sense of astrocytic proliferation in response to a partial injury to CNS tissue, is distinguished from this by having an underlying cause (e.g. death of nerve cells, blood–brain barrier deficiency or demyelination), and by not being a progressive change. The distinction may, however, not be fundamental. Very little is known about the immediate causes of gliosis, and even less about those of astrocytoma; it is reasonable to suppose that the former is induced by chemical or hormonal influences arising in the area of damage, which cease to operate when the damage is repaired, and that the abnormal persistence of a similar hormone might account for the astrocytoma. In this connection it is worth mentioning the not-infrequent reports of gliomas arising in proximity with an older plaque of MS.

Returning from the theoretical to the practical, the diagnosis of astrocytoma on a biopsy specimen — especially on a smeared preparation — should always be guarded. We know of instances where the surgeon, on the evidence of angiograms or air encephalograms, has diagnosed a temporal lobe glioma; and the presence of an excess of astrocytes in the biopsy seemed to confirm the diagnosis. Later it has emerged that the temporal lobe was oedematous and gliotic

as a consequence of a middle fossa meningioma. This counsel of hesitancy still applies even when many of the astrocytes appear abnormally large, or possess bizarre, polyploid nuclei. Bizarre astrocytes may be found in a variety of conditions, including hepatic failure, PML and acute MS. Before leaving this topic we should stress that difficulty in distinguishing between reactive and neoplastic astrocytes is not merely a pitfall for beginners. An experienced neuropathologist, examining the outskirts of a frankly malignant glioma post mortem, will not always be able to say whether the astrocytes in the border zone represent reaction or infiltration.

Microscopically, the commonest cell type in astrocytomas is the *fibrillary astrocyte* and its reactive form, the *gemistocyte*. Astrocytomas in which fibrillary astrocytes predominate are moderately cellular and are composed of cells diffusely arranged or displayed as bundles of elongated cells with ill-defined cell borders. In 'piloid' astrocytomas the processes are aligned in the direction of underlying nerve fibre tracts (Fig. 12.4). The cell processes are well shown with the PTAH stain (Fig. 12.5), or with antibodies to GFAP (Fig. 4.26). They may contain condensations of material forming hyaline PTAH-positive, elongated or globular bodies called *Rosenthal fibres* (Fig. 12.6), or more rounded granular bodies. Small foci of calcification may be seen in blood vessel walls or scattered in the fibrillary matrix. The cell bodies are usually inconspicuous and spindle-shaped, and the nuclei round or oval and moderately dense. Mitotic figures are rare or absent in well-differentiated tumours of this type. Slight variation in nuclear size is common, and provides a useful feature distinguishing a sparsely cellular astrocytoma from reactive gliosis (Fig. 12.7). Some tumours have a microcystic background matrix which, if present, also helps to distinguish benign astrocytoma from gliosis.

In contrast to astrocytomas containing mainly fibrillary

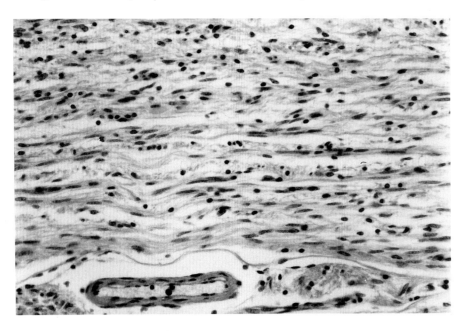

Fig. 12.4. Diffuse astrocytoma in which the bipolar neoplastic astrocytes are aligned parallel to the direction of the infiltrated fibre tract. H&E, ×175.

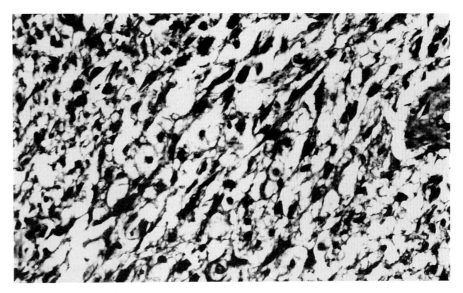

Fig. 12.5. Fibrillary astrocytoma stained with PTAH to show up the processes as well as the cell bodies of the tumour cells. ×400.

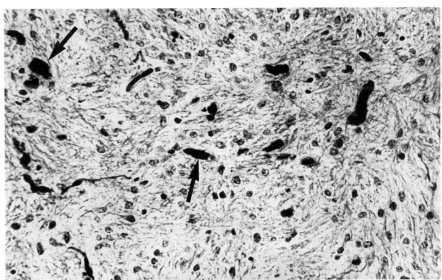

Fig. 12.6. Rosenthal fibres in a fibrillary astrocytoma, examples arrowed. PTAH, ×340.

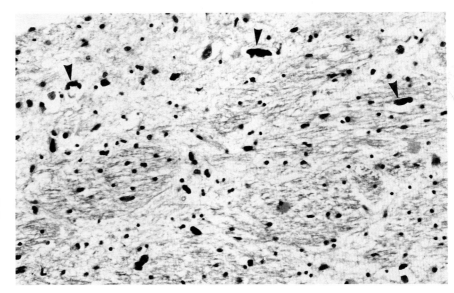

Fig. 12.7. Diffuse astrocytoma infiltrating cerebral white matter. The overall cellularity is hardly increased, but the presence of neoplasia is revealed by the pleomorphism of some of the nuclei (arrow heads). Note, however, that there are other conditions giving rise to pleomorphic astrocyte nuclei (see p.74). H&E, ×160.

astrocytes are rarer tumours in which *protoplasmic astrocytes* predominate. These tumours have a low or moderate degree of cellularity and are composed of cells with multiple, fine processes which form a delicate network frequently interspersed with microcystic spaces containing eosinophilic fluid (Fig. 12.8). The fine processes take the PTAH stain. Nuclei show some variation in size. Mitotic figures are usually absent.

Gemistocytic tumour astrocytes have a distinctive microscopic appearance. They are large cells with a prominent, rounded cell body containing pale eosinophilic cytoplasm and an eccentric nucleus (Fig. 12.9). Short processes are given off from the margins of the cells and these stain with PTAH or with GFAP antibody. Many astrocytomas contain foci of gemistocytic astrocytes, but it is rare for a tumour to be composed solely of cells of this type. However, they may predominate in a biopsy specimen. Their presence in an astrocytic tumour is generally associated with a poor prognosis.

The distinctive *astrocytic gliomas* arising in the *cerebellum*

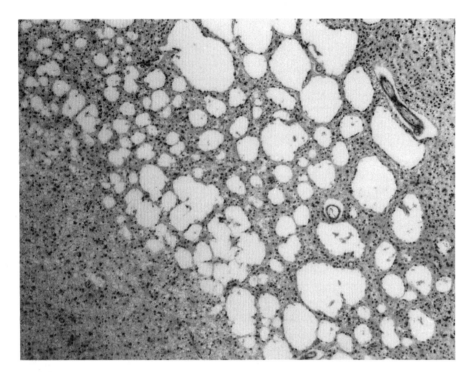

Fig. 12.8. Low-power view of a section of a protoplasmic astrocytoma containing microcysts. H&E, ×90.

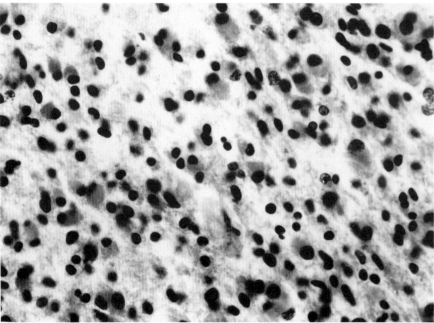

Fig. 12.9. Gemistocytic astrocytoma composed of cells with abundant, eosinophilic cytoplasm and eccentrically placed nuclei. The processes of these cells are inconspicuous, but can be shown up with the PTAH stain. H&E, ×300.

have already been referred to. Most contain intermingled areas of fibrillary astrocytes and microcystic foci in which the cell bodies of the neoplastic cells cluster around blood vessels and project fine processes to form a sketchy, web-like pattern interspersed among the cysts. Foci of calcification and haemosiderin deposition are common, and a moderate degree of vascular hyperplasia may be present without the implied malignant potential that this feature imparts to cerebral astrocytomas (see p.178). Leptomeningeal invasion is also common and does not influence the usually benign outcome following removal of this tumour. Features that are correlated with a poor outcome are only rarely seen and consist of a high overall degree of cellularity and frequent mitotic figures (Fig. 12.10). Nuclear pleomorphism may be found even in benign tumours.

Subependymal giant cell tumours may occur in subjects with tuberous sclerosis (p.262), *formes frustes* of that condi-tion, and in a number of cases in isolation. These tumours occur around the lateral ventricles and are relatively slow-growing and circumscribed (Fig. 16.17b). Microscopically they contain conspicuous large cells with abundant cytoplasm and short processes. Nuclei are large, often bizarre, and are eccentrically situated (Fig. 12.11). Some of the cells resemble gemistocytic astrocytes, but others are larger and may have two or more nuclei. Foci of calcification are frequently present. These tumours are considered to be related to the bizarre astrocytes found in the cortex in tuberous sclerosis, and their immuno reactions (often GFAP-negative, usually NSE-positive, sometimes NF-positive) suggest an origin from dysplastic cells related both to neurons and astrocytes. The unwary may take these tumours for glioblastomas, but they differ from these in the absence or rarity of mitotic figures, and absence of necrosis and of endothelial hyperplasia (p.188).

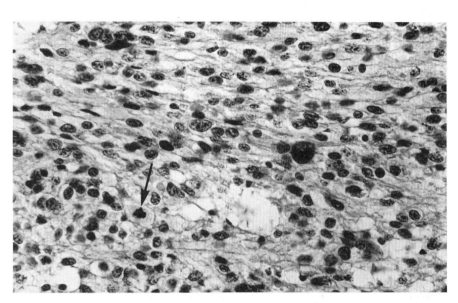

Fig. 12.10. Malignant cerebellar astrocytoma showing a high degree of cellularity, nuclear pleomorphism and mitoses (example arrowed). H&E, ×340.

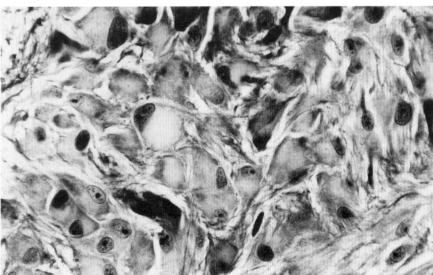

Fig. 12.11. Subependymal tumour from a case of tuberous sclerosis. The cells are large, closely packed and contain several processes. Nuclei are large and pleomorphic, often with prominent nucleoli. Mitoses are not a regular feature of these tumours. H&E, ×370.

Foci of anaplastic change may occur in an otherwise better-differentiated astrocytoma. Microscopically, *anaplastic astrocytoma* is hard to differentiate from glioblastoma and, in terms of clinical outcome, the distinction is of no real value. Compared with well-differentiated astrocytoma, anaplastic tumour shows greater overall cellularity, and fewer recognizable astrocytic features, though gemistocytic astrocytes may be present. The tumour cells are haphazardly arranged, and nuclei are pleomorphic (Fig. 12.12). Mitotic figures are present, and there is endothelial cell enlargement and hyperplasia, and a high degree of vascularity in most tumours. Small areas of necrosis may be present. When infiltrating the cortex these tumours characteristically produce clusters of cells around neuron cell bodies, mimicking the satellitosis seen sometimes in the deep cortex late in life (Fig. 12.13).

An unusual variant of astrocytic glioma, warranting recognition because of its relatively good prognosis compared with other variants of pleomorphic astrocytoma, is the *pleomorphic xanthoastrocytoma*. This is a tumour found superficially situated in the cerebrum in young adults. It is distinguished by the presence of lipid in the cytoplasm of many of the tumour cells (Fig. 12.14), and by the presence of reticulin around them (Fig. 12.15).

Well-differentiated astrocytoma reacts immunohistologically with antibodies to GFAP (Fig. 4.26). A variable proportion of tumour cells in anaplastic astrocytoma do likewise (Fig. 4.27). However, this reaction is not specific

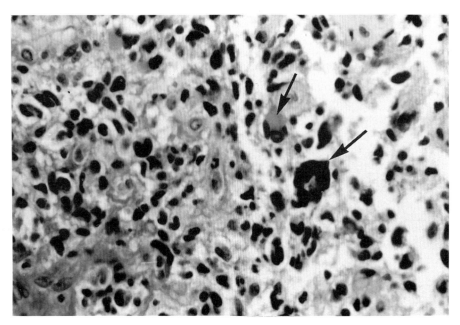

Fig. 12.12. Anaplastic astrocytoma showing closely packed cells of varying size and shape, some with multiple nuclei (arrowed). Nuclei are hyperchromatic and pleomorphic. H&E, ×300.

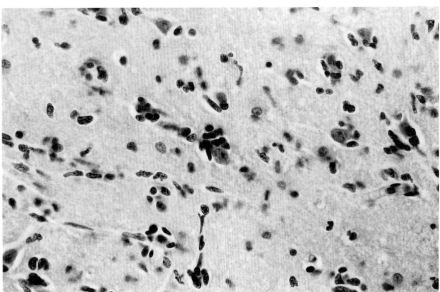

Fig. 12.13. Cerebral cortex adjacent to an anaplastic astrocytoma of the white matter. Clusters of astrocytes surround neuron cell bodies, producing an appearance resembling satellitosis. H&E, ×280.

for astrocytoma, since ependymoma, glioblastoma and oligo-dendroglioma may also show some GFAP-immunoreactivity. Even haemangioblastoma, medulloblastoma and choroid plexus papilloma may contain a few tumour cells reactive with GFAP antibodies. The majority of astrocytic tumours also react with anti-Leu 7 (NK cell) monoclonal antibody, but again this is not a specific reaction (see Table 4.2). Astrocytomas also contain vimentin, and some investigators have found an inverse relation between the intensity of staining for vimentin and the degree of differentiation of the astrocytoma.

Gliomas composed predominantly of oligodendrocytes

Tumours of oligodendrocytes are more often than not associated with astrocytoma. In their purer forms they are usually fairly well circumscribed, expanding rather than infiltrating, and tending to grow slowly (Fig. 18.4). They occur almost exclusively in the cerebral hemispheres. Peculiar features are, first, their tendency to evoke calcification (often visible on radiographs) in the surrounding brain tissue, and second, a way of fungating into the subarachnoid space, without widespread subarachnoid seeding. Some have associated cysts, whereas others do not.

Microscopically, these tumours are composed of diffusely arranged uniform cells with a centrally situated, more or

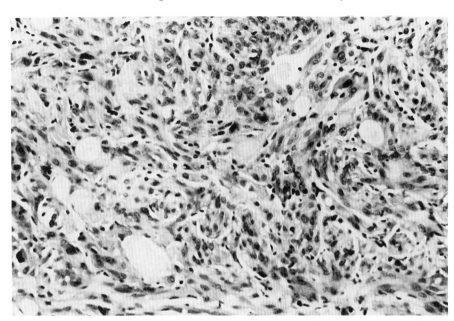

Fig. 12.14. Pleomorphic xanthoastrocytoma. The cells are haphazardly arranged and show considerable nuclear pleomorphism. Some cells possess pale, swollen cytoplasm containing lipid droplets. H&E, ×220.

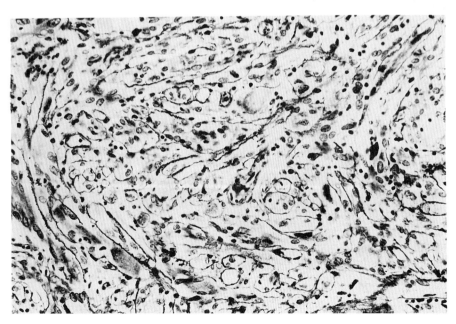

Fig. 12.15. Adjacent section to that shown in Fig. 12.14, stained for reticulin. There is an abundant reticulin network throughout the tumour. ×220.

less round nucleus, with coarse, stippled chromatin and small nucleolus. The surrounding cytoplasm is often swollen and empty looking (Fig. 12.16). The appearance of such cells has been aptly likened to that of fried eggs. Some areas of the tumours lack the cytoplasmic swelling, and then the cells appear more closely packed (Fig. 12.17). Processes are not visible on the cells with routine stains, but can be shown up on some cells with silver stains. Calcospherites and calcification of blood vessel walls in and just beyond the tumour are common findings. Occasionally bone may form. There is an abundance of capillaries in most oligodendroglial tumours and these characteristically form a prominent network dividing the tumour cells into clusters (Fig. 12.18), or parallel rows. Endothelial hyperplasia may be seen in otherwise benign-appearing tumours. Nuclei usually show little pleomorphism and mitotic figures are rare in most tumours. Mucinous degeneration may occur in clusters of tumour cells and spill over into the background matrix of the tumour. As indicated above, mixed gliomas composed of oligodendrocytes and astrocytes are more common than tumours composed solely of oligodendrocytes. Malignant oligodendrogliomas are also well recognized. They have a higher cell

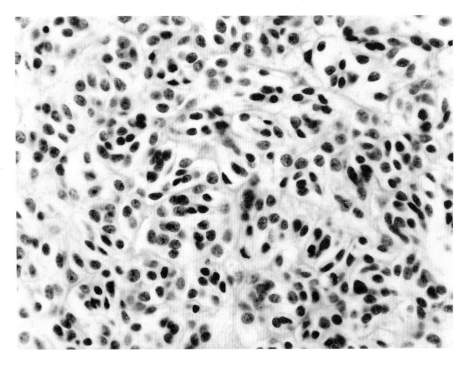

Fig. 12.16. Microscopic appearances of an oligodendroglioma. Cells are uniform, polygonal or cuboidal, and have centrally placed, regular nuclei. The cells are divided into clusters by a delicate, vascular stoma. H&E, ×470.

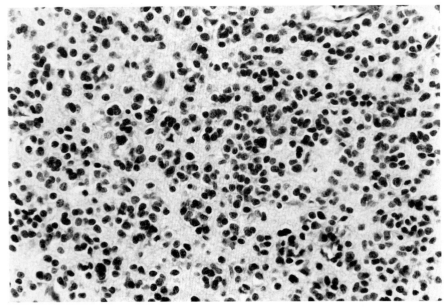

Fig. 12.17. Microscopic appearance of an oligodendroglioma infiltrating cerebral cortex. The tumour cells are less swollen and their cytoplasm less 'empty' looking than those in Fig. 12.16. H&E, ×340.

density, greater nuclear pleomorphism and more numerous mitotic figures than the more benign tumours (Fig. 12.19).

Immunohistologically, oligodendrocytes are mainly characterized by the absence rather than the presence of recognizable antigens. They give negative reactions with antibodies to neurofilaments, epithelial membrane antigen and cytokeratins. However, they usually show some reaction with antibodies to GFAP (Fig. 4.29) and S-100 protein, and with the monoclonal antibody Leu 7.

Gliomas composed predominantly of ependymal cells

Ependymomas may arise wherever there are ependymal cells; in practice, they are commonest in the fourth ventricle (including Luschka's foramina). Other common sites are the so-called central canal of the spinal cord, the filum terminale, the third ventricle and the aqueduct. They are generally slow growing, although malignant varieties occur. In the third and fourth ventricles and aqueduct their main effect is to produce hydrocephalus by obstructing the flow of CSF. In the spinal cord the effect is to compress the surrounding tissues (Fig. 11.9) and in the filum terminale to compress the roots of the cauda equina (Fig. 12.20). The fourth-ventricle tumours are surgically accessible; if they arise from the roof of the ventricle a complete removal may be achieved, but if they arise from, or are closely adherent to, the floor of the ventricle, this is not practicable. Spinal ependymomas can sometimes be shelled out from behind, and those of the filum terminale can be dissected away entire.

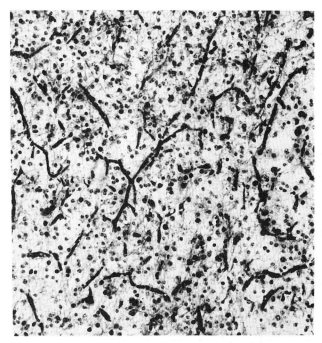

Fig. 12.18. The capillary network in an oligodendroglioma, shown up here by the staining of red cells in congested vessels. PTAH, ×110.

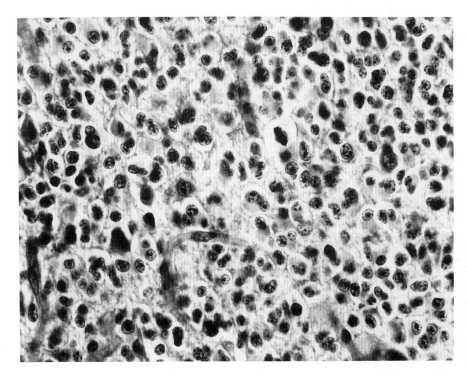

Fig. 12.19. Malignant oligodendroglioma. The tumour cells are packed closely together, are less uniform than those of a benign oligodendroglioma, and have pleomorphic nuclei. A few foci of capillary calcification are present. H&E, ×19420.

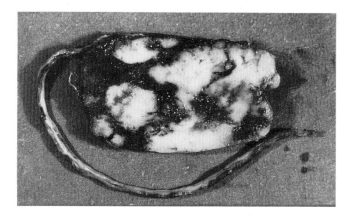

Fig. 12.20. Section across an ependymoma of the filum terminale.

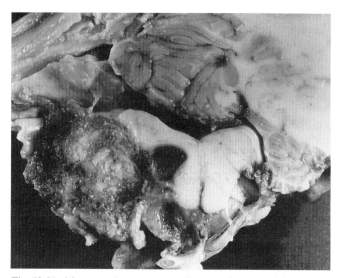

Fig. 12.21. Macroscopic appearance of an ependymoma arising in the left foramen of Luschka. After incomplete surgical removal of the tumour there was a 6-year survival. The tumour is seen spilling out into the subarachnoid space, and invading the medulla.

Macroscopic appearances vary, but most tumours appear greyish in colour and are granular in texture. They are sometimes cystic and are usually circumscribed, but not encapsulated. They tend to spill irregularly, or in lobulated form, into the ependymal-lined cavity from which they arise (Fig. 12.21). Seeding of tumours into the CSF can give rise to metastatic CNS deposits.

Microscopic appearances show wide variation, but certain features usually allow *typical ependymomas* to be easily identified. The most characteristic of these is the occurrence of rosettes of cells arranged around a central space (Fig. 12.22), recalling the appearance of reactive ependymal cells buried beneath the ventricular surface. Sometimes the central spaces of the rosettes are enlarged to form microscopic or macroscopic cysts, and the arrangement of the tumour cells may then be papillary (Fig. 12.23). Even more common than rosettes are pseudorosettes, formed by elongated bipolar tumour cells orientated around blood vessels (Fig. 12.24). Nuclei of the tumour cells are placed well away from the vessel, the space between being occupied by the radially directed processes of the ependymal cells. These processes appear poorly defined and eosinophilic with H&E, but are better appreciated with the PTAH stain. The PTAH stain will also sometimes reveal clusters of cytoplasmic bodies, blepharoplasts, the basal bodies to which the shafts of cilia are attached. Cilia themselves may be visible, but blepharoplasts are more widespread. At the ultrastructural level, microvilli occupy the central space in the rosettes and gap junctions can be found, reflecting the epithelial character of the cells. The nuclei of ependymoma cells are oval or round and darkly stained. They usually show little pleomorphism, and mitotic figures are rare or absent.

Myxopapillary ependymomas are virtually confined to the cauda equina region, where they appear to arise from the

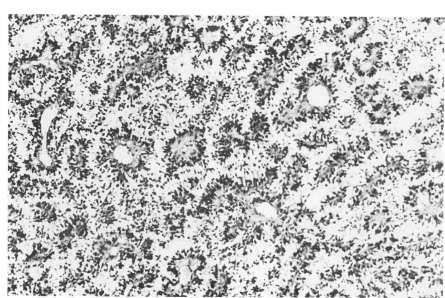

Fig. 12.22. Ependymoma. Low-power view showing a pattern chiefly of pseudorosettes, with tumour cells orientated around blood vessels. H&E, ×100.

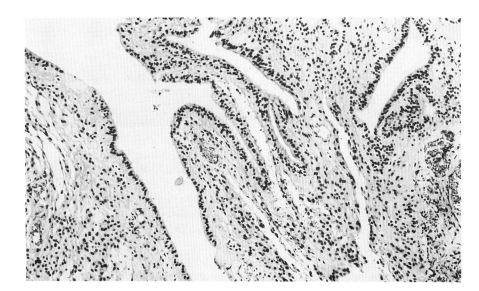

Fig. 12.23. Papillary pattern of growth in a cystic ependymoma. H&E, ×100.

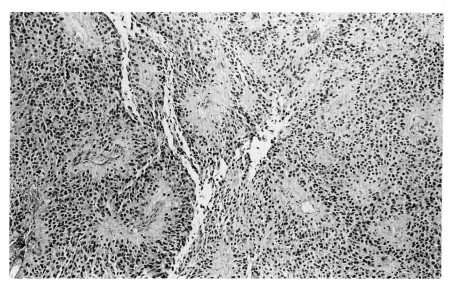

Fig. 12.24. Pseudorosettes in an ependymoma. Vessels are surrounded by a pale zone containing processes of tumour cells, which separate the vessel wall from the cell nuclei. H&E, ×100.

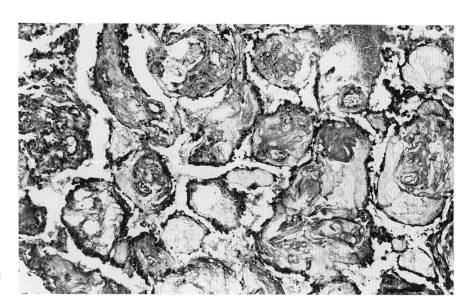

Fig. 12.25. Myxopapillary ependymoma of the cauda equina. The tumour is composed of cores of myxoid stroma surrounding blood vessels, and covered by a layer of flattened cuboidal epithelial cells. The epithelium appears as a dark layer enveloping the myxoid cores. H&E, ×100.

filum terminale. They form sausage-like, slightly irregular, discrete masses surrounded by compressed nerve roots. The microscopic appearance of these tumours is unusual and distinctive. They are composed of flattened cuboidal epithelial cells covering connective tissue cores containing blood vessels and abundant acellular, hyaline, matrix material (Fig. 12.25). The matrix reacts with stains for mucin. Nuclei are small and uniform, without mitoses. The prognosis for these tumours is usually very good, but occasionally they exhibit malignant behaviour.

A not uncommon tumour composed of an intimate mixture of ependymal cells with fibre-forming astrocytes, called *subependymoma*, occurs mainly in the fourth ventricle, where it may be an incidental post mortem finding (Fig. 12.26). For the most part these tumours belong to the benign end of the glioma spectrum.

Ependymomas with malignant features (patchy necrosis, invasive tendencies, pleomorphism and frequent mitoses; Fig. 12.27) occur most commonly in children, and are usually situated in the fourth ventricle. The differential diagnosis of such tumours includes malignant choroid plexus tumour, glioblastoma and medulloblastoma. At the malignant end of the spectrum is the ependymoblastoma, a rare childhood variant combining cellular anaplasia, a high mitotic incidence and a characteristic ependymal pattern.

In their immunohistological reactions, ependymomas usually show foci of positive reactivity for GFAP and to a lesser extent for Leu 7 antigen. Epithelial membrane antigen is focally expressed by the more benign forms, but not by malignant ones, a distinction of some diagnostic value (Fig. 4.25).

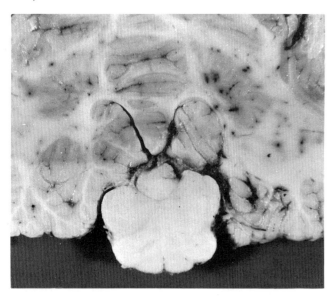

Fig. 12.26. A subependymoma arising in the floor of the fourth ventricle, which was discovered as an incidental finding at post mortem examination. The tumour is almost filling the cavity of the fourth ventricle, and might have been expected to cause hydrocephalus eventually.

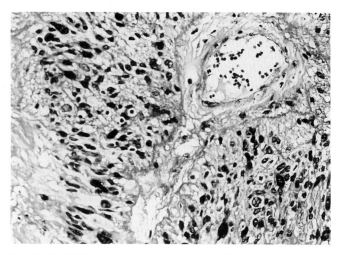

Fig. 12.27. Malignant ependymoma showing a disorganized, but still recognizable, pseudorosette pattern. Nuclei are pleomorphic. H&E, ×210.

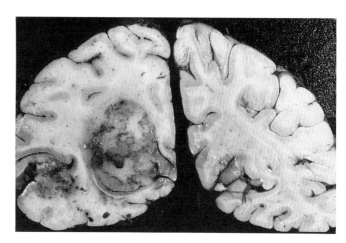

Fig. 12.28. Glioblastoma of the left temporoparietal region. The main tumour mass occupies the white matter, but it extends into lateral occipital cortex also. Note variegated, partially necrotic, cut surface appearance and relatively sharp margin to the tumour.

Glioblastomas

The commonest kind of glioma lies, alas, at the most malignant end of the spectrum. Although the various cell types seen in this tumour bear little, if any, resemblance to embryonic glial cells, the tumour is generally known as glioblastoma (the adjective 'multiforme', which is traditionally attached to this term, is redundant, as it does not differentiate one type of glioblastoma from another). The most striking macroscopic feature is its variegated appearance on slicing, which is largely due to: scattered haemorrhages which show dark or red-brown; patches of necrosis showing yellow or white; and multiple, small cystic cavities, containing yellowish fluid, which coagulates on fixation and even on standing (Fig. 12.28). On palpation there is a similar variety, ranging from slimy through mushy, soft and rubbery, to tough and gristly. The tumours are commonest in elderly people, and arise most often in one or' other cerebral hemisphere, but may occupy both hemispheres as so-called 'butterfly tumours', with a connection through the corpus callosum (Fig. 12.29). Their effect on the brain is exerted in three ways: they destroy, they expand, and they give rise to cysts. Some glioblastomas seem, from the clinical and pathological evidence, to have been malignant and fast growing from the start. The illness lasts six months or less; on slicing the brain, the tumour is separated from more or less normal brain tissue by a margin only a centimetre or less wide, of infiltrated tissue. In other cases, with a longer history — a year or more — one finds a large area of diffuse astrocytoma containing a malignant patch (Fig. 12.30). Such tumours are sometimes referred to as 'astrocytoma-gone-bad'. Similarly, one may come across cases, again with somewhat longer clinical histories, of 'oligodendroglioma-gone-bad' and 'ependymoma-gone-bad'. The malignant areas in these are hardly distinguishable from 'bad-from-

the-start' tumours. In a few cases glioblastomas appear to arise in more than one focus; they may then be misinterpreted clinically and in scans or radiographs as metastatic tumours.

Microscopic appearances in glioblastomas are varied. In some tumours there are foci of clearly recognizable astrocytes, fibrillary or gemistocytic, or of oligodendrocytes. In other areas there are densely packed, haphazardly arranged, nondescript, small cells with scanty wisps of cytoplasm and darkly staining nuclei (Fig. 12.31). Some fields contain markedly pleomorphic, larger cells with conspicuous, lobulated or multiple nuclei, and in a few tumours multinucleate cells are numerous (Fig. 12.32). Other fields consist of frankly necrotic debris. A very characteristic appearance, best appreciated at low power, is of 'pseudopalisading' of dense rows of nuclei around irregular or serpiginous patches of necrosis (Fig. 12.33). Some of these nuclei are those of tumour cells, but others belong to macrophages. Mitotic figures in the tumour cells are frequent, but are not always conspicuous, and may need to be carefully sought. The

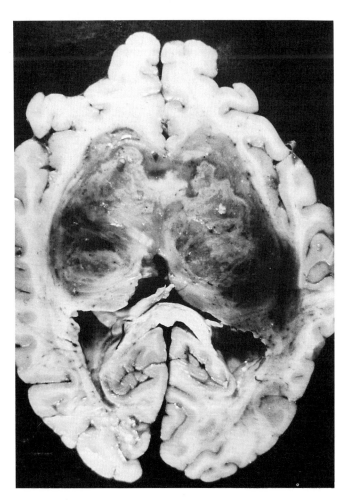

Fig. 12.29. Horizontal slice through a 'butterfly'-shaped glioblastoma massively expanding both cerebral hemispheres and the corpus callosum.

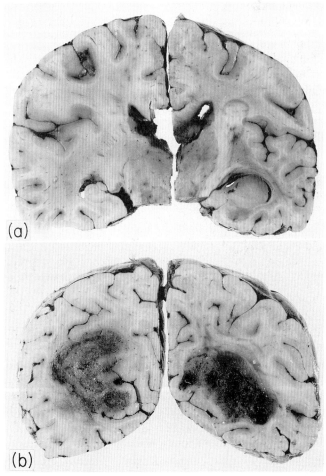

Fig. 12.30. Diffuse cerebral astrocytoma expanding the right hippocampus in the more rostral slice (a). A glioblastoma has arisen in this tumour more posteriorly (b).

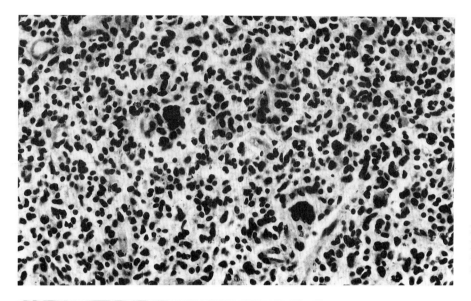

Fig. 12.31. Glioblastoma composed of densely packed, small cells with dark-stained nuclei and scanty cytoplasm, with wispy processes. Several multinucleate cells are present. H&E, ×200.

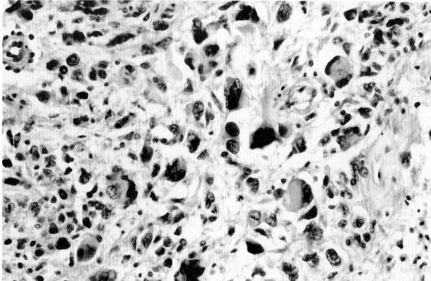

Fig. 12.32. Glioblastoma in which many of the tumour cells are large and multinuleate. H&E, ×250.

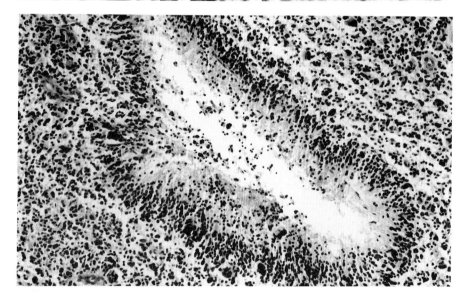

Fig. 12.33. 'Pseudopalisade' of nuclei surrounding a focus of necrosis in a glioblastoma. H&E, ×150.

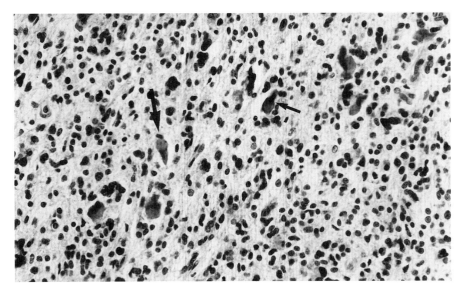

Fig. 12.34. Surviving brain stem neurons (arrowed) surrounded by a dense infiltrate of tumour cells in a rare glioblastoma arising in the medulla. H&E, ×220.

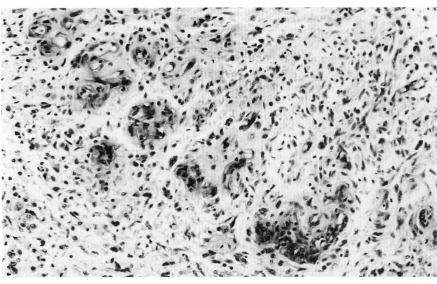

Fig. 12.35. Zone of hyperplastic blood vessels at the growing margins of a glioblastoma. H&E, ×120.

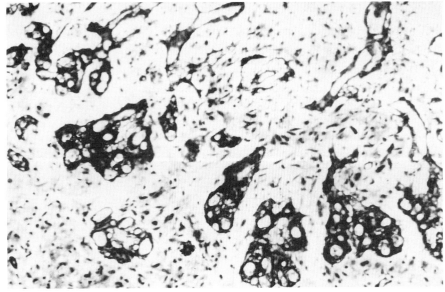

Fig. 12.36. Adjacent section to that shown in Fig. 12.35, stained to show the heavy reticulin deposition associated with the hyperplastic blood vessels. ×120.

PTAH stain reveals positively stained neuroglial fibrils to a variable extent in the cells of a glioblastoma. Remnants of surviving neural structure, such as neurons and axons, are encountered in some tumours, testifying to the infiltrating character of the tumour growth (Fig. 12.34). The vasculature is striking. There are large, thin-walled, congested vessels, usually with evidence at some point of haemorrhage or thrombosis or both. The small vessels, particularly the capillaries, show a characteristic hyperplastic change which makes them appear tortuous, with thickened walls composed of enlarged endothelial cells, some containing mitotic figures, increased reticulin and reduplicated basal lamina. Zones of hyperplastic change in small vessels are frequently prominent at the advancing edge of the tumour (Figs 12.35 and 12.36), and explain the high degree of enhancement seen in CAT scans at the margin of these tumours when the patient has been given contrast medium (Fig. 12.37). In some tumours this hyperplastic change becomes neoplastic (see section on gliosarcomas below). The factor responsible seems to be the production of an endothelial growth factor by the tumour cells.

Immunohistologically, glioblastomas usually contain only a few GFAP-positive cells and processes, reflecting the low

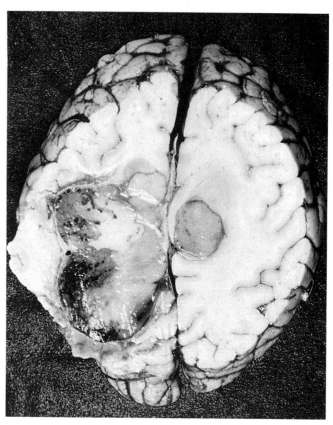

Fig. 12.38. Macroscopic appearance of a gliosarcoma in a high horizontal slice through the cerebral hemispheres. The bulk of the glioblastoma component is in the left cerebral hemisphere. The sarcomatous element, which appears pale and felt tough, surrounds the medial aspects of the tumour in the left hemisphere, and extends into the right hemisphere.

degree of astrocytic differentiation. Vimentin and Leu 7 antigen are also usually detectable in these tumours, and there may be a focal reaction for cytokeratins.

Gliosarcomas

A gliosarcoma is a malignant tumour containing both glial and mesenchymal neoplastic elements. The glial element has features of a glioblastoma, and the mesenchymal component appears to be derived from the hyperplastic vascular structures seen in typical glioblastomas or from the lepto-meninges. Up to 10% of tumours in published glioblastoma series have a sarcomatous element and the prognosis is unaffected. Macroscopically, these tumours are frequently seen reaching the meninges, and the sarcomatous areas are tough and (being relatively avascular) pale (Fig. 12.38). Microscopically, there are swathes of spindle cells with pleomorphic nuclei and mitotic figures, with reticulin and collagen deposition in the sarcomatous areas (Figs 12.39 and 12.40). Very occasionally, differentiation of the mesenchymal elements towards muscle or cartilage may be found.

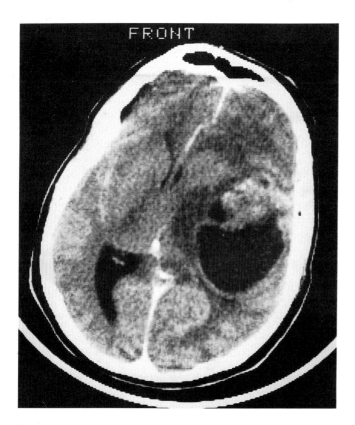

Fig. 12.37. CAT scan of a predominantly right-sided cerebral glioblastoma after the patient had been given intravenous contrast medium. There is contrast enhancement, reflecting the abundant blood flow in hyperplastic vessels, around the low-density area which consists of a zone of central tumour necrosis.

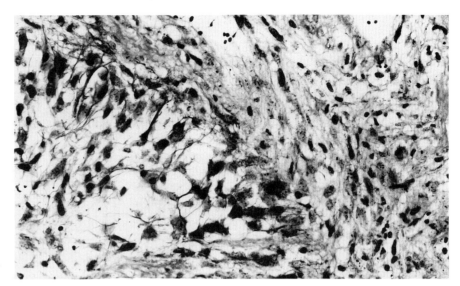

Fig. 12.39. Microscopic appearance of a gliosarcoma, with intermingled areas of glioma (left) and sarcoma (right), PTAH, ×220.

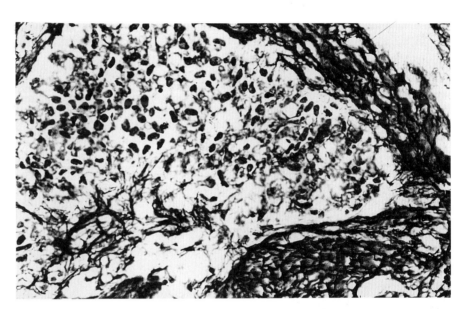

Fig. 12.40. Adjacent section to that shown in Fig. 12.39, stained to show the dense reticulin network in the sarcomatous regions of the tumour only. ×220.

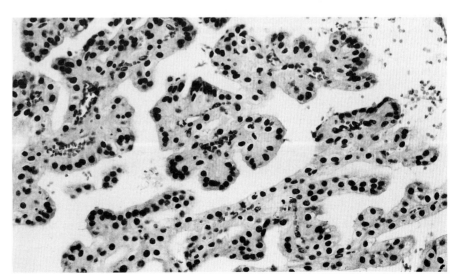

Fig. 12.41. Choroid plexus papilloma. The papillary growth pattern is well developed, and the resemblance to choroid plexus easily appreciated. H&E, ×140.

Choroid plexus tumours

Choroid plexus tumours are rare, occurring mainly in infants and children. Benign papillomas form discrete, papillary growths projecting into a ventricular cavity, most commonly the fourth ventricle. There may be associated hydrocephalus, attributable either to obstruction or to excess production of CSF. Microscopically, the pattern of growth of the papillae resembles that of normal choroid plexus, only the profusion of cells and a slight raggedness of the pattern distinguishing the tumour (Fig. 12.41). There are ribbons of cuboidal epithelial cells covering vascular stalk-like projections or papillae. Nuclei are regular and without mitoses. Some mucus production or cilia may be seen. Even such benign-appearing neoplasms may give rise to recurrent local or distant tumour on account of the readiness with which tumour cells seed into the CSF.

Anaplastic or malignant choroid plexus tumours still bear a resemblance to normal choroid plexus. In contrast to benign papillomas, there tends to be a heaping up of epithelial cells into layers more than one cell thick. The fronds of cells are more disordered, nuclei more variable in size and staining properties, and mitotic figures are much more easily found than in benign papillomas (Fig. 12.42).

Immunohistological reactions of choroid plexus papillomas are mixed. They show some foci of positivity with antibody Leu 7, antibodies to epithelial membrane antigen, GFAP and carbonic anhydrase 2.

Medulloblastomas

These are malignant, radiosensitive tumours arising in the cerebellum, usually in childhood. The cells of origin are believed to be those of the fetal external granular layer or their forerunners. Cells in this layer normally migrate into the cerebellum during the first year of postnatal life, and have the capacity to differentiate into neurons of the granule cell layer of the cortex, or into cortical neuroglia. The tumours arise near the midline or, less commonly, in a hemisphere (Fig. 12.43). They appear soft, pink-grey or purple, and are friable. They extend into the fourth ventricle, where seedling deposits are frequently released and become transported to the subarachnoid space, there to establish metastases which tend to re-invade the brain or spinal cord.

Microscopically these tumours are densely cellular and composed of diffusely arranged small cells with scanty, ill-defined cytoplasm and dark, hyperchromatic nuclei (Fig. 12.44). Occasional rosette formations may be seen (Fig. 12.45). There are frequently small foci of necrosis, and mitotic figures are plentiful. Most medulloblastomas have a scanty, vascular stroma, but a few extend into the subarachnoid space, where they may provoke a dense, collagenous reaction, giving rise to an abundant stroma which divides the cells into clusters. This is termed a 'desmoplastic' reaction. Neuroblastic differentiation may be discernible in a small proportion of medulloblastomas in preparations stained with silver, and more frequently if antigenic markers of neural cells (e.g. neurofilaments, neuron-specific enolase) are sought with appropriate antibodies. Evidence of glial differentiation is also sometimes present, as reflected in the expression of GFAP. Rare, related tumours to medulloblastomas are a melanin-containing papillary neuro-ectodermal tumour and a medulloepithelioma, details of which can be found in Russell & Rubinstein (1989) and Becker & Hinton (1986).

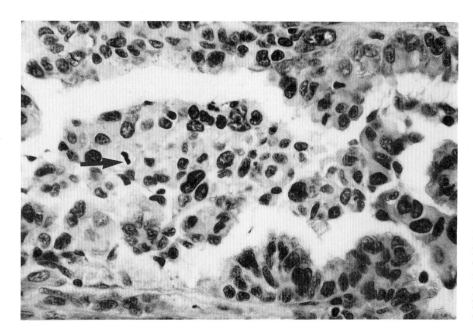

Fig. 12.42. Malignant choroid plexus papilloma. The papillary pattern is still discernible, but the cellular arrangement is much more dishevelled than in a benign papilloma. Cell nuclei are also more pleomorphic and there are frequent mitoses (arrowed). H&E, ×400.

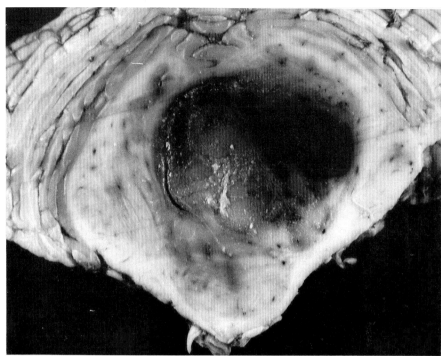

Fig. 12.43. Macroscopic appearance of a medulloblastoma. Some terminal haemorrhage has occurred.

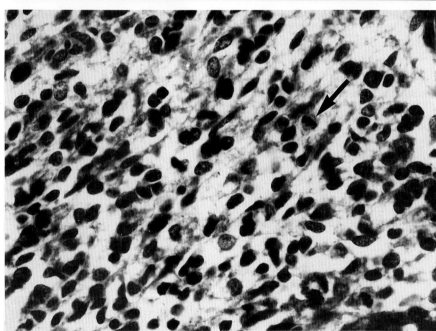

Fig. 12.44. Medulloblastoma composed of small cells with dark-stained nuclei with mitoses (arrowed), and barely discernible cytoplasm. Cells are arranged diffusely, with little intervening stroma. H&E, ×360.

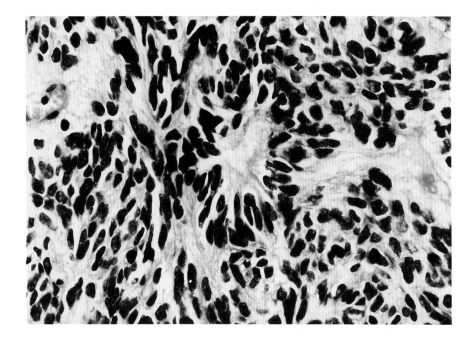

Fig. 12.45. Rosette formation (centre) in a medulloblastoma. H&E, ×490.

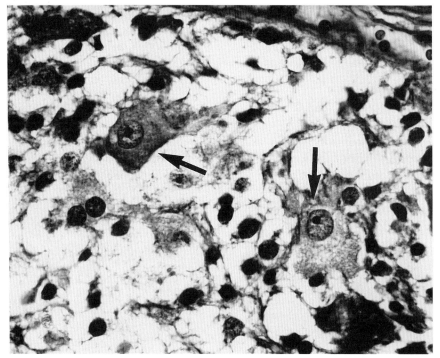

Fig. 12.46. Two large, abnormal neurons (arrowed) in a tumour removed from the pituitary fossa of a patient with acromegaly. The tumour contained some areas of gangliocytoma, of which this was a small part, and other areas of eosinophil adenoma, which were reactive for growth hormone. H&E, ×400.

Tumours containing neurons

Tumours containing mature neurons are rare in the CNS, and uncommon elsewhere. In the CNS they must be distinguished from the much more common finding of neurons surviving in an area of neural parenchyma extensively infiltrated by a glioma (Fig. 12.34). Neurons forming part of the neoplastic process are found rarely in the CNS in neuro-

blastomas, gangliocytomas and ganglioneuromas, and in the peripheral nervous system in neuroblastomas and ganglioneuromas.

Neuroblastomas have been described as rarely arising in the cerebral hemispheres in infants and children. These malignant tumours are generally quite well circumscribed and firm, and are sometimes cystic. Microscopically they are composed of dense collections of small cells with dark-staining nuclei, resembling those of a medulloblastoma. Rosette formations may be present and mitotic figures are plentiful. A well-developed fibrous connective tissue stroma is usually present, dividing the tumour cells into lobules. Some mature or immature ganglion cells may be identifiable in these tumours. These are large, polygonal cells with vesicular nuclei and prominent nucleoli. Cell processes may be detectable if silver stains are used.

Gangliocytomas and gangliogliomas are tumours composed predominantly of mature neurons in a stroma of non-neoplastic glia (gangliocytoma) or neoplastic glia (ganglioglioma). Such tumours outside the CNS have a stroma of Schwann cells and a few fibroblasts (ganglioneuroma). To identify such a tumour, it is necessary to be convinced of the neoplastic nature of the neurons. Indications of neoplasia include abnormal cellular morphology and occurrence at sites not normally harbouring ganglion cells (Fig. 12.46). Mitotic figures are not seen in the neurons. Astrocytes contribute to the stroma and may be frankly neoplastic, as in a fibrillary astrocytoma.

Certain other space-occupying lesions, not clearly neoplastic in nature, are occasionally seen. These include hamartomas in the region of the mamillary bodies or tuber cinereum (p.378), which are a cause of precocious puberty in children, a curious, expanding cerebellar lesion found in Lhermitte−Duclos disease (p.264), and the cortical tubers found in tuberous sclerosis (p.262).

Primary CNS lymphomas

Lymphomas are encountered in neuropathological practice at two main sites: in the brain, usually as a primary lymphoma, or as extradural metastases from an extracranial tumour. The primary CNS lymphomas are rare, but have an increased incidence in immunosuppressed individuals, including those with AIDS. They have a varied naked-eye appearance, which can mimic glioblastoma, metastatic carcinoma, or a brain stem glioma (Fig. 12.47). Those in the cerebrum often form soft, ill-defined grey masses with a granular texture (Fig. 12.48). They occur in any part of the brain, most commonly in the cerebrum or around the lateral and third ventricles. Microscopically they are composed of medium or large, round or polygonal cells, which tend to cluster densely in the Virchow−Robin spaces as well as spilling out in sheets into the brain parenchyma. Wide areas of necrosis occur. Beyond the edge of the main tumour, lymphoid cells are found in perivascular spaces in a remarkably wide

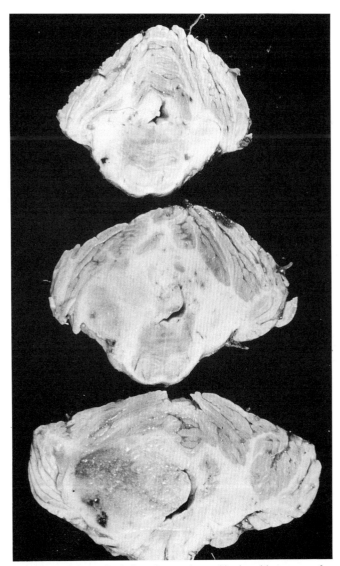

Fig. 12.47. Primary brain lymphoma, situated in the white matter of the left cerebellar hemisphere, causing compression of the brain stem and fourth ventricle. The margins of the tumour are ill-defined, and its texture granular.

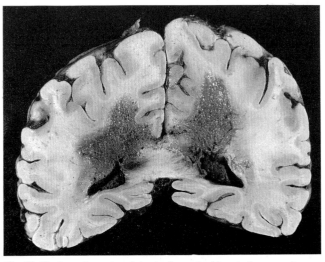

Fig. 12.48. Lymphoma involving both cerebral hemispheres, and showing some macroscopic resemblance to a glioma.

distribution (Fig. 12.49). The abnormal cells have scanty cytoplasm and large, lobulated nuclei with prominent nucleoli and frequent mitoses (Fig. 12.50). Reticulin is increased in infiltrated perivascular spaces (Fig. 12.51). Investigation of these tumours with antibodies to leucocyte antigens shows that the great majority of them are derived from B-lymphocytes, and very few of them carry antigenic markers specific for macrophages, belying the former term 'micro-gliomatosis'. However, lymphoma of the brain is accompanied by the widespread occurrence of increased numbers of reactive microglial cells in the surrounding neuropil.

Another rare form of lymphoma involving the CNS is that of a B-cell lymphoma in which the tumour cells are

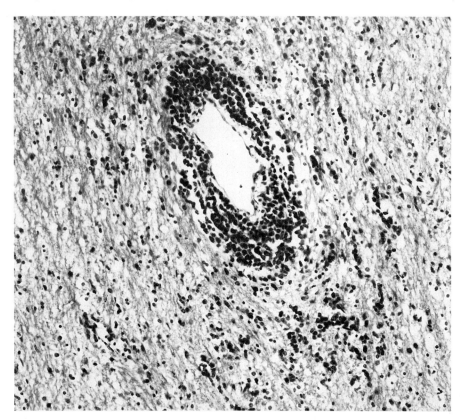

Fig. 12.49. Lymphoma cells occupying a perivascular space, and spilling over into surrounding white matter distant from the main tumour mass. H&E, ×100.

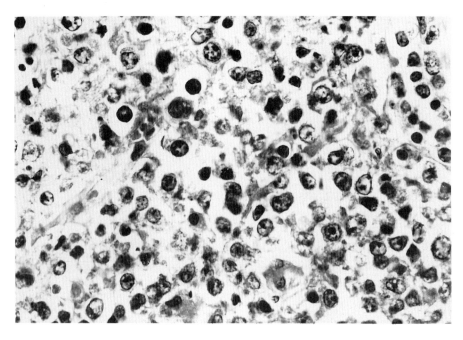

Fig. 12.50. High-power view of the cells of a primary cerebral lymphoma. H&E, ×350.

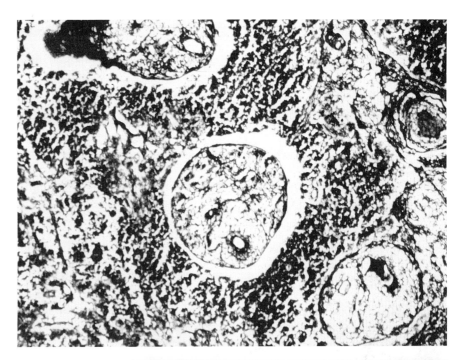

Fig. 12.51. Reticulin deposition in infiltrated perivascular spaces in a cerebral lymphoma. ×100.

predominantly found in blood vessels, and the symptoms produced are due to ischaemia rather than to space occupation (Figs 12.52 and 12.53). This is referred to as an *angiotropic lymphoma*. Some cases of so-called malignant angioendotheliomatosis now appear to fall into this category.

Haemangioblastomas

These tumours occur usually in the cerebellum, less commonly in the spinal cord, and very rarely elsewhere. In some subjects there is associated angiomatosis of the retina, (von Hippel's disease), non-neoplastic renal or pancreatic cysts, or renal tumours. This constellation of abnormalities is known as Lindau's syndrome. It may be familial, as may be isolated haemangioblastomas. An interesting feature of these tumours is the occurrence in some cases of polycythaemia, which disappears after removal of the tumour. Tumours with an identical appearance to the cerebellar haemangioblastoma also rarely occur around the spinal cord, outside the spinal dura and in the supratentorial meninges, where they are classed as haemangioblastic meningiomas. The classical cerebellar tumours form discrete but unencapsulated masses, frequently cystic, with the tumour appearing as a firm, dark-red nodule in or near the edge of the cyst. The cyst fluid may be rusty-coloured from previous haemorrhage. The tumour has a rich vascular supply, with prominent draining veins.

Microscopically the tumour appears to be composed of two elements, one being endothelial cells forming well-defined capillary channels, and the other intervening stromal cells with pale, foamy, fat-laden cytoplasm (Fig. 12.54).

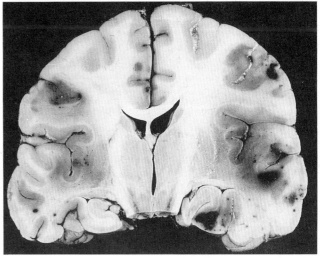

Fig. 12.52. Macroscopic appearance of the cerebrum in a case of B-cell angiotrophic lymphoma. There was a 6-month history of dementia and focal neurological deficits, which at post mortem seemed to be largely attributable to infarcts and haemorrhages, scattered throughout the cortex and white matter.

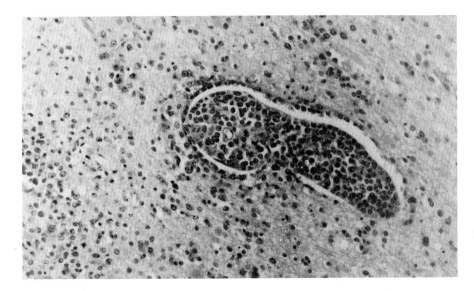

Fig. 12.53. Angiotropic B-cell lymphoma. Neoplastic cells occupy the lumen of a small vein, and a few extend into neighbouring white matter. H&E, ×200.

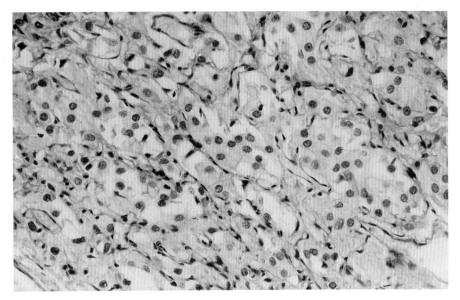

Fig. 12.54. Pale, lipid-laden stromal cells of a haemangioblastoma. Nuclei are small and regular, without mitoses. H&E, ×360.

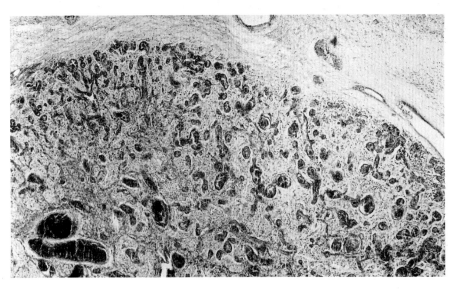

Fig. 12.55. Low-power view of a section of haemangioblastoma showing the abundant capillary spaces that comprise one element of this tumour. H&E, ×70.

Stromal and capillary elements are irregularly intermixed in varying proportions (Fig. 12.55). The two types of cell appear quite uniform, though there may be nuclear pleomorphism in the stromal cells. Mitotic figures are rarely seen. Abundant reticulin surrounds the capillaries, and may also be seen between the stromal cells. The tumours are slow growing, but recur if incompletely removed, and very occasionally metastasize in the CNS. Multiple cerebellar tumours may occur successively. The origin of the stromal cells in haemangioblastomas is not clear. Some tumours have been shown ultrastructurally to contain neurosecretory granules, suggesting an origin from a neurosecretory cell. In immunohistological reactions most tumours give a focally positive reaction with GFAP antibodies.

Further reading

Becker LE, Hinton D. 1986. Pathology of neoplasia in children and adolescents. In Finegold M (Ed.) *Major Problems in Pathology*. WB Saunders, Philadelphia, **18**, 397−418.

Burger PC, Vogel FS. 1982. *Surgical Pathology of the Nervous System and its Coverings*. John Wiley, New York, 2nd edn.

Kernohan JW, Mabon RF, Svien HJ, Adson AW. 1949. Symposium on a new and simplified classification of gliomas. *Proc Mayo Clin* **24**, 71.

Rorke LB, Gilles FH, Davis RL, Becker LE. 1985. Revision of the WHO classification of brain tumours for childhood brain tumours. *Cancer* **56** (Suppl), 1869−86.

Rubinstein LJ. 1982. *Armed Forces Institute of Pathology Atlas of Tumour Pathology*, Fascicle 6, second series, Washington.

Rubinstein LJ. 1985. Embryonal central neuroepithelial tumours and their differentiating potential. *J Neurosurg* **62**, 795−805.

Russell DS, Rubinstein LJ. 1989. *Pathology of Tumours of the Nervous System*, 5th edn. Edward Arnold, London.

WHO Histological classification of tumours of the central nervous system. International Histological Classification of Tumours No. 21. WHO, Geneva, 1979.

Zulch KJ. 1986. *Brain Tumours, their Pathology and Biology*. Springer, Heidelberg.

Chapter 13
Other Tumours Affecting the Nervous System

Nerve sheath tumours

In the past there has been impassioned debate about the cells of origin of nerve sheath tumours, and consequently about how they should be named. For our part, we are content to follow Russell & Rubinstein (1977) in recognizing two types: one, derived from Schwann cells, called *schwannoma*, and another derived from perineurial fibroblasts, called *neurofibroma*. The fact that both types of tumour occur in von Recklinghausen's disease, and that both kinds of tissue can sometimes be seen together in a single tumour, suggests that the two are in some way related. Terms now deemed to be objectionable, but still in use, are *neurinoma* and *neurilemmoma*. Tumours of the eighth cranial nerve are commonly referred to by neurosurgeons as *acoustic neuromas*. The objection here is that *neuroma* is also the name of a non-neoplastic tangle of regenerating nerve fibres arising from a severed nerve — a lesion sometimes giving rise to discomfort, or worse, in an amputation stump (Figs 22.7 and 22.8).

Schwannomas

These tumours arise on cranial and spinal nerve roots, and on peripheral nerves. In the cranial cavity, the eighth (vestibulo-acoustic) nerve is by far the commonest site. Schwannomas occurring on both acoustic nerves usually indicate that the patient is suffering from an inherited condition similar to, but distinct from, *von Recklinghausen's disease*. In von Recklinghausen's disease itself, multiple nerve sheath tumours occur in the dermis, attached to deep nerves and on cranial and spinal nerve roots. Both *bilateral acoustic neurofibromatosis* and von Recklinghausen's disease

are transmitted by dominant inheritance, whereas solitary nerve sheath tumours are more often sporadic. These tumours are slow growing, encapsulated, firm, discrete masses of variable size (Fig. 11.13). Large acoustic schwannomas may distort and indent the brain stem (Fig. 13.1). Smaller ones occupy the angle between the pons, medulla and cerebellum. The cut surface of the tumour shows a yellow or white, whorled, sometimes partially cystic appearance. There may be evidence of old haemorrhages in the form of foci of rusty discoloration.

Microscopically, schwannomas display intermingled areas containing bundles of compact, interweaving, elongated spindle cells, alternating with areas of looser texture. The

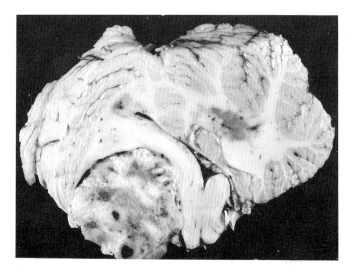

Fig. 13.1. Schwannoma of the left acoustic nerve, compressing, but not invading, the left cerebellar hemisphere and brain stem. Areas of old and fresh haemorrhage are visible on the cut surface of the tumour.

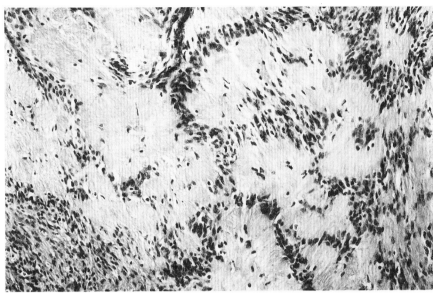

Fig. 13.2. Area of a schwannoma in which the nuclei of the elongated, bipolar tumour cells are aligned in rows ('palisading'). H&E, ×110.

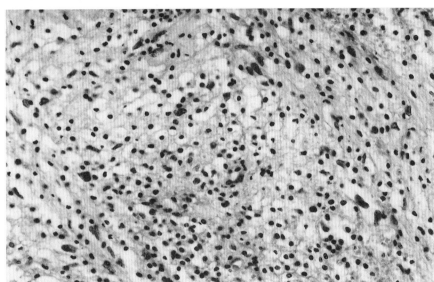

Fig. 13.3. Area of a schwannoma showing the more open, microcystic appearance of Antoni B tissue. H&E, ×180.

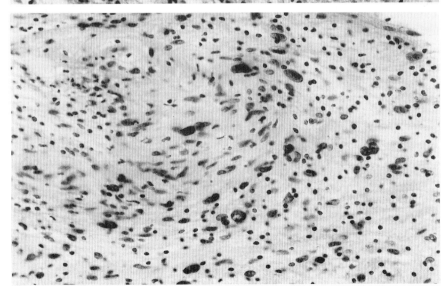

Fig. 13.4. Nuclear pleomorphism in a schwannoma — a feature that does not have sinister implications in these tumours. H&E, ×160.

former are known as Antoni A and the latter as Antoni B tissues. Overall these tumours show a sparse to moderate degree of cellularity. Antoni A areas show some degree of alignment of nuclei in parallel rows or clusters, referred to as palisading (Fig. 13.2), while in Antoni B areas the cells are haphazardly arranged, have ill-defined boundaries and are set in a microcystic matrix (Fig. 13.3). Mitotic figures are not usually found, though nuclei may show considerable variation in size, shape and staining properties (Fig. 13.4). Blood vessels in schwannomas are notable for the frequent presence of degenerative change with hyaline thickening and fibrin deposition. Haemosiderin deposition is also fairly common in schwannomas. Nerve fibres are not seen coursing through the tumour, but may be seen as a group of compressed fascicles at one margin of the tumour.

Schwannomas at the cerebellopontine angle may need to be differentiated from meningiomas, which can also occur at this site. Points of distinction in their histology are: the alternating types of tissue (Antoni A and B); palisading of nuclei and degenerative changes in the blood vessel walls in schwannomas; and the presence of psammoma bodies in some meningiomas, which at this site are often of the fibroblastic type (p.205).

Neurofibromas

These rarely occur as single tumours, but are common and sometimes very numerous in subjects with von Recklinghausen's disease. Most tumours that develop as part of this disease do so in the peripheral nervous system, though paradoxically those subjects who develop the more serious proximal nerve root or CNS tumours often have little in the way of peripheral disease. Tumours are liable to develop on the cranial and spinal nerve roots (Fig. 13.5). The tumours are schwannomas, neurofibromas or a mixture of the two. Some undergo malignant change. Patients with von Recklinghausen's disease also suffer from an increased incidence of gliomas (especially those involving the optic system), meningiomas, and phaeochromocytomas of the adrenal gland. Neurofibromas usually form an ill-defined expansion of the nerve in which they occur. Microscopically they are sparsely cellular and composed of spindle-shaped cells with narrow, elongated, darkly staining nuclei (Fig. 13.6). Mitotic figures are not usually present. There is an abundance of collagen and reticulin in a structureless matrix which is rich in mucopolysaccharides. Matrix fibres and spindle cells pursue a characteristically wavy course through this matrix. Nerve fibres can be found scattered singly or in small groups throughout the tumour (Fig. 13.7). Over-wrapping of nerve bundles with Schwann cells and fibroblasts may be found in some subjects with von Recklinghausen's disease, even in apparently normal lengths of nerve.

Malignant schwannomas and neurofibromas

Malignant nerve sheath tumours are uncommon, and occur chiefly on the spinal roots, where they often form dumb-bell-shaped tumours expanding inward and outward from an intervertebral foramen. Others occur on deeply situated peripheral nerves. At least half of them occur in subjects

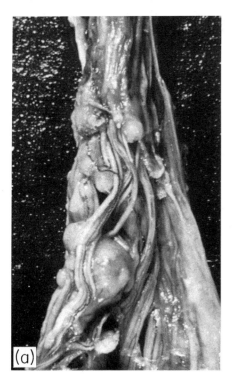
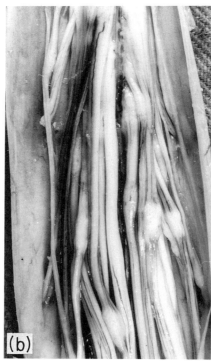

Fig. 13.5. (a) Neurofibromas attached to individual roots of the cauda equina from a case of von Recklinghausen's disease. (b) Small nodules of metastatic carcinoma in the same location. In this case each tumour frequently involves more than one nerve root.

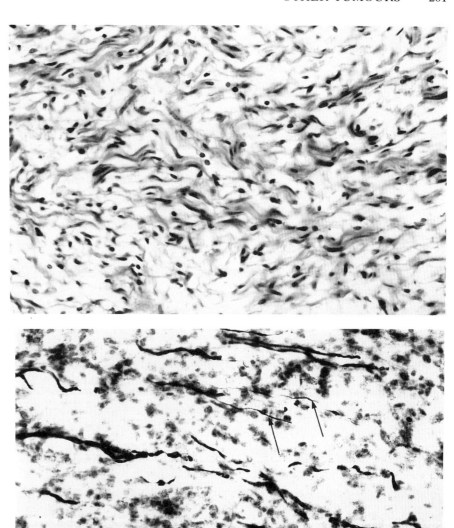

Fig. 13.6. Microscopic appearance of a neurofibroma. The tumour cells are relatively sparse and separated by a pale intercellular matrix. The cells are elongated, with wavy processes and elongated or oval nuclei. H&E, ×250.

Fig. 13.7. Schofield silver stain on a frozen section of a spinal neurofibroma from a patient with von Recklinghausen's disease. Nerve fibres (arrowed) are scattered within the tumour. ×200.

with von Recklinghausen's disease. The cell of origin in most cases is thought to be the Schwann cell. The tumours are circumscribed, but may be large — as much as 6 cm across — when first discovered. They are demonstrably related to a peripheral nerve or nerve root. The microscopic appearance is highly cellular, the tumour being composed of interlacing bundles of spindle cells with sausage-shaped nuclei showing pleomorphism and mitotic figures (Fig. 13.8). Foci of necrosis are usually present. Reticulin is widely distributed throughout the tumour. The tumours that occur peripherally can be difficult to distinguish microscopically from other malignant spindle cell tumours of soft tissue. Immunostaining can be helpful, particularly with antibody Leu 7, which can be applied to paraffin sections, and gives a positive reaction with most malignant as well as benign nerve sheath tumours. However, it should be noted that this antibody gives positive reactions with many other CNS

tumours. Antibodies to S-100 protein react positively with benign nerve sheath tumours but only rarely do so with their malignant counterparts. They also react with certain other tumours, so again the reaction cannot be regarded as specific for nerve sheath tumours.

Meningiomas

Meningiomas arise in the meningeal coverings of the brain and spinal cord. The main cells of origin are thought to be the arachnoid cap cells (p.56; Figs 3.25 and 3.26), particularly those that contribute to the formation of arachnoid villi in the dura. The tumours present chiefly in middle and late adult life. Small ones, often calcified and resembling small stones, are commonly found incidentally at post mortem, usually over the convexities of the cerebral hemispheres. Occasionally meningiomas show evidence of hormone de-

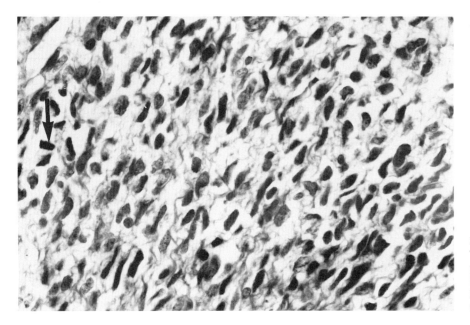

Fig. 13.8. Malignant nerve sheath tumour. There is a high cell density, and nuclei are pleomorphic. Mitotic figures are present (arrowed). The matrix retains the wavy longitudinal pattern seen in more benign tumours. H&E, ×340.

pendency, growing rapidly during pregnancy. Most meningiomas have an attachment to the dura, particularly adjoining the sagittal sinus at the convexity, the sphenoidal ridges, olfactory grooves or tuberculum sellae. Other attachments and locations are well recognized, intracranially in the leptomeninges or in a lateral ventricle attached to choroid plexus. They also occur in the petrous bone, and rarely extracranially, from presumed ectopic arachnoid cap cells, at sites around the head and neck. The spinal meninges, particularly over thoracic segments of the cord, give origin to spinal meningiomas which occupy the intradural compartment.

Macroscopically, meningiomas appear encapsulated, firm, smooth or slightly lobulated (Fig. 13.9). The majority can be readily shelled out from the tumour bed. Benign meningiomas indent, but do not invade, the underlying brain or spinal cord (Fig. 11.2). However, some meningiomas, particularly those arising around the base of the brain, have a tendency to wrap themselves around neighbouring structures, such as major cerebral arteries or cranial nerves (Plate 2.4). Meningiomas that display this creeping pattern of growth to a marked extent are sometimes referred to as meningioma 'en plaque'. The adjacent bone, particularly over the convexities, is occasionally obviously thickened, and nearby venous sinuses may commonly be invaded by tumour, even a benign one. On the cut surface meningiomas usually have a whorled or streaky appearance and feel firm and granular. Frequently they are gritty. They are grey or pink in colour.

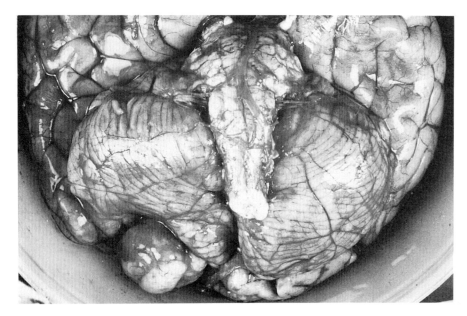

Fig. 13.9. Small meningioma indenting the surface of the right cerebellar hemisphere. Note the clear plane of cleavage between the encapsulated tumour and the brain.

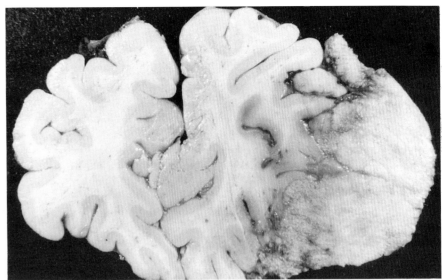

Fig. 13.10. Right frontal meningioma displaying an invasive pattern of growth in which there is no clear plane of demarcation between the tumour and brain, or well-defined pia-derived capsule (cf. Fig. 11.2). There is cingulate subfalcine herniation from right to left.

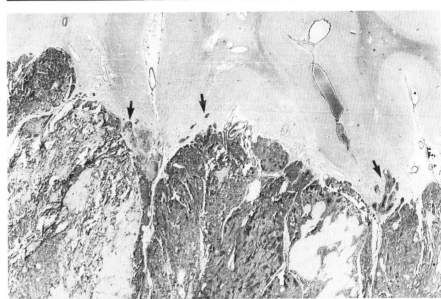

Fig. 13.11. Low-power view of a section taken at the interface between the frontal lobe and tumour shown in Fig. 13.10. Finger-like projections of tumour are seen invading the brain at the sites indicated by arrows. H&E, ×40.

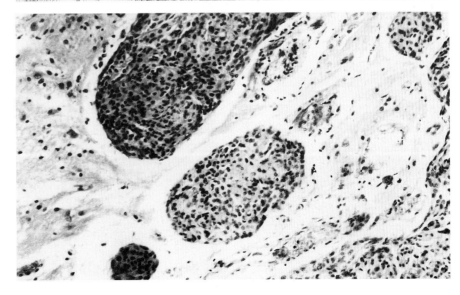

Fig. 13.12. Projections of meningioma into superficial cortex in a surgical biopsy. H&E, ×90.

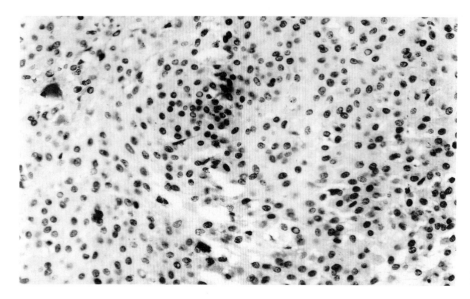

Fig. 13.13. Histological pattern of a syncytial meningioma. H&E, ×160.

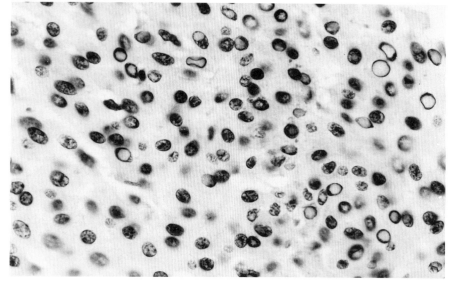

Fig. 13.14. Glycogen vacuolation of nuclei in a syncytial meningioma. H&E, ×360.

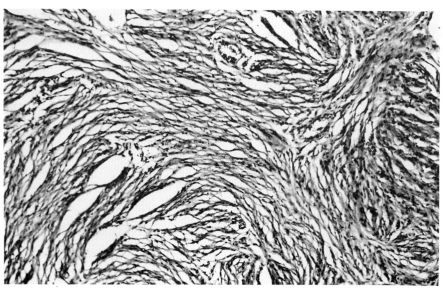

Fig. 13.15. Low-power view of a fibroblastic meningioma to show the swirling, interlacing bundles of strap-like tumour cells. H&E, ×100.

Those that have undergone xanthomatous degeneration contain yellow areas.

Microscopically there is considerable variation in the appearances of meningiomas. Six basic patterns are recognized among benign forms: syncytial, fibroblastic, transitional, psammomatous, haemangioblastic and angiomatous. Histology of more than one type may be displayed in a single tumour, and the features defining the separate types overlap to some extent, so that the classification is somewhat imprecise. Although most meningiomas displaying features of these subtypes behave as benign tumours, some are more aggressive. Invasion of neighbouring bone or venous sinuses does not indicate aggressive behaviour, but invasion of underlying brain does (Figs 13.10 and 13.11); this feature should be carefully looked for microscopically, in biopsy specimens (Fig. 13.12). High mitotic activity is found in malignant tumours, but not in slow-growing ones. The latter may, however, contain small, pyknotic nuclei, which should not be mistaken for mitoses.

Syncytial meningiomas are composed of cells with ill-defined cell boundaries. The nuclei appear as if embedded in a sheet-like syncytial cytoplasmic matrix (Fig. 13.13). There may be an impression of a swirling growth pattern in the matrix. The nuclei are pale and small- to medium-sized, and frequently contain glycogen vacuoles (Fig. 13.14). Collagen and reticulin are sparse and are related to the vascular stroma. Mitotic figures are rare or absent.

Fibroblastic meningiomas are composed of better defined, elongated spindle cells with narrow, rod-like nuclei. The cells are arranged in interlacing bundles, and a tendency to a whorling pattern can usually be seen (Fig. 13.15). Occasional *psammoma bodies* may be present. These are calcified, spherical particles, approximately 30–80 μm across

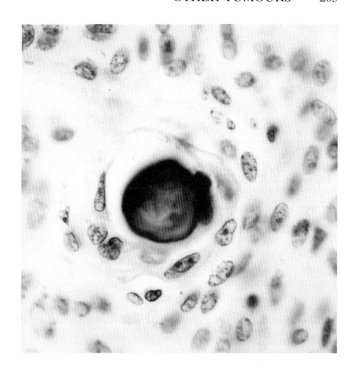

Fig. 13.16. Calcified psammoma body at the centre of a whorl in a meningioma. H&E, ×450.

(Fig. 13.16). There is an abundance of collagen and reticulin in fibroblastic meningiomas. Few or no mitotic figures are present.

Transitional meningiomas derive their name from the presence of some features of both fibroblastic and syncytial types. Whorls are well developed (Fig. 13.17). They consist of groups of plump, imbricated spindle cells. Psammoma bodies, often found at the centres of whorls, are also easily

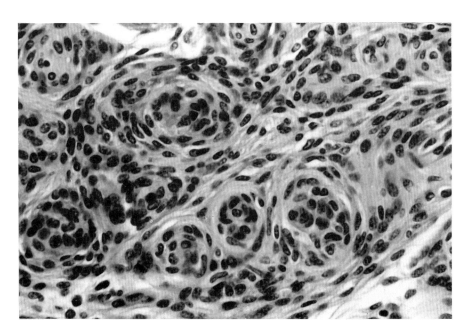

Fig. 13.17. Whorl formations in a transitional meningioma. H&E, ×280.

found in this type of meningioma. Nuclei are oval, generally pale, and often have some glycogen vacuolation (Fig. 13.14). They are occasionally aligned in palisades reminiscent of schwannomas. Mitoses are rare or absent. Moderate amounts of reticulin and collagen are present. *Psammomatous meningiomas* closely resemble transitional meningiomas, but contain large numbers of psammoma bodies. They are very common among spinal meningiomas, and are very slow-growing tumours.

Many meningiomas are highly vascular tumours containing an abundance of capillaries. In the *angiomatous* type there are many less well-defined sinusoidal blood spaces. These tumours otherwise share features of the types described above. A further benign, and highly vascular, form of meningioma appears virtually identical microscopically to the cerebellar haemangioblastoma, with groups of vacuolated cells lying in pockets of reticulin which separate them from the thin-walled, abundant capillaries. This is sometimes referred to as the haemangioblastic type of meningioma.

Benign forms of meningioma may undergo various forms of secondary degeneration which considerably alter the overall histological appearance of the tumour. Common forms of degeneration are hyaline, collagenous degeneration and xanthomatous change, in which sudanophilic lipid accumulates focally in groups of cells, giving them a vacuolated appearance in paraffin sections (Fig. 13.18). Less common are myxomatous change and cystic degeneration. Some meningiomas contain hyaline bodies which take the PAS stain.

The final three variants of meningiomas are the least typical in appearance and the most aggressive in their behaviour: the haemangiopericytic, papillary and anaplastic

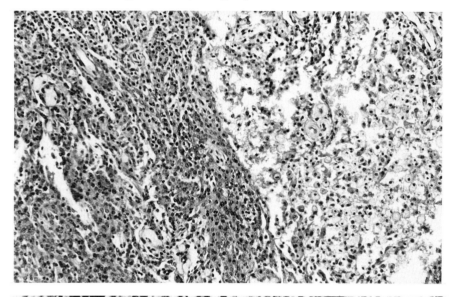

Fig. 13.18. Focus of xanthomatous degeneration in a meningioma (right). The cytoplasm of cells in this area are paler than those on the left. H&E, ×100.

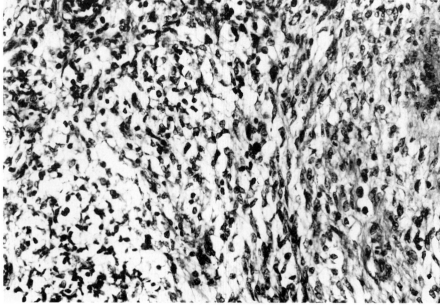

Fig. 13.19. Haemangiopericytic meningioma. Polygonal and spindle cells separated by cleft-like spaces. H&E, ×200.

types. They are likely to recur, and occasionally metastasize. *Haemangiopericytic meningiomas*, formerly commonly regarded as variants of angioblastic meningiomas, closely resemble haemangiopericytomas arising in other parts of the body. The tumour cells bear an intimate relation to the lining cells of the sinusoidal blood spaces. The cells are polygonal or angular, rather than spindle shaped (Fig. 13.19). Mitotic figures are invariably present. An intricate reticulin network extends around each of the tumour cells as well as around the closely related blood spaces (Fig. 13.20). Whorls and psammoma bodies are not present.

Papillary meningiomas are rare, malignant tumours. Parts of the tumour may resemble syncytial or transitional forms, but other areas show a distinctly papillary pattern of growth with a striking degree of nuclear pleomorphism and a much less well-differentiated cellular appearance (Fig. 13.21).

Most of the cells are large and well defined, with plentiful, eosinophilic cytoplasm and vesicular or hyperchromatic nuclei. Mitoses are frequent. Distinction from metastatic carcinoma may prove difficult in biopsies if areas of better-differentiated meningioma are not present.

Anaplastic meningiomas are meningeal tumours in which the histological pattern shows no more than a faint resemblance to one of the better-differentiated forms. There are frequently features suggestive of malignancy, such as invasion of the brain by fingers of tumour (Figs 13.10–13.12), necrosis, and poor cytological differentiation. The tumour cells are spindle shaped, with some tendency to whorl formation (Fig. 13.22). There is a variable collagen and reticulin content. Mitotic figures are numerous. Nuclei are pleomorphic and frequently bizarre, but it should be noted that this feature on its own is not necessarily indicative of

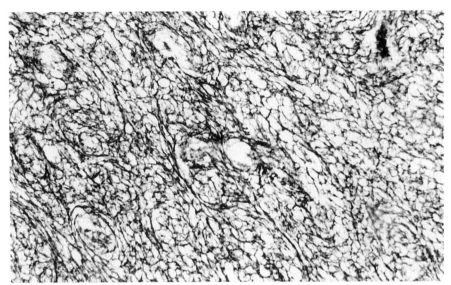

Fig. 13.20. Reticulin pattern of a haemangiopericytic meningioma. There is an intricate network of reticulin around individual tumour cells. ×100.

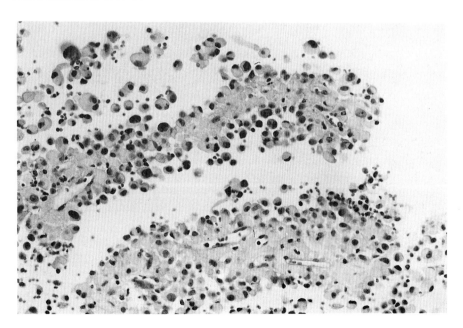

Fig. 13.21. Meningioma with a papillary growth pattern, rounded cell outlines and nuclear pleomorphism — all features that make differentiation of this tumour from carcinoma difficult. H&E, ×250.

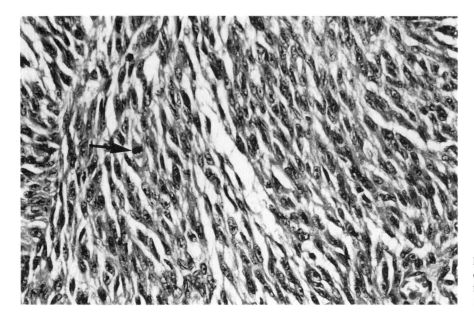

Fig. 13.22. Malignant meningioma composed of elongated, densely-packed spindle cells with frequent mitotic figures (arrowed). H&E, ×350.

malignancy in a meningioma. Anaplastic features can occur focally in a large meningioma. Since their presence influences the prognosis they should be carefully sought by wide sampling of different areas in a large tumour.

With regard to their immunohistological characteristics, meningiomas show variable patterns of reactivity. Most give a positive reaction for vimentin, S-100 protein and epithelial membrane antigen, while some, particularly those that contain PAS-positive hyaline bodies, show focal expression of cytokeratin (Fig. 4.24). These tumours therefore show reactions that are characteristic of both epithelial and mesenchymal tumours.

Meningeal sarcomas

Spindle-celled meningeal tumours with malignant features in which no resemblance to benign meningiomas is apparent in any part of the tumour are regarded as primary meningeal sarcomas, and have a histological pattern closely resembling that of fibrosarcoma.

Meningeal melanomas

These are rare tumours with an attachment to the pia mater, though they may burrow deeply into the brain or

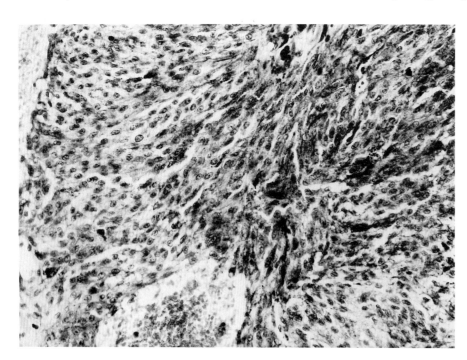

Fig. 13.23. Spindle-celled, heavily pigmented melanoma, found at post mortem to have arisen in the leptomeninges. H&E, ×175.

spinal cord. They usually remain confined to the CNS. They arise more commonly from the leptomeninges overlying the spinal cord than from the brain. Histologically, they resemble the commoner melanomas that are metastatic to the CNS (Fig. 13.23). They are not the only melanin-containing tumours arising in the CNS. Occasional meningiomas, schwannomas, ependymomas, medulloblastomas and choroid plexus papillomas contain melanin.

Craniopharyngiomas (suprasellar cysts, Rathke's pouch tumours, adamantinomas)

These are cystic, or cystic and solid, lesions occurring in the suprasellar or parasellar region, with a presumed origin from epithelial remnants of the embryonic Rathke's pouch.

They present usually in childhood, or early adult life, with symptoms related to compression of the pituitary stalk or gland, or by obstructing the third ventricle, and causing hydrocephalus (Fig. 13.24). The cyst grows slowly, but never undergoes malignant transformation, and does not metastasize. The cyst fluid is usually brown or yellow and contains glistening cholesterol crystals. It has an irritant effect, producing a chemical meningitis if it reaches the subarachnoid space. The wall of the cyst is composed of epithelial cells, and tends to adhere to surrounding structures. When in contact with the brain the lesion excites a dense glial reaction. Microscopically the cyst wall contains stratified epithelium, in some areas flattened and in others focally thickened to form irregular cords or islands (Fig. 13.25). Mitotic figures are not seen. The basal cuboidal layer rests

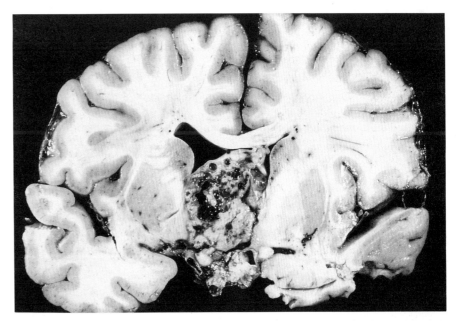

Fig. 13.24. Craniopharyngioma occupying and expanding the third ventricle, and causing compression of the right lateral ventricle and obstructive dilatation of the left lateral ventricle. There are cystic and solid, partly calcified, regions in this tumour. Damage to the right temporal lobe was due to previous surgery.

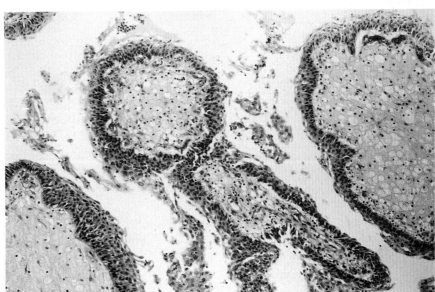

Fig. 13.25. Epithelial cyst wall of a craniopharyngioma. H&E, ×100.

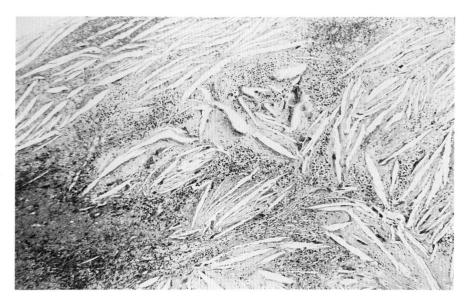

Fig. 13.26. Low-power view of a section of part of the wall of a craniopharyngioma containing numerous cholesterol clefts, scattered multinucleated foreign-body giant cells and an infiltrate of mononuclear inflammatory cells. H&E, ×40.

on basement membrane, and elicits a fibrotic and glial reaction where it abuts on the leptomeninges and brain. In the collagenous and glial layers there are frequently cholesterol clefts, calcification, flakes of keratin, multinucleate foreign-body giant cells and other inflammatory cells (Fig. 13.26). Biopsy specimens may contain no epithelial tissue, but the diagnosis can usually be made by exclusion, after discussion of the possibilities with the surgeon.

Dermoid and epidermoid cysts (pearly tumour, 'cholesteatomas')

These are simple cysts, thought to be derived from heterotopic inclusions of epidermal cells. Dermoid cysts are found most frequently in the posterior fossa, particularly in the vermis, or, intraspinally, at the lumbosacral level. Epidermoid cysts occur mainly in the middle and posterior cranial fossae, and occasionally in the cerebral hemispheres and spinal cord. A dermal sinus may be identifiable, connecting a dermoid cyst with an overlying dimple in the skin, and both types of cyst may be associated with local congenital skeletal defects. Macroscopically the cysts are of variable size and are smooth or slightly nodular and encapsulated. The capsule may be partly calcified. The contents of a dermoid cyst appear thick and yellowish, with some hairs included, while those of an epidermoid cyst are white, waxy or flaky (Fig. 13.27). Microscopically the wall of a dermoid cyst is composed mainly of simple squamous epithelium with variable additional skin appendages such as hair follicles, sebaceous glands and sweat glands. Epidermoid cysts lack the skin appendages but are otherwise similar. Foreign-body giant cells are commonly found in relation to keratin inclusions in connective tissue deep to the epithelium.

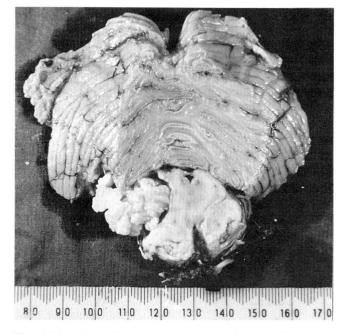

Fig. 13.27. Epidermoid cyst at the cerebellopontine angle. The contents of the cyst are white, flaky and friable.

Pituitary adenomas

Most of the tumours removed from the pituitary fossa are adenomas. Many adenomas are received as surgical specimens, and some are found incidentally or unexpectedly at post mortem. With regard to the management of surgical specimens, EM can be helpful in classifying these tumours, and we recommend that small blocks of tissue be fixed and embedded for EM. Ultrathin sections may not need to be examined from the most straightforward cases, but the material is then available, if required. The remainder can be fixed for routine light microscopy. H&E and Orange G/PAS, or a similar stain for distinguishing between eosinophil, basophil and chromophobe cells, are used routinely, and the reticulin stain is useful if there is doubt about whether a sample consists of tumour or pituitary gland. The anterior part of the gland has a distinctive reticulin network which is absent from adenomas (Figs 13.28 and 13.29). A Congo Red stain may show the presence of small amounts of amyloid in some adenomas. Haemosiderin is frequently seen in pituitary adenomas, and occasionally frank haemorrhage and necrosis are found, particularly in tumours from patients with 'pituitary apoplexy'. Simple epithelial-lined cysts may also be encountered in some tumours or occasionally as space-occupying lesions in their own right (Rathke's

pouch cyst). Very small cysts occur as an incidental finding in 'normal' pituitary glands.

Immunohistology using antisera to pituitary hormones is certainly helpful in diagnosis, and can be carried out on paraffin sections. Antisera to the major pituitary hormones are commercially available, those to growth hormone (GH), adenocorticotrophic hormone (ACTH), prolactin (PRL), and the β subunits of thyroid stimulating hormone (TSH), luteinizing hormone (LH) and follicle stimulating hormone (FSH) being probably the most used. As the antisera are expensive and can be used most economically by treating batches of 10–12 tumours at once, our practice is to issue a report on the nature of the tumour based on the light-

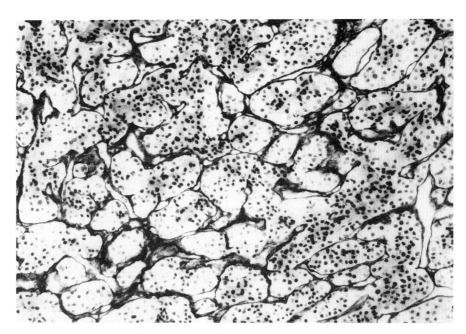

Fig. 13.28. Reticulin pattern of the anterior pituitary gland, showing epithelial cells in clusters, enclosed by reticulin strands. ×100.

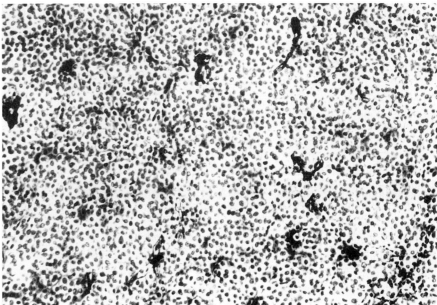

Fig. 13.29. Reticulin pattern of a pituitary, prolactin-secreting chromophobe adenoma. The amount of reticulin is much reduced compared to that of the anterior pituitary gland. ×100.

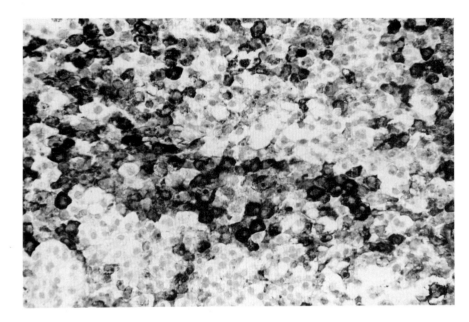

Fig. 13.30. Reaction for growth hormone in a pituitary adenoma associated with acromegaly. A varying intensity of reaction is found in different tumour cells. Immunoperoxidase, counterstained with haematoxylin, ×200.

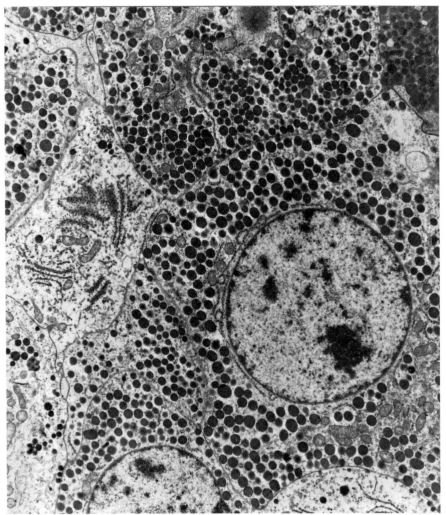

Fig. 13.31. Heavily-granulated cells of a growth-hormone-secreting pituitary adenoma. Uranyl acetate and lead citrate, ×6630.

microscopical appearances in stained sections, and to follow this up with a supplementary report describing the immunohistological findings and EM. In the initial report the traditional classification of adenomas into eosinophil, basophil or chromophobe is used. Although simplistic and largely superseded by classifications based on the hormone content of the tumours, use of this classification does at least assure the surgeon in the initial report that the tumour is indeed a pituitary adenoma and not some other type of tumour. In the supplementary report the tumour is classified according to its hormone content. The main categories of pituitary adenoma are summarized below. A more detailed classification is recommended by some authorities, details of which may be found in the several recent monographs and reviews listed at the end of the chapter.

Growth-hormone-containing adenomas

Acromegaly or gigantism is evident clinically in patients with these tumours. Routine stains on paraffin sections show an eosinophil or mixed chromophobe and eosinophil tumour composed of medium-sized, polygonal epithelial cells usually arranged diffusely (Plate 6.2). Immunohistology shows some reaction for GH in most or all of the tumour cells, the intensity of the reaction varying from cell to cell (Fig. 13.30). Some PRL-containing cells may be interspersed among those containing GH, but reactions for other hor-

mones are usually negative. EM shows cells with medium- or large-sized granules in the cytoplasm (Fig. 13.31). Another ultrastructural feature present in the cells of some GH tumours is the 'fibrous body'. This occupies perinuclear cytoplasm and is composed of intermingled tubules and filaments (Fig. 13.32).

Occasionally a GH tumour and a ganglioneuroma occur together in the pituitary fossa.

Prolactin-containing adenomas

Symptoms of hyperprolactinaemia are likely to have been detected in premenopausal women with these tumours. Men and elderly women have less overt hormone-related symptoms, and present usually with a space-occupying lesion. The tumours appear chromophobe or weakly eosinophil with routine stains. The cells are small- or medium-sized, oval or polygonal in shape, and usually arranged diffusely or with a perivascular orientation (Plate 6.3). Some contain small, scattered calcospherites. PRL-containing tumours which are removed after a prolonged period of bromocriptine treatment are likely to show a reduction in size of the tumour cells and a considerable increase in the collagen and reticulin present between the tumour cells (Fig. 13.33). Immunohistology shows a uniform pattern of PRL-reactivity, often accentuated in the perinuclear cytoplasm, throughout the tumour (Plate 6.3). There is less positive reaction in

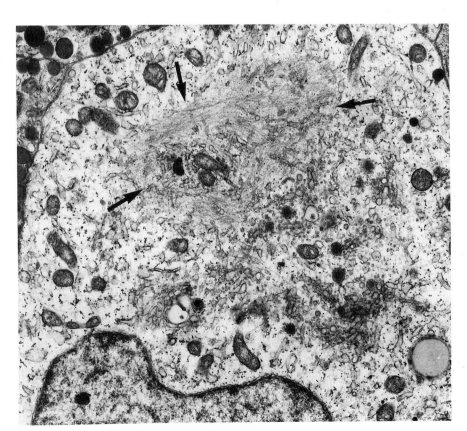

Fig. 13.32. Electron micrograph showing perinuclear cytoplasm from a growth-hormone-secreting pituitary adenoma. A fibrous body, consisting of intermingled filaments (11 nm diameter) and microtubules, is present (arrowed). Uranyl acetate and lead citrate, ×15 440.

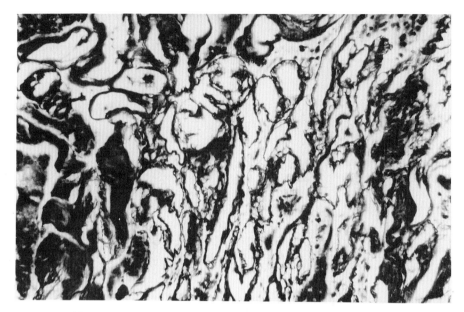

Fig. 13.33. Marked increase in collagen and reticulin content of a prolactin-secreting pituitary adenoma from a patient treated preoperatively with bromocriptine for 36 weeks (compare with Fig. 13.29). ×200.

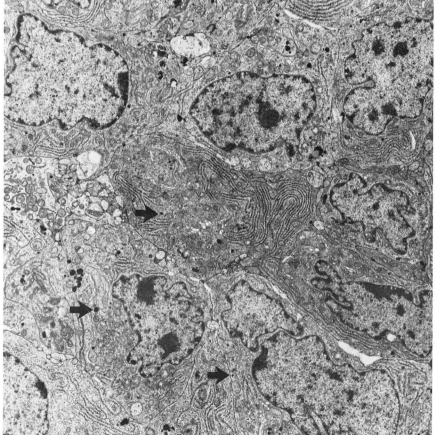

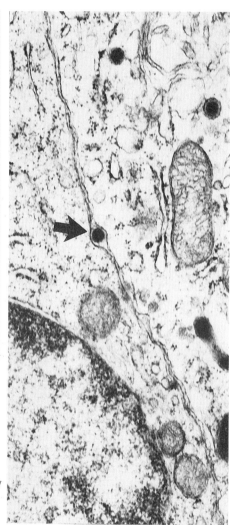

Fig. 13.34 (*above*). Low-power electron micrograph of a prolactin-secreting pituitary adenoma. Tumour cells contain abundant rough endoplasmic reticulum and sparse, medium-sized secretory granules in the cytoplasm (arrowed). Uranyl acetate and lead citrate, ×4500.

Fig. 13.35 (*right*). Higher power electron micrograph of a prolactin-secreting pituitary adenoma showing a secretory granule (arrowed) situated between the adjacent cytoplasmic boundaries of two tumour cells ('misplaced exocytosis'). Uranyl acetate and lead citrate, ×37 600.

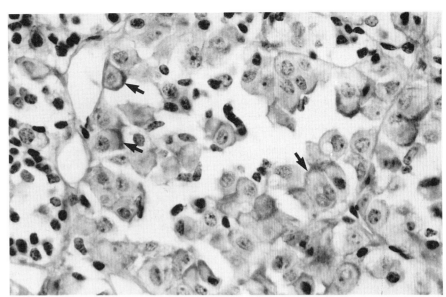

Fig. 13.36. Group of basophil cells showing Crooke's hyaline change in the anterior pituitary gland from a subject with Cushing's disease. Granules are displaced to the margin of the cells (arrowed), and the perinuclear cytoplasm is pale. Orange G/PAS, ×400.

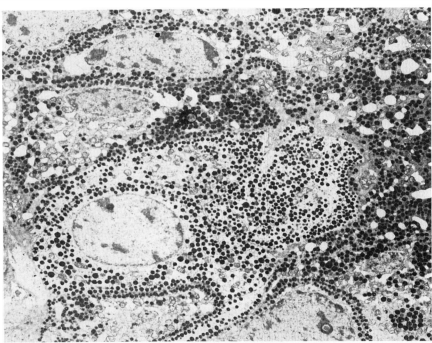

Fig. 13.37. Low-power electron micrograph of an ACTH-secreting pituitary adenoma. Abundant, large secretory granules are present in tumour cell cytoplasm, and show some tendency to be aligned adjacent to cell membranes. Uranyl acetate and lead citrate, ×3000.

tumours that have been treated with bromocriptine. Occasionally a few GH-containing cells are present. Ultrastructurally the tumour cells contain abundant amounts of rough endoplasmic reticulum and sparse medium-sized secretory granules scattered throughout the cytoplasm (Fig. 13.34). Occasional granules are seen lying between the cell membranes of adjacent cells, a feature referred to as misplaced exocytosis (Fig. 13.35).

ACTH-containing adenomas

In most cases of Cushing's disease occurring as a consequence of pituitary malfunction, an adenoma can be identified in surgical specimens. The tumour cells are medium- or large-sized, slightly elongated or polygonal and arranged diffusely or in a pseudopapillary pattern (Plate 6.4). Crooke's hyaline change may be seen in the tumour cells and in basophils of adjacent gland fragments (Fig. 13.36). The tumour cells are basophil or chromophobe. Immunohistology shows uniformly-positive reactions for ACTH in all the tumour cells. Reactions for other pituitary hormones are usually negative. EM shows tumour cells containing medium or large secretory granules scattered throughout the cell cytoplasm or aligned near the cell margins (Fig. 13.37). Fine 7 nm diameter filaments lying in bundles may be seen in perinuclear cytoplasm (Fig. 13.38).

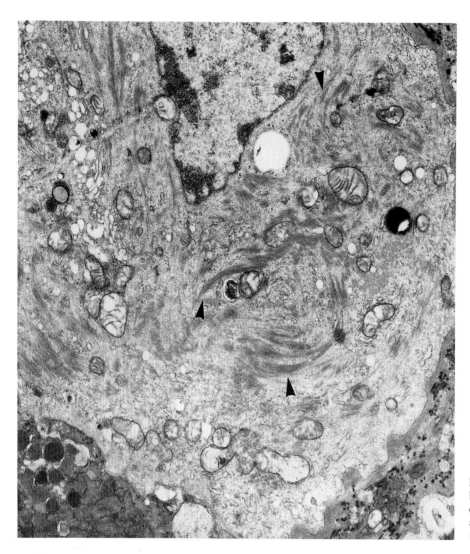

Fig. 13.38. Bundles of microfilaments (arrow heads) in perinuclear cytoplasm of a tumour cell from an ACTH-secreting pituitary adenoma. Uranyl acetate and lead citrate, ×13 730.

The appearances of tumours removed from cases of Nelson's syndrome show the same features as those described above. In some cases of Cushing's disease, despite evidence of over-production of ACTH by the pituitary gland, there is no identifiable tumour in the surgical specimen. Many ACTH-containing basophils may be found lying adjacent to fragments of neurohypophysis. This is considered by some authorities to represent hyperplasia of ACTH-producing cells. However, the diagnosis of basophil hyperplasia in small surgical fragments of pituitary gland is difficult when it is remembered that normal glands frequently contain sizeable clusters of ACTH-containing basophils in this region.

Non-functioning adenomas

Space-occupying pituitary tumours which produce no clinical evidence of hormone secretion have a variable histological appearance, with cells arranged around sinusoids, or diffusely (Plate 6.5). Routine staining shows the cells to be chromophobe or eosinophil. Immunohistological reactions may be entirely negative, but in quite a number of the tumours there are found to be scattered groups of cells which react for βFSH, βLH or both. Such tumours and a few others which are negative with these antisera give a positive reaction for the α subunit of the glycoprotein hormones (Fig. 13.39). Some other non-functioning tumours contain small numbers of cells reactive for several different hormones. Ultrastructurally these tumours contain small secretory granules which may be aligned close to the cell membranes or scattered more diffusely in the cytoplasm (Fig. 13.40). Some also contain many mitochondria (oncocytic change; Fig. 13.41) or multivesicular bodies.

Other pituitary adenomas

Rare examples occur of TSH-containing and other pituitary adenomas, details of which can be found in Robert & Martinez (1986).

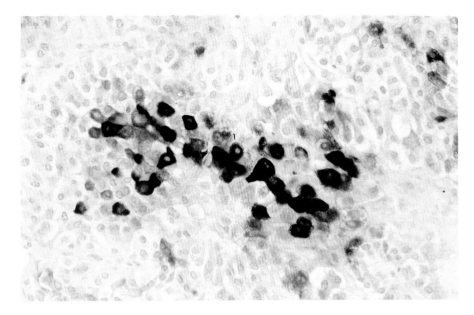

Fig. 13.39 (*right*). Reaction for α subunit of the glycoprotein pituitary hormones in a cluster of cells in a non-functioning, chromophobe pituitary adenoma. Immunoperoxidase with haematoxylin counterstain, ×250.

Fig. 13.40 (*below*). Low-power electron micrograph of a non-functioning chromophobe pituitary adenoma. The cell cytoplasm contains stacks of rough endoplasmic reticulum, and moderate numbers of different-sized secretory granules. Uranyl acetate and lead citrate, ×4320.

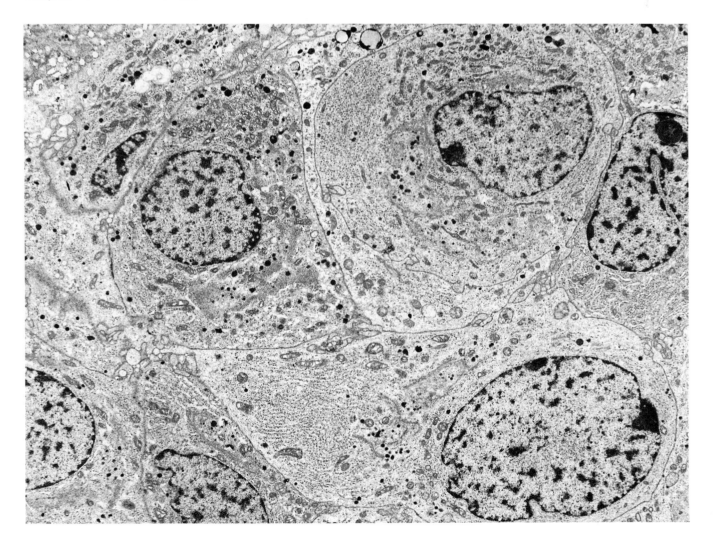

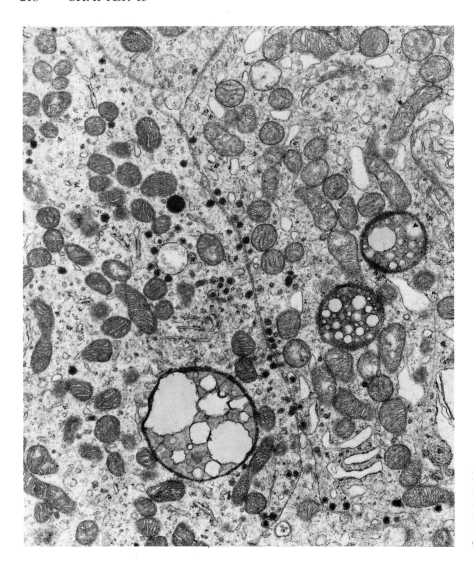

Fig. 13.41. Cytoplasm of tumour cells from a non-functioning pituitary adenoma. Note the abundant mitochondria, multivesicular bodies and very small secretory granules, lying close to the cell membrane. Uranyl acetate and lead citrate, ×29 700.

Malignant or invasive pituitary adenomas

A few pituitary tumours, among both hormonally active and inactive ones, show an invasive local growth pattern and even metastasize. Such tumours are generally not distinguishable histologically from their benign counterparts. Cytological features of nuclear pleomorphism and high mitotic activity are seen in a minority of pituitary adenomas, and are certainly worth noting in reports, but have not been clearly shown to relate to clinical behaviour of the tumours.

Post mortem examination on cases of pituitary tumour

At post mortem it is not uncommon to find incidental adenomas of the pituitary gland. Most of these are no more than a few millimetres across, but a few are larger and extend out of the pituitary fossa (Fig. 13.42). In these cases it is convenient to remove a block of sphenoid bone con-

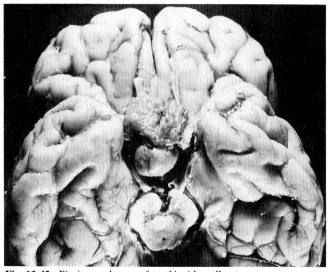

Fig. 13.42. Pituitary adenoma found incidentally at post mortem examination, projecting upward to compress the optic chiasm.

taining the pituitary fossa together with the tumour for detailed examination after fixation (see p.3). Most are found to be of the non-functioning type, or to contain PRL. If the tumour has produced GH or ACTH there will be features in the rest of the body attributable to the excess hormone. Occasionally the relentless expansion of a pituitary adenoma, or sudden acute expansion due to haemorrhage into the tumour, causes death. In these cases the extent of the tumour needs to be determined by inspection of the sphenoid and other paranasal sinuses for growth downward. Sideways extension of the tumour is likely to involve the sphenoid bone, cavernous sinus, and neighbouring cranial nerves and internal carotid arteries. Upward extension of the tumour occupies the suprasellar region around the floor of the third ventricle, and there may be obstructive hydrocephalus if the ventricle itself is distorted or occluded. Suprasellar extension of pituitary tumours also causes compression of the medial aspect of the optic chiasm and tracts (Fig. 13.42). The optic nerves may be surrounded by tumour and destroyed, and the temporal and frontal lobes of the brain indented, though rarely actually invaded by tumour. Optic nerves, tracts and lateral geniculate bodies should always be examined histologically from cases of this type. Extension of the tumour into middle and posterior cranial fossae can also occur, and in exceptional cases there is found to be metastatic spread of tumour outside the cranial cavity.

Non-adenomatous pituitary tumours

Craniopharyngiomas (p.209), simple pituitary cysts, including those derived from remnants of Rathke's cleft, meningiomas (p.201), germinomas (p.220), metastatic tumours (p.223)

and, rarely, glial tumours of the infundibular region of the brain or posterior pituitary gland (Fig. 13.43), may all present as space-occupying lesions in or near the pituitary fossa. Another rare tumour occurring at this site is the granular cell myoblastoma, or choristoma. This is a benign, sparsely cellular tumour composed of spindle-shaped or polygonal cells with abundant, granular, eosinophilic cytoplasm and small, dark, regular nuclei (Fig. 13.44). Fibrosarcoma arising in the suprasellar region has been described as occurring as a late complication of irradiation to the pituitary fossa.

Pineal tumours

'Pinealomas'

Confusion over the use of this term, which has not yet altogether subsided, is attacked in Chapter 7 of Russell & Rubinstein (1977). Up to about 1945, the term was generally applied to the most commonly encountered tumour of the pineal region, which is now generally classed, along with seminoma of the testicle, dysgerminoma of the ovary and other rare malignancies, as a primitive germ-cell tumour, under the label 'germinoma'. The term 'ectopic pinealoma', which used to be applied to similar tumours arising at the base of the brain, especially the pituitary region, is now regarded as obsolete; likewise the term 'atypical teratoma', used by Dorothy Russell (1944, 1954), who early recognized the tumour's affinity with other teratoid tumours. It should be noted that teratomas within the head tend to occur in the midline; and that malignant germinoma tissue may be found mixed with the more benign components of a typical teratoma. Because of past confusions, it is still advisable to avoid

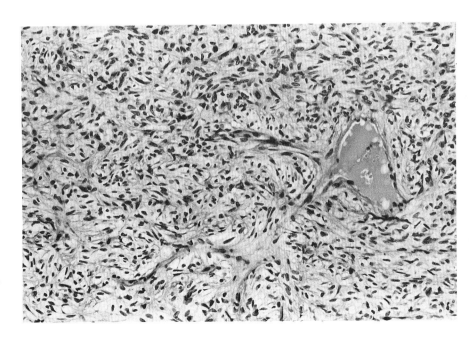

Fig. 13.43. Pituitary tumour arising in the posterior part of the gland and composed of bipolar cells orientated around blood vessels, showing histological appearances closely resembling those of pituicytes (modified astrocytes). H&E, ×100.

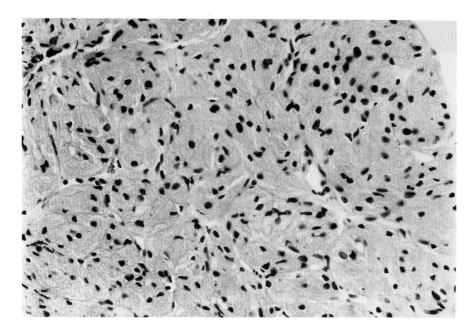

Fig. 13.44. Granular cell myoblastoma of the posterior pituitary. The tumour cells have pale, granular cytoplasm and regular, dark-staining nuclei. H&E, ×220.

the use of the term 'pinealoma', and to use the term 'pineocytoma' for the benign growths arising from the pineal tissue, and 'pineoblastoma' for the malignant ones.

Teratomas

The pineal gland and the parapineal region are the commonest sites for intracranial teratomas. These tumours are rare, and occur almost exclusively in young males. They are well-defined, often partially cystic, and contain such varied elements (hair, bone and cartilage, glands, etc.) as are found in teratomas elsewhere. The less well-differentiated examples are not recognizable with the naked eye. Microscopically they show epithelial elements in the form of well-

defined tubules or papillae, or layers of squamous epithelium, smooth muscle, collagen and, in some cases, cartilage and bone. Less well-differentiated tumours resemble embryonal carcinoma or choriocarcinoma, or contain areas of germinoma (see below). The poorly differentiated tumours contain many mitotic figures and are invasive, with the potential for metastatic spread.

Germinomas (formerly 'atypical teratomas', 'ectopic pinealomas')

This is a rare tumour, found most frequently in or near the pineal gland, or in the suprasellar region. Boys in the second or third decade are those most often affected.

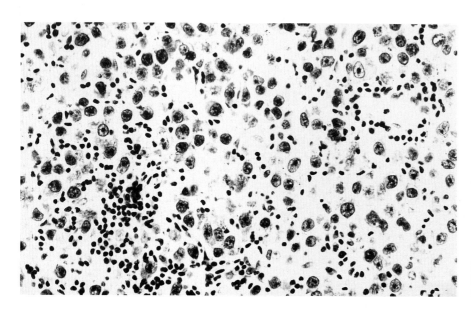

Fig. 13.45. Germinoma, showing intermingled large tumour cells and small stromal lymphocytes. H&E, ×220.

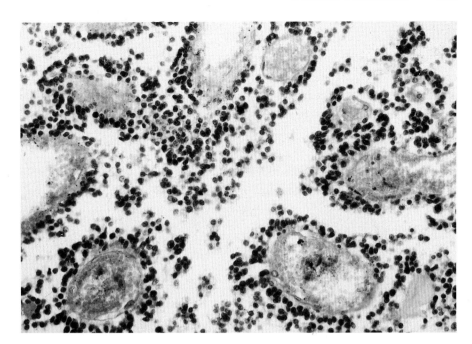

Fig. 13.46. Arrangement of tumour cells in a well-differentiated pineal tumour (pineocytoma) in which there are rosettes of cells orientated around a central pale area. H&E, ×220.

Germinomas are locally invasive and therefore appear poorly circumscribed, and have a pink colour and soft texture. They may produce hydrocephalus by exerting pressure on the tectum of the midbrain. Microscopic appearances are quite distinctive. The tumour is composed of groups of large polygonal cells with eosinophilic cytoplasm and vesicular nuclei with prominent nucleoli. The cell boundaries are well defined and rounded, without processes. The stroma contains blood vessels, collagen and a striking number of small lymphocytes (Fig. 13.45). Occasionally a granulomatous reaction may be seen. Small areas may contain epithelial-lined tubules. Tumour with typical appearances of a germinoma may be an ingredient of a typical teratoma. No glial elements are detectable. Mitotic figures are plentiful in the large, polygonal cells. These tumours are malignant and have a capacity to metastasize in the subarachnoid space.

Pineal parenchymal tumours

These are rare tumours arising from the cells of the pineal gland itself. Well-differentiated tumours of this type are known as *pineocytomas*, and the poorly differentiated forms as *pineoblastomas*. There is, however, no very clear dividing line between them. Most of these tumours are locally invasive and ill defined, appearing as grey or pink, soft, partly necrotic tumours. The microscopy of the better-differentiated tumours bears a resemblance to that of the pineal glandular elements, with orientation of the cells as large rosettes around a central pale area (Fig. 13.46). This area contains argyrophilic fibrils resembling neuronal processes (Fig. 13.47). This feature is regarded as evidence of neuronal differentiation, and has been shown to correlate with a relatively slow growth rate of the tumour. Occasionally astrocytic

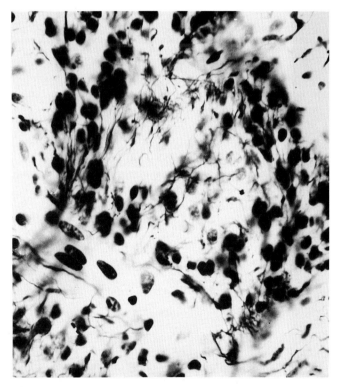

Fig. 13.47. Silver stain (Glees) to demonstrate cell processes in a pineocytoma. ×440.

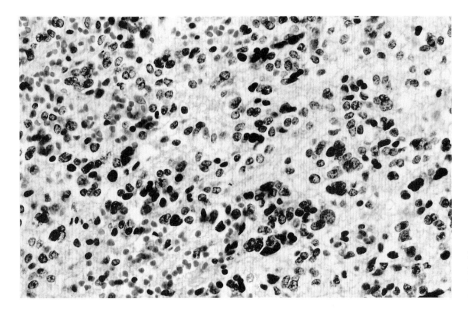

Fig. 13.48. Poorly differentiated pineoblastoma. The cells retain some tendency to a radial grouping around a central, pale area. H&E, ×250.

rather than neuronal differentiation is evident and these cases have a less certain outcome. Pineal parenchymal tumours that lack evidence of any differentiation are more rapidly growing and tend to have a poor outcome. They are composed of diffusely arranged, poorly differentiated cells, or cells arranged in a lobular pattern (Fig. 13.48). Nuclei are dark and lack visible nucleoli. Mitotic figures are usually present in all these pineal tumours, but are only numerous in the poorly differentiated pineoblastomas.

Pineal cysts

Occasional simple, space-occupying cysts occur in the pineal region. These are lined by cuboidal or columnar epithelium, probably related to ependyma. Some large cysts are lined by glial fibres which may contain Rosenthal fibres (p.174; Fig. 12.6).

Tumours extending locally to involve the CNS

There are many tumours which arise in and around the skull and vertebral column and involve the CNS by direct extension. Some of those arising in the eye are, indeed, derived from the CNS itself. Apart from pituitary adenomas, which have already been described, most of these tumours will be familiar to the general pathologist and will not be described here. They include:

1 Carcinomas arising in the paranasal sinuses, the ear, upper nasopharynx, skin of the face and parotid gland.
2 Orbital tumours.
3 Skull and vertebral column tumours: osteogenic sarcomas (especially arising in association with Paget's disease), osteomas, osteochondromas, chondromas, chondrosarcomas, chordomas, fibromyxosarcomas, fibrosarcomas and malignant giant cell tumours of bone, and myelomas.

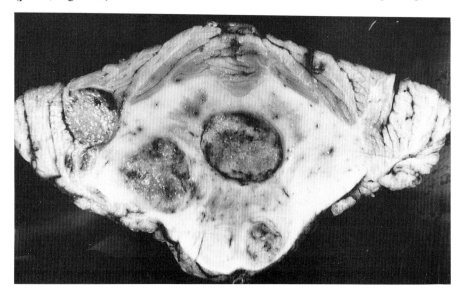

Fig. 13.49. Multiple carcinoma deposits in the cerebellum, fourth ventricle and pons from a primary gastric carcinoma. The tumours appear deceptively well demarcated from surrounding brain, but they are not encapsulated, and are very difficult to remove entire.

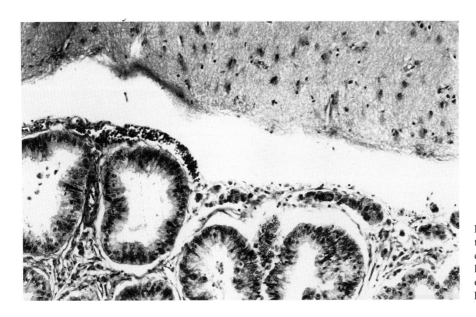

Fig. 13.50. Adenocarcinoma cells (below) in the subarachnoid space around the cerebral cortex from a case with carcinomatosis of the leptomeninges. The molecular layer of the cortex (top) contains reactive astrocytes. H&E, ×85.

4   Tumours invading the spinal extradural space from the retroperitoneum, especially lymphomas and soft-tissue sarcomas.

5   Glomus jugulare tumours, which can arise from chemoreceptor cells in the jugular bulb and invade the posterior fossa or compress the lower cranial nerves.

6   Olfactory neuroblastomas.

One practical point is that the neuropathologist may be required to become familiar with the appearances of these tumours in smear preparations or frozen sections, since they may be biopsied by the neurosurgeon under circumstances that demand rapid diagnosis. Illustrations of some of these tumours as they appear in smears can be found in Chapter 4.

Metastatic tumours

Malignant tumours metastatic to the CNS are fairly common. They are blood-borne and frequently multiple. Their size varies from microscopic to 6 cm or more across. Carcinomas are the commonest tumours to metastasize to the CNS. They usually produce spherical masses in the brain, and much less commonly in the spinal cord. Nerve roots may also be affected (Fig. 13.5b). They may occupy or project into a ventricle and cause hydrocephalus (Fig. 13.49). Uncommonly adenocarcinomas spread as a thin layer, barely discernible by the naked eye, in the subarachnoid space (Fig. 13.50). The solid tumours appear relatively well circumscribed, firm and white or yellowish. Areas of necrosis are usually obvious to inspection and there may also be haemorrhages. In some cases there is severe surrounding oedema (Fig. 11.4a). Primary tumours particularly liable to metastasize to the CNS include oat cell and other lung carcinomas (by far the commonest source), breast, stomach, colon, kidney, thyroid, chorio- and testicular carcinomas,

and melanomas. Metastatic lymphoma may produce a mass lesion in the CNS or diffuse infiltration in the subarachnoid space and around nerve roots. One rare form of lymphoma occupies small cerebral blood vessels and causes ischaemic lesions in the brain. This was formerly known as malignant angio-endotheliomatosis (p.194). Metastatic lymphoma or carcinoma also commonly invades the spinal extradural space. The lymphomas that do this include both Hodgkin's and non-Hodgkin's types. Involvement of the CNS by leukaemia usually takes the form of diffuse subarachnoid, perivascular and nerve root infiltration. Multiple myeloma and bony metastatic carcinoma deposits can spread secondarily from the vertebral column to the spinal extradural space.

Microscopic appearances of metastatic neoplasms reflect the nature of the primary tumour to a variable extent. It is not uncommon for a malignant tumour to manifest itself for the first time as a CNS metastasis whose biopsy provides an opportunity for the pathologist to hazard an opinion as to the likely primary site. Although such an opinion can frequently be given, it is inadvisable to be too dogmatic. Tumours that can be diagnosed with considerable confidence from the appearances seen in CNS metastases or locally invading deposits include melanomas, renal clear cell carcinomas, squamous carcinomas (usually from the lung), thyroid carcinomas, chondrosarcomas, chordomas, myelomas and some lymphomas. Suggestive appearances are seen with gastrointestinal, prostatic and breast carcinomas. Tumours that are particularly difficult to identify are small-celled anaplastic tumours and some lymphomas, which can also be difficult to differentiate from malignant CNS neoplasms. Use of a panel of antibodies and immunohistology can be of considerable help in this context (p. 79).

Remote effects of carcinoma on the nervous system are discussed on p. 160.

Further reading

Pituitary tumours

Robert F, Martinez AJ. (Eds) 1986. Pituitary tumours. *Seminars in Diagnostic Pathology*. (Series ed Santa Cruz DJ) Grune and Stratton, New York, vol. 3 pt. 1.

Russell DS. 1944. Pinealoma: its relationship to teratoma. *J Path Bact* **56**, 145.

Russell DS. 1954. 'Ectopic pinealoma': its kinship to atypical teratoma of the pineal gland. *J Path Bact* **68**, 125.

Scheithauer BW. 1984. Surgical pathology of the pituitary: the adenomas. In Sommers SC, Rosen PP (Eds) *Pathol Annu* **19**, pt. 1, pp. 317–74, and pt. 2, pp. 269–329.

Scheithauer BW. 1985. Pathology of the pituitary and sellar region: exclusive of pituitary adenomas. In Sommers SC, Rosen PP, Fechner RE (Eds) *Pathol Annu* **20**, pt. 1, pp. 67–155.

WHO Histological classification of tumours of the central nervous system. *International Classification of Tumours* No. 21. WHO, Geneva, 1979.

Chapter 14
Multiple (Disseminated) Sclerosis (MS)

In a typical case of MS the lesions, which are confined to the CNS, are so obvious that a confident diagnosis can be made by naked eye alone. In some cases they are apparent as soon as the brain is taken out, in the form of irregular grey patches on the normally whitish surface of the pons (Fig. 14.1), or on the cut surfaces of the upper cervical cord and optic nerves (Fig. 14.2). If the brain is incised fresh (a step which we do not recommend except when fresh plaque tissue is required, e.g. for chemical or histochemical examination), sharply-demarcated grey or pinkish-grey patches may be met with. These, the so-called *plaques*, are firmer to the touch than the surrounding brain tissue. In the fixed state, the difference in texture is hardly appreciable. In the spinal cord, for reasons given below, the plaques, though generally obvious, are sometimes less clearly demarcated. Since they are grey in colour, the plaques are less eye-catching in grey matter than in white; but grey matter is not spared. The greyness of the plaque is of course due to destruction of myelin.

Histologically, the lesions show *demyelination*, as defined on p.58, also known as 'primary demyelination'. (It should be noted that MS is not the only cause of primary demyelination in the CNS (Table 14.1)). Axons, on entering a plaque, lose their myelin sheaths and run naked to the far side, where their sheaths are restored. Within the plaque, nerve cells appear healthy and stain normally (Fig. 14.3). The axons — most of them at least — maintain their integrity, though their ability to conduct nerve impulses is impaired. Thus, vision of poor quality may be preserved in spite of total demyelination of the optic nerves.

During the life of most sufferers MS remains a clinical diagnosis without pathological confirmation. There are no absolutely specific diagnostic tests for the disease, though

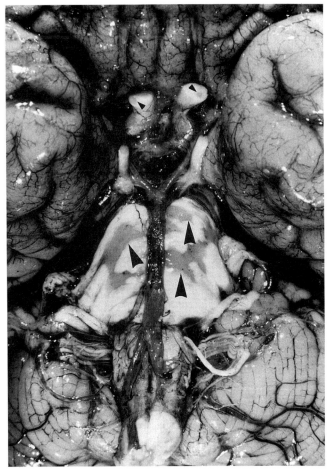

Fig. 14.1. Surface of the pons from a case of MS. There are irregular grey patches (large arrow heads) contrasting with the normal white appearance. Small plaques can also be seen in both optic nerves (small arrow heads).

diagnostic imaging, particularly using nuclear magnetic resonance, has now developed to a point at which a very high level of suspicion of MS can be sustained (Fig. 14.4). Biopsy of the CNS is normally only performed if some other disease has been suspected, and it is still the case that post

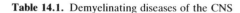

Table 14.1. Demyelinating diseases of the CNS

Multiple sclerosis and its variants (Schilder, Devic, Balò)
Perivenous encephalomyelitis (PVEM) (see p.154)
Prolonged cerebral oedema (see p.165)
Central pontine myelinolysis (see p.305)
Marchiafava–Bignami disease (see p.305)
Progressive multifocal leucoencephalopathy (see p.150)
Subacute sclerosing panencephalitis (see p.149)
Encephalopathy in AIDS (see p.153)
Vitamin B$_{12}$ deficiency (see p.318)
Genetically determined metabolic diseases of white matter
  (leucodystrophies) (see p.296)

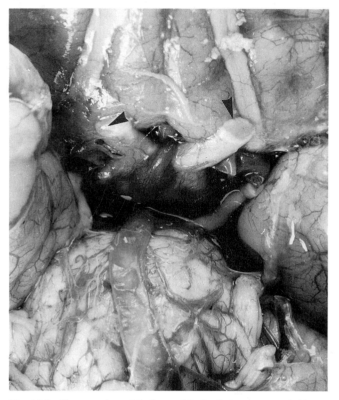

Fig. 14.2. Close-up view of the base of the brain from a case of MS. The whole of the cut surface of the left optic nerve (situated on the right in the figure) and part of the cut surface of the right optic nerve appear grey (arrow heads).

mortem examination of the CNS provides the only opportunity to confirm the diagnosis and obtain tissues for research investigations.

When a post mortem is carried out on a suspected case of MS it is necessary to remove not only the brain but also the spinal cord and optic nerves for examination. In a few cases of MS it is difficult or impossible to identify lesions in the brain, whereas the cord may show devastatingly severe lesions. If the spinal cord from such cases is not examined, doubt will remain about the diagnosis.

Macroscopic appearance of the CNS in MS

After slicing the fixed brain and spinal cord the full extent of the myelin damage in a case of MS becomes readily apparent. The plaques appear as foci of grey discoloration varying in size from that of a pinhead to vast lesions that occupy most of a cerebral hemisphere. The term 'plaque' is not really appropriate for the large irregular lesions which often extend to involve much of the ventricular surfaces. Although nowhere in the CNS is exempt, certain sites are at particularly

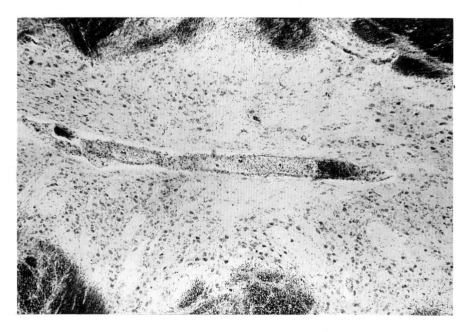

Fig. 14.3. Low-power view of a perivenous MS plaque in the pons. Neurons in pontine nuclei in the demyelinated area remain healthy. LBCV, ×75.

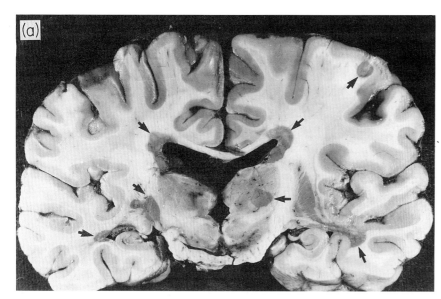
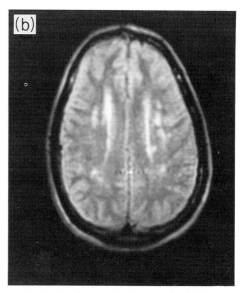

Fig. 14.4. (a) Coronal slice through the cerebrum from a case of severe MS. There are many sharply defined areas of grey demyelination in grey and white matter, including the lateral margins of the lateral ventricles, particularly their inferior horns (arrowed). (b) NMR imaging of MS plaques during life; spin echo sequence, showing high signal intensity (bright) areas in the periventricular regions. (Courtesy NMR Unit, Hammersmith Hospital, London.)

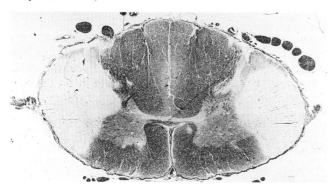

Fig. 14.5. Transverse myelin-stained section of cervical spinal cord (C7) from a case of MS. Demyelination affects lateral white matter on both sides.

high risk for the development of plaques in MS: all subependymal regions, especially the lateral angles of the lateral ventricles (Fig. 14.4), optic nerves and spinal cord. In the spinal cord plaques tend to be most numerous at the cervical level, where the lateral columns are particularly commonly affected (Fig. 14.5). Small plaques often surround small veins (Fig. 14.6) or may be found adjacent to the subarachnoid space, where their shape often suggests an origin close to the surface (Fig. 14.7). Long-standing chronic plaques appear sharply demarcated with a smooth edge. Recent ones are less well-demarcated because of the presence of oedema, and because myelin may still be in the process of breaking down at the margins. In severe, acute MS the

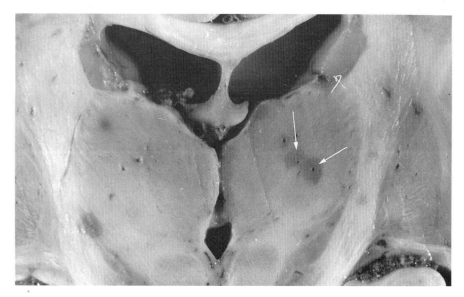

Fig. 14.6. Close-up view of perivenous MS plaques. The vein is visible in the plaques marked with arrows.

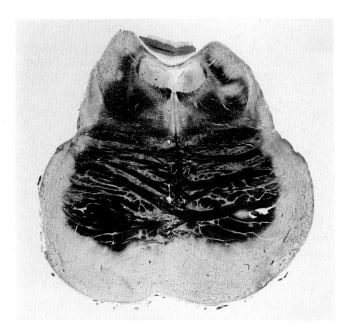

Fig. 14.7. Extensive demyelination of subpial margins of the pons from a case of severe, acute MS.

oedema may be quite generalized, and when the spinal cord or the optic nerves are affected the local blood supply may be compromised because of their close investment, by the pia in the case of the spinal cord, and by the bony canals that encircle the optic nerves. Plaques examined in three dimensions often appear almond-shaped, with a vein running in the centre of the long axis, or they follow the sinuous curves of the veins they surround (Fig. 14.8). They may have irregular perivenous finger-like projections from the main lesion ('Dawson's fingers').

In most cases of MS it is possible to identify upward of a dozen or so plaques with ease. Exceptionally there may be massive, bilateral plaques in the centrum ovale with or

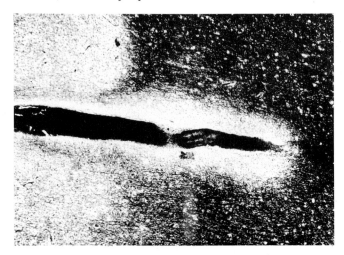

Fig. 14.8. Low-power view of perivenous extension of an established MS plaque. Inflammatory cells lie alongside the vessel. LBCV, ×35.

without more typical, smaller plaques elsewhere (Fig. 14.9). These are the characteristic appearances in the Schilder type of MS, which is an acute form of the disease occasionally encountered in young people. In the past there has been some confusion in the use of the term 'Schilder's disease'. The main source of confusion was Schilder himself, who between 1912 and 1924 published, under the common name of 'encephalitis periaxalis diffusa', three cases of what are now recognized as totally different diseases. One of these was almost certainly a case of adrenoleucodystrophy (p.298); one was probably a case of SSPE (p.149); whereas the 1912 paper described the case of a 14-year-old girl who died after a 19-week progressive illness from what was clearly an acute attack of MS, causing massive lesions in the cerebral hemispheres. This case is the prototype for what has been called the *Schilder type of MS*. To avoid renewed confusion, it is advisable to eschew the term 'Schilder's disease', and the equally imprecise label of 'diffuse sclerosis'.

In *Balò's type of MS* there are curious, concentric, laminated demyelinated zones separated by intervening

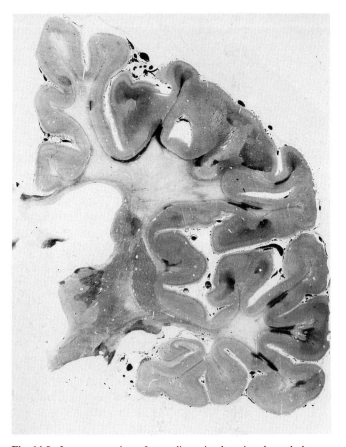

Fig. 14.9. Low-power view of a myelin-stained section through the right cerebral hemisphere from a case of long-standing MS, showing very extensive demyelination of most of the white matter of frontal and temporal lobes. Vestiges of myelin remain in the immediately subcortical zones. There is shrinkage of the tissue, with marked narrowing of the corpus callosum and dilatation of the lateral ventricle.

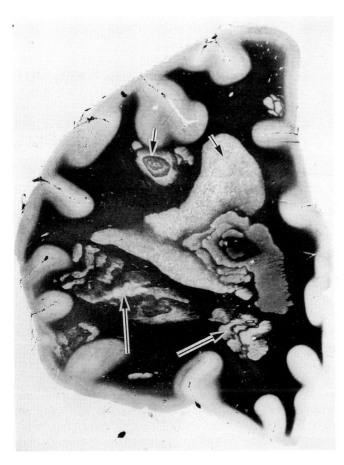

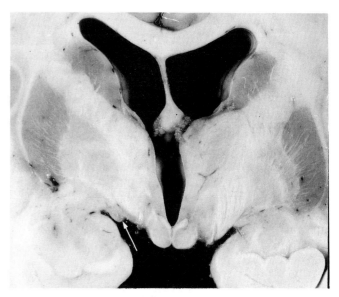

Fig. 14.11. Coronal section of the cerebrum at the level of the mamillary bodies from a case of MS. The optic tracts (left one indicated by arrow) are shrunken and discoloured as a consequence of severe, long-standing demyelination in the optic nerves (cf. Fig. 2.8a).

Fig. 14.10. Low-power view of section through the left frontal lobe from a case of the Balò type of MS. There are well-demarcated areas of myelin loss within which islands of preserved myelin remain. The large centrally situated lesions, and the smaller one in the white matter of the middle frontal gyrus (short arrows) show approximately concentric bands of demyelination. These bands are sharply defined at their outer margins, but less so at their inner ones. The more ventral lesions (long arrows) show more irregular zones of demyelination. A vein can just be seen at the centre of the concentric middle frontal gyrus lesion. Myelin stain.

bands of preserved myelin (Fig. 14.10). In *Dévic's type of MS* severe lesions are found in the optic nerves and spinal cord. These variants of MS are not always totally distinct pathologically from the more classical lesions and do not therefore warrant consideration as distinct diseases, as they have sometimes been considered in the past.

In severe, long-standing MS with extensive cerebral lesions there is usually a degree of cerebral atrophy, with compensatory enlargement of the lateral ventricles. In cases with severe involvement of the optic nerves the optic tracts show shrinkage and discoloration (Fig. 14.11). A severely affected spinal cord appears shrunken and grey. Extensive lesions in which there has been severe oedema may show a post-oedematous cystic state (Fig. 11.8). At the other end of the spectrum of severity that MS displays are cases in which a few small, chronic plaques are found incidentally at post

mortem examination in a patient who had no history of neurological disease. Such incidental plaques are most likely to be found at the lateral angles of the lateral ventricles (Fig. 14.12). Very occasionally gliomas have been found in brains of subjects with MS and some appear to have arisen in a plaque.

In any individual case of MS, correlation of the siting of plaques with clinical symptomatology is often possible, for example when the lesions are situated in the optic nerves, brain stem or spinal cord. Cerebral plaques tend to be harder to correlate with clinical features, but are often extensive in patients with prominent mental changes. In every case note should be taken of the particular clinical features that were present and an attempt made to discover lesions that account for them.

Microscopy of MS: dating of lesions

Many patients with MS eventually die several decades after the onset of their disease. There is often little evidence of disease progression clinically in the latter years, and death may be due to a disease quite unrelated to MS, or to complications resulting from a static neurological deficit, as for example when a patient dies from renal failure secondary to repeated urinary tract infections precipitated by loss of bladder control, or from pneumonia consequent on immobility. The MS lesions in such patients are mainly of a type regarded as inactive, or showing no evidence of recent demyelination. Microscopically these lesions appear less cellular than the surrounding tissue (Fig. 14.13), and in general the chronicity of the lesions is inversely related to

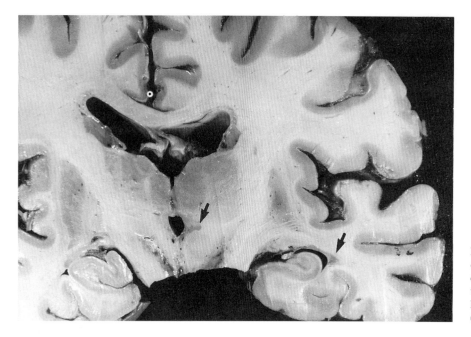

Fig. 14.12. Incidental finding of small, chronic demyelinated plaques in a patient dying of carcinoma of the colon. These are situated at the margin of the inferior horn of the right lateral ventricle, and in the right thalamus (arrowed).

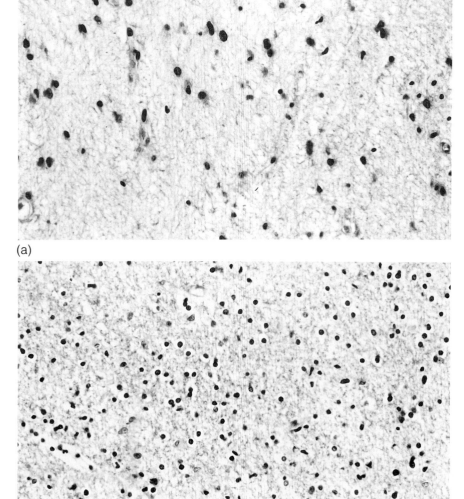

(a)

(b)

Fig. 14.13. Comparison of nuclei in a chronic MS plaque (a), and normal white matter (b). In the plaque nuclei are fewer in number, less regularly distributed, and most clearly belong to astrocytes. In normal white matter most of the nuclei are smaller, more uniform and rounded, with appearances of oligodendrocyte nuclei. This population of cells is severely depleted in chronic MS plaques. H&E, ×250.

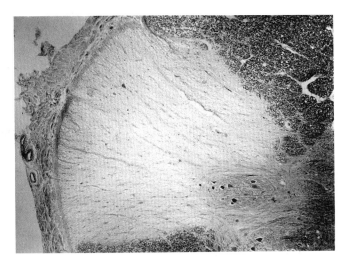

Fig. 14.14. Low-power view of myelin stained section of a lateral column chronic MS plaque in the spinal cord. The border of the plaque is sharply defined. LBCV, ×18.

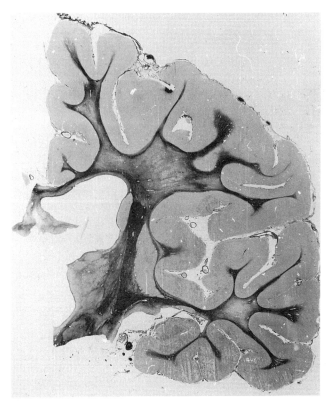

Fig. 14.15. Adjacent section to that shown in Fig. 14.9, stained by the Holzer technique to show glial fibres. The whole demyelinated area is densely gliotic.

cellularity. There is abrupt loss of myelin as one moves into the plaque (Fig. 14.14), and oligodendrocyte nuclei are reduced in numbers or abolished in the plaque (Fig. 14.13). Axons are for the most part preserved, and there is a dense felt-work of glial fibres forming scar tissue. This is clearly seen with a Holzer stain (Figs 3.15 and 14.15). Inflammation is sparse, and macrophages few·or absent in the lesion. Neutral fat cannot be demonstrated in more than an occasional cell. Partially myelinated axons, lying in groups, are frequently found inside or just beyond the margins of chronic plaques, and as these regions stain palely with myelin stains they are termed areas of 'shadow' plaque (Figs 3.15, 14.16 and 14.17). Many of these areas probably represent

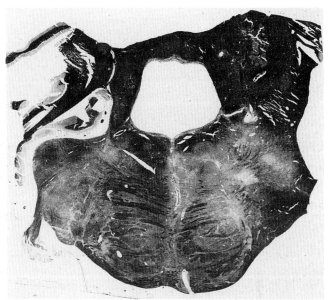

Fig. 14.16 Section of pons containing inactive, 'shadow' plaques. Myelin stain, ×2.

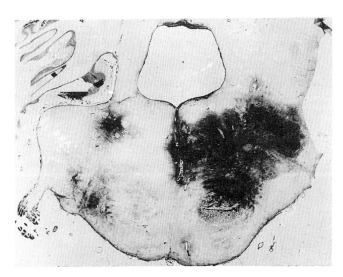

Fig. 14.17. Adjacent section to that shown in Fig. 14.16, showing gliosis within the plaques. Holzer, ×2.

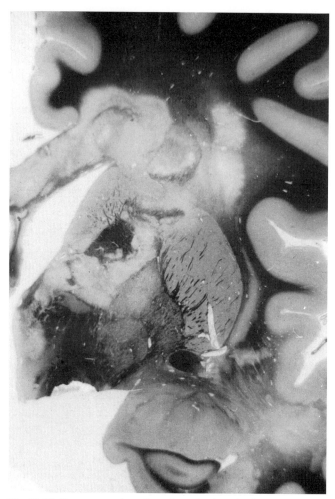

Fig. 14.18. Low-power view of myelin-stained section from a case of acute MS. Margins of the irregular, demyelinated zone appear blurred on account of oedema. Note also some residual myelin remaining adjacent to, and within the corpus callosum.

areas of remyelination, though in other contexts, for example in acute plaques, areas of myelin pallor may in contrast be due to incomplete demyelination, or to oedema (Fig. 14.18). Extensive chronic plaques are often associated with some wallerian degeneration due to loss of chronically demyelinated axons. The site at which such secondary degeneration can be demonstrated will vary according to the site of the plaques. For example, chronic plaques in the cervical spinal cord may be associated with wallerian degeneration in the lateral corticospinal tracts at lower levels of the cord.

Intermingled with the inactive plaques described above there may be other plaques whose centres appear inactive, but whose edges are hypercellular (Fig. 14.19). These are thought to be plaques at the margins of which demyelination is intermittently continuing. The increased cells at the margins consist of macrophages, a few lymphocytes, astrocytes and possibly increased numbers of oligodendrocytes. Some of the macrophages may contain neutral fat, representing breakdown products of degenerate myelin (Plate 2.3 and Fig. 14.20). Areas of shadow plaque may also be present in the vicinity. These marginal zones probably represent areas where demyelination and partial remyelination alternately occur.

Patients occasionally die with a relatively short history of MS, or during a relapse. The brain and spinal cord of such patients contain lesions that show evidence of active demyelination. Many of them are small and intensely cellular (Fig. 14.21). They show loss of myelin, though this may not be complete, and contain many macrophages, some of which have ingested fragments of myelin which still react with myelin stains. Reactive astrocytes with enlarged cell bodies may be present, but glial fibres are lacking. Lymphocytes and a few plasma cells are present not only in

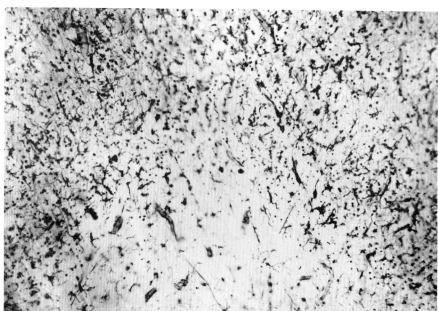

Fig. 14.19. Margin of MS plaque (below), showing increased numbers of microglial cells at the margin. Weil–Davenport, ×140.

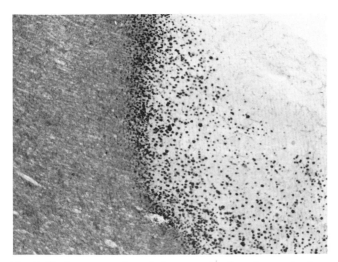

Fig. 14.20. Low-power view of a frozen section from the margin of a MS plaque (right), stained to show neutral fat. At the interface with normally myelinated white matter (left) there are many lipid-containing phagocytes. Oil red-O, ×25.

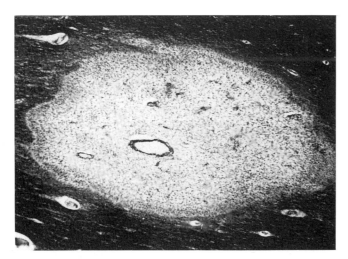

Fig. 14.21. A small, acute perivenous plaque showing intense cellularity. LBCV, ×35.

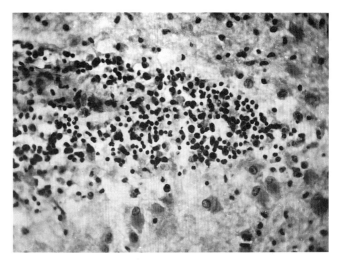

Fig. 14.22. Perivenous and parenchymal mononuclear inflammatory cells in an acute MS plaque. Note also many plump-bodied astrocytes. H&E, ×180.

perivascular spaces but also in the plaque parenchyma (Figs 14.22 and 14.23). Interstitial oedema is present in and immediately around the plaque (Fig. 14.18). Axons for the most part remain intact, though some may show swelling (Fig. 14.24). Neuron cell bodies in grey matter plaques appear entirely unscathed (Fig. 14.3). Beyond the edge of acute plaques microglial cells appear enlarged and increased in number, and perivascular lymphocytes and macrophages are conspicuous.

The lesion in Balò's type of MS consists microscopically of alternating concentric zones of preserved and destroyed myelin around a central vein (Fig. 14.25). Occasionally the pattern resembles crazy paving rather than concentric circles of preserved and destroyed myelin. Other, more conventional, MS lesions are usually present elsewhere. The outer margins of the demyelinated zones are less sharply defined than the inner ones. The zones themselves do not seem to relate to any orientation of anatomical tracts or of vascular territories.

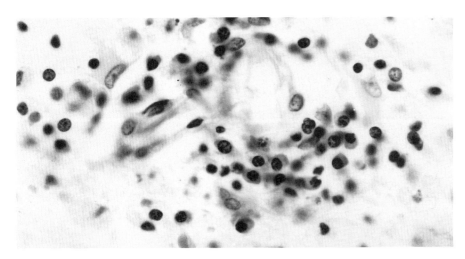

Fig. 14.23. Plasma cells surrounding a small vein in an acute MS plaque. H&E, ×400.

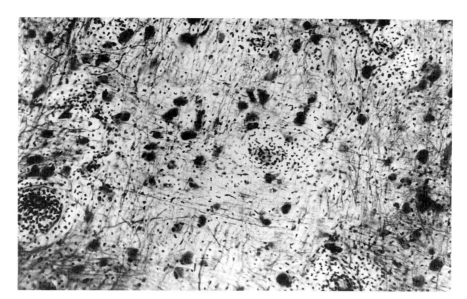

Fig. 14.24. Subacute MS plaque showing perivascular inflammation, surviving axon cylinders and the cell bodies of reactive astrocytes. Hortega double impregnation, ×125.

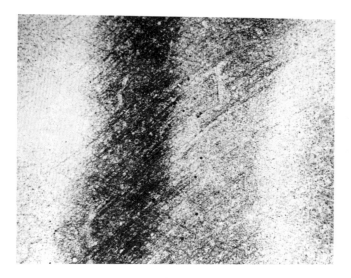

Fig. 14.25. Successive bands of partial and complete demyelination in a Balò type lesion of MS. These are unrelated to the direction of the nerve fibres, which run obliquely across the field. Three densities of myelin staining intensity are apparent. Myelin stain, ×38.

EM is not routinely carried out on MS tissues, though this method has certainly contributed much to the understanding of the pathogenesis of MS lesions when it has been undertaken as a research investigation. Similarly, analysis of T-lymphocyte subsets is not necessary for diagnosis, but is valuable in trying to understand the pathogenesis of MS.

The differential diagnosis of acute MS lesions includes other inflammatory and demyelinating conditions. The absence of damage to neurons distinguishes MS from most forms of viral encephalitis, but acute MS lesions can be difficult to distinguish from those of acute PVEM (p.154). MS lesions usually have more bulk, extending further from the vein walls than the narrow sleeves of demyelination found in PVEM, and they are less uniformly distributed throughout the neuraxis. Occasionally cases occur in which lesions that can properly be described as characteristic of both MS and PVEM can be found (Fig. 10.45). The focal demyelinating lesions of PML (p.150) do not usually give rise to confusion, because this latter disease, unlike MS, arises against a background of immunosuppression, inflammation is usually minimal or lacking in PML, and MS lacks the oligodendroglial nuclear inclusion bodies and gross astrocytic nuclear pleomorphism (Figs 10.31 and 10.32) that are seen in PML (see Chapter 10). Recent and older MS plaques sometimes need to be distinguished from small, sharply-defined arteriolar infarcts in white matter (Fig. 7.10), a distinction readily made by examining a section stained for axons, which shows preserved axons in MS plaques (Fig. 14.24), and severe damage to axons, or their loss, in infarcts.

Ideally, the neuropathologist should not rest content with a simple post mortem diagnosis of MS. There remains the question why a particular episode of demyelination occurred in a particular place on a particular date. In most instances this question will have to remain unanswered; but a convincing answer in only a few cases may give a lead to better understanding of a very mysterious disease.

Further reading

Allen IV. 1984. Demyelinating diseases. In Adams JH, Corsellis JAN, Duchen LW (Eds) *Greenfield's Neuropathology*, 4th edn. Edward Arnold, London, pp. 338–84.

Hallpike JF, Adams CWM, Tourtellotte WW. 1983. *Multiple Sclerosis: Pathology, Diagnosis and Management*. Chapman and Hall, London.

McDonald WI, Silberberg DH. 1986. *Multiple Sclerosis*. Butterworths, London.

Prineas JW. 1985. The neuropatholgoy of multiple sclerosis. In Vinken PJ, Bruyn GW (Eds) *Handbook of Clinical Neurology*, Elsevier, Amsterdam, **3**, 213–57.

Raine CS. 1985. Demyelinating diseases. In Davis RL, Robertson DM (Eds) *Textbook of Neuropathology*. Williams and Wilkins, Baltimore, pp. 468–547.

Chapter 15
Neuronal Decay

Definitions

There are many different causes for progressive loss of nervous functions. Some of these are at least partially understood; for instance, various types of lipidosis and leucodystrophy are known to be related to specific enzyme deficiencies, though the therapeutic application of this knowledge lies in the future. In a few cases — for example, subacute combined degeneration of the cord, Wilson's disease, and Wernicke's encephalopathy — the disease can be arrested, and even reversed. But there remains a depressingly large residuum of diseases of which the causes are completely unknown, apart from the fact that some of them, are familial. These are the primary, or idiopathic, *neuronal degenerations*.

The common clinical characteristic of this group of diseases is the unremitting *progression* (which may be rapid or slow) of the patient's disability. Their common pathological process is a steady loss of nerve cells, in many instances beginning at the distal ends of their axons, with glial response. This cell loss is *systematic*, not regional, and quite independent of vascular supply or drainage. In motor neuron disease, cells are lost from the anterior horns of the spinal cord, while the dorsal (Clarke's) nuclei remain intact. The reverse of this occurs in Friedreich's ataxia. In one form of multiple system atrophy Purkinje cells are lost. The rest of the cerebellar cortex, and the dentate nuclei, are spared. In Friedreich's ataxia the dentate nuclei are affected, but not the Purkinje cells. In general, the lesions tend to be symmetrical; but some cases of Parkinson's disease and of motor neuron disease show a marked lateral asymmetry.

Table 15.1 shows the main clinical and pathological features of five relatively common degenerative conditions. All five diseases vary somewhat in their manifestations, but are sufficiently constant to merit separate names. Many others have been named, but are comparatively rare. Beyond these, there is a great array of very rare conditions, some confined to a single known family, for which names are not available, and not really needed. Not included in this table are those degenerative conditions whose principal manifestation is dementia. These, which include Alzheimer's and Pick's diseases and Creutzfeldt−Jakob disease, are dealt with in Chapter 17.

Procedures

At post mortem, when there are clinical grounds for suspecting the presence of a neurodegenerative disease, the brain and spinal cord should be taken routinely. One is however faced with an immediate decision on whether to immerse all the material in formalin, or whether to reserve certain parts in the deep freeze for later biochemical investigations. The decision will depend largely on whether a working relationship has already been established with research workers in the fast-growing field of neurochemistry. Some of the centres where such research is carried out are listed in Appendix B (p.393). Guidance can also be sought from the various societies concerned with the collection and spread of information on particular diseases. Some of these are also listed in Appendix B.

In many degenerative conditions *peripheral nerves* are involved. These include motor neuron disease, Friedreich's ataxia, peroneal muscular atrophy (Charcot−Marie−Tooth disease) and some types of multiple system atrophy. In a few, visceral organs are affected. In 'classical' Friedreich's ataxia, for example, the *heart* is affected; thus in any case of

Table 15.1. The main clinical and pathological features of five relatively common degenerative conditions

Disease	Main clinical features	Naked-eye changes	Histological changes
Motor neuron disease 'Classical' form	Usual onset in sixth and seventh decades. Rarely familial. Progressive weakness and wasting of skeletal muscles, excluding ocular muscles	Muscle wasting and pallor. Wasting of anterior spinal roots. Medullary pyramids may be wasted	Loss of motor cells from anterior grey horns, and from cranial motor nuclei V, VII, (X), XI, XII. Denervation changes in muscles. Pyramidal tract degeneration
Werdnig–Hoffmann disease	Onset in late fetal life onwards. Recessive inheritance. 'Floppy baby'	Muscle wasting and pallor. Wasting of anterior spinal roots	Loss of motor cells. Denervated muscles. Pyramidal tracts not affected
Paralysis agitans (Parkinson's disease, idiopathic parkinsonism)	Usual onset in seventh and eighth decades. Not familial. Bradykinesia, resting tremor, 'cogwheel' rigidity, festination, mask-like facies, etc. Autonomic failure in some cases	Loss of pigment from substantia nigra and locus ceruleus. Basal ganglia appear normal	Loss of pigmented cells from substantia nigra and locus ceruleus; intracytoplasmic inclusions (Lewy bodies) in cells of these nuclei, nucleus basalis (substantia innominata) and elsewhere. No striatal cell loss. Intermediolateral column cell loss in some cases
Multiple system atrophy Striatonigral type*	Usual onset in fifth to seventh decades. Parkinsonism (not responding to L-dopa). Autonomic failure (Shy–Drager syndrome) in some cases	Atrophy and discoloration of putamen. Loss of pigment from substantia nigra and locus ceruleus	Cell loss and gliosis in putamen, substantia nigra, locus ceruleus, intermediolateral columns
Pontocerebellar type*	Progressive ataxia and dysarthria	Atrophy of pons, olives, cerebellar cortex and white matter, middle and inferior cerebellar peduncles	Cell loss and gliosis in pontine nuclei, olives, Purkinje cells. (Different selection of lesions in different cases. Motor cells and sensory ganglia occasionally affected, but mildly. Likewise pyramidal tracts)
Friedreich's ataxia	Onset in first and second decades. Progressive ataxia, beginning in lower limbs. Mild sensory changes. Signs of cardiomyopathy, with abnormal ECG. Death commonly from heart failure	Atrophy of posterior spinal roots, spinal cord, brain stem, superior cerebellar peduncles; in some cases atrophy of globus pallidus, subthalamic nuclei, optic nerves. Cerebral infarcts rather common. Hypertrophy and fibrosis of heart	Cell loss from sensory ganglia (lower cord segments), dorsal and accessory cuneate nuclei, and dentate nuclei. Loss of axons in sensory nerves, posterior columns, pyramidal and spinocerebellar tracts, superior cerebellar peduncles, etc. Chronic myocarditis

* These two types are often combined.

progressive ataxia coming on in early life, a careful examination of several regions of the heart should be carried out.

In any case of suspected neuronal degeneration, samples of peripheral nerve, sensory and autonomic ganglia, and muscles from neck and upper and lower limbs should be taken. In selecting muscles, it should be borne in mind that the final state of muscles which have undergone severe neurogenic atrophy is practically indistinguishable from that of muscles affected by dystrophy or other myopathies. For this reason, it is advisable to take samples of mildly affected, and of apparently unaffected, muscles. In any denervating condition pallor of the muscle, due to loss of myoglobin, is a

rough naked-eye indication of the degree of denervation. Samples of muscles supplied by cranial nerves should be taken in any case suspected of motor neuron disease. A procedure for obtaining these is described on pp.5–6.

The choice of blocks for histological examination should depend on a careful reading of the clinical notes.

Motor neuron diseases

A small to moderate degree of motor cell loss occurs in a variety of degenerative conditions, including multiple system atrophy. To make a diagnosis of 'classical' motor neuron disease (*amyotrophic lateral sclerosis*) one must not only demonstrate motor cell loss in the anterior horns of the cervical and lumbar enlargements, and in the hypoglossal nuclei, but also show that there is no obvious degeneration in other parts of the CNS — in particular, the basal ganglia, the cerebellar system and the sensory pathways. In most cases of motor neuron disease a certain amount of degeneration is also seen in the corticospinal (pyramidal) tracts. This may be apparent, in myelin preparations, over the full extent of the tracts, from Rolandic cortex to the sacral segments of the cord. In other cases, it may be detectable only in the lowest cord segments. It was Charcot's (1874) observation of greyness of the crossed pyramidal tracts in sections of the cord that gave rise to the term 'lateral sclerosis'. Strictly speaking, the diagnosis of 'amyotrophic lateral sclerosis' is inappropriate for cases of motor neuron disease not showing this feature. The process is one of 'dying back'; that is, it begins at the distal ends of the axons, and works its way back to the cells of origin. As the axon dies, its myelin sheath breaks down, and the fatty degradation products can be selectively stained by the Marchi method (p.59), which gives positive evidence of tract degeneration when the negative evidence provided by the myelin stain is inconclusive (see Figs 3.28 and 3.29).

When the process has reached up to midbrain level, myelin and Marchi preparations show it to be confined to the middle thirds of the cerebral peduncles (Fig. 2.29). Above this, it can be traced, through the posterior limb of the internal capsule and the centrum ovale, to the Rolandic (precentral and postcentral) cortex, where most of the tract originates. When the process has reached thus far, a further band of degeneration may be detected, running between the Rolandic areas on the two sides via the corpus callosum (Fig. 15.1).

For detecting *motor cell loss*, Nissl staining should be carried out on thick (20 µm or more) sections of brain stem and spinal cord, and the sections compared with normal controls (Fig. 15.2). Appropriate levels for brain stem motor nuclei are shown in Fig. 2.26. Since cranial nerve nuclei have a limited up-and-down extent, and since it may be important to distinguish between left and right sides, the blocks should be clearly marked to indicate which surface is to be cut (see p.39). For assessing the degree of cell loss, it is essential that the sections should be of the same thickness as the control sections; and it is desirable to examine several adjacent sections, both of the block under scrutiny and of the control block, since there are often considerable variations in neuron population between one section and its neighbour. The identification of motor neurons in Nissl preparations is usually fairly easy (Plate 1.5); but it may be rendered difficult, or even impossible, if the tissue has undergone agonal ischaemic changes. The staining of nerve

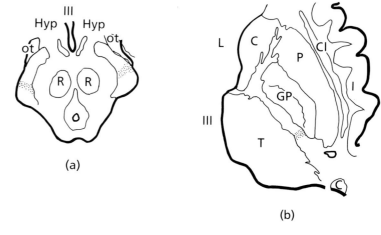

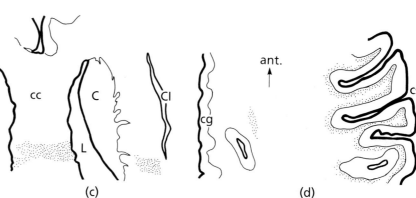

Fig. 15.1. Camera lucida tracings from Marchi preparations on horizontal sections of (a) upper midbrain, (b) basal nuclei, (c) centrum ovale and corpus callosum, and (d) superior frontoparietal region. The stippled areas indicate positive Marchi degeneration. C = caudate nucleus; cc = corpus callosum; cg = cingulate gyrus; Cl = claustrum; cs = central sulcus; GP = globus pallidus; Hyp = hypothalamus; I = insula; L = lateral ventricle; ot = optic tract; P = putamen; R = red nucleus; T = thalamus; III = third ventricle.

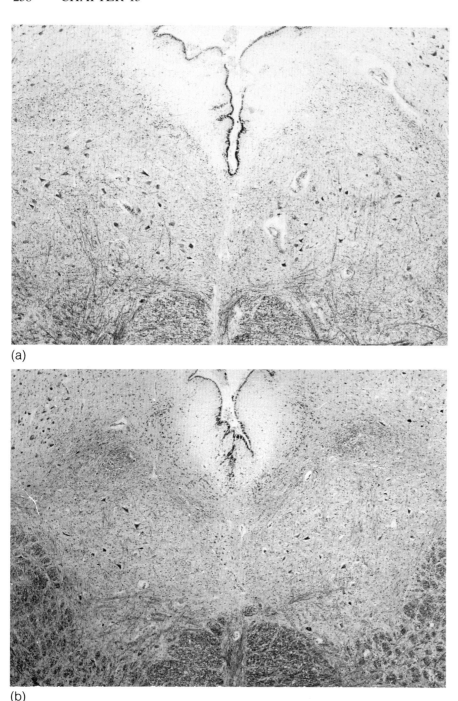

(a)

(b)

Fig. 15.2. (a) Normal hypoglossal nucleus. 20 μm section. Klüver–Barrera stain. (b) Same area, same stain. Case of motor neuron disease. There is a severe depletion of motor cells. (c) Normal cord, level C6. 20 μm section. Klüver–Barrera stain. (d) Same level, same stain. Case of motor neuron disease. Severe depletion of motor cells. Pallor of crossed and uncrossed pyramidal tracts.

fibres, on the other hand, is unaffected by ischaemia. It is often easier to assess loss of spinal motor neurons by examining transverse sections of anterior nerve roots in silver-impregnated sections. A useful block may be obtained by tying a piece of thread around the lower end of the cord, along with the roots of the cauda equina. In a Holmes, Palmgren or similar preparation, there may be a striking difference between the axon densities of anterior and posterior nerve roots.

Types of motor neuron disease

The classical form of motor neuron disease has its onset for the most part in the sixth and seventh decades of life, and has a mean duration of under three years, though some cases survive ten years or more. The commonest causes of death are respiratory failure and aspiration pneumonia, attributable to weakness of the muscles of respiration and deglutition. The clinical labels of 'progressive (distal) mus-

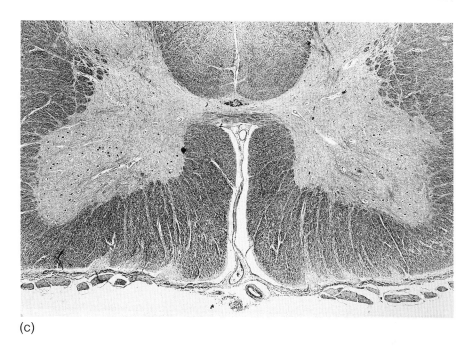

(c)

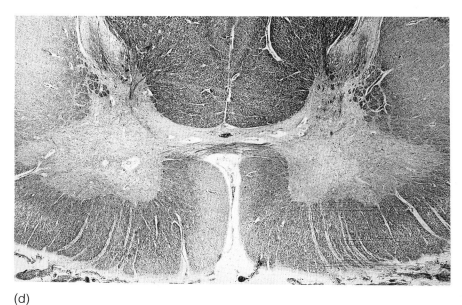

Fig. 15.2. (*continued*)   (d)

cular atrophy' and 'progressive bulbar palsy' are generally appropriate only in the early stages of the disease. By the time of death, the lesions are generally widespread. The condition is only rarely familial.

In marked contrast, there is a rather common form of motor neuron disease, with recessive inheritance, affecting infants, including the newborn. Multiparous mothers of such children are reported as having noticed feebleness of fetal movements. This condition — *Werdnig–Hoffmann disease* — is one of the causes of the 'floppy baby' syndrome. It is rapidly fatal: in general, the earlier the onset, the sooner the child dies. The main pathological findings are of motor cell loss, atrophy of anterior spinal roots, and denervation atrophy of muscles. The pyramidal and other long tracts are unaffected.

Apart from these two life-threatening types of motor neuron disease — the classical and the Werdnig–Hoffmann types — there is a range of comparatively rare types, with onset in later childhood or adolescence, a few of which have acquired eponyms, such as *Kugelberg–Welander disease*. Again, the general rule is that the later the onset the more benign is the course of the disease. They do not appear to form a continuum with classical motor neuron disease. For the most part they show autosomal recessive inheritance.

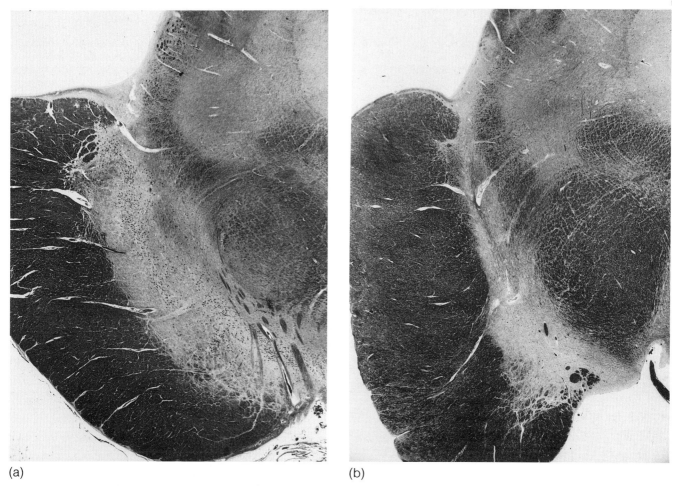

(a)   (b)

Fig. 15.3. (a) Substantia nigra, showing a normal population of large pigmented cells. Klüver–Barrera stain. (b) Same area, in a case of Parkinson's disease. There is severe depletion of pigmented cells, and the whole area is shrunken. (c) Similar depletion and shrinkage in a case of multiple system atrophy.

Parkinsonism

The commonest cause of the syndrome of bradykinesia, resting tremor, cogwheel rigidity, weakness, immobile facies, and 'festinant' gait is *paralysis agitans*, or *Parkinson's disease*. The second commonest is probably the use of drugs of the phenothiazine series. Little is known of the histopathology of drug-induced parkinsonism. Since the condition is generally reversed by withdrawal of the drug, it is not to be expected that gross changes would be observed. However, if cases of this kind come to post mortem, it would be advisable to preserve the brain (or at least parts of it) in cold storage for eventual neurochemical and histochemical studies on the pigmented nuclei and basal ganglia.

Some of the clinical features of parkinsonism may occur in patients with diffuse cerebrovascular disease: the term 'arteriosclerotic parkinsonism' is sometimes used to refer to this condition. The brains from cases of this kind frequently show 'lacunes' (small areas of rarefaction) in the lentiform nuclei (see p.116); but so do the brains of many old people

not afflicted by tremor. Progressive parkinsonism, with added features such as dementia, psychosis and oculogyric crises, was a common sequela in cases of *encephalitis lethargica* (von Economo's encephalitis; see p.161) acquired during the epidemics of 1918 and 1926. Postencephalitic parkinsonism probably still occurs, rarely and sporadically; but further epidemics are always possible. The characteristic findings are of a devastating loss of cells from the substantia nigra, scattered small gliotic scars in the basal nuclei and upper brain stem, and neurofibrillary tangles (similar in form and staining properties to those of Alzheimer's disease) in large cells in these and other areas.

Paralysis agitans

In paralysis agitans (Parkinson's disease, idiopathic parkinsonism) the main features are (i) loss of pigmented cells from the substantia nigra, locus ceruleus and nucleus basalis, most marked in the middle third of the substantia nigra (Figs 2.17 and 15.3) and (ii) the presence of intracytoplasmic

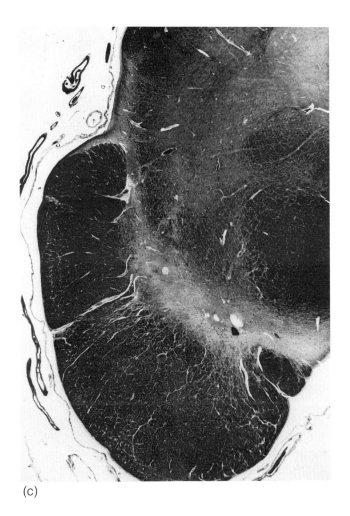

(c)

inclusions (*Lewy bodies*; Plate 1.4) in remaining pigmented cells, and in non-pigmented cells in other places, including the nucleus basalis. Without finding such inclusions, it would be hard to sustain a diagnosis of paralysis agitans. They may occasionally be found in brains not showing loss of pigmented cells from patients not afflicted with parkinsonism. In such cases, one may reasonably conjecture that the disease was present, but still in a subclinical, or preclinical, phase. Incidentally, Lewy bodies are not easily seen in a Nissl stain, but are well displayed by H&E, and still better by Lendrum's phloxine−tartrazine method.

Striatonigral degeneration

A much rarer condition, which may give rise to a clinical picture indistinguishable from that of paralysis agitans, but which does not respond to treatment with L-dopa, is striato-nigral degeneration. This condition forms part of the wide spectrum of *multiple system atrophy*, which includes most (possibly all) cases of pontocerebellar atrophy, and most cases of progressive autonomic failure (*Shy−Drager syndrome*). In multiple system atrophy the following structures are at risk: striatum (particularly the putamen), substantia nigra, locus ceruleus, pontine nuclei, inferior olives, Purkinje cells of the cerebellar cortex, cranial and spinal motor cells, and thoracic and sacral intermediolateral columns (pre-ganglionic autonomic efferent cells) (Figs 15.4−15.9). Doubtless other structures, hitherto unidentified, share the risk. These may include parts of the nucleus ambiguus, supplying the posterior crico-arytenoid muscle, which is frequently found to be selectively wasted in cases of the

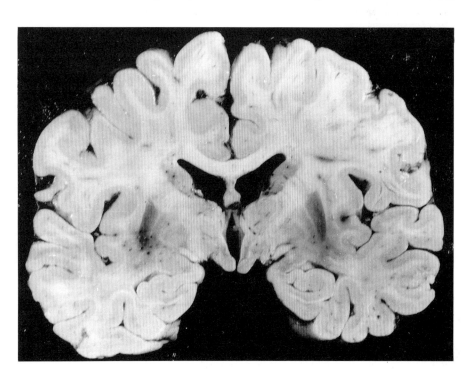

Fig. 15.4. Multiple system atrophy. Coronal slice at level A1 from a woman aged 66, suffering from parkinsonism, ataxia, and autonomic failure. The putamen is shrunken and discoloured on both sides.

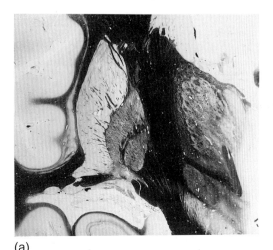

(a)

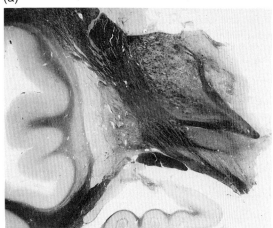

(b)

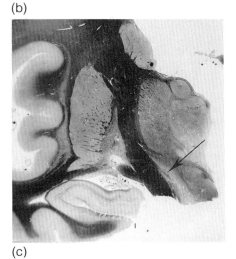

(c)

Fig. 15.5. (a) Normal lentiform nucleus. Coronal section, level P1. Klüver–Barrera stain. (b) Same area, same stain. Woman, aged 58, with multiple system atrophy. Note the pallor and shrinkage of the putamen. The minor degree of pallor and shrinkage in the globus pallidus is mainly due to loss of myelinated axons coming from the putamen. (c) Same area, same stain. Woman, aged 71, with progressive supranuclear palsy. The putamen, and its myelinated bundles, appear normal, but the globus pallidus is grossly atrophic, and the subthalamic nucleus (arrowed) is shrunken and pale.

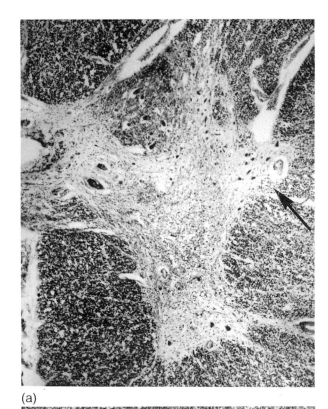

(a)

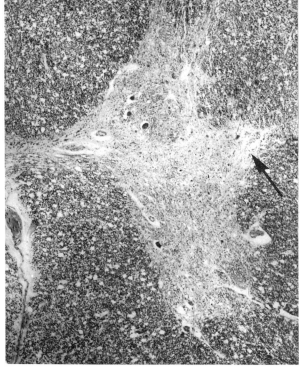

(b)

Fig. 15.6. (a) Anterior and lateral horns, at mid-thoracic level. 20 μm section, Klüver–Barrera stain. There is a normal number of cells in the intermediolateral column (arrowed). (b) Same area and stain, in a man aged 58, suffering from multiple system atrophy, with autonomic failure. Only one nerve cell is visible in the intermediolateral column.

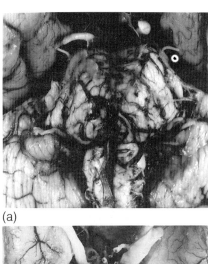

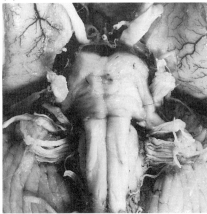

Fig. 15.7. (a) Surface view of normal pons and medulla. (b) Same view, in a case of multiple system atrophy. The leptomeninges have been stripped away. The pons and olives are greatly shrunken. Woman aged 76, suffering from parkinsonism and ataxia.

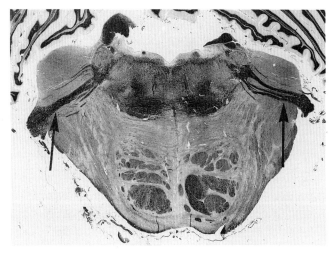

Fig. 15.8. Multiple system atrophy. Section of pons, stained for myelin, showing atrophy of the basis pontis and middle cerebellar peduncles, with normal-looking tegmentum, superior cerebellar peduncles and corticospinal tracts. The entering roots of the trigeminal nerves (arrowed) are conspicuously preserved. Woman of 54 with parkinsonism, ataxia and autonomic failure.

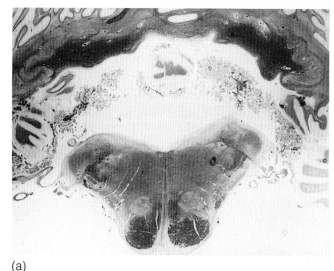

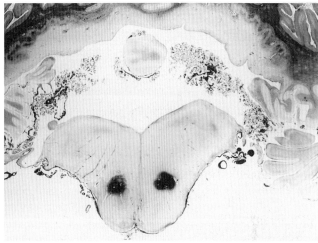

Fig. 15.9. Multiple system atrophy. Sections of upper medulla stained (a) for myelin and (b) for fibrous gliosis (Holzer). The fourth ventricle is enlarged because of cerebellar atrophy. The inferior olives are shrunken and densely gliotic, and there is heavy gliosis of the cerebellar white matter, but not of the superior cerebellar peduncles. Man, aged 62. Main complaint, ataxia. Familial case.

Shy–Drager syndrome, with the added symptom of nocturnal stridor. Although it seems that any combination of lesions may occur, some combinations are more frequent than others; for instance, it would be rare to find atrophy of the putamen, or loss of intermediolateral cells, in the absence of cell loss in the substantia nigra. A curious overlap between paralysis agitans and striatonigral degeneration, which are generally regarded as quite separate diseases, is that in both of them loss of pigmented cells may be associated with loss of intermediolateral cells in the thoracic and sacral cord, and the clinical features of progressive autonomic failure (orthostatic hypotension, loss of sweating, loss of bladder control, sexual impotence in men, etc.). For a fuller discussion see Oppenheimer (1984).

The most striking naked-eye change in striatonigral degeneration is symmetrical shrinkage and brown discoloration of the putamen (Figs 15.4 and 15.5). The caudate nucleus and globus pallidus are little, if at all, involved, except that myelinated bundles of fibres from the putamen, passing through the globus pallidus, are reduced or lost. There is an obvious loss of pigment from the *substantia nigra*, affecting all parts. Histological sections show the usual features of neuronal degeneration — cell loss and gliosis — in the affected structures, but Lewy inclusion bodies are not seen. Although parkinsonism, with or without autonomic failure, may have been the predominant clinical feature, one may expect to find minor changes in other structures at risk.

In any case with clinical features of parkinsonism, part of the following structures should be examined histologically: putamen, thalamus, nucleus basalis (see Fig. 2.25), midbrain, upper pons (for locus ceruleus) and lower medulla (for pigmented cells of the dorsal vagal nuclei). If striatonigral degeneration is suspected, parts of the cerebellar system (see below) should be examined.

Ataxia

In addition to various toxic or metabolic disorders causing ataxia, there is a wide range of degenerative (i.e. unexplained) diseases affecting the cerebellum and its connections. Many attempts to classify these have ended in frustration, or at best in tables with a residuum labelled 'unclassified'. Here, we shall merely draw attention to three main types of cerebellar system disease, it being understood that many cases of progressive ataxia do not fit readily into any of these three. For toxic and other causes of ataxia see p. 370.

Cerebellar cortical (cerebello-olivary) degeneration

This has its onset in middle age, does not appreciably shorten life, and shows autosomal recessive inheritance. The pathological changes consist of loss of Purkinje cells and cells of the inferior olives, with shrinkage and gliosis of their efferent fibre tracts in the cerebellar white matter and inferior cerebellar peduncles. The cerebellar cortex tends to be affected mainly in the superior aspects of the vermis and hemispheres. Cells of the dentate and pontine nuclei, and afferent tracts, appear intact. The associated degeneration of the inferior olives may well be a secondary phenomenon. The affected parts are those which send their axons to affected areas of cerebellar cortex. Retrograde degeneration of olivary cells commonly is seen in cases with focal traumatic, ischaemic or other lesions of the cerebellum.

Pontocerebellar (olivopontocerebellar) atrophy

This is a relatively common type of degeneration causing ataxia. In spite of heroic attempts to sort out the various forms of this condition, it is still not clear whether it is one disease or several. Most cases are sporadic, but some show dominant, others recessive, inheritance. Some, at least, belong to the group referred to above (p.241) under the heading *multiple system atrophy*, and are liable to show major or minor lesions in the putamen, pigmented nuclei and/or intermediolateral columns. Parts of the cerebellar system involved — sometimes severely — are the pontine nuclei and their efferent tracts in the middle cerebellar peduncles, the inferior olives and their efferents in the inferior cerebellar peduncles, and the Purkinje cells (all areas of cerebellar cortex may be affected). In consequence the cerebellar white matter is shrunken and gliotic, leaving an enlarged fourth ventricle (Figs 8.11 and 15.9); and the dentate nuclei, although there is no appreciable cell loss, are gliotic because of loss of incoming Purkinje axons. Additional lesions — not usually severe — may be found in sensory ganglia, anterior horn cells, dorsal (Clarke's) nuclei, and in spinocerebellar and/or corticospinal tracts.

Friedreich's ataxia

Some clinicians apply this term indiscriminately to any form of progressive familial ataxia; but since the 'classical' type of Friedreich's disease is exceptionally constant in its clinical and pathological manifestations, it is better to confine the eponymic title to more or less typical cases.

The onset of the disease is at some time in the first two decades of life, with a peak at ten years of age. The first symptom is ataxia of the lower limbs; later, the arms become ataxic, and finally the bulbar musculature is involved, and the patient's speech becomes dysarthric. A further symptom, not giving rise to much distress, is loss of common sensation, again affecting the legs before the arms, and rarely involving the face. A few patients suffer progressive visual or auditory loss. Outside the nervous system, the *heart* is almost always affected. The ECG is abnormal, the heart enlarges, and heart failure is the commonest immediate cause of death. Cerebrovascular accidents, attributable to emboli from the heart, are fairly common.

The most striking naked-eye changes include atrophy of the posterior roots in the lumbosacral region and cauda equina, and of the spinal cord and brain stem. Histological sections of lower spinal posterior roots and their ganglia show loss of ganglion cells and of their axons. In the cord there is well-marked degeneration of the posterior columns, affecting the gracile more than the cuneate funiculus, and of the pyramidal and spinocerebellar tracts, accounting in large measure for the overall shrinkage of the cord (Figs 15.10 and 15.11). Anterior and lateral horn cells are preserved, but there is severe loss of cells in the dorsal (Clarke's column) nuclei. In the brain stem, cell loss is seen in the accessory cuneate nuclei (the cephalic homologues of the dorsal nuclei) and in the gracile nuclei in long-standing cases — presumably due to transneuronal degeneration. In the cerebellum, the dentate nuclei are nearly always severely affected, and the superior cerebellar peduncles correspondingly shrivelled (Figs 15.12 and 15.13). Purkinje cells and inferior olives are generally unaffected; when they are involved, it is probably as a result of ischaemia sustained in episodes of heart failure. At higher levels, some cases show symmetrical cell loss in the globus pallidus and subthalamic nucleus, and in some there is shrinkage and loss of fibres in the optic nerves and tracts. The usual findings in the heart are of chronic myocarditis, with fibrosis.

Ataxia–telangiectasia

Progressive ataxia, starting in childhood, is not always due to Friedreich's disease. An alternative cause is ataxia–telangiectasia (Louis–Bar syndrome). This is a familial condition, probably with autosomal recessive inheritance. Ataxia develops in early childhood, and is followed by the appearance of telangiectatic areas in the conjunctivae and

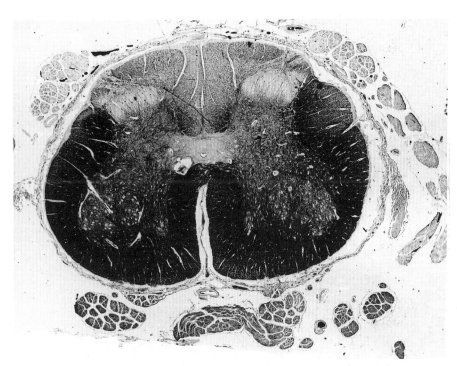

Fig. 15.10. Friedreich's ataxia. Boy, aged 10 years at death. Onset of ataxia at age 6. Lower lumbar cord and surrounding nerve roots, stained for myelin. The posterior roots, and the posterior columns, are pale and shrunken.

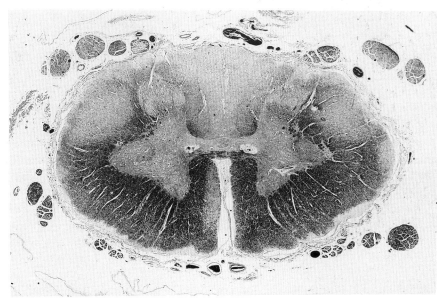

Fig. 15.11. Friedreich's ataxia. Man, aged 31. Onset of ataxia at age 10. 8th cervical segment, stained for myelin. Posterior roots are less affected than in Fig. 15.10. The gracile funiculi are more affected than the cuneate. Both dorsal and ventral spinocerebellar tracts, and the corticospinal tracts, are severely affected. (Note that there is no uncrossed pyramidal tract on the right side of the picture: and that the areas of the crossed pyramidal tract on the right and the uncrossed tract on the left add up to the area of the crossed tract on the left. This type of asymmetry, due to partial decussation at the lower end of the medulla, is very common.)

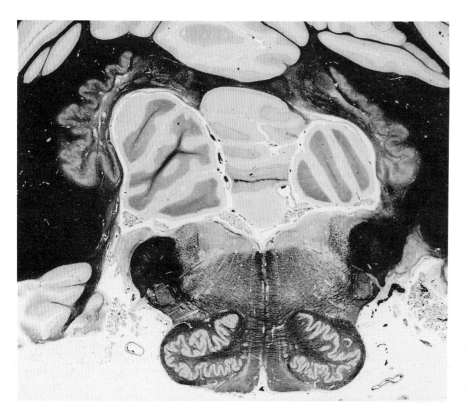

Fig. 15.12. Friedreich's ataxia. Upper medulla and cerebellum, stained for myelin. There is severe shrinkage and pallor of the pyramids, and of the hila of the dentate nuclei. The solitary tracts are almost invisible. In contrast with the cases of multiple system atrophy illustrated above, the cerebellar white matter and inferior olives appear normal.

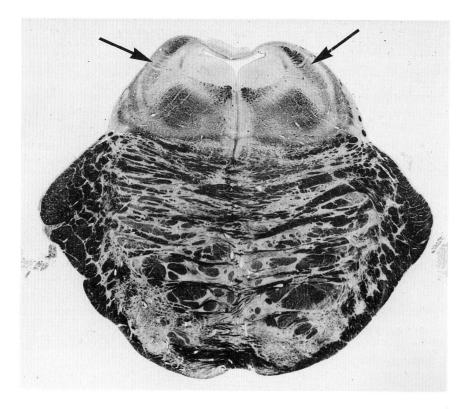

Fig. 15.13. Same case as in Fig. 15.12. The basis pontis and tegmentum appear normal; but there is shrinkage and pallor of the superior cerebellar peduncles (arrowed), due to cell loss in the dentate nuclei.

elsewhere. The victims are unduly prone to respiratory infections. Bodily growth is retarded, and mental deterioration may occur in the later stages of the disease. There is an enhanced liability to develop malignant growths, particularly lymphomas; these, along with recurrent infections, account for most of the patients' deaths. Laboratory findings include low levels of IgA in serum and other fluids, defective responses of blood lymphocytes to phytohaemagglutinin and, in many cases, lymphopenia. Post mortem findings include hypoplasia, or even absence, of the thymus, general reduction of lymphoid tissue, hypoplastic gonads and widespread infiltration of viscera by large cells with bizarre nuclei. The telangiectases consist of dilated, tortuous venules. In the CNS, there is atrophy of the cerebellar cortex, with extensive loss of both Purkinje and granule cells, and retrograde cell loss in the inferior olives. Some cases show degeneration of the posterior columns, especially of the gracile funiculus. Posterior root ganglia show a deficiency of satellite cells, and of the larger ganglion cells; and in some cases there is drop-out of motor neurons, with consequent atrophy of muscles.

Correlation of clinical and anatomical changes

There is at present no body of knowledge connecting particular types of ataxic disturbance with lesions in particular components of the cerebellar system. The same can be said of the state of knowledge connecting particular kinds of abnormal movement, such as chorea or athetosis, with focal lesions in the basal ganglia. An exception is the frequent, but not invariable, association of *hemiballism* with lesions of a *subthalamic nucleus*.

Huntington's chorea

This is the best-known example of a dominantly-transmitted neuronal degeneration. It presents, usually during the third to fifth decades of life, with a combination of movement disorders and mental disturbances. Of these two, either may precede the other; occasionally, one does not occur at all. The movement disorder progresses from a slightly fidgety behaviour to frank chorea. The mental disorders are variable, and include dementia and schizophrenia. Some patients spend years in a psychiatric hospital before neurological signs develop. Since the threat posed by the disease is usually known to the whole family before it shows itself, it is not surprising that anxiety and depression are listed among the mental disturbances suffered by patients; and as it is common knowledge that there is no effective treatment, it is not surprising that many sufferers fail to consult a doctor. An uncommon variant of the disease, with onset in the second decade, is characterized by muscular rigidity rather than chorea, with epilepsy as an additional feature.

The characteristic naked-eye change is a severe sym-

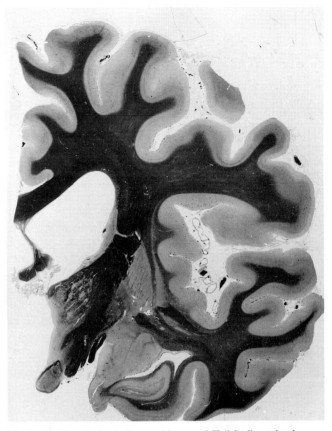

Fig. 15.14. Huntington's disease. Man, aged 52. Myelin-stained section at level A1. The dilatation of the anterior horn of the lateral ventricle is due mainly to shrinkage of the caudate nucleus, and to a lesser extent of the lentiform nucleus. Note the normal size of the inferior (temporal) horn of the lateral ventricle.

metrical shrinkage of the *corpus striatum* (lentiform and caudate nuclei), with compensatory dilatation of the anterior horns of the lateral ventricles (Figs 8.9 and 15.14). A similar striatal atrophy occurs in some cases of Pick's disease, but in these there is a concomitant atrophy of the temporal lobes (Figs 8.10 and 15.15). There may also be a slight generalized thinning of the cortical ribbon. Under the low power of the microscope, one finds a devastating loss of small neurons in the caudate nucleus and putamen, with relative sparing of the large cells, and loss of the myelinated fibre bundles passing through the pallidum. The atrophied regions are densely gliotic. Apart from the corpus striatum, cell loss of varying severity may be found in the cerebral cortex, thalamus, hypothalamus, substantia nigra, cerebellar cortex, dentate nuclei, olives, and other brain stem nuclei. Further details, including electron microscopic and neurochemical abnormalities, are given by Tomlinson & Corsellis (1984).

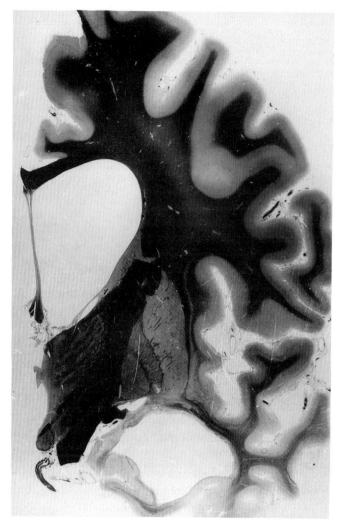

Fig. 15.15. Pick's disease. Man, aged 57. As in Fig. 15.14, the caudate nucleus is atrophic: the obvious difference lies in the extreme atrophy of the temporal lobe in this case, with compensatory dilatation of the inferior horn of the lateral ventricle.

Progressive supranuclear palsy

This rare condition was first reported by Steele, Richardson and Olszewski in 1964. The onset is in the fifth to seventh decades of life, and men are twice as often affected as women. The disease is not familial. Clinical disturbances include paralysis of upward gaze, dysarthria, and muscular rigidity, which is most marked in the muscles of the neck. The most striking naked-eye change is a symmetrical atrophy of the globus pallidus and subthalamic nucleus (Fig. 15.5c). Microscopically, there is cell loss and gliosis in these nuclei, and in the red nuclei, substantia nigra, tectum of the upper brain stem, and the dentate nuclei of the cerebellum. A further peculiarity is the presence of neurofibrillary tangles in neurons in many areas, including some where cell loss is

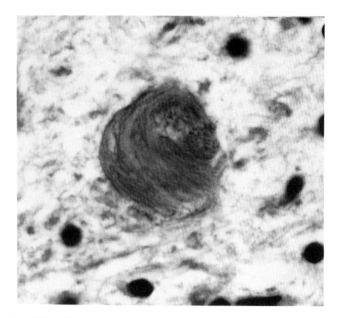

Fig. 15.16. Progressive supranuclear palsy. Same case as in Fig. 15.3c. Neurofibrillary tangle in brain stem. H&E, ×1200.

not apparent (Fig. 15.16). These tangles differ from those of Alzheimer's disease, Down's syndrome, the parkinsonism–dementia of Guam and post-encephalitic parkinsonism, which are very similar to each other, in their electron microscopic features (for references, see Oppenheimer 1984).

Dentato–rubro–pallido–luysian atrophy (DRPLA)

Another rare disease, reported mainly but not exclusively from Japan, is dentato-rubro-pallido-luysian atrophy (DRPLA). In this condition (or group of conditions) the clinical features are very variable, even when the pathological findings are closely similar. The main disturbances consist of involuntary movements, variously described as ataxic, athetotic, choreic, ballistic or myoclonic. The condition is reviewed by Iizuka *et al.* (1984).

Peroneal muscular atrophy (Charcot–Marie–Tooth disease)

This condition is generally classed as a progressive neuropathy, along with a number of other familial neuromuscular disorders. It does not appear to differ in any important respect from the CNS degenerations discussed above. There is loss of anterior horn cells and their axons, as in motor neuron disease, and of sensory ganglion cells and their processes, similar to that occurring in Friedreich's ataxia. In practice, the neuropathologist has the task of examining both the central and the peripheral nervous systems.

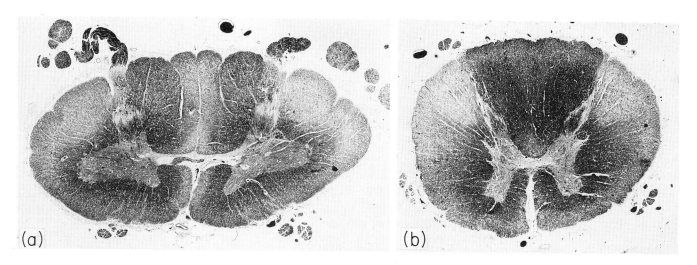

Fig. 15.17. Strümpell's disease (familial spastic paraplegis). Man aged 67. Onset of weakness in legs during adolescence: little change since then. (a) Section of cervical cord, stained for myelin, showing diffuse pallor in the lateral white columns, and specific fibre loss in the crossed and uncrossed pyramidal tracts and gracile funiculi. (b) Thoracic cord from the same case. Degeneration of the crossed pyramidal tracts is more marked, but the posterior columns at this level appear intact.

Doubtfully degenerative conditions

There are at least two conditions generally classed as progressive degenerations, probably incorrectly. One is Strümpell's *familial spastic paraplegia*. This has its onset in the second decade of life, but normally remains static after bodily growth ceases. It does not shorten life. In most cases, paraparesis is a fairer description than paraplegia. The lesions are found in the spinal cord. In the cervical region, the posterior columns and spinocerebellar tracts are thinned; in the lumbosacral segments the pyramidal tracts are affected (Fig. 15.17). The other doubtful degeneration is the Brown–Vialetto–van Laere disease (*pontobulbar palsy with deaf-ness*). The condition is often familial. It presents at any age, but most commonly in early life. The onset is sudden, with total hearing loss developing over a period of a few hours, accompanied or followed by paralysis of some or most of the muscles supplied by the lower cranial nerves. After this, the patient's condition may remain static for some years, or for the rest of her life (most of the patients are female); or another episode of rapid deterioration may follow. This is not the pattern of relentless progression seen in most cases of primary neuronal degeneration. Histological features include loss of cells from the lower cranial motor nuclei, and of acoustic nerve fibres, with degeneration of the ventral cochlear nuclei (Fig. 15.18).

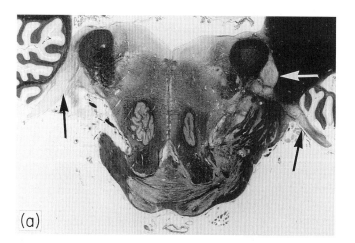
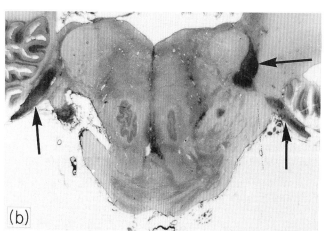

Fig. 15.18. Pontobulbar palsy with deafness. Boy aged 23 months. Sections of the junction of pons and medulla, stained (a) for myelin and (b) for fibroglia. The cut is slightly asymmetrical, with a higher level on the right side of the picture. Severe loss of myelin is seen in both acoustic nerves and ventral cochlear nuclei (arrowed), with corresponding gliosis.

Table 15.2. Sites of selective cell loss in various conditions

Site	'Degenerative'	Metabolic, etc.	Toxic
Hippocampus		Hypoxia Epilepsy	
Sensory, visual and auditory cortex			Organic mercury (p.313)
Motor cortex (Betz cells)	MND FA		
Striatum	Hunt MSA CJD	Wilson's disease (p.293) Hepatic failure (p.302)	Methyl alcohol (p.313) Manganese (p.313)
Pallidum	DRPLA PSP FA	Hallervorden—Spatz disease (p.296)	Manganese (p.313)
Subthalamic nuclei	DRPLA PSP FA	Wilson's disease (p.293)	Manganese (p.313)
Substantia nigra	PA MSA		MPTP (p.314)
Locus ceruleus	MSA PA		
Pontine nuclei	MSA		
Inferior olives	MSA CCD Hunt		clioquinol (p.311)
V, VII and XII motor nuclei	MND PBP		
Dorsal nucleus X	MSA PA		
Dentate nuclei	FA PSP DRPLA	Wilson's disease (p.293)	
Purkinje cells	MSA CCD AT	Hypoxia Epilepsy Carcinoma	Ethyl alcohol (p.309) Methyl alcohol (p.313)
Cerebellar granule cells	CJD AT		Ethyl alcohol (p.309) Methyl alcohol (p.313) Organic mercury (p.313)
Spinal cord Motor cells	MND, WHD CMTD, CJD	Poliomyelitis	
Autonomic (intermedio-lateral)	MSA PA		
Dorsal (Clarke's column) nuclei	FA		
Sensory ganglia	FA CMTD	Avitaminoses Tabes dorsalis Carcinoma Hereditary sensory neuropathy	

AT   Ataxia—telangiectasia (p.245)
CCD   Cerebellar cortical degeneration (p.244)
CJD   Creutzfeldt—Jakob disease (p.274)
CMTD   Charcot—Marie—Tooth disease (p.248)
DRPLA   Dentato-rubro-pallido-luysian atrophy (p.248)
FA   Friedreich's ataxia (p.244)
Hunt   Huntington's disease (p.247)
MND   Motor neuron disease (p.236)
MSA   Multiple system atrophy (pp.241, 244)
PA   Paralysis agitans (Parkinson's disease) (p.240)
PBP   Pontobulbar palsy (p.249)
PSP   Progressive supranuclear palsy (p.248)
WHD   Werdnig—Hoffmann disease (p.239)

'Abiotrophy'

The idea that the neuronal degenerations represent a premature ageing of nervous tissue ('abiotrophy'), proposed by Gowers in 1902, is still current. It would, in any case, be difficult to disprove. It is also difficult to see how this idea, even if true, helps with our understanding of these diseases. Certain changes do undoubtedly take place in the CNS with advancing years. One such, which is easily confirmed by cell counting, is a tendency to thinning-out of the Purkinje cells in the cerebellum. They are also thinned out in several of the diseases discussed above; but in other conditions they survive, while other cell types disappear. It is often stated in print that after the age of 15 (or perhaps 25, or 35) the brain loses cells at the rate of 1000 (or 30 000, or 100 000) a day.

These statements, we believe, belong to the realm of scientific journalism rather than of scientific research.

Sites of selective cell loss in various 'degenerative', toxic and metabolic diseases are shown in Table 15.2.

Further reading

Iizuka R, Hirayama K, Maebara K. 1984. Dentato-rubro-pallido-luysian atrophy. *J Neurol Neurosurg Psychiat* **47**, 1288–98.

Oppenheimer DR. 1984. Diseases of the basal ganglia, cerebellum and motor neurons. In Adams JH, Corsellis JAN, Duchen LW (Eds) *Greenfield's Neuropathology*, 4th edn. Edward Arnold, London, Chapter 15.

Tomlinson BE, Corsellis JAN. 1984. Ageing and the dementias. In Adams JH, Corsellis JAN, Duchen LW (Eds) *Greenfield's Neuropathology*, 4th edn. Edward Arnold, London, Chapter 20.

Chapter 16
Malformations of the Central Nervous System

Causes of malformations

Knowledge of the causes of CNS malformations is at present rather sketchy. There has been a good deal of experimental work on teratogenesis in animals, and a little is known about factors affecting human embryos. These include genetic traits, intoxications, nutritional defects, maternal infections and irradiation. In this chapter we shall confine ourselves to the description of some of the commoner developmental anomalies. The conditions mentioned here are without doubt heterogeneous, since we know of no sure means of distinguishing between malformations due to genetic or 'idiopathic' causes and those due to toxic or metabolic disturbances. Further information on these matters is to be found in Keeling (1987) and Larroche (1984).

Malformations of the spinal cord

The most commonly encountered of these are associated with *spina bifida*, i.e. failure of the spines and laminae of certain vertebrae to fuse in the midline, leaving a gap through which the spinal meninges may protrude. The lumbar vertebrae are the ones most often affected. In a *meningocele* the dura and arachnoid are ballooned backwards, and lie immediately beneath a layer of thinned-out skin; underneath, there is a sac containing CSF and nerve roots. In a *meningomyelocele* part of the spinal cord is included, and nerve roots are found stuck to the walls of the sac. The cord itself is usually malformed in this region. Muscles of the lower limbs, normally supplied by the affected nerve roots, are more or less denervated, wasted and useless. The sac is present at birth. If it is not treated

surgically, the thin overlying skin is apt to become ulcerated, and infection sets in. Purulent meningitis is a common, and commonly fatal, outcome. At post mortem a sample of the contained fluid should be withdrawn for bacteriological examination. In *spina bifida occulta* there is a less capacious sac, with similar involvement of nerve roots, but no obvious protrusion on the surface. In some cases there is a dimple in the skin over the affected vertebra, marking the position of a dermal track, which leads to the spinal meninges. In all cases of spina bifida, it is best to take the entire vertebral column at post mortem. If this is not done, a careful dissection of the region should be carried out when the spinal cord is removed.

Other malformations, sometimes but not always associated with a spina bifida, are *diastematomyelia*, in which the left and right sides of the cord are separated by a space, or by a layer of connective tissue, and *diplomyelia*, in which two more or less complete cords lie side by side. Some degree of *hydromyelia* (expanded central canal) is a common finding in all these types of malformation.

Malformations of the brain stem and cerebellum

Chiari malformations, types 1 and 2

In Chiari's type 1 malformation there is elongation of one or both cerebellar tonsils, which dangle through the foramen magnum into the upper part of the spinal canal (Fig. 16.1). This deformity may cause no symptoms until, for one reason or another, intracranial pressure is increased. Since the capacity of the cisterna magna is reduced, the risk of foraminal herniation, with impaction, is enhanced. The patient may, for example, die suddenly in the course of an

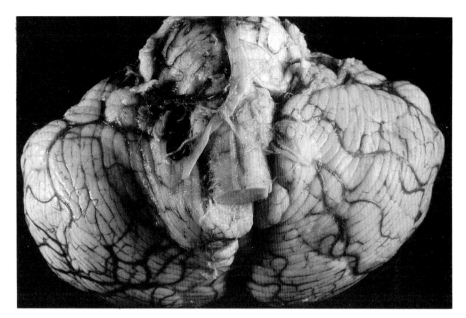

Fig. 16.1. Chiari malformation, type 1. Incidental finding in a man aged 62. No other malformations present. The lower end of the medulla has been cut away to display the elongated right cerebellar tonsil (on the left of the picture).

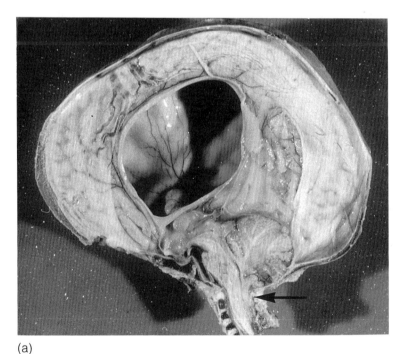

(a)

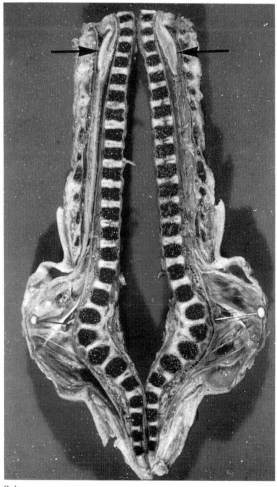

(b)

Fig. 16.2. Chiari malformation, type 2. The brain and spinal column have been removed by the method described on p.8. Infant, aged 4 months, with congenital hydrocephalus and meningomyelocele. (a) A midline cut shows an enormous lateral ventricle, a paper-thin falx cerebri, and a malformed hindbrain, with the cerebellar tonsils (arrowed) extending far down into the spinal canal, accompanied by a downward extension of the fourth ventricle. (b) A midline cut shows a misshapen spinal column, with a lumbar kyphus instead of lordosis, and deficient lumbar and sacral bony arches. Above (arrowed), the downward extension of the medulla oblongata appears to be folded over the spinal cord. Below, the roots of the cauda equina are attached to the walls of a large meningocele.

acute feverish illness. In a case of this kind examined in our department, the patient had suffered a series of episodes, with signs and symptoms referable to the lower brain stem, which were very reasonably ascribed to MS.

Chiari's type 2 malformation (commonly referred to as the *Arnold–Chiari malformation*) is unfortunately far commoner, and is the commonest cause of congenital hydrocephalus. The principal features of this condition are as follows (see Figs 16.2 and 16.3):

1 The vault of the skull varies in size from large to enormous. The fontanelles are very wide, and do not close. The posterior fossa is small and shallow.

2 Enlargement of the skull is caused by, and corresponds with, enlargement of the lateral and third ventricles. The aqueduct is usually patent, but the fourth ventricle is not enlarged.

3 The outer surfaces of the cerebral hemispheres are flattened, with virtual obliteration of the cerebral sulci and disappearance of the subarachnoid space. The cortex and underlying white matter are thinned; in a severe case, the distance between the pia and lateral ventricle may be less than a centimetre throughout.

4 The tentorium and falx cerebri are paper-thin, and often fenestrated.

5 The anatomy of the thalamus, basal ganglia and upper brain stem is more or less normal.

6 The cerebellum, lower brain stem and fourth ventricle are grossly deformed. The cerebellar tonsils are prolonged for a distance of 10 cm or so into the spinal canal, and are accompanied by an irregularly folded medulla oblongata and an elongated fourth ventricle.

7 There is a lumbar spina bifida, with a protruding meningomyelocele. The lower end of the spinal cord is splayed open, and its emergent nerve roots are embedded in the wall of the sac.

8 Lower limb muscles supplied by these nerve roots show varying degrees of denervation atrophy.

One or more of these features may be lacking in individual cases. How many of them are causally linked, and whether they can all be traced to a single mishap in early development, are still subjects of debate, which we shall not attempt to pursue here.

To display the features of either type of Chiari malformation, one should avoid the conventional method of removing the brain at post mortem, as this entails cutting through the herniated cerebellar tonsils when the brain stem is separated from the spinal cord. For the type 2 malformation, the technique described on p.8 gives a good display (see Figs 16.2 and 16.3). Unless it is intended to carry out a detailed study of the disordered brain stem anatomy, the whole specimen can be divided in the midline, and mounted as a museum specimen. For the type 1 malformation, a transverse cut can be made through the upper cervical cord from behind, before extracting the

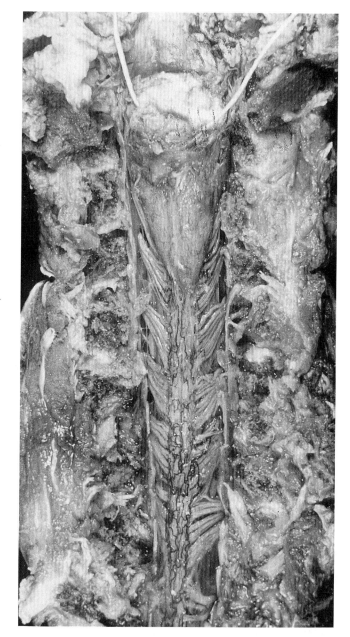

Fig. 16.3. View from behind of a cord with the Chiari type 2 malformation. As in the last example, the medulla extends far down into the spinal canal. The posterior spinal nerve roots, which normally slope downward from the cord, here slope upward, and undergo a sharp bend downward at the points where they penetrate the dura. The patient was a boy aged 18 years, with spina bifida and a lumbar meningomyelocele. He was mentally normal. He died of a purulent meningitis.

brain from the skull (the diagnosis has often been made radiologically before death).

Cerebellar hypoplasia

The cerebellum as a whole may be abnormally small, or parts of it may be hypoplastic, or even missing. When one cerebellar hemisphere is hypoplastic, the inferior olive and pontine nuclei on the opposite side also tend to be under-developed. In *pontoneocerebellar hypoplasia* the lateral lobes of the cerebellum, pontine nuclei and middle cerebellar peduncles are reduced in size (Fig. 16.4), whereas the vermis and flocculi are of more or less normal size. In other cases, the lateral lobes may be normal, while the vermis is hypoplastic or absent. In the *Dandy–Walker malformation* the vermis is partially or completely replaced by a large ependyma-lined cyst (Fig. 16.5); and there is often an associated hydrocephalus, and agenesis of the corpus callosum.

Disorderly development of patches of cerebellar cortex gives rise to a condition variously known as *pachygyria* or *microgyria* (the same two terms are used for two quite distinct types of malformation of cerebral cortex). In the cerebellar condition, the cellular elements — Purkinje cells, granule cells and the rest — in a number of adjacent folia are jumbled up, and divisions between folia are lost. The condition is said to be rare, but tiny areas of similar cellular

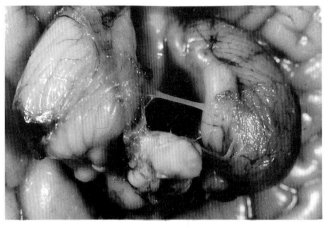

Fig. 16.5. Dandy–Walker malformation in a week-old infant with patent ductus arteriosus. The cerebellar vermis is replaced by a large cavity.

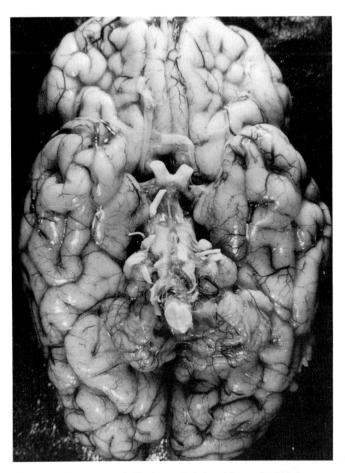

Fig. 16.4. Pontoneocerebellar hypoplasia in a 14-month-old infant. Total brain weight 658 g; hindbrain alone, 21g. Cerebrum, pyramidal tracts and cerebellar vermis more or less normal. Pontine nuclei, middle cerebellar peduncles and hemispheres tiny. Incomplete cell loss in dentate nuclei and olives.

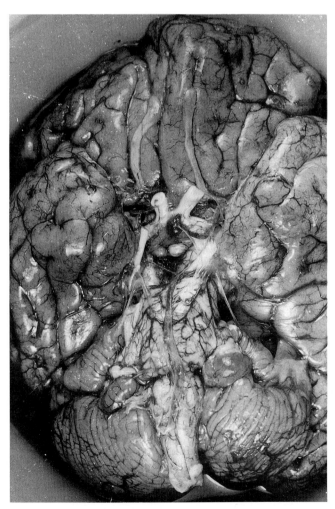

Fig. 16.6. Cerebrocerebellar degeneration in a woman aged 62. Left spastic hemiparesis, epilepsy and mental defect since infancy. Cause not known. Right cerebral hemisphere shrunken: areas of ulegyria. Shrinkage and scarring of right side of brain stem and left cerebellar hemisphere.

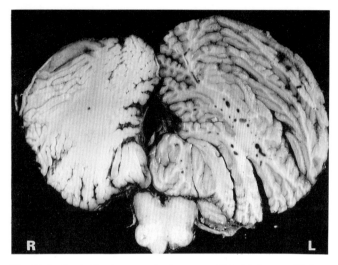

Fig. 16.7. Cerebellar degeneration in a man of 25 with Sturge–Weber disease (see p.262) affecting mainly the left cerebral hemisphere. Epilepsy, mental defect and right hemiplegia from infancy. Left hemispherectomy at age 16, with good results. Deterioration for 1 year before death, due to intracranial bleeding. Post mortem: superficial haemosiderosis, and gross atrophy of left side of brain stem and right side of cerebellum, with extensive loss of cortical neurons and dense gliosis. Dilated veins in the left cerebellar hemisphere are part of the original disease.

disorder are quite commonly seen in the neighbourhood of the foramina of Luschka as incidental findings. Less commonly, areas of ectopic cortical cells are found within the cerebellar white matter.

In *cerebrocerebellar (crossed cerebellar) atrophy* smallness of one cerebellar hemisphere is associated with smallness of the opposite cerebral hemisphere (Figs 16.6 and 16.7). The primary lesion in such cases, which may be one of a great

variety of prenatal or postnatal mishaps, is to be found in the cerebrum. The affected cerebellar hemisphere may be histologically more or less normal. More often, there is loss of cells and glial scarring, which in many cases can be plausibly attributed to the effects of repeated epileptic attacks.

Malformations of the cerebral hemispheres

In this, as in the preceding sections, we wish to make it clear that most of the italicized words/headings are not the names of diseases, but merely labels attached, for convenience, to certain naked-eye and microscopic appearances. The diseases causing them remain for the most part unknown. We hope, and indeed expect, that a more satisfactory nomenclature will emerge in the course of the next ten or twenty years. An analogous process has taken place in the naming of the lipidoses. At first they were known by the names of their original describers. Next, they were subdivided according to their clinical and histological characteristics. Now, they are generally referred to in terms of missing enzymes (Table 19.1).

Microencephaly and megalencephaly

Microencephaly and megalencephaly do not seem to us to be very useful terms. The weights of normally-functioning brains vary within wide limits; they may even weigh less than 1 kg or more than 2 kg without causing trouble. Very large and very small brains often show abnormalities, gross or histological, apart from size; and it is these abnormalities which determine the diagnosis.

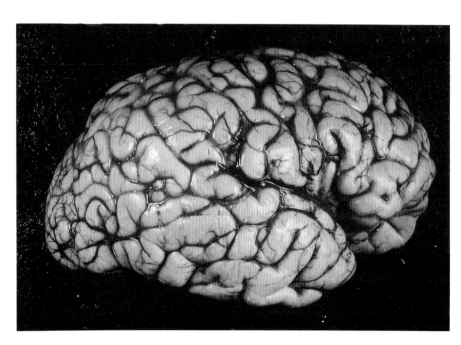

Fig. 16.8. Down's syndrome. Man, aged 43. The brain is generally small (weight 1035 g) and short from back to front. The superior temporal gyrus is relatively narrow.

Down's syndrome

In Down's syndrome (Mongolism) the brain is usually of below average size, with relative smallness of the hind-brain. The cerebrum appears short from front to back, with a small parietal lobe; and there is often a hypoplasia of the superior temporal gyri (Fig. 16.8). Various histological abnormalities have been described, but none peculiar to Down's syndrome, with the possible exception of a minor malformation of the thoracic cord, described by Benda (1947), consisting of fusion across the midline of the dorsal (Clarke's) nuclei. It has also been observed that patients reaching middle age tend to show numerous cortical plaques and neurofibrillary tangles, resembling those seen in Alzheimer's disease, in cortical nerve cells.

Other trisomies

Down's syndrome is usually associated with trisomy 21. There is also a wide range of malformations associated with trisomy of the 13−15 group. The simplest of these is *ar-rhinencephaly*, i.e. absence of the olfactory parts of the

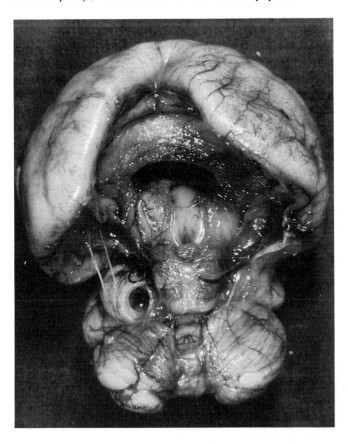

Fig. 16.9. Holoprosencephaly. Brain of neonate, seen from behind. There is a single forebrain cavity, covered partly with a rudimentary cortex and partly with a thin membrane. Here the membrane has been torn, giving an indecent exposure of the thalamus and basal ganglia, which have a relatively normal structure.

forebrain. This may be combined with the rather common major malformation of *holoprosencephaly*. In this, the hemispheres are not separated, and there is a single large cavity replacing the lateral ventricles (Fig. 16.9). The skull and facial bones are malformed, and in some cases there is *cyclopia*, i.e. a single, malformed, centrally-placed eye. Trisomy 18 is found in some cases of this type. For a fuller discussion see Laurence (1987).

Disorders of cell migration

In fetal life these are held responsible for two types of malformation: *heterotopias* and *lissencephaly* (Fig. 16.10). In the former, heterotopic (or ectopic) masses of grey matter are found in unexpected places, such as the centrum ovale, or the cerebellar white matter. In the latter, there seems to be a generalized failure of outward migration of cells from the mantle layer to the cerebral cortex. As a result of this, the normal pattern of cortical gyri and sulci, and the normal six-layered cortex, fail to develop. Externally, the hemispheres show either a grossly simplified convolutional pattern, with a few broad gyri (*pachygyria*), or a lack of sulci other than a shallow depression representing the lateral fissure (*agyria, lissencephaly*). On slicing, the hemispheres are separate, with normally-placed, but dilated, lateral and third ventricles; the centrum ovale, though normally myelinated, is much reduced in bulk; and outside this is a layer, 2 cm or so thick, of grey matter in which the cells, though showing lamination of a kind, are not readily equated with the six layers of normal cortex. Passing through the abnormal cortex are radial bundles of myelinated fibres. Associated abnormalities in the CNS include defective development of the corpus callosum, heterotopic grey matter in the cerebellum, and malformations of the inferior olives. Malformations may also be present in viscera such as heart and kidneys. Some cases are familial.

Agenesis of the corpus callosum

Partial or total absence of the corpus callosum may be part of a complex of cerebral anomalies, or it may occur in isolation, in the absence of clinically-observed defects (Fig. 16.11). The pattern of sulci on the medial aspects of the hemispheres is commonly abnormal, lacking a cingulate sulcus.

Schizencephaly

In this condition there is a cleft, extending from the lateral surface of one hemisphere (or more commonly both) to the ependyma of the lateral ventricle (Fig. 16.12). The lips of the cleft may be apposed, or separated by a subarachnoid space. The cortex lining the cleft is commonly malformed, and there may be heterotopic masses of grey matter. In

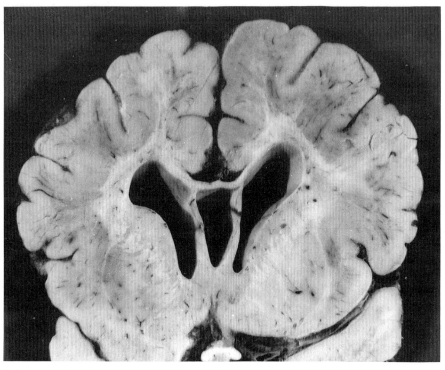

(a)

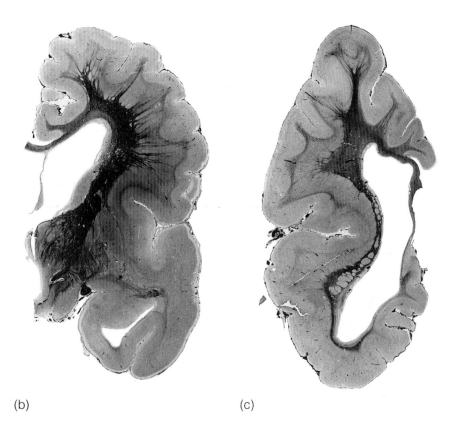

(b)   (c)

Fig. 16.10. Pachygyria (lissencephaly) in a 5-month-old girl with multiple congenital defects. (a) Coronal slice at the level of the optic chiasm, showing a somewhat simplified convolutional pattern, with an abnormally wide cortical ribbon and a corresponding paucity of central white matter. The corpus callosum is present, but thin. The lateral ventricles are large, and there is a conspicuous cavum septi pellucidi. (b) A myelin-stained section at anterior thalamic level shows relatively normal thalamus and corpus striatum, and normal myelination of the deeper white matter. Between this and the cortex proper there is a zone within which bundles of myelinated fibres are mixed with cells which have failed to migrate outward. Sulci between convolutions are very shallow. (c) Posteriorly, ectopic islands of grey matter lie in the periventricular white matter.

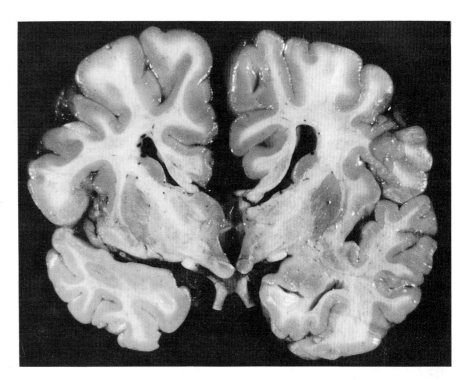

Fig. 16.11. Agenesis of the corpus callosum in a 2-year-old child with polymicrogyria and aqueduct stenosis.

some cases the Rolandic cortex and corticospinal tracts are lacking. These clefts are distinguished from so-called *poren-cephalic cysts* by the fact that there is no sign of tissue destruction during the prenatal or perinatal periods.

Encephaloceles

These are protrusions of cerebral tissue through defects in the cranium. They occur most commonly through an occipital defect, or, more rarely, through a gap between the frontal

and ethmoid bones (anterior meningocele or encephalo-meningocele). The latter condition is said to be rare in Europe, but relatively common in South East Asia. Posterior encephaloceles can become very large, and may contain an extension of the posterior horn of the lateral ventricle.

Cavum septi pellucidi

This, on its own, barely qualifies as a malformation, though it may be combined with more serious deformities, as in

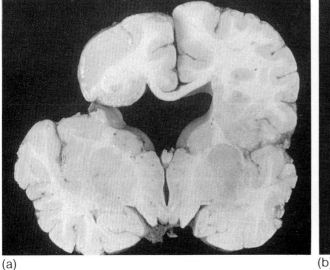

(a)

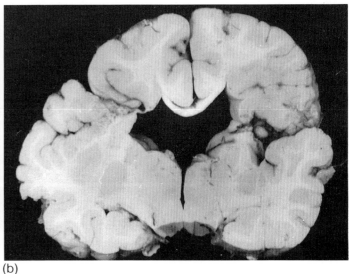

(b)

Fig. 16.12. Schizencephaly in a girl aged 6 years, described as 'spastic'. Coronal slices at levels A1 (a) and P1 (b) show bilateral clefts, extending from the pial surface to the ependyma of the lateral ventricles. There are foci of ectopic grey matter in the centrum ovale on both sides, and scattered areas of malformed cortex (polymicrogyria).

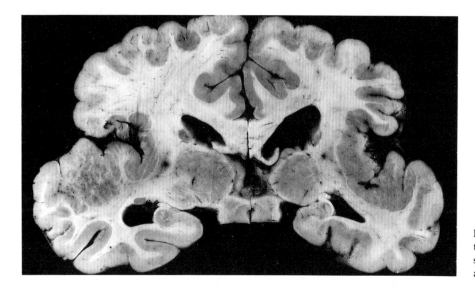

Fig. 16.13. Polymicrogyria, affecting mainly the superior temporal gyri and insulae on both sides, in a mentally defective 'spastic' youth aged 16.

Fig. 16.10. It is normally present in fetal life, and may persist. A cavum septi is also said to be a characteristic acquired feature in the brains of professional boxers.

Polymicrogyria

This is a condition affecting large or small, generally asymmetrical, areas of cerebral cortex. The pathogenesis is still uncertain, but there is often a history suggesting a toxic, infective or hypoxic episode occurring at some time before the sixth month of fetal life. The external appearance has been compared to the surface of a cauliflower or of a peeled chestnut. Slicing (Figs 16.12 and 16.13) shows a much-wrinkled cortical ribbon, with pia mater covering multiple tiny wrinkles, not dipping between them. Within the ribbon, it is usually possible to distinguish four layers, of which the first (outer) and third are sparsely populated, while the second and fourth are richly supplied with neurons. A detailed description, with discussion of the theoretical aspects of the condition, is given by Larroche (1984). The condition is not uncommon. Mental defect and epilepsy are common in affected patients; but small lesions may be clinically silent.

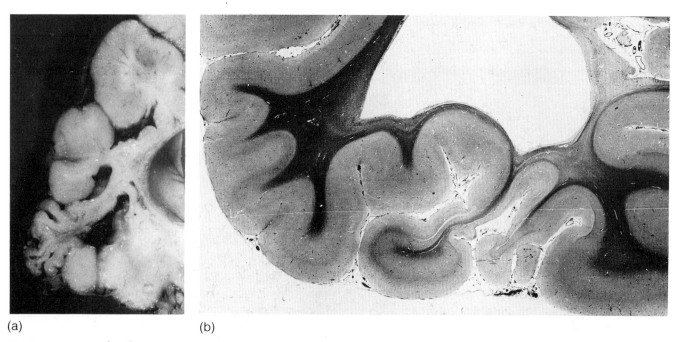

(a)   (b)

Fig. 16.14. Ulegyria. Operation specimen from the right occipital lobe of a mentally defective, blind, epileptic man aged 35. (a) Macroscopic view of sliced specimen, showing various degrees of cortical scarring; (b) myelin-stained section, showing areas of normal cortex on each side, with ulegyric cortex between, and secondary degeneration in the underlying white matter.

Ulegyria

This is a type of cortical scarring dating from early life. It is not, as is sometimes suggested, confined to lesions acquired before or at the time of birth; it has been seen, for instance, in material removed in the operation of hemispherectomy for epilepsy consequent upon infantile hemiplegia, when the original vascular mishap occurred at the age of 12 months or more. On the surface of the hemisphere there may be little sign of damage. On section, the affected gyri show cell loss, shrinkage and gliosis in the depths of sulci, whereas the crowns of the gyri appear intact (Fig. 16.14). The condition is discussed on pp.106 and 325.

Anencephaly

This is said to be the commonest fetal malformation of the head. The skull is grossly abnormal, and the brain is replaced by a mass of vascular connective tissue. The causes are not known. *Hydranencephaly*, in spite of the name, is a totally different condition, attributed to perinatal cerebral ischaemia. It is discussed by Larroche (1984).

General recommendation

In any case of CNS malformation, the pathologist should search the clinical notes for clues to the aetiology: in particular, he should look for records of maternal infections (such as rubella), intoxications, or episodes of hypoxia or hypotension.

Vascular malformations

These are classified according to the predominant structural component. The commonest and least clinically important are *capillary telangiectases*, which may be found incidentally at post mortem, particularly in the pons or cerebral cortex and subjacent white matter. These are usually solitary lesions composed of a cluster of dilated, congested capillary channels. They rarely bleed spontaneously.

Cavernous angiomas

These occur at similar sites, are usually solitary but occasionally multiple, and are rather larger than capillary telangiectases, measuring up to 4 cm across. They appear dark red, and may show evidence of having bled. They are composed of thin-walled, blood-filled spaces of variable size, some very large in comparison with the thinness of their walls. The walls contain a single endothelial layer and a thin rim of collagen. Gliotic brain parenchyma lies between these blood-filled spaces, and may contain haemosiderin-laden macrophages, testifying to former leakage of red blood cells. Occasionally cavernous angiomas give rise to haemorrhage, and those in or close to the cerebral cortex may be associated with epilepsy.

Arteriovenous malformations

These types of vascular malformation are of greatest clinical importance (Figs 16.15 and 16.16). They may give rise to

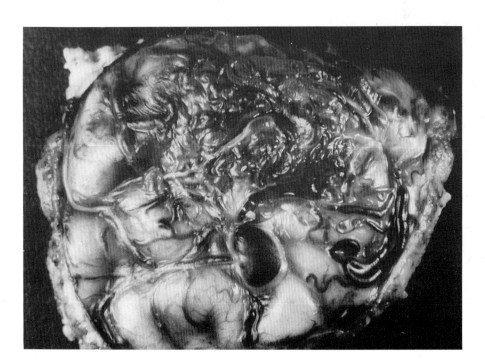

Fig. 16.15. Arteriovenous malformation. Operation specimen from the right frontal lobe of a boy aged 12, who presented one month earlier with an epileptic fit.

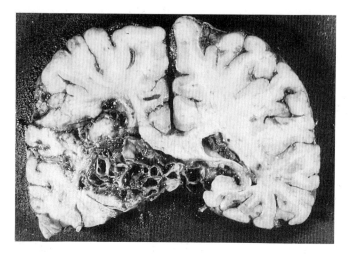

Fig. 16.16. Arteriovenous malformation. Coronal slice, at level P3, from a 70-year-old woman with a 43-year history of uncontrollable epilepsy. There is a massive tangle of blood vessels in the left cerebral hemisphere.

symptoms (i) by bleeding, (ii) by provoking epileptic attacks, (iii) by enlarging and so acting as compressing lesions, or (iv) by diverting blood from neighbouring structures, which are thereby rendered ischaemic. In the brain they are commonest in the cerebrum, and are usually related to a leptomeningeal or ependymal surface. They form a more or less circumscribed tangle of vessels, some of which, on microscopic examination, are found to be arteries, and others veins. In the arteries there is frequently reduplication of elastic tissue and irregularity in width of the media. Aneurysmal dilatation, with gross thinning of the wall, may be seen. The veins show collagenous thickening of their walls, with some admixed smooth muscle. The veins are particularly prominent in spinal arteriovenous malformations, which are discussed on p.31.

Sturge–Weber disease (encephalofacial angiomatosis)

In this rare condition there is an extensive, diffuse capillary and venous malformation in the leptomeninges of one cerebral hemisphere, and an associated cutaneous 'port wine' naevus in the ipsilateral trigeminal distribution. Over the affected cerebral hemisphere the leptomeninges are thickened and contain a multitude of fine-calibre blood vessels. The underlying cortex is frequently atrophic and contains numerous calcified fine vessels. The parenchyma is usually gliotic, with variable neuronal loss.

There is an interesting twilight zone in which the category of congenital (sometimes hereditary) malformations merges into that of neoplasia. Two of the better-known conditions in this area are the syndromes of Lindau and Bourneville.

Lindau's syndrome

This comprises haemangioblastoma of the cerebellum (more rarely of the cord), haemangioblastoma of the retina (von Hippel's disease), a relatively benign tumour of the kidney ('benign hypernephroma') and cysts, thought to be congenital, in pancreas and kidneys. The syndrome affects only a minority of patients with a cerebellar haemangioblastoma, but is commoner in patients with (i) a family history of such tumours, and (ii) multiple tumours in the cerebellum. In making a post mortem examination on *any* case of cerebellar haemangioblastoma, the pathologist should look carefully at the *spinal cord*, both *kidneys*, and *pancreas*. For histological details of the tumour, see p.195.

Tuberous sclerosis complex (Bourneville's disease)

Clinically, this disorder comprises epilepsy, mental defect, adenoma sebaceum of the face, other skin lesions, and haematuria. The associated structural lesions include 'tubers' in the brain, rhabdomyomas of the heart muscle, and angiomyolipomas of the kidney. The condition, when familial, is said to be transmitted by an autosomal dominant gene. Within an affected family, its expression is very variable, with one member exhibiting the full disease, while another merely shows a benign kidney tumour.

The brain lesions occur in two main sites: cerebral cortex and the ependyma of the lateral ventricles. On the surface, the cortical tubers are firm to the touch (more noticeably so before fixation), pale in colour, and appear as focal expansions of the gyri in which they occur (Fig. 16.17). Under the microscope they show a disorderly arrangement of cells, with loss of the normal lamination, dense gliosis, and numerous bizarre giant cells (Fig. 16.18), which are not easily classified as neurons or glial cells. The paraventricular lesions, described as 'candle-gutterings' by a generation familiar with the behaviour of candles, are elongated nodules, projecting into the ventricular cavity, composed of a variety of glial cells, among which large gemistocytic types of astrocyte are conspicuous. It is these lesions that on occasion give rise to expanding neoplasms, which are described on p.177. As a rule, neither the cortical nor the paraventricular lesions become neoplastic. As specimens from both types of lesion may turn up unexpectedly as biopsies, or even smears, it is important not to confuse them with malignant gliomas — a mistake facilitated by the presence of bizarre giant cells.

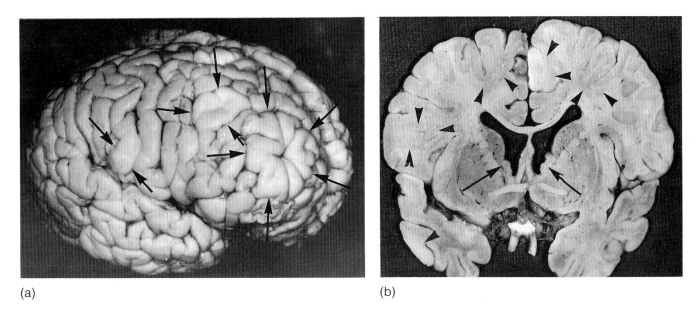

(a)   (b)

Fig. 16.17.   Tuberous sclerosis. Girl, aged 10 months. Epileptic, with malformed heart and polycythaemia. Brain weight 900 g. (a) Right lateral view, showing cortical tubers (arrowed). (b) Coronal slice at level A2, showing cortical tubers (arrow heads) and 'candle-gutterings' (arrowed) in the walls of the lateral ventricles. (Courtesy of Dr Betty Brownell.)

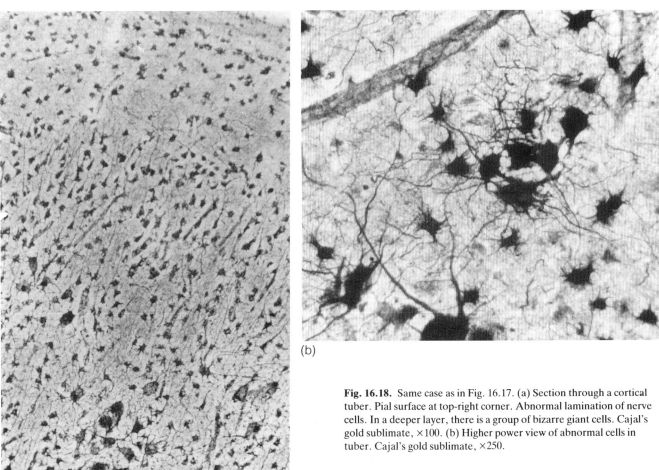

(b)

Fig. 16.18.   Same case as in Fig. 16.17. (a) Section through a cortical tuber. Pial surface at top-right corner. Abnormal lamination of nerve cells. In a deeper layer, there is a group of bizarre giant cells. Cajal's gold sublimate, ×100. (b) Higher power view of abnormal cells in tuber. Cajal's gold sublimate, ×250.

(a)

Chapter 17
Dementia

In this chapter we discuss the pathological diagnosis in cases of progressive dementia with onset in adult life. Dementia, in which there is loss of previously intact mental faculties, needs to be distinguished from mental defect, in which these faculties may never have developed normally. Dementia in childhood is due to a different range of diseases from those found in adults. There are many diseases in which dementia may occur in adults as part of the clinical picture, for example in cases of MS, diffuse cerebral tumour or PML. These cases are not our primary concern here, though they may be expected to turn up as occasional causes of unexplained progressive dementia. So too may conditions giving rise to confusion, memory loss or aphasia (Chapter 25), which may be mistakenly diagnosed clinically as dementia. Progressive supranuclear palsy (p.248) is sometimes regarded as a dementing condition, but the cognitive impairment in that disease is due more to slowed reactions than to a true dementia. A fixed, rather than progressive, dementia dating from an acute onset may occur following severe head injury or a hypoxic insult to the brain. Most adult cases in which the clinical disease is dominated by progressive mental deterioration will be found to be suffering from one of the conditions dealt with in this chapter.

The pathologist usually becomes involved with the diagnosis of cases of dementia after patients have died, but there are some medical centres that undertake cerebral biopsy as part of the investigation of cases of dementia. If a biopsy is taken, it is desirable that part of it be submitted for biochemical assay of choline acetyltransferase activity, which is selectively reduced in the cerebral cortex in Alzheimer's disease. The remainder is examined by light and electron microscopy (p.83). It is recommended that the sample for biochemistry is snap-frozen in liquid nitrogen or at −70°C and stored until microscopy has been carried out on the remainder of the sample. In this way a diagnosis of Creutzfeldt—Jakob disease (CJD) can usually be excluded before any biochemical investigation is undertaken.

Precautions regarding the agent responsible for Creutzfeldt—Jakob disease

Cases of progressive dementia on which a post mortem examination has been carried out may occasionally be found (when sections for microscopy become available), contrary to expectation, to be cases of CJD. CJD is a horrible, and at present untreatable, disease. It is also the subject of unsettled controversy. It is certain that transmission has been effected inadvertently, via penetrating electro-encephalogram (EEG) electrodes, a corneal graft and most recently by injections of pituitary extract administered to growth-hormone-deficient children. There is also strong evidence for occurrence of a closely related condition, the Gerstmann—Sträussler syndrome, as an autosomal dominant disease, and there have been transmissions from such familial cases to experimental animals. Strict precautions have been recommended, most recently by the Committee on Health Care Issues of the American Neurological Association (1986), for the post mortem handling of tissues from suspected cases; but the actual risks involved are quite unknown. Over 50 years elapsed between Jakob's description of the disease and the demonstration that it could be transmitted to animals. During this time cases were examined without precautions, yet there are still no recorded cases of CJD in pathologists or mortuary attendants, though two cases have recently been reported in laboratory technicians. On the other hand,

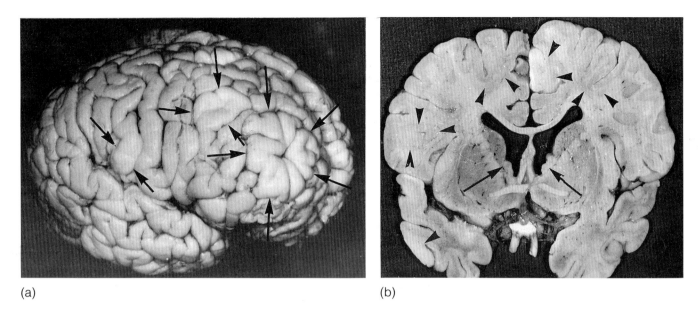

(a)   (b)

Fig. 16.17. Tuberous sclerosis. Girl, aged 10 months. Epileptic, with malformed heart and polycythaemia. Brain weight 900 g. (a) Right lateral view, showing cortical tubers (arrowed). (b) Coronal slice at level A2, showing cortical tubers (arrow heads) and 'candle-gutterings' (arrowed) in the walls of the lateral ventricles. (Courtesy of Dr Betty Brownell.)

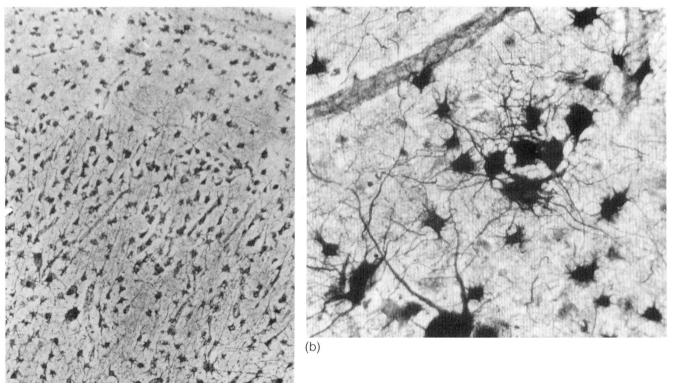

(b)

(a)

Fig. 16.18. Same case as in Fig. 16.17. (a) Section through a cortical tuber. Pial surface at top-right corner. Abnormal lamination of nerve cells. In a deeper layer, there is a group of bizarre giant cells. Cajal's gold sublimate, ×100. (b) Higher power view of abnormal cells in tuber. Cajal's gold sublimate, ×250.

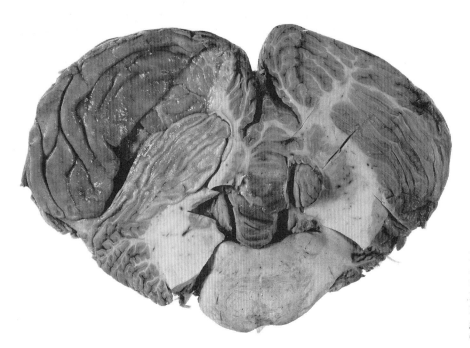

Fig. 16.19. Lhermitte–Duclos disease. Man, aged 43. Previously well. He developed a headache and the next day was found dead. Large brain (2210 g), with right tonsillar herniation. Right cerebellar hemisphere grossly enlarged with widely expanded folia. (Courtesy of Dr John Clark.)

Lhermitte–Duclos disease

An even rarer condition belonging to the twilight zone between malformation and neoplasia is the Lhermitte–Duclos disease. This presents clinically as an expanding cerebellar tumour. The cerebellar lesion, exposed at operation or post mortem, consists of an area in which the folia are expanded and pale (Fig. 16.19). On section, the tissue is found to consist of two layers: an outer one, occupied by myelinated nerve fibres, and an inner one composed of rather large abnormal nerve cells (Fig. 16.20). At the margins of the abnormal tissue, the outer layer is seen to be continuous with the molecular layer, and the inner one with the granule cell layer. Silver impregnations show that the myelinated fibres in the outer layer have the orientation of normal granule cell axons, running vertically outward, bifurcating, and then running horizontally, parallel with the axis of the folium. In the affected area there is a total loss of Purkinje cells, and of central white matter. Outside the area, where normal-looking granule and Purkinje cells are present, there may be areas in which some of the granule cell axons are myelinated, with attendant oligodendrocytes.

The fact that the lesion behaves as an expanding tumour has led some authors to classify it as a neoplasm, under a title such as *gangliocytoma dysplasticum*; against this view is the fact that there is no sign of cellular proliferation. If the cells are what they appear to be — that is, hypertrophic granule cells — their numbers are *reduced*; the expansion of the tissue is due to the enormous increase in size of the individual cells. It is presumably the resulting increased pressure that accounts for the disappearance of the central white matter. Nothing is known of the causes of the disease; but in one instance it affected a mother and her son. In

examining a proven case post mortem, we would recommend paying particular attention to the margins of the lesion, and to seemingly normal areas of cerebellum, and looking for hamartomatous lesions elsewhere in the brain and in the rest of the body.

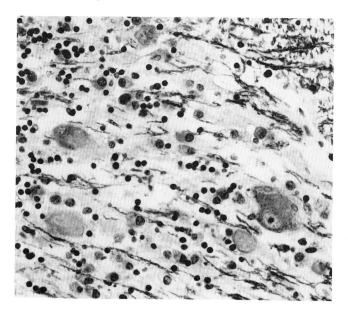

Fig. 16.20. Lhermitte–Duclos disease. Same case as in Fig. 16.19. The picture shows a transition-zone between a normal-looking granule cell layer and an area in which the cells are all grossly enlarged. At this point all stages between normal and hypertrophic granule cells can be seen; also their abnormally myelinated axons. Klüver–Barrera, ×250.

General comments

Malformations of the CNS vary greatly in their consequences. Some, such as anencephaly and holoprosencephaly, are fatal shortly after birth. Others, including encephaloceles and meningoceles, may be successfully patched up by the surgeon. Here, the main risk to life is a purulent meningitis. Minor malformations, such as polymicrogyria or agenesis of the corpus callosum, may give rise to epilepsy, 'cerebral palsy', and/or varying degrees of mental defect in childhood and after. As a general rule, minor malformations cause inconvenience or distress to the patient, whereas major ones, if they are compatible with continued life, are responsible for years of misery suffered by members of patients' families. They also constitute a drain on the resources of the social services. Research into the causes of malformations is well worth while, both for the light it may throw on embryological processes, and in the hope that better understanding may, in at least some of these conditions, suggest preventive measures.

Further reading

Benda C E. 1947. *Mongolism and Cretinism*. Grune and Stratton, New York.

Keeling JW (Ed.). 1987. *Fetal and Neonatal Pathology*. Springer, Berlin, Chapter 23.

Larroche J-C. 1984. Malformations of the nervous system. In Adams JH, Corsellis JAN, Duchen LW (Eds) *Greenfield's Neuropathology*, 4th edn. Edward Arnold, London, Chapter 10.

Chapter 17
Dementia

In this chapter we discuss the pathological diagnosis in cases of progressive dementia with onset in adult life. Dementia, in which there is loss of previously intact mental faculties, needs to be distinguished from mental defect, in which these faculties may never have developed normally. Dementia in childhood is due to a different range of diseases from those found in adults. There are many diseases in which dementia may occur in adults as part of the clinical picture, for example in cases of MS, diffuse cerebral tumour or PML. These cases are not our primary concern here, though they may be expected to turn up as occasional causes of unexplained progressive dementia. So too may conditions giving rise to confusion, memory loss or aphasia (Chapter 25), which may be mistakenly diagnosed clinically as dementia. Progressive supranuclear palsy (p.248) is sometimes regarded as a dementing condition, but the cognitive impairment in that disease is due more to slowed reactions than to a true dementia. A fixed, rather than progressive, dementia dating from an acute onset may occur following severe head injury or a hypoxic insult to the brain. Most adult cases in which the clinical disease is dominated by progressive mental deterioration will be found to be suffering from one of the conditions dealt with in this chapter.

The pathologist usually becomes involved with the diagnosis of cases of dementia after patients have died, but there are some medical centres that undertake cerebral biopsy as part of the investigation of cases of dementia. If a biopsy is taken, it is desirable that part of it be submitted for biochemical assay of choline acetyltransferase activity, which is selectively reduced in the cerebral cortex in Alzheimer's disease. The remainder is examined by light and electron microscopy (p.83). It is recommended that the sample for biochemistry is snap-frozen in liquid nitrogen or at $-70°C$ and stored until microscopy has been carried out on the remainder of the sample. In this way a diagnosis of Creutzfeldt–Jakob disease (CJD) can usually be excluded before any biochemical investigation is undertaken.

Precautions regarding the agent responsible for Creutzfeldt–Jakob disease

Cases of progressive dementia on which a post mortem examination has been carried out may occasionally be found (when sections for microscopy become available), contrary to expectation, to be cases of CJD. CJD is a horrible, and at present untreatable, disease. It is also the subject of unsettled controversy. It is certain that transmission has been effected inadvertently, via penetrating electro-encephalogram (EEG) electrodes, a corneal graft and most recently by injections of pituitary extract administered to growth-hormone-deficient children. There is also strong evidence for occurrence of a closely related condition, the Gerstmann–Sträussler syndrome, as an autosomal dominant disease, and there have been transmissions from such familial cases to experimental animals. Strict precautions have been recommended, most recently by the Committee on Health Care Issues of the American Neurological Association (1986), for the post mortem handling of tissues from suspected cases; but the actual risks involved are quite unknown. Over 50 years elapsed between Jakob's description of the disease and the demonstration that it could be transmitted to animals. During this time cases were examined without precautions, yet there are still no recorded cases of CJD in pathologists or mortuary attendants, though two cases have recently been reported in laboratory technicians. On the other hand, the condition has until very recently been regarded as very rare, and has therefore been rarely diagnosed. As the incubation period is said to be over a year, the connection between infection and the development of symptoms would be easy to miss. It should be remembered that formalin fixation is insufficient to destroy the transmissible agent. However, the procedures recommended will sterilize tissue and other materials so there is no good reason to avoid examination of biopsy or post mortem material on safety grounds, provided these recommendations are followed.

We have found it convenient to adopt the practice of assuming that *any case of progressive dementia in which survival from onset of symptoms to death is less than one year is a case of CJD until proved otherwise.* Also, cases with a disease duration of longer than one year in which a clinical diagnosis of CJD has been made are similarly treated. Since most cases of CJD die within a few months of the onset of dementia, and cases of progressive dementia due to other causes usually live well over a year from onset, this provides a reliable rule of thumb to apply when deciding whether it is necessary to adopt the precautions recommended for dealing with cases of CJD (Howie 1978; Committee on Health Care Issues of the American Neurological Association 1986). These precautions advise the following:

1 For removal of the brain at post mortem the skull is opened with a manual saw.

2 A gown and gloves are worn while handling tissues.

3 Dissecting instruments, the body and potentially contaminated working surfaces are sterilized by exposure to 1N sodium hydroxide for at least one hour (more effective than bleach, which was formerly recommended).

4 Histopathology specimens are fixed in formalin to which is added phenol to a final concentration of 10%.

5 Particular care is taken to avoid cuts, and if they occur they are washed thoroughly with water and treated with disinfectant.

6 The fixed brain is sliced and processed in a separate small laboratory equipped with a microbiological safety cabinet with an external extraction system (Howie 1978).

7 Knives used for cutting sections are either discarded if disposable, or chemically sterilized and then steam auto-claved at 134°C for at least 18 min after use.

Provision of post mortem material for research purposes

It has been realized during the last 20 years that brain samples obtained post mortem from cases of dementia provide a valuable source of research material. Many enzymes retain activity after death provided the body is refrigerated rapidly. Arrangements are made by some laboratories to collect deep-frozen material from pathologists able to supply it. Relatives of the deceased must be consulted, and usually give ready consent. As with biopsy

Table 17.1. Guide to the examination of the brain in cases of adult progressive dementia

Macroscopic appearance	Probable significance	Blocks recommended
Foci of softening	MID (but AD may also be present)	Softened foci, temp/hippo to exclude AD
Normal, or mild, generalized atrophy	Probably AD; other possibilities CJD (especially if illness < 1 yr), MID (micro-infarcts), schizophrenia	AD blocks (see text); CJD blocks (see text); cortex/white matter for MID
Marked atrophy of cortex (focal/ generalized) and comp. vent. dil.	Possible AD; Pick's disease (post 2/3 of sup. temp. gyrus spared); CJD with long survival; syphilis (meninges thick)	Pick's disease blocks (see text); AD blocks (see text); CJD blocks (see text); frontal lobe/ventricular surface for syphilis
Atrophy of caudate with normal or atrophic cortex and comp. vent. dil.	Huntington's chorea; milder caudate atrophy — Pick's disease; AD	See p.247 for Huntington's chorea; Pick's disease blocks (see text); AD blocks (see text)
Enlarged ventricles without atrophy	'Normal pressure' or obstructive hydrocephalus	Leptomeninges and outlet of 4th ventricle; temp/hippo to exclude AD
Cerebral white matter discoloration/ softening; cortex preserved	Binswanger's disease; also consider AIDS (see p.153)	Foci of softening/ discoloration; temp/hippo to exclude AD; for AIDS see p.153
Pale SN	PD with dementia; prog. supranuc. palsy with dementia	Midbrain, pons, AD blocks (see text); for prog. supranuc. palsy see p.248
Chronic subdural haematoma	If small, probably secondary to atrophy; if large, may be cause of dementia	If small, look for disease causing atrophy (see above)
Cerebellar atrophy	If mainly vermis, alcoholism; CJD	For alcoholism see p.309; CJD blocks (see text)

AD Alzheimer's disease; CJD Creutzfeldt−Jakob disease; MID multi-infarct dementia; SN substantia nigra; temp/hippo temporal lobe and hippocampus; comp. vent. dil. compensatory ventricular dilatation; prog. supranuc. palsy progressive supranuclear palsy; sup. temp. gyrus superior temporal gyrus.

samples, it is essential on safety grounds that the diagnosis of CJD should have been excluded by the pathologists for any case from which material is supplied for such purposes. The exact manner in which the specimens are taken from the fresh brain to be deep frozen is a matter for agreement between the pathologist and research worker, but one practical, convenient and usually acceptable procedure is to divide the brain into right and left halves by cutting through the corpus callosum, thalamic connection, floor of the third ventricle and hindbrain. One-half of the brain is deep frozen while the other half can be fixed by suspension if the basilar artery is retained with it. As the diseases that are likely to be responsible for progressive dementia virtually always involve both sides of the brain, there is very little danger of missing the diagnosis by adopting this procedure.

Naked-eye examination of the brain (Table 17.1)

Although the list of pathological diagnoses in cases of dementia is very long, in practice most cases are accounted for by a small number of conditions, and it is only when such conditions have been excluded, or one is confronted with the macroscopic evidence, that one needs to consider the rare alternatives. Most of the responsible conditions require only that the brain, and not other parts of the nervous system, be examined in detail. But if CJD is suspected, it is desirable to examine the spinal cord as well.

The macroscopic appearance of the brain is of considerable help in distinguishing between likely causes of dementia. Findings in other parts of the body may also be important, particularly the state of the heart and blood vessels, the possible presence of tumours in viscera, and the state of the reticuloendothelial system. In multi-infarct dementia the brain is likely to show multiple areas of softening due to infarction (Fig. 17.1), and the cardiovascular system is likely to show advanced atheromatous disease. Occasionally, however, multi-infarct dementia occurs in the absence of gross lesions, there being innumerable tiny infarcts, barely visible to the naked eye, or an extensive cribriform state of the white matter. In most such cases, and in those in which there is more diffuse damage to white matter associated with a predominantly dementing illness, as occurs in Binswanger's disease, there is usually evidence of long-standing hypertension. In Alzheimer's disease, which is much the commonest cause of progressive dementia in adults, the naked-eye appearances of the brain are variable; occasionally it appears grossly atrophic, with narrowed cortical gyri, gaping sulci and enlarged subarachnoid spaces (Fig. 17.2), but more often it is only mildly atrophic, or within normal limits for the age of the patient. Cortical atrophy is more readily seen if the leptomeninges are stripped from the surface of the brain. In brain slices, cases of Alzheimer's disease show variable dilatation of the lateral

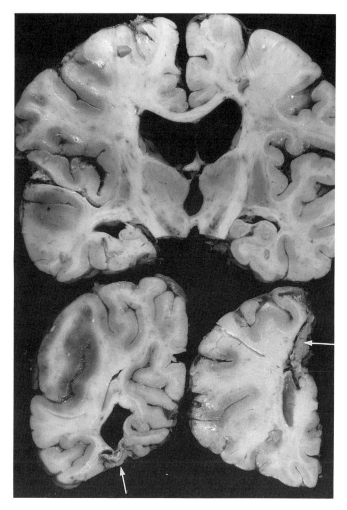

Fig. 17.1. Cerebral hemisphere slices from a case of multi-infarct dementia. Old infarcts (arrowed) are present in the left superior frontal gyrus (below right) and left fusiform gyrus (below left). There is also ischaemic atrophy of the left hippocampus (top), and a terminal infarct in territory supplied by the left middle cerebral artery. Lateral ventricles are dilated.

ventricles, with narrowing of the corpus callosum. Some cases show mild atrophy of the caudate nuclei and others, particularly very elderly cases, focal atrophy of the hippocampus, amygdala, and temporal lobe, with compensatory dilatation of the inferior horns of the lateral ventricles (Fig. 17.3). In Pick's disease there is focal, quite often asymmetrical, or generalized cerebral cortical atrophy, often of severe degree (Figs 8.10, 15.15 and 17.4). The posterior two-thirds of the superior temporal gyri are characteristically spared. In slices, the brain may show atrophy of the caudate nuclei, and marked dilatation of the lateral ventricles (Fig. 8.10). In Parkinson's disease with dementia, pallor of the substantia nigra is usually evident (Fig. 2.17), and in 'normal pressure hydrocephalus' there is marked ventricular dilatation, particularly of the lateral ventricles (see p.124).

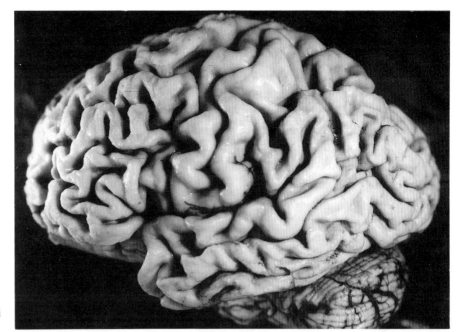

Fig. 17.2. Unusually severe, generalized, cortical atrophy in Alzheimer's disease. The leptomeninges have been stripped to show the narrowing of cortical gyri and widening of sulci (cf. Fig. 2.2).

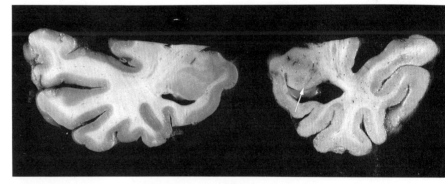

Fig. 17.3. Comparison of normal temporal lobe and amygdala (left) with the same area from an elderly case of Alzheimer's disease (right). The latter shows atrophy of the amygdala (arrowed), with compensatory dilatation of the inferior horn of the lateral ventricle. In addition, the temporal lobe cortex and white matter are reduced in volume in Alzheimer's disease. (cf. Fig. 2.5, level A1.)

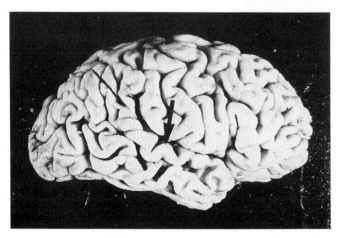

Fig. 17.4. Lateral view of the cerebrum in Pick's disease. The lateral aspect of the temporal lobe is severely atrophied. Note relative sparing of the posterior part of the superior temporal gyrus (arrowed).

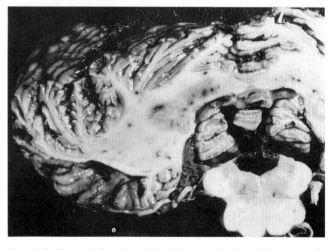

Fig. 17.5. Coronal slice through the left cerebellar hemisphere, vermis and medulla from a case of CJD. There is marked atrophy of the cerebellar folia.

Evidence of obstruction to CSF flow should be sought, but cannot always be found. Most commonly it occurs in the subarachnoid space as a consequence of leptomeningeal thickening. In Huntington's chorea there is severe atrophy of the caudate nuclei and putamen (p.247; Figs 8.9 and 15.14), and in Binswanger's disease grey discoloration, possibly with foci of softening, in white matter of the centrum ovale (Figs 7.21 and 7.22). In CJD the brain usually appears normal to naked-eye examination, but in cases with exceptionally long survival, there may be marked atrophy of the cerebrum and/or cerebellar cortex (Fig. 17.5). In dementia associated with alcoholism the lesions of Wernicke's encephalopathy, or of cerebellar degeneration, may be visible to the naked eye (p.316).

Microscopic examination of the brain

The choice of blocks for microscopy depends on the clinical diagnosis and the range of possible pathological diagnoses that present themselves once the brain has been examined with the naked eye. Table 17.1 provides a guide to procedures, taking as the starting point the macroscopic appearance of the brain. Summarized alphabetically below are the specific microscopic findings which should be identified in order to diagnose the most important diseases causing dementia. These represent minimum diagnostic requirements. Obviously in the context of many research projects there may be an indication to examine more widespread sites.

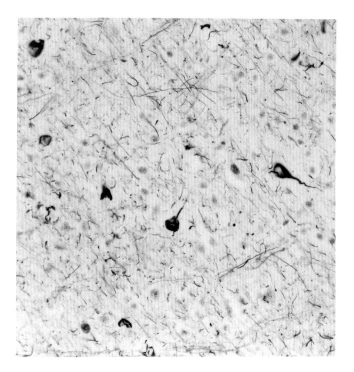

Fig. 17.6. Neurofibrillary tangles shown in a paraffin section stained by Cross' modification of the Palmgren stain (Appendix 1), ×200.

AIDS encephalopathy

This is a recently encountered cause of dementia in adults who may or may not be known to be suffering from AIDS at the time that psychiatric or neurological symptoms appear. The features found in the brain in AIDS encephalopathy, and the blocks recommended for examination if this is suspected, are described on p.153.

Alzheimer's disease

The characteristic microscopic findings are the following:
1 The presence of numerous argyrophilic plaques in the hippocampus, neocortex (cortex outside the hippocampus and its immediate surroundings) and some subcortical nuclei, particularly the amygdala.
2 The presence of numerous neurofibrillary tangles in hippocampal pyramidal neurons and neurons of the subiculum, entorhinal region and parahippocampal gyrus, and of some neurofibrillary tangles in neurons of the neocortex, amygdala, nucleus basalis, raphé nuclei of the midbrain and certain other subcortical nuclei. The neocortex is not uniformly affected by tangle formation in Alzheimer's disease; for example, areas of association cortex tend to be severely affected, whereas primary sensory areas, apart from the olfactory cortex, are relatively spared, as is the primary motor cortex. Figures 2.25d and 2.31 show where the structures affected by tangle formation in Alzheimer's disease can be found.
3 The presence of granulovacuolar degeneration in hippocampal pyramidal neurons. The same neurons may also contain Hirano bodies (Plate 6.6).
4 Amyloid deposits in small leptomeningeal and cortical blood vessels (Plate 7.1).
5 Some neuron cell loss, not usually very conspicuous, at the sites that contain neurofibrillary tangles.

Argyrophilic plaques are foci of degeneration in neural parenchyma containing abnormal neuritic processes and sometimes having at their centre a core of amyloid. The abnormal neurites are argyrophilic, and are more or less condensed into discrete, shrubby masses 20–200 μm across (Fig. 3.11). Neurofibrillary tangles are abnormal collections of argyrophilic, congophilic fibrillary material in neuron cell bodies (Figs 3.10, 17.6 and 17.7). Ultrastructurally, tangles are composed of bundles of helically wound, paired filaments (Fig. 17.8). A few filaments of the same type can also be found in the neurites in argyrophilic plaques (Fig. 17.9). These two structures, plaques and tangles, occurring together, are the most diagnostically useful pathological features of Alzheimer's disease. Plaques are not generally visible in H&E-stained sections, but can be seen with the PAS stain and are best shown with an appropriate silver method, such as that of von Braunmühl (p.391), or with a stain for amyloid which shows up the core. Neurofibrillary tangles can be

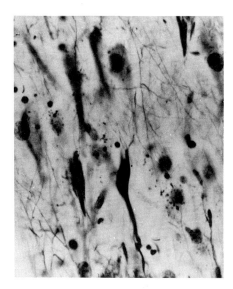

Fig. 17.7 (*above*). Neurofibrillary tangles in a frozen section of the hippocampus in Alzheimer's disease. von Braunmühl, ×700.

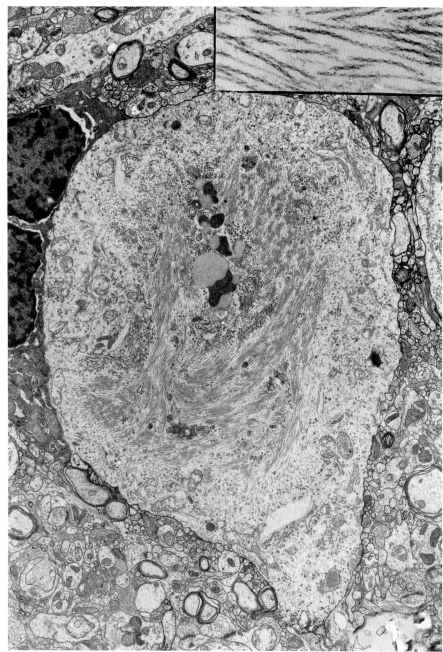

Fig. 17.8 (*right*). Electron micrograph of a cortical pyramidal neuron containing a neurofibrillary tangle in a biopsy sample from a case of Alzheimer's disease. The bundles of paired helical filaments occupy the centre of the cell, where they are admixed with some lipofuscin. Uranyl acetate and lead citrate, ×6250. Inset top right: high-power view of the paired helical filaments, ×47 000. (Courtesy of Dr J.J. Sloper.)

seen with H&E but are much easier to detect with silver stains, of which the best, in our hands, is Cross' modification of the Palmgren stain (see Appendix A). An amyloid stain demonstrates tangles quite well, and tangles also react with some neurofilament antibodies (Fig. 17.10). Granulovacuolar degeneration is the accumulation of abnormal argyrophilic granules in small, cytoplasmic spaces in neuron cell bodies (Fig. 17.11), and Hirano bodies are rod-shaped eosinophilic structures lying adjacent to neuron cell bodies (Plate 6.6). Both these structures are well seen with the H&E stain.

Cases of Alzheimer's disease occurring before the age of 65 years are easy to confirm pathologically because all the structures described above are usually present in profusion, whereas in normal brains of the same age they are present in no more than trivial numbers. In elderly cases of Alzheimer's disease, particularly those over 80 years, the microscopic changes of the disease are not so clearly distinguished from those found in 'normal' ageing, because all the features described above may occur to some extent in aged, undemented individuals. We do not intend to imply by this statement that the pathological features of Alzheimer's disease are an inevitable consequence of ageing; rather that very mild, locally restricted, clinically trivial, Alzheimer's lesions are exceedingly common in the very

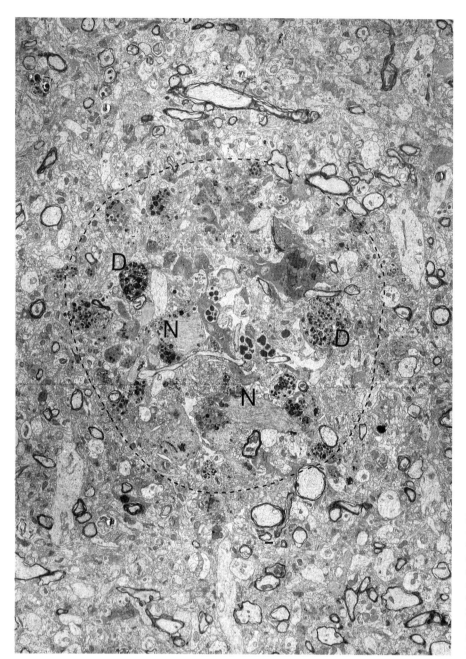

Fig. 17.9. Low-power electron micrograph of a cortical plaque in a biopsy sample from a case of Alzheimer's disease. The area occupied by the plaque is outlined by the dotted line. Details of the plaque structure cannot be displayed at this magnification, but clearly recognizable are expanded, dystrophic nerve endings containing dense bodies (D) and neuritic processes containing paired helical filaments (N). Uranyl acetate and lead citrate, ×3200. (Courtesy of Dr J.J. Sloper.)

old. The pathologist needs to beware of attributing clinically evident dementia to the presence of some plaques in the cerebral cortex and some tangles in the hippocampal and related regions of the brain shown in Figs 2.25d and 2.31. A definition of Alzheimer's disease in the very old becomes a matter of quantitative distinction (Khatchachurian 1985). However, there is one feature which almost never occurs in 'normal' ageing, and that is the presence of tangles in the neocortex – that is, cortex outside the hippocampus and related entorhinal and parahippocampal regions. This we regard as the most useful single distinguishing feature of Alzheimer's disease in old age. Tangles are also greatly increased in number in the hippocampus and para-

hippocampal/subicular regions in Alzheimer's disease, but detection of this increase above that found in normal ageing requires experience of tangle numbers that the pathologist may not have had the opportunity to acquire. In Alzheimer's disease in the very elderly, cortical tangles are not as widespread as in younger cases and are largely confined to temporal lobe neocortex. For this reason a block of temporal lobe cortex is the best place in which to search for the features of Alzheimer's disease in the very old. One or two additional areas of cortex should also be examined, e.g. frontal and parietal cortex, and the hippocampus should be examined for granulovacuolar degeneration and Hirano bodies. Plaques tend to be most numerous in the outer

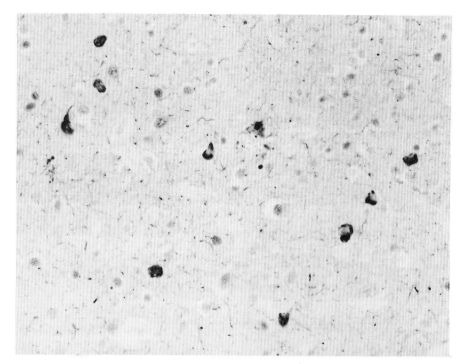

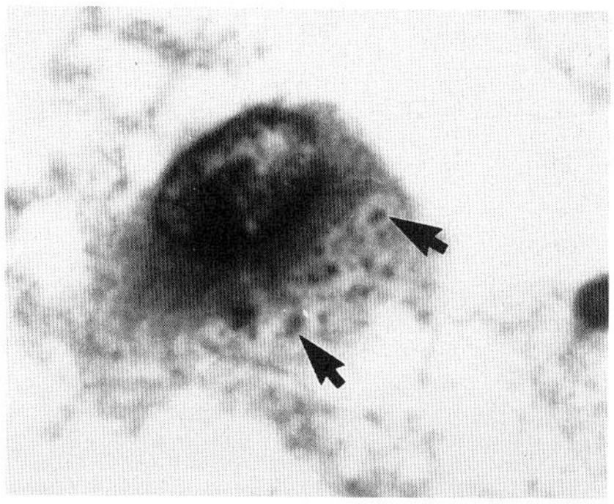

Fig. 17.11. Granulovacuolar degeneration in a hippocampal pyramidal neuron from a case of Alzheimer's disease. Multiple, small cytoplasmic vacuoles contain basophilic granules (arrowed.) H&E, ×670.

Fig. 17.10. Cortical pyramidal neurons showing an abnormal reaction with neurofilament monoclonal antibody RT97. An adjacent section stained with silver showed reactive neurons contained neurofibrillary tangles. Counterstained with haematoxylin, ×200.

three layers of the cortex, while tangles tend preferentially to occur in pyramidal cells of cortical layers 3 and 5. It is important to realize that most of the microscopic features that occur in Alzheimer's disease (albeit with slight modifications in the case of plaques) also occur in other diseases (Table 17.2), and it is the combination of all or most of them together in the same brain, and in the characteristic locations, that is diagnostic of Alzheimer's disease.

Chronic subdural haematoma

This condition may arise following a head injury or develop apparently spontaneously in the elderly. Usually there is some headache or clouding of consciousness, but occasionally dementia is the main presenting feature. Fluctuation in clinical state is usually obvious. There may be a chronic subdural haematoma membrane over one or both cerebral hemispheres (Fig. 11.1) (see also p.97). The underlying brain is frequently mildly oedematous, or may show evidence of recent or earlier ischaemic/hypoxic damage.

Table 17.2. Other diseases showing one of the microscopic features of Alzheimer's disease

Argyrophilic plaques
  Normal ageing*
  Down's syndrome (from early middle age)
  Familial cerebral amyloid angiopathy (p.104)
  Gerstmann−Sträussler syndrome (p.276)

Neurofibrillary tangles
  Normal ageing†
  Postencephalitic parkinsonism (p.240)
  Post-traumatic brain injury in boxers (p.93)
  Parkinson−dementia complex of Guam
  Subacute sclerosing panencephalitis (p.149)
  Progressive supranuclear palsy (p.248)
  Down's syndrome (from early middle age)
  Familial cerebral amyloid angiopathy (p.104)

Granulovacuolar degeneration
  Normal ageing*
  Pick's disease
  Parkinson−dementia complex of Guam
  Down's syndrome

Hirano bodies
  Normal ageing*
  Parkinson−dementia complex of Guam
  Down's syndrome
  Many other conditions (see Tomlinson & Corsellis 1984)

* small to moderate numbers compatible with normal mental state in old age.
† limited to hippocampus and parahippocampal gyrus/subiculum in normal old age.

Creutzfeldt–Jakob disease (CJD)

This is a rare disease associated with the presence in the brain of an, as yet, incompletely characterized transmissible agent. The agent, and the pathology it produces, closely resemble those found in another even rarer human disease, 'kuru', and in two animal diseases: scrapie in sheep and mink encephalopathy. The agents responsible for CJD and scrapie, on which most work has been done, have unusual biological and chemical properties; the diseases they produce have unusually long incubation periods, measured in months or years, the agents themselves are resistant to most (but not all) physical and chemical agents that inactivate pathogens, and their infectivity is closely associated with the presence of a glycoprotein which tends to accumulate after extraction as amyloid-like fibrils. This associated protein is host derived — a fact that may explain another odd feature of these diseases, the lack of any agent-specific immune reaction.

When selecting blocks for microscopy from cases of suspected CJD it is preferable on safety grounds to avoid the use of formalin-frozen sections and to rely instead solely on paraffin sections. Three or four blocks of cerebral cortex, two or three of deep grey matter, and one or two of the

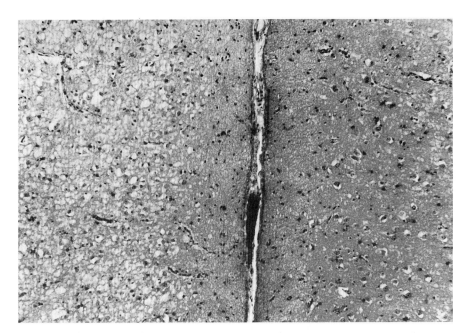

Fig. 17.12. Foci of spongy change (left) in the cerebral cortex from a case of CJD. The gyrus on the right is not affected. PTAH, ×100.

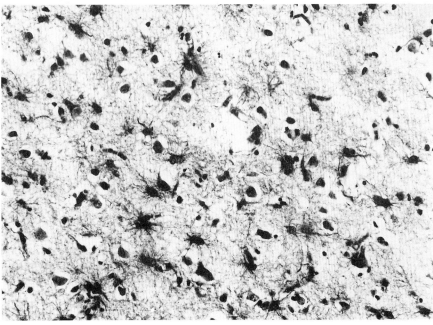

Fig. 17.13. Cerebral cortex from a case of CJD showing depletion of neurons and a marked excess of reactive astrocytes. PTAH, ×295.

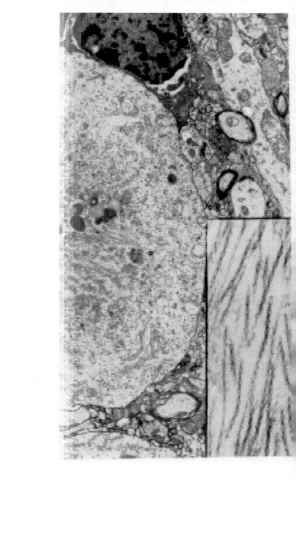

cerebellar cortex should provide sufficient evidence with which to confirm or refute the diagnosis of CJD. The characteristic microscopic features of the disease are spongy change (status spongiosus), neuron loss, and reactive gliosis (Figs 17.12 and 17.13). A few cases also show amyloid plaques, which differ from Alzheimer plaques in their lack of peripheral neuritic processes, and in their common location in the cerebellar as well as in cerebral cortex (Fig. 17.14). The spongy change is the most useful diagnostic feature, as the others are entirely non-specific. Spongy change is readily seen with the H&E stain, but is more impressive in a PTAH-stained section, which also shows the astrocytic re-

action clearly. In most cases of CJD, spongy change, cell loss and gliosis are all quite widespread in the cerebral cortex, though they vary in severity from lobe to lobe, and the hippocampus tends to be relatively spared. Cerebellar cortex is also regularly affected, and shows mainly loss of the granule cells and spongy change in the molecular layer (Fig. 17.15). Deep grey matter involvement is variable, with the putamen liable to be affected and brain stem nuclei usually spared. In some cases there is loss of anterior horn motor neurons in the spinal cord. Reactive gliosis in CJD occurs not only at sites that have lost neurons, but also at sites whose afferent innervation has been destroyed (Fig.

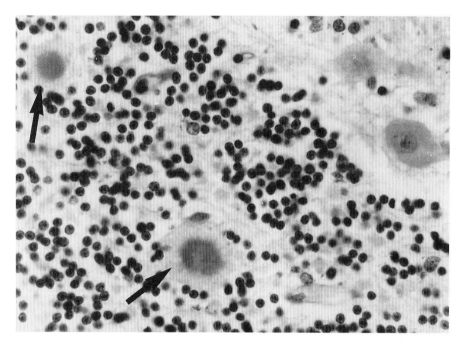

Fig. 17.14. Amyloid plaques in the granule cell layer of the cerebellum in CJD (arrowed). Two Purkinje cells are seen on the right. PAS, ×560. (Courtesy of Prof. J.H. Adams.)

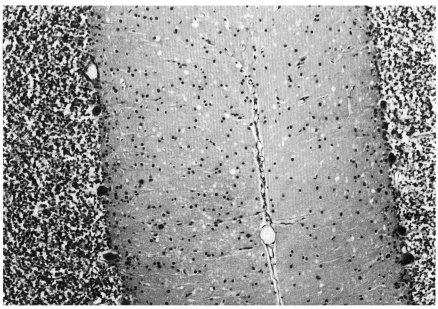

Fig. 17.15. CJD. Spongy change in the molecular layer of the cerebellum. H&E, ×95.

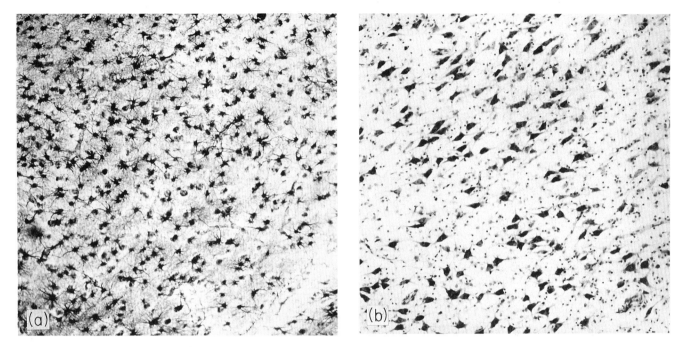

Fig. 17.16. Adjacent sections from the hippocampus from a case of CJD showing the marked gliosis (a) that may occur despite preservation of the neurons (b). The gliosis in this case was attributable to loss of afferent fibres to the region. (a) Cajal, (b) Nissl, ×140.

17.16). Neuron loss is usually, but not always, severe enough to be appreciated by inspection of sections (Fig. 17.14). Care must be taken to distinguish the spongy state of CJD from artefactual vacuole formation which may occur following dehydration during processing, particularly of oedematous brain. A useful point of distinction is that artefactual vacuoles surround neurons or small blood vessels, whereas the spongy state of CJD consists of empty vacuoles 5–50 μm across, located mainly in grey matter parenchyma. A condition known to be closely related to CJD, and capable of being transmitted to animals, is the Gerstmann–Sträussler syndrome, an inherited disease characterized by progressive dementia and ataxia. Spinocerebellar tracts show degeneration in this disease, and there are amyloid plaques in cerebral and cerebellar cortex, together with neuron loss and gliosis in the same areas. Spongy change is, however, not a feature of this disease.

General paralysis of the insane

This formerly common dementing disease, due to infection of the brain by *Treponema pallidum*, and a manifestation of tertiary syphilis, has fortunately become rare with the widespread availability of penicillin. It produces marked atrophy of the brain, particularly of the frontal lobes, with thickening of the overlying leptomeninges. The ventricles are moderately dilated, and their surfaces covered with tiny warts composed of glial fibres (Fig. 9.9). Microscopically, the affected parts of the cortex in untreated cases show an overall increase in cellularity and diffuse neuron loss. The extra cells are microglial cells, perivascular inflammatory cells and reactive astrocytes. Small blood vessels are also unusually prominent and endothelial cells hypertrophied. Iron deposits are found in microglial and endothelial cells. *Treponema* is found in untreated cases using appropriate stains, in groups or scattered singly in the neuropil of the cerebral cortex, in endothelial cells, and ingested in microglia. The overlying meninges in chronic cases show fibrosis and mild inflammation.

Multi-infarct dementia

Cases of dementia due to cerebrovascular disease, the second most common cause of dementia in old age, are usually distinguishable clinically from those due to Alzheimer's disease. At post mortem examination the brains of such cases contain infarcts of various sizes ranging from grossly visible extensive areas of softening to numerous microscopic infarcts, or areas of white matter rarefaction around hyalinized cerebral arterioles. Binswanger's disease, in which the latter changes are accompanied by more diffuse damage to cerebral white matter, is also thought to be due to an attenuated blood supply in patients with long-standing hypertension (Figs 7.21 and 7.22). Occasionally there are numerous small cortical infarcts and tiny haemorrhages associated with extensive amyloid deposition in leptomeningeal and cortical blood vessels (Plate 7.1). This may be associated with evidence of occlusion of some of the affected vessels, sometimes with re-canalization, or with an inflammatory reaction around them. Such cases are almost always

Plate 7

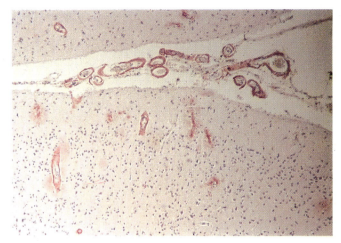

7.1. Amyloid deposits in leptomeningeal and cortical blood vessels in Alzheimer's disease. Congo Red, ×50.

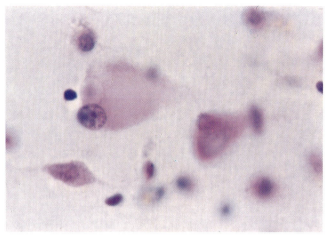

7.2. Swollen neuron cell body with pale cytoplasm (Pick cell) in the temporal lobe cortex from a case of Pick's disease. Nissl, ×800.

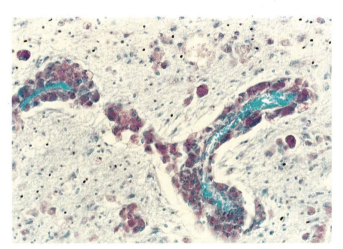

7.3. Krabbe's leucodystrophy. Globoid cells in perivascular spaces and brain parenchyma. LFB/PAS, ×400.

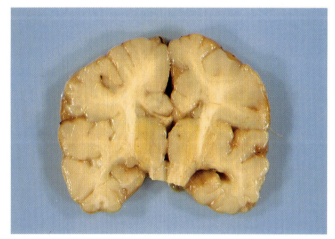

7.4. Coronal slice through the cerebrum from a case of severe neonatal jaundice with kernicterus.

associated with some plaque and tangle formation, though this may not be sufficiently extensive to warrant a diagnosis of Alzheimer's disease. Conversely, although cerebrovascular amyloid deposition is a characteristic feature of Alzheimer's disease, it is not, in most cases, associated with cortical infarction of the type described above. However, it is not uncommon for the features of Alzheimer's disease to coexist along with cerebral infarction due to atheroma or embolism in elderly subjects, and it is therefore necessary, in cases of possible multi-infarct dementia, to exclude coexisting Alzheimer's disease by examining a temporal lobe/hippocampal section for the features of this disease as well as examining sections of softened areas to confirm the presence of infarction and to try to identify the pathology of the underlying vascular disease (see Chapter 7). Arteritis or lymphomatous blockage of small vessels are among the rarer causes of multi-infarct dementia.

Parkinson's disease with dementia

The lesions responsible for the development of dementia in a minority of cases of Parkinson's disease are not clearly established. The lesions of Parkinson's disease, neuron loss and Lewy body formation (p.240), though principally located in the pigmented nuclei of the brain stem, are not confined to these sites, but are also found in the nucleus basalis and occasionally in the cerebral cortex. It is possible that damage to these structures provides an explanation of the dementia in some cases of Parkinson's disease, and these sites should be examined microscopically in such cases (see Fig.

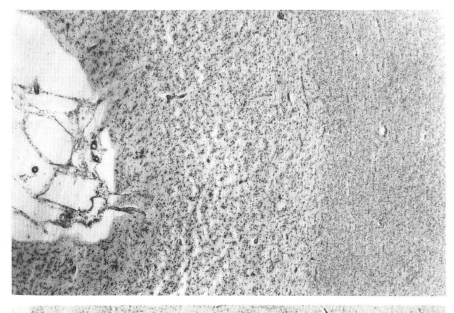

Fig. 17.17. Low-power view of cerebral cortex from a severely affected temporal lobe in Pick's disease (above), with control (below). The width of the cortex in Pick's disease is approximately halved, and larger neurons, which are just detectable at this power in the control, are almost entirely absent in Pick's disease. LBCV, ×25.

2.25d for the location of the nucleus basalis). Features of Alzheimer's disease should also be sought, as some cases show pathological features of both Parkinson's disease and Alzheimer's disease. It is possible that dementia in Parkinson's disease is attributable to damage to structures such as the nucleus basalis by the process responsible for Parkinson's disease, summating with plaque and tangle formation which is of a degree that would, on its own, be insufficient to produce clinical dementia.

Parkinsonism—dementia complex of Guam

Symptoms of progressive dementia, parkinsonism and motor neuron disease occurring in combination in the same subject or in different members of one community are remarkably common among the Chamorro tribe of the Mariana Islands in the Pacific. The pathology of this condition is reviewed by Hirano & Llena (1986).

Pick's disease

This rare autosomal dominant (occasionally sporadic) disease produces distinctive appearances in the brain, with severe focal cerebral atrophy most commonly confined to the frontal and temporal poles (Figs 8.10, 15.15 and 17.4), but sometimes occurring in a more widespread distribution (Fig. 8.10). A characteristic feature is sparing of the posterior two-thirds of the superior temporal gyrus. The cortex displays the most marked atrophy, but there may also be atrophy of the caudate nuclei and loss of cerebral white

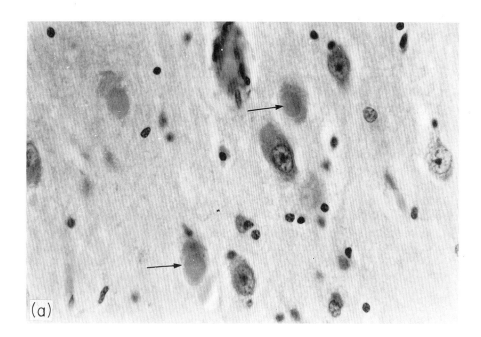

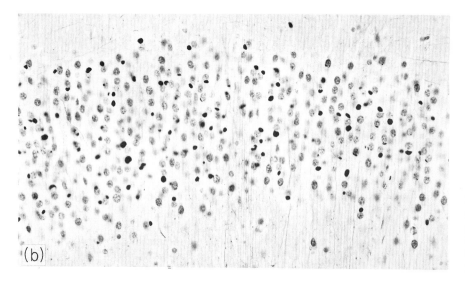

Fig. 17.18. Pick bodies: rounded cytoplasmic, argyrophilic inclusions (a) in hippocampal pyramidal neurons (arrowed), (b) in the dentate fascia granule cells in Pick's disease (stained black). (a) H&E, ×250; (b) Cross' modification of Palmgren, ×150.

matter. Microscopy should be performed on sections of atrophic cortex, less severely affected cortex, hippocampus and brain stem. The worst affected areas show severe neuron loss (Fig. 17.17), with reactive astrocytosis and fibrillary gliosis of underlying white matter. Some neuron cell bodies are greatly expanded by argyrophilic collections of neurofilaments (Pick cells) (Plate 7.2). Others contain collections of neurofilaments (Pick bodies) that do not actually expand the cell body (Fig. 17.18). Pick cells may be focally plentiful, but can be difficult to find in cortex that has been largely depleted of neurons. Pick bodies can usually be found in the dentate granule cell and pyramidal cell layers of the hippocampus (Fig. 17.18). Granulovacuolar degeneration also occurs in the hippocampus, and occasional cases show other features of Alzheimer's disease, including plaques and tangles.

Cases of dementia without specific pathology

In around 5—8% of cases in published series with well-documented histories of dementia, no specific pathology has been found within the brain. Particular groups of such patients are recognized:

1 Those with dementia and symptoms of motor neuron disease: such cases show the pathology of motor neuron disease (p.238), but no more than slight spongy change in layer 2 of the cortex (precentral motor cortex and elsewhere) to account for their dementia.

2 Chronic alcoholics who were demented may show lesions of Wernicke's encephalopathy (p.316), or those of repeated head injury (p.89), but some show none of these lesions, and in these cases the cause of dementia may remain undefined.

3 Chronic schizophrenics who become demented (see p.379).

4 Those with 'toxic' dementia (e.g. dialysis dementia).

5 Very old subjects who may show a mild degree of plaque and tangle formation that is insufficient to justify a diagnosis of Alzheimer's disease.

Such cases may also have small areas of vascular or hypoxic damage to the brain, which may precipitate development of symptoms of dementia in people who would otherwise remain asymptomatic.

Further reading

Committee on Health Care Issues of the American Neurological Association 1986. Precautions in handling tissues, fluids and other contaminating materials from patients with documented or suspected Creutzfeldt—Jakob disease. *Ann Neurol* **19**, 75—7.

Hirano A, Llena J. 1986. Neuropathological features of Parkinsonism—Dementia complex of Guam: reappraisal and comparative study with Alzheimer's disease and Parkinson's disease. In Zimmerman HM (Ed.) *Progress in Neuropathology*. Raven Press, New York, **6**, 17—31.

Howie Report. 1978. *Code of Practice for the Prevention of Infection in Clinical Laboratories and Post Mortem Rooms*. HMSO, London.

Khatchachurian ZS. 1985. Diagnosis of Alzheimer's disease (Conference Report). *Arch Neurol* **42**, 1097—104.

Roth M, Iversen LL. (Eds) 1986. Alzheimer's disease, and related disorders. *Br Med Bull* **42**, No. 1. Churchill Livingstone, Edinburgh.

Tomlinson BE, Corsellis JAN. 1984. Ageing and the dementias. In Adams JH, Corsellis JAN, Duchen LW (Eds) *Greenfield's Neuropathology*, 4th edn. Edward Arnold, London, 951—1025.

Chapter 18
Epilepsy

Epilepsy is an episodic disorder due to excessive synchronous electrical discharges by groups of neurons. Isolated epileptic fits occurring in the context of a generalized metabolic disorder are not included in the definition, and do not give rise to specific cerebral pathology in most cases. It is the task of the pathologist to attempt to identify pathological changes occurring in the brain of an epileptic subject in material examined either after surgical removal or at post mortem. The pathological changes associated with epilepsy range from gross lesions such as large tumours to minute or even microscopic irregularities, the significance of which is often doubtful. In some instances there may be dispute as to whether the lesions are the cause or the effect of the patient's fits. In about two-thirds of cases in published series an acceptable cause for epilepsy can be identified, though the exact proportion varies with age and with duration of epilepsy. In the remaining third of the cases no structural lesion can be identified. It should be pointed out that most of the literature on the pathology associated with epilepsy is concerned with severe cases, and the proportion of mild cases in which lesions can be identified is probably much lower.

In those cases in which a structural lesion is present, the mechanism that allows the excessive electrical discharge which generates the fit to occur is obscure. It is thought likely that interference with normal inhibitory influences acting upon pyramidal cortical neurons, particularly those mediated by the neurotransmitter gamma-aminobutyric acid (GABA), is involved. In those cases of epilepsy in which no structural lesion can be identified there may be an important genetic predisposition to epilepsy (McKusick 1983), but the structural basis for such a predisposition, if any, is unknown.

The commonest brain lesions thought to play a causative

role in epilepsy are, in children, birth and neonatal injuries (Chapter 21), a preceding febrile convulsion (especially if prolonged), vascular accidents, head injuries (Chapter 5) and malformations (Chapter 16). The ultrastructural observation that in young monkeys an episode of hypoxia results in degeneration of predominantly symmetrical, inhibitory synapses in the cerebral cortex may be relevant to the pathogenesis of epilepsy in infants suffering perinatal brain damage (Sloper, Johnson & Powell 1980). In adults the commonest related conditions are cerebral tumours (Chapters 11 and 12) or head injury (Chapter 5), followed by infections of the brain and its coverings — bacterial, viral or parasitic (Chapters 9 and 10) — and in later life, degenerative diseases such as Alzheimer's disease (Chapter 17) or cerebrovascular disease (Chapter 7). Table 18.1 lists a number of conditions giving rise to epileptic fits.

Post mortem examination of the body of a known epileptic is sometimes required in circumstances that make it unclear whether epilepsy was responsible for the terminal event. For example, the subject may have been found dead at home unexpectedly. In these cases it is necessary to search for evidence of a recent fit, such as incontinence or tongue-biting. Not infrequently there is evidence of inhalation of vomit while unconscious. Clues of this sort are more likely to establish a cause of death in such cases than an examination of the brain.

When examining the brain of an epileptic patient post mortem the areas of special interest are the cerebral cortex, hippocampus and cerebellum. It is factors acting on the cerebral cortex that tend to initiate epilepsy, and these factors are most likely to be epileptogenic if they are situated near the central sulcus. The two most characteristic lesions in the brains of epileptics are cell loss and gliosis in

Table 18.1. Some major causes of epilepsy

Focal intracranial lesions
   Tumour
   Abscess
   Angioma

Inflammatory conditions
   Meningitis
   Encephalitis

Trauma
   Perinatal brain injury
   Head injury
   Operative neurosurgery

Congenital abnormalities and malformations

Degenerations and inborn errors of metabolism
   Neuronal storage disorders
   Leucodystrophies
   Pick's disease
   Alzheimer's disease
   Creutzfeldt–Jakob disease

Vascular disorders
   Infarction
   Haemorrhage
   Hypertensive encephalopathy
   Eclampsia
   Autoimmune disorders (e.g. systemic lupus erythematosus)
   Intracranial aneurysm

Intoxications

No apparent cause (idiopathic)

the hippocampus and cerebellar cortex. These are now generally regarded as effects rather than causes of fits. These two areas are well known to be vulnerable to hypoxia, however caused; similar lesions can be produced in animals subjected to experimental seizures. There is increasing support for the view that the hippocampal lesion may result from the toxic effect of excess excitatory neurotransmitter. Cerebral hypoxia during prolonged fitting may also contribute. According to one view, the hippocampal lesion (commonly referred to as Ammon's horn sclerosis) may itself act as an epileptic focus, and a sequence has been suggested in which febrile convulsions in childhood lead to Ammon's horn sclerosis, which leads to temporal lobe epilepsy in later life.

Naked-eye appearance of the brain

Appearances of the brain in epileptics will obviously differ, depending on the cause. The external surface should be carefully inspected for focal cortical lesions such as a tumour (Fig. 18.1), or malformation, such as polymicrogyria (Fig. 16.13) or tuberous sclerosis (Figs 16.17 and 16.18). There may be evidence of acute or chronic meningitis, subdural empyema, old contusions due to head injury, or venous thrombosis.

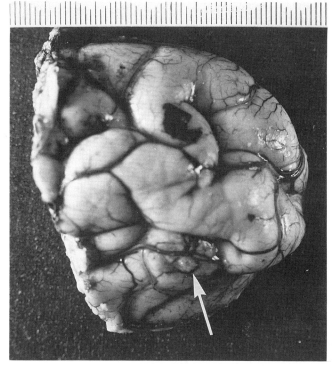

Fig. 18.1. Temporal lobectomy specimen illustrating the external appearance of a small, superficial oligodendroglioma (arrowed).

Caution is needed in attributing epilepsy to contusions, as they may also be a consequence of falls suffered during fits (Fig. 18.2). Convincing evidence linking head injury causally to epilepsy has however come from follow-up studies during life of head injury victims. They have shown a particularly high risk of epilepsy developing if there has been an open head injury, i.e. one in which the skull was fractured and the dura breached. The prevalence in these conditions reaches 40% by 5 years after injury, whereas after a closed injury the equivalent figure is 10%. The important pathological lesion would appear to be a pial tear and mechanical damage to the underlying cortex (contusion). Slightly more than half of those developing epilepsy after a head injury do so after an interval of months or years, and there may be a similar delay before epilepsy develops following an infection such as a brain abscess. The reason for this delay is said to be the gradual evolution of an epileptogenic scar at the site of the lesion.

Tumours causing epilepsy can be fully assessed and described after the brain has been fixed and sliced. They are variable in size. Large tumours are almost certain to have been detected clinically (Fig. 18.3), but small ones sometimes escape clinical detection (Fig. 18.4). Slowly growing tumours are particularly liable to cause epilepsy. They are usually situated above the tentorium, and frequently impinge directly on the cortex. Common tumour types responsible for epilepsy are gliomas, metastases, meningiomas, angiomas, hamartomatous lesions and tuberous sclerosis (Chapter 16).

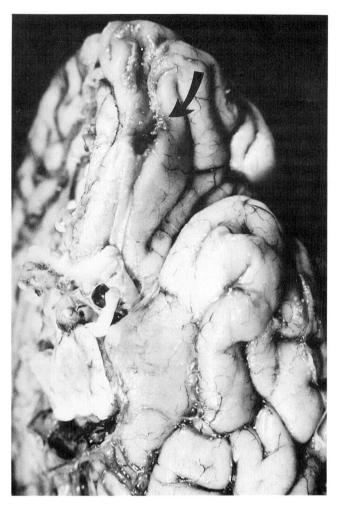

Fig. 18.2. Undersurface of the left frontal lobe from a young woman who had suffered from epilepsy since early childhood. She had no history of trauma preceding the onset of epilepsy, but had suffered frequent falls during her fits. There are old, cortical scars attributable to these (arrowed).

Of infective causes of epilepsy, abscesses and granulomas are likely to be evident macroscopically, as is herpes simplex encephalitis and meningitis. Other infections may require microscopy for identification.

Vascular causes of epilepsy include cerebral arterial and venous infarction, subarachnoid and intracerebral (especially lobar) haemorrhage, and perinatal vascular insults. They are usually readily visible externally or when the brain is sliced.

Some of the lesions that result from epilepsy can be detected by careful naked-eye inspection of the brain. They include cerebral hemiatrophy (Fig. 16.6) in which the whole or most of one cerebral hemisphere, the ipsilateral thalamus and contralateral cerebellar hemisphere are smaller than on the other side. Also detectable by inspection are laminar cortical necrosis (Fig. 7.4), and atrophy of the hippocampus

on one or, rarely, both sides (Fig. 7.6), which may be accompanied by atrophy of the ipsilateral fimbria and mamillary body.

Microscopic examination of the brain

In selecting blocks any lesions visible macroscopically should be included in the samples. It is also recommended that bilateral hippocampal blocks and a block of cerebellar cortex should be examined microscopically whether or not they show macroscopic lesions. Whether to take more blocks, if the brain appears normal macroscopically, is more problematic. We favour taking at least one additional block from the amygdala and another to include neocortex from an arterial boundary-zone territory, as damage to the neocortex, if present, tends to be maximal in such regions. It is also worth examining any parts of the neocortex which were known to have exhibited abnormal electrical activity on EEG recording, and in cases of Jacksonian epilepsy the appropriate part of the motor cortex should be examined.

Surgical specimens removed from subjects with epilepsy are likely to be either a tumour resection, which should be treated as discussed in Chapter 4, or an anterior temporal lobe resection performed for the relief of temporal lobe epilepsy. The latter is best sliced coronally, blocks for microscopy being taken to include any macroscopic lesions and, even in their absence, from each slice. If well-preserved temporal lobectomy specimens are regularly received in a department, it is likely that special investigations will be undertaken on them, since they are a scarce and valuable source of material that can be studied to advance understanding of human cortical organization in general and epilepsy in particular. Golgi studies, histochemistry and EM are all techniques of value for use on such material, but their choice depends on local interest and expertise, and they are not essential for routine diagnostic purposes.

Occasionally a hemispherectomy operation is performed for severe and intractable epilepsy. The surgical specimen received from this resection includes the cerebral cortex and white matter of all the main lobes from one cerebral hemisphere, together with variable portions of the amygdala and hippocampus. The specimen is usually sliced coronally after fixation and blocks for microscopy prepared from macroscopically abnormal areas from each slice, or from representative samples from each slice if no naked-eye lesions are visible. Small samples of tissue for special investigations, such as those outlined above for temporal lobe specimens, can be taken immediately after arrival of the specimen in the laboratory. Hemispherectomy specimens commonly show gross lesions such as ulegyria (p.261; Fig. 16.14). The operation is sometimes complicated by postoperative bleeding and the development of superficial siderosis (p.105; Fig. 6.15 and Plate 2.5), which may be found in patients dying after an interval of years.

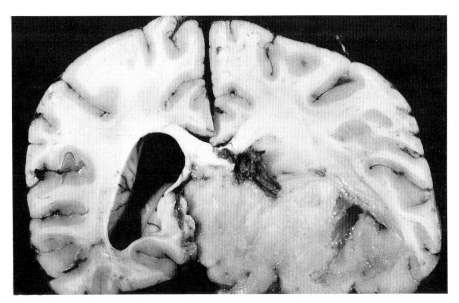

Fig. 18.3. Right temporo-occipital astrocytoma from a case in which epilepsy, including psychomotor fits, dominated the clinical course.

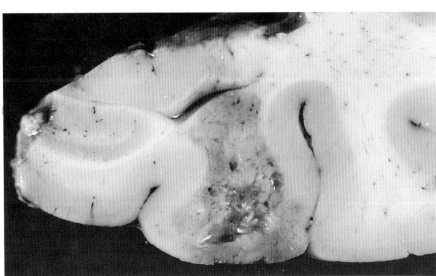

Fig. 18.4. A small, superficial oligodendroglioma from a patient with psychomotor epilepsy. This is the cut surface appearance of the tumour shown in Fig. 18.1.

In the absence of a macroscopic lesion in an epileptic brain, Nissl-stained sections are useful in searching for abnormalities in neuron populations or abnormal cyto-architecture in the cerebral cortex. A glial stain, particularly the Holzer stain, is also useful to detect areas of focal gliosis. Loss of neurons and gliosis should be searched for in the hippocampus, neocortex and cerebellum. Small degrees of cell loss will be missed unless quantitative studies are undertaken, but this is more appropriate for research than for routine investigation. The sites most likely to show cell loss and gliosis in the hippocampus are the Sommer sector of the pyramidal cell layer (H1) (Fig. 7.6) and the end folium (H4) (Fig. 18.5). The granule cells for the dentate fascia are also reduced in some cases. The H2 region is characteristically preserved. The hippocampal atrophy that results from the loss of these neurons and their fibres causes focal dilatation of the neighbouring inferior horn of the

lateral ventricle. There may also be cell loss in the amygdala and temporal cortex, particularly in the fusiform, inferior and middle temporal gyri. The cell loss in the temporal lobe cortex is often accentuated at the depths of sulci, and it is usually laminar in distribution, affecting principally layers 2 and 3. It may extend outside the temporal lobe to arterial boundary zones in frontal, parietal and occipital lobes, or may involve the entire hemisphere and produce hemi-atrophy. *Mesial temporal sclerosis* is a term used for the hippocampal and related pathology. It is interesting that in the great majority of cases it is a unilateral lesion. Similar lesions can be induced in experimental animals by focal injection of kainic acid, and investigations of these lesions suggest that the hippocampal damage may be produced by neurotoxic effects of excess release of the excitatory neuro-transmitter glutamate.

The cerebellar Purkinje cells, and to a lesser extent the

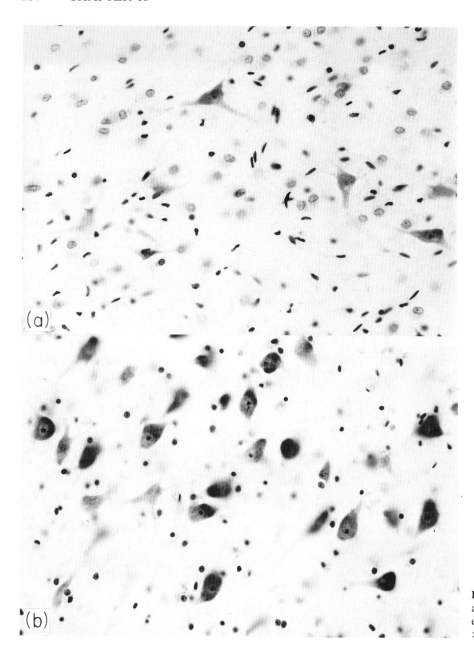

Fig. 18.5. Loss of neurons in the end folium in a case of long-standing epilepsy (a). Normal end folium for comparison (b). (a) and (b) ×250.

granule cells, are susceptible to damage in epilepsy (Fig. 18.6). They may be affected together with, or independently of, the neocortical and hippocampal pathology. Prolonged seizures appear to cause physiological changes that are sufficient to reproduce similar experimental damage in animals. Although phenytoin, used extensively in the treatment of epilepsy, gives rise to cerebellar malfunction as a toxic side-effect, it is not certain whether it can give rise to cell loss of the type and extent seen in the cerebellum in some long-term epileptics.

Temporal lobe (psychomotor) epilepsy

The commonest lesion found in temporal lobe specimens surgically resected for the relief of temporal lobe epilepsy is mesial temporal sclerosis, which is present in 50−60% of cases (Meldrum & Corsellis 1984). Small glial or vascular tumours, scars due to previous head injury, old vascular lesions, inflammatory lesions and cortical dysplasia are also described, and in about 20% of cases no lesion is identifiable. Prognosis for cessation of fits following surgery is best if the lesion identified is mesial temporal sclerosis or a benign, completely resected tumour. The fact that removal of the focus of damage, which mesial temporal sclerosis constitutes, can frequently lead to cessation of temporal lobe

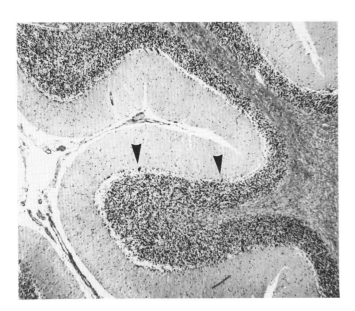

Fig. 18.6. Low-power view of the cerebellar cortex from a case of long-standing epilepsy. Very few Purkinje cells remain (two examples are indicated by arrows), and the granule cell layer is somewhat reduced in width. The patient had received high doses of phenytoin for many years. H&E, ×35.

(psychomotor) fits supports the view that this lesion, or one closely related to it, can itself act as an initiator or perpetuator of temporal lobe fits.

Status epilepticus

Epileptic fits lasting longer than an hour carry an appreciable mortality. Deaths in acute cases, particularly in adults, may be accompanied by no specific neuropathological changes. In most cases the brain appears swollen and congested and there may be a few petechial haemorrhages. Histological examination of the brain should include sampling the hippocampus on both sides, neocortex, thalamus and cerebellum. Quite frequently there is ischaemic cell change in a patchy or laminar distribution in the cortex, in the Sommer sector of the hippocampus, and in the thalamus and cerebellum. After several days' survival, neuron loss and a microglial and astrocytic reaction are likely to be found at the same sites.

Myoclonic epilepsy

Myoclonus may occur as a symptom in a number of different diseases (Fahn *et al*. 1986). As a principal feature it occurs together with epilepsy in a rare, familial, metabolic condition, *Lafora body disease*. In this disease, which can be diagnosed during life on the basis of appearances in a liver or muscle biopsy, there is an abundance of concentric microscopic inclusions occurring in neuronal cytoplasm, axons and dendrites, and lying free in the neuropil of the brain. The Lafora bodies are most numerous in the thalamus, globus pallidus, substantia nigra, superior olives, brain stem reticular formation, lateral geniculate bodies, dentate nuclei and pre- and postcentral gyri. Blocks for microscopic examination, if this condition is suspected, should be prepared from these sites. The inclusions are intensely stained by PAS and stains for acid-mucopolysaccharides. They appear basophilic with haematoxylin, a point of distinction from Lewy bodies, which they otherwise resemble. They closely resemble corpora amylacea (see p.62; Plate 2.1).

Occasionally severe myoclonus occurs in the absence of Lafora bodies. Such cases may show features of a system degeneration, such as dentatorubral atrophy, or there may be predominantly cerebellar pathology. Myoclonus may occur as one of a number of features in other diseases, such as SSPE (Chapter 10), sialidosis type 1, Creutzfeldt–Jakob disease, or Alzheimer's disease (Chapter 17).

Further reading

Corsellis JAN, Bruton CJ. 1983. Neuropathology of status epilepticus in humans. In Delgado-Escueta AV, Wasterlain CG, Treimen D, Porter RJ (Eds) *Status Epilepticus: Mechanisms of Brain Damage and Treatment*. Raven Press, New York, pp. 129–39.

Dam AM. 1980. Epilepsy and neuron loss in the hippocampus. *Epilepsia* **21**. 617–29.

Fahn S, Marsden CD, van Woert MH (Eds). 1986. Myoclonus. *Advs in Neurology* **43**. Raven Press, New York.

Jennett WB. 1965. Predicting epilepsy after blunt head injury. *Br Med J* **1**, 1215–16.

Jennett WB, Lewin W. 1960. Traumatic epilepsy after closed head injury. *J Neurol Neurosurg Psychiat* **23**, 295–301.

McKusick R. 1983. *Mendelian Inheritance in Man*, 6th edn. William Heinemann, London.

Meldrum BS, Corsellis JAN. 1984. Epilepsy. In Adams JH, Corsellis JAN, Duchen LW (Eds) *Greenfield's Neuropathology*, 4th edn. Edward Arnold, London, pp. 921–50.

Russell WR, Whitty CWM. 1952. Studies in traumatic epilepsy. 1 Factors influencing the incidence of epilepsy after brain wounds. *J Neurol Neurosurg Psychiat* **15**, 93–8.

Sloper JJ, Johnson P, Powell TPS. 1980. Selective degeneration of interneurons in the motor cortex of infant monkeys following controlled hypoxia: a possible cause of epilepsy. *Brain Res* **198**, 204–9.

Chapter 19
Metabolic Diseases of the Nervous System

These are a diverse group of diseases, many of them rare and complex, whose nomenclature has undergone radical revision during the last few years. Many started off with eponymous names, or were classified according to the type of pathology they produced (e.g. lipidoses). Biochemical clarification of the nature of some of them then led to classifications based on underlying enzyme deficiencies, and at present many of them are referred to by several different names. Table 19.1 lists alternative names for some of these conditions.

Recognition of those metabolic diseases that are inherited is important not only for the patient but also for the family, since the genetic implications need to be spelt out once the diagnosis has been confirmed pathologically and biochemically. Diagnosis of inherited metabolic diseases during life has been greatly aided by the development of enzyme assays which can be performed on non-nervous tissues requiring, in some cases, no more than a sample of blood (Table 19.2). Tests which can be performed on other family

Table 19.1. Alternative nomenclature of metabolic diseases of the nervous system

Older/eponymous name	Alternative name	Name based on biochemical defect
Tay–Sachs', Sandhoff's diseases	—	GM_2 gangliosidosis
—	—	GM_1 gangliosidosis
Amaurotic idiocies (includes Batten's, Kufs', Haltia–Santavuori and Jansky–Bielschowsky diseases)	Familial cerebral lipidoses	Neuronal ceroid lipofuscinosis
Niemann–Pick disease	—	Sphingomyelinase deficiency
Gaucher's disease	Glucosylceramide lipidosis	Glucocerebrosidase deficiency
Hurler's syndrome	Mucopolysaccharidosis type IH	α-L-iduronidase deficiency
Scheie's syndrome	Mucopolysaccharidosis type IS	α-L-iduronidase deficiency
Hunter's syndrome	Mucopolysaccharidosis type II	α-L-idurona-2-sulphate sulphatase deficiency
Sanfilippo syndrome A	Mucopolysaccharidosis type IIIA	Heparan sulphaminidase deficiency
Sanfilippo syndrome B	Mucopolysaccharidosis type IIIB	N-acetyl-α-D-glucosaminidase deficiency

Table 19.1. (*continued*)

Older/eponymous name	Alternative name	Name based on biochemical defect
Sanfilippo syndrome C	Mucopolysaccharidosis type IIIC	α-glucosaminide-N-acetyl-transferase deficiency
Sanfilippo syndrome D	Mucopolysaccharidosis type IIID	α-N-acetyl-α-D-glucosaminide-6-sulphate sulphatase deficiency
Morquio–Brailsford A	Mucopolysaccharidosis type IVA	chondroitin sulphate sulphohydrolase deficiency
Morquio–Brailsford B	Mucopolysaccharidosis type IVB	β-galactosidase deficiency
Maroteaux–Lamy disease	Mucopolysaccharidosis type VI	Arylsulphatase deficiency
Sly disease	Mucopolysaccharidosis type VII	β-glucuronidase deficiency
—	—	Mannosidosis
—	—	Fucosidosis
—	—	Aspartylglycosaminuria
Fabry's disease	Hereditary dystrophic lipidosis	α-galactosyl-lactosyl ceramidosis
Farber's disease	Lipogranulomatosis	Ceramidase deficiency
Wilson's disease	Hepatolenticular degeneration	—
Menkes' kinky hair disease	Trichopoliodystrophy	—
Porphyria	—	—
Leigh's encephalopathy	Infantile subacute necrotizing encephalopathy	—
Hallervorden–Spatz disease	—	—
Zellweger's cerebrohepatorenal syndrome	—	—
Metachromatic leucodystrophy	Sulphatide leucodystrophy	Arylsulphatase A deficiency
Krabbe's leucodystrophy	Globoid cell leucodystrophy	Galactocerebrosidosis
Included among cases of Schilder's disease	Adrenoleucodystrophy	—
Pelizaeus–Merzbacher disease	—	—
Canavan's diffuse sclerosis	Spongiform leucodystrophy	—
Cockayne's syndrome	—	—
Cerebrotendinous xanthomatosis	—	—
Bassen–Kornzweig syndrome	Abetalipoproteinaemia	Low-density lipoprotein deficiency
Tangier disease	Hypoalphalipoproteinaemia	High-density lipoprotein deficiency
Reye's syndrome	—	—
Alexander's disease	—	—
Central pontine myelinolysis	—	—
Marchiafava–Bignami disease	—	—

members and on the fetus *in utero* are becoming increasingly available and provide a valuable basis for offering advice to affected families. Such tests always require the services of a specialized laboratory. In this chapter we have taken the course of dividing the diseases into two main groups according to whether the grey or the white matter of the CNS is predominantly involved. We believe such a division can be helpful in the initial stages of the neuropathological diagnosis of difficult cases (Table 19.3). Detailed description of the individual diseases is not given here, but may be obtained from current textbooks of neuropathology such as *Greenfield's Neuropathology* (1984). In examining cases of inherited metabolic disease it is very important to reserve some fresh tissue for biochemical and histochemical study before fixing the remainder of the tissue. Tissues should also be taken for EM.

Inherited metabolic diseases chiefly affecting grey matter

Lysosomal disorders

The gangliosidoses

These are a group of disorders with autosomal recessive inheritance in which excess amounts of gangliosides of normal chemical structure are present in the brain, and, in some cases, in other organs as well. Two main groups are recognized:

The GM_2 gangliosidoses. These include infantile, juvenile and adult forms. Affected individuals are usually normal at birth but, in the infantile form, fail to achieve developmental

Table 19.2. Diagnostic procedures for metabolic CNS diseases

Condition	Useful investigations outside CNS	Definitive biochemical investigation	Tissues
GM_2 gangliosidosis	HCh + EM on suction rectal bx	Assay hexosaminidases A and B	WBC, CF, AFC
GM_1 gangliosidosis	HCh + EM on suction rectal bx	Assay β-galactosidase	WBC, CF, AFC
Neuronal ceroid lipofuscinosis	HCh + EM on skin, conjunctiva, blood	None	
Niemann–Pick disease (A, B)	HCh + EM on suction rectal bx, conjunctiva, bone marrow	Assay sphingomyelinase	WBC, CF, AFC
Gaucher's disease	HCh + EM on bone marrow	Assay β-glucocerebrosidase	WBC, CF, AFC
Mucopolysaccharidoses	HCh + EM on bone marrow	Mucopolysaccharide analysis; assay for suspected enzyme defect in light of findings in urine	WBC, CF, AFC
Mannosidosis	HCh + EM on bone marrow, blood, suction rectal bx	Assay α-mannosidase	WBC, CF, AFC
Fucosidosis	HCh + EM on bone marrow, blood, suction rectal bx	Assay α-fucosidase	WBC, CF, AFC
Aspartylglycosaminuria		Assay aspartylglycosylamine amidohydrolase, urinary metabolites	WBC, urine, CF, AFC
Fabry's disease	HCh + EM on skin biopsy	Examine urine for excess ceramide hexosides; assay lysosomal α-galactosidase A	Plasma, tears, urine, CF, AFC
Leigh's encephalopathy	Some cases show mitochondrial abnormalities in EM of muscle bx	Pyruvate metabolism and respiratory chain enzymes; blood lactate usually elevated	Variable; e.g. muscle, liver, cultured fibroblasts
Metachromatic leucodystrophy	HCh + EM on skin and nerve biopsies	Examine urine sediment for metachromatic granules, assay arylsulphatase A	Urine, serum, WBC, CF, AFC
Krabbe's leucodystrophy	—	Assay lysosomal galactocerebroside β–galactosidase	Serum, WBC, CF, AFC
Adrenoleucodystrophy	EM on adrenal cortex	Assay very-long-chain fatty acids	Serum, CF, AFC

EM electron microscopy; WBC white blood cells; CF cultured fibroblasts; HCh histochemistry; AFC cultured amniotic fluid cells (for prenatal diagnosis); bx biopsy.

Table 19.3. Guide to neuropathological diagnosis of diseases in which there is abnormal stored material in the CNS (see Table 19.2 for confirmatory biochemical investigations)

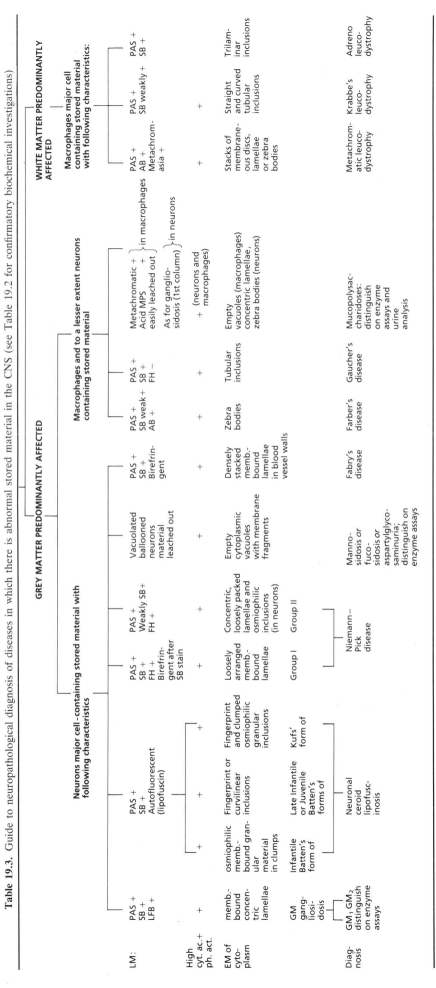

	GREY MATTER PREDOMINANTLY AFFECTED									**WHITE MATTER PREDOMINANTLY AFFECTED**		
	Neurons major cell-containing stored material with following characteristics					Macrophages and to a lesser extent neurons containing stored material				Macrophages major cell containing stored material with following characteristics		
LM:	PAS + SB + LFB +	PAS + SB + Autofluorescent (lipofuscin)	PAS + SB + FH + Birefringent after SB stain	PAS + Weakly SB + FH +	Vacuolated ballooned neurons material leached out	PAS + SB + Birefringent	PAS + SB weak+ AB +	PAS + SB + FH −	Metachromatic + Acid MPS easily leached out } in macrophages; As for gangliosidosis (1st column) } in neurons	PAS + AB + Metachromasia +	PAS + SB weakly +	PAS + SB +
High cyt. ac. ph. act.	+	+	+	+		+	+	+	+ (neurons and macrophages)	+	+	
EM of cytoplasm	memb.-bound concentric lamellae	osmiophilic memb.-bound granular material in clumps; Fingerprint or curvilinear inclusions; Fingerprint and clumped osmiophilic granular inclusions	Loosely arranged memb.-bound lamellae	Concentric, loosely packed lamellae and osmiophilic inclusions (in neurons)	Empty cytoplasmic vacuoles with membrane fragments	Densely stacked memb.-bound lamellae in blood vessel walls	Zebra bodies	Tubular inclusions	Empty vacuoles (macrophages) concentric lamellae, zebra bodies (neurons)	Stacks of membraneous discs, lamellae or zebra bodies	Straight and curved tubular inclusions	Trilaminar inclusions
Diagnosis	GM gangliosidosis (GM₁, GM₂ distinguish on enzyme assays)	Neuronal ceroid lipofuscinosis — Infantile Batten's form of; Late Infantile or Juvenile Batten's forms of; Kufs' form of	Niemann–Pick disease (Group I)	Niemann–Pick disease (Group II)	Mannosidosis or fucosidosis or aspartylglycosaminuria; distinguish on enzyme assays	Fabry's disease	Farber's disease	Gaucher's disease	Mucopolysaccharidoses: distinguish on enzyme assays and urine analysis	Metachromatic leucodystrophy	Krabbe's leucodystrophy	Adrenoleucodystrophy

LM light microscopical appearance; FH ferric haematoxylin; cyt. ac. ph. act. cytoplasmic acid phosphatase activity; AB Alcian blue; EM electron microscopical appearance; MPS mucopolysaccharide; PAS periodic acid schiff; SB Sudan black; LFB Luxol-fast blue.

milestones from a few months of age and develop blindness and progressive neurological abnormalities. A cherry-red spot is present at the macula on ophthalmological examination. At post mortem examination the brain may be normal in size, enlarged or atrophic. There is loss of a clear distinction between grey and white matter, and the cortical ribbon may be narrowed. All parts of the brain show microscopic abnormalities, the most striking being ballooning of neuronal cytoplasm, with compression of the nucleus to one margin of the cell. Large neurons are affected more than small ones, and neurons of sensory and autonomic ganglia are not exempt. In microscopic sections, in addition to the ballooning of neurons and a foamy appearance to their cytoplasm, there is an increase in number and size of microglial cells, which contain excess PAS-positive material. Stored material in neurons stains positively with Sudan black and Luxol fast blue. The ganglioside is found in increased numbers of large lysosomes, which can be demonstrated histochemically using the acid phosphatase reaction. EM of the stored material shows membrane-bound lysosomal structures filled with concentric lamellae. The enzyme which is deficient is hexosaminidase A, or, in Sandhoff's disease, hexosaminidase A and B.

GM₁ gangliosidosis. This presents in infants, young children or, rarely, in adults. In the infantile form there is hypotonia at birth, developmental delay, skeletal deformities, failure to thrive and hepatosplenomegaly. The brain at post mortem may be macroscopically normal or may show cortical atrophy. Microscopically it shows ballooned neurons alongside normal ones in all areas (Fig. 19.1), and similar changes are present in the myenteric and submucosal plexuses of the gut. Appearances resemble those seen in GM₂ gangliosidosis, but the enzyme that is deficient is the lysosomal enzyme, β-galactosidase.

Neuronal ceroid lipofuscinosis

There are various forms of this condition, which differ in clinical features, age of onset and pathology, particularly at the ultrastructural level. The infantile form of Batten's disease presents from about 8 months with rapidly progressive motor and mental retardation, visual loss, ataxia and hypotonia. Death occurs at 3–10 years. Late infantile Batten's disease has its onset between 18 months and 4 years. Progressive mental and motor retardation with visual disturbance occur, with death eventually supervening at 4–10 years. In juvenile Batten's disease the initial presentation is with visual impairment in later childhood, followed by fits, gait disturbance and weakness, leading to death in the second or third decade. In the adult form (Kufs' disease) onset of symptoms may occur in childhood or adult life, with progressive dementia, ataxia, epilepsy and extrapyramidal movement disturbance. Most forms are recessively inherited.

In all forms of the disease the brain is found post mortem to be very atrophic and covered by thickened leptomeninges, and the skull is also thickened. The cerebral and cerebellar cortex are greatly narrowed and the white matter firm and gliotic. In general the changes are most severe in the infantile form. Microscopic sections show neuron loss, reactive gliosis and macrophage infiltration in many areas. All surviving neurons in infantile Batten's disease, and most in the other forms, contain prominent granular material with the histochemical characteristics of lipofuscin (PAS and Sudan black positivity and strong autofluorescence). Excess

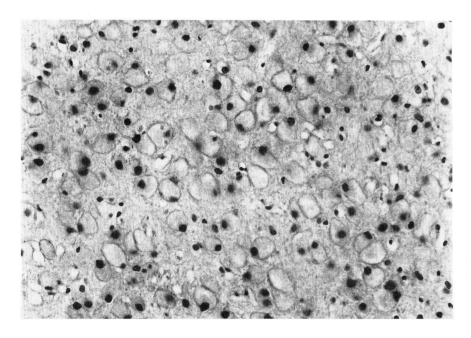

Fig. 19.1. GM₁ gangliosidosis. Appearance of swollen neurons in pontine nuclei. The cytoplasm is pale, and many of the nuclei are displaced from the centre of the cell. PAS, ×170.

acid phosphatase activity can be demonstrated histochemically. Ultrastructural examination shows inclusions of differing type in the different forms of the disease. In infantile Batten's disease they consist of osmiophilic, granular, clumped material surrounded by a unit membrane. In late infantile Batten's disease they are curvilinear in form, in the juvenile disease fingerprint bodies are described and in Kufs' disease there are fingerprint and clumped osmiophilic inclusions. Outside the CNS stored material is present in neurons in peripheral ganglia, and in viscera, endothelium and muscle. The chemical nature of the stored material has not been identified, nor an enzyme defect uncovered.

Niemann–Pick (and related) disease

Two major subgroups of this disease are recognized: group 1, with sphingomyelinase deficiency, in which clinical forms with and without CNS involvement, in addition to visceral involvement, are distinguishable; and group 2, with normal sphingomyelinase activity, in which, again, there may or may not be early neurological involvement. All forms show enlargement of liver and spleen, and, in infants, failure to thrive. Infants in group 2 may also suffer severe neonatal jaundice. Childhood and adult cases, as well as infantile ones, occur in both groups. In group 1 cases with neurological involvement, the brain is slightly atrophic and the white matter firm. Neurons and glial cells are ballooned (Fig. 19.2), and white matter demyelinated, gliotic and infiltrated with foamy macrophages containing stored material. Similar macrophages, 20–90 μm across, infiltrate lymphoreticular tissue, and can be found also in most organs. These cells contain sphingomyelin and give a positive reaction in cryostat or frozen sections with Sudan black and ferric haematoxylin. The cytoplasmic deposits are also PAS-positive and show red birefringence under polarized light after Sudan black staining. The acid phosphatase reaction is strongly positive around the foamy vacuoles. By EM the neuronal inclusions contain loosely arranged lipid lamellae in membrane-bound vacuoles. There is a demonstrable deficiency of lysosomal sphingomyelinase in many tissues, including white blood cells and cultured fibroblasts. In group 2 cases with CNS involvement there may be slight cerebral atrophy and the white matter is gliotic, but not demyelinated. Ballooning of neuronal cytoplasm is present in all regions, and is accompanied by some axonal swelling. The stored material in neurons is not sphingomyelin, and in frozen sections is only weakly sudanophilic and stains positively with ferric haematoxylin and PAS. Spleen foam cells, however, do contain sphingomyelin, with the histochemical properties described above for group 1 cases. The neuronal stored material consists at the EM level of concentric, membrane-bound, loosely packed lamellae accompanied by dense osmiophilic inclusions. The enzymatic basis of the group 2 defect is not known.

Gaucher's disease

This is a rare autosomal recessive disease with three recognized forms, in two of which neurological involvement occurs in the form of psychomotor delay in infancy or intellectual deterioration followed by further neurological deficits in childhood. Hepatosplenomegaly, failure to thrive and bone fractures also occur. Macroscopically the brain appears normal at post mortem in all forms of the disease, but microscopically there are found to be collections of Gaucher's cells in cerebral cortex, basal ganglia, brain stem and cerebellum. These are large macrophages, some of which may be multinucleate, measuring 20–100 μm across and containing coarsely fibrillar or striated, pale material. The nucleus is eccentrically placed. The stored material is PAS-positive, but negative for fat and with ferric haematoxylin. Acid phosphatase activity in the cells is high. EM shows cytoplasmic twisted tubular inclusions. Slight neuron loss may be evident in the cerebral cortex and more severe loss, with gliosis and

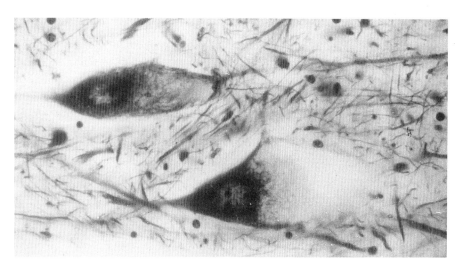

Fig. 19.2. Appearance of ballooned neuronal cytoplasm in Niemann–Pick disease. The lower neuron is clearly more affected than the upper one. Holmes/Luxol fast blue, ×530.

slight swelling of neuronal cytoplasm, may be seen in the basal ganglia and brain stem. Lymphoreticular tissue contains numerous Gaucher's cells. The stored material consists of glucocerebroside and there is a deficiency of lysosomal glucocerebrosidase which can be demonstrated in leucocytes and cultured fibroblasts.

The mucopolysaccharidoses

A number of different types of the mucopolysaccharidoses are recognized, in some of which there is involvement of the brain. Affected infants are usually normal at birth but develop mental retardation, characteristic facial and skeletal deformities, and excessive hair towards the end of the first year. Most forms have an autosomal recessive pattern of inheritance. At post mortem the brain usually appears normal macroscopically except for the presence of perivascular 'pitting', empty spaces around vessels which may be visible in brain slices. These are due to leaching out of highly water-soluble acid mucopolysaccharides from perivascular macrophages. Microscopically this material can be demonstrated in snap-frozen cryostat sections using a metachromatic stain. In addition to collections of perivascular macrophages the brain may show some neuronal swelling in the cerebral cortex, hippocampus, basal ganglia and thalamus. This material is not mucopolysaccharide but consists of gangliosides (Table 19.3). In some forms neuronal storage material accumulates in peripheral neurons as well as in the brain. Ultrastructurally the perivascular macrophages contain numerous empty cytoplasmic vacuoles with a few fragments of membranes, while the neuronal storage material resembles that found in the gangliosidoses. Specific enzyme defects have been identified in the various forms of mucopolysaccharidosis and all result in abnormal excretion of mucopolysaccharides in the form of dermatan, heparan or keratan sulphates in the urine. Enzyme assays can be performed on blood leucocytes or cultured fibroblasts.

Mannosidosis and fucosidosis

Clinically resembling the mucopolysaccharidoses are two further autosomal recessive diseases, mannosidosis and fucosidosis. These are due to deficiency of lysosomal mannosidase and α-fucosidase activity respectively. The urine contains excess quantities of mannose- or fucose-rich substances. The nervous system may be affected in both diseases. Routine microscopy shows swollen vacuolated neurons, from which stored material has leached out. In snap-frozen cryostat sections PAS-positive material may be found in the vacuoles, and acid phosphatase activity is increased in cell cytoplasm. In both conditions EM shows empty vacuoles containing only a few membrane fragments in affected cytoplasm. The enzyme defect in both conditions can be demonstrated in leucocytes or cultured fibroblasts.

Aspartyl glycosaminuria

This very rare disease may cause psychomotor retardation in childhood. The brain appears normal to the naked eye but in routine microscopic sections vacuolated neurons are found in the cerebral cortex and basal ganglia. Stored material cannot be detected, even in snap-frozen cryostat sections, but excess acid phosphatase activity is demonstrable in the cytoplasm of affected cells. There is a deficiency of the lysosomal enzyme aspartylglycosylamine amidohydrolase, and this can be demonstrated in blood leucocytes.

Fabry's disease

This is a multi-system, X-linked disease presenting in late childhood with a rash and episodes of severe pain in the limbs, chest and abdomen. Corneal opacities are found on slit-lamp examination. There is widespread vascular pathology with endothelial cells and smooth muscle cells in vessel walls appearing swollen and containing stored material which can be shown in snap-frozen cryostat sections to be PAS-positive, sudanophilic and birefringent. The acid phosphatase reaction in affected cells is strongly positive. Storage material with the same characteristics is also present in swollen neurons in the amygdala, hypothalamus, brain stem, intermediolateral column and Onufrowicz' nucleus neurons in the spinal cord, and peripheral sensory and autonomic ganglia. The brain may also show ischaemic lesions related to the vascular pathology, and peripheral nerves show loss of small-diameter myelinated nerve fibres. Stored material is present in peripheral nerves in perineurial and endoneurial cells. EM of stored material shows densely stacked lamellae and occasional tubular inclusions. These consist of ceramide di- and tri-hexosides, substances which also appear in the urine. There is deficiency of α-galactosidase activity, which can be demonstrated in cultured fibroblasts.

Farber's disease

This very rare disease of infants causes painful subcutaneous nodules, respiratory and feeding problems, and severe motor and mental retardation from within a few weeks of birth. There is neuronal storage of ceramide and G ganglioside, which are PAS-positive, Alcian blue-positive, weakly sudanophilic and birefringent. Neuron loss and gliosis may also be present. The subcutaneous nodules contain foam cells laden with storage material, and similar cells are found in the lymphoreticular tissues. Affected cells show excess acid phosphatase activity. EM shows empty vacuoles or membrane-bound inclusions, the nature of which differ from one tissue to another, but in neurons they appear as zebra bodies. There is a deficiency of the enzyme lysosomal ceramidase, which is demonstrable in cultured fibroblasts.

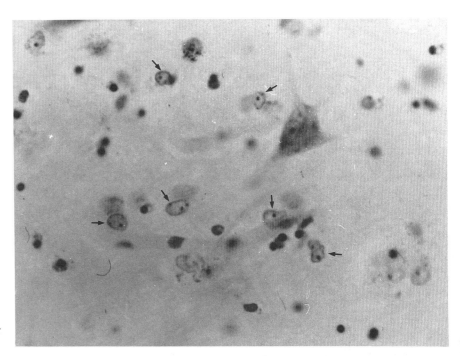

Fig. 19.3. Cerebral cortex in hepatic encephalopathy. Enlarged astrocyte nuclei (arrowed) with prominent nucleoli (Alzheimer type 2 glia) are present. H&E, ×350.

Wilson's disease (hepatolenticular degeneration)

This autosomal recessive disorder of copper metabolism produces degeneration principally in the corpus striatum of the brain. At post mortem the brain appears normal externally, but on slicing there is found to be shrinkage and brownish discoloration of the putamen and caudate nuclei. The putamen may contain cysts, and central white matter may also be softened and cystic. Microscopic examination should include sections of the putamen, caudate nucleus, thalamus, subthalamic nucleus, red nucleus, cerebral white matter and cortex, brain stem and cerebellum. Most marked changes are present in the putamen, which shows loss of neurons of various sizes and an abundance of astrocytes, which are remarkable for their enlarged, vesicular nuclei and prominent nucleoli (Fig. 19.3). In contrast, the astrocyte cytoplasm is inconspicuous. These cells are called Alzheimer type 2 glia. There may also be occasional larger, multinucleate glial cells (Alzheimer type 1 glia) (Fig. 19.4). Macrophages are present in and around any cystic or softened areas and in nearby perivascular spaces. They frequently contain fat and iron. Petechial haemorrhages or their residua are common, and capillaries appear prominent. Perivascular and parenchymal granular deposits of copper are demonstrable using the rhodanine or rubeanic acid stains. Similar changes to those seen in the putamen, though generally less severe, are found in the globus pallidus, thalamus and subthalamic nuclei. Opalski cells may also be seen in these regions. These are large cells with rounded cytoplasmic outline, granular cytoplasm, sometimes vacuolated, and small, darkly stained nucleus. Further sites of variable cell

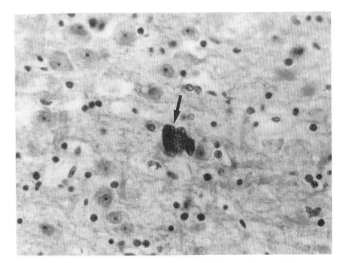

Fig. 19.4. Hepatolenticular degeneration (Wilson's disease). Section showing much enlarged, multilobular glial nucleus (arrowed) in the lateral geniculate body (Alzheimer type 1 glia). H&E, ×310.

loss and gliosis are the dentate nuclei and cerebral cortex. Calcification may occur in the floor of the fourth ventricle (Fig. 19.5). These pathological lesions may be modified following treatment with penicillamine. Some of the changes that are seen in Wilson's disease occur also in acquired forms of hepatic encephalopathy, but the copper deposition and the topographic emphasis of the pathology described above are particularly characteristic of Wilson's disease.

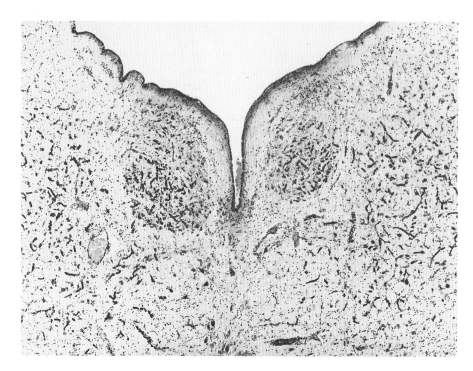

Fig. 19.5. Low-power view of a section of the medulla from a case of hepatolenticular degeneration (Wilson's disease). Capillaries in medullary nuclei in the floor of the fourth ventricle appear prominent because their walls are calcified. H&E, ×22.

Menkes' kinky hair disease (trichopoliodystrophy)

Unusual neuropathological changes are described in this rare, X-linked inherited disorder of copper metabolism. It presents in early infancy with failure to thrive, pallor and brittleness of the hair, hypothermia, mental retardation, and myoclonic epilepsy. The cerebrum at post mortem is atrophic and shows neuron and white matter loss with fibrillary gliosis. The most characteristic abnormality is in the cerebellum, where the Purkinje cells have expanded and distorted dendritic processes. Ultrastructurally there are abnormal mitochondria in muscle, and activity of the mitochondrial enzyme, cytochrome oxidase, is reduced.

Porphyria

There are no very specific changes in the brain in porphyria, though there are often non-specific foci of softening, considered to be ischaemic in origin. There is also a peripheral neuropathy, with 'dying back' of large axons and chromatolysis in anterior horn motor neurons. The spinal cord also shows degeneration of posterior column fibres.

Leigh's encephalopathy (infantile subacute necrotizing encephalopathy)

This is a rare condition resulting from a number of different biochemical defects, most of them as yet ill-defined, affecting mitochondrial function. This is reflected in a raised blood lactate level. It is usually familial, disease presenting in most cases in infancy or childhood, but occasionally in later

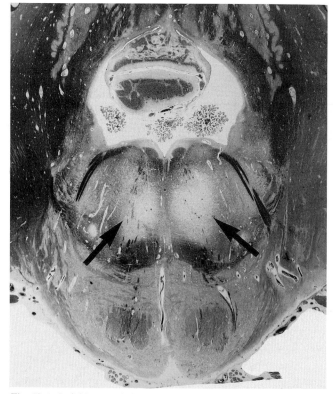

Fig. 19.6. Leigh's encephalopathy. Myelin-stained section of the lower pons showing symmetrical, focal areas of tissue rarefaction in the tegmentum (arrowed). ×2.5.

life. A wide range of neurological abnormalities occur, including hypotonia and respiratory disturbances. Post mortem the brain may appear normal macroscopically, or may show multiple small, symmetrical areas of softening with brownish discoloration. Microscopic sections should include cerebral cortex and white matter, deep-grey matter, brain stem, cerebellum and spinal cord. Of these, the brain stem is the most constantly affected part, and it should be examined in sections taken from at least four levels. The microscopic lesions are usually symmetrical, and predominate in the deep grey matter and brain stem (Fig. 19.6). They may also occur in the cerebral cortex and cerebellum. They closely resemble the lesions of Wernicke's encephalopathy (p.316), though their distribution is different, most notably in the way in which they spare the mamillary bodies. There is capillary proliferation and dilatation, well displayed with the PAS stain (Fig. 19.7), pericapillary haemorrhages and oedema. These vascular changes appear to antedate the neural ones. In the more chronic lesions there is haemosiderin deposition and pericapillary fibrosis (Fig. 19.8). In the most severe lesions there is some neuron loss, reactive astrocytosis, and a macrophage and microglial reaction. These foci differ from micro-infarcts in containing preserved neurons and in their different topography. Ultrastructural studies have shown abnormal mitochondrial structure in some cases in skeletal muscle and, in a few cases, in the brain.

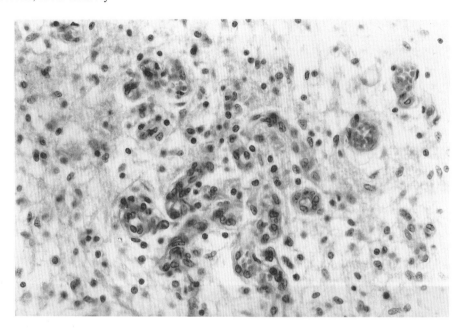

Fig. 19.7. Proliferated capillaries, with hyperplastic endothelium in an acute lesion from a case of Leigh's encephalopathy. PAS, ×235.

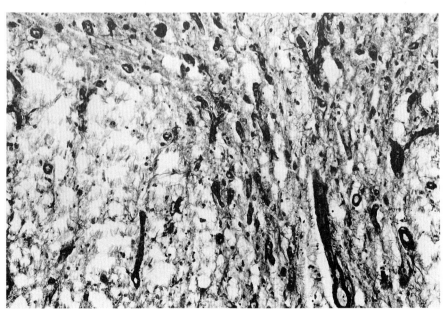

Fig. 19.8. Microscopic appearance of the lesion shown in Fig. 19.6. This is a long-standing lesion in which pericapillary fibrosis is prominent, and there is some rarefaction of the neuropil (left). In more recent lesions the nerve cells tend to be fairly well preserved. Holzer, ×100.

Hallervorden–Spatz disease

This is a rare, familial, slowly progressive disorder in which one noteworthy macroscopic change is found in the brain at post mortem: rusty-brown discoloration of the globus pallidus and reticular zone of the substantia nigra. In microscopic sections this can be seen to be due to deposition of brownish-yellow pigment in the cytoplasm of nerve cells, microglia and astrocytes. Extracellular pigment deposits are also present, particularly around blood vessels in the same areas. These deposits give a strong reaction for iron and are PAS-positive and Sudan-black-positive. Neurons are depleted in the globus pallidus and reticular zone of the substantia nigra and in some cases in the subthalamic nuclei and cerebellum (Purkinje cell layer and dentate nuclei), and reactive gliosis occurs at the same sites. A characteristic finding is of axonal swellings, appearing as round or oval bodies in a widespread distribution. The spinal cord may show pyramidal tract and posterior column fibre loss.

Neuro-axonal dystrophies are rare degenerative diseases in which axonal swellings similar to those seen in Hallervorden–Spatz disease are found widely distributed in the central and peripheral nervous system. These cases lack the pigment deposition characteristic of Hallervoden–Spatz disease.

Zellweger's cerebrohepatorenal syndrome

This is an uncommon autosomal recessive disorder of infancy in which there is a characteristic facial appearance and hepatomegaly progressing to cirrhosis, renal cysts and severe neurological abnormalities. The brain may show developmental abnormalities such as polymicrogyria, pachygyria or grey matter heterotopias (Chapter 16). There is also accumulation of neutral fat in astrocytes. EM studies of the liver in this condition show a deficiency of peroxisomes, and there is absence of certain peroxisomal enzymes, such as acyl CoA dihydroxyacetone phosphate acyltransferase in cultured fibroblasts.

Inherited metabolic diseases chiefly affecting white matter

In inherited white matter disorders there is diffuse and widespread, though not universal, degeneration of myelin. Fibres lying just below the cortex tend to be spared, and elsewhere the damage is seldom uniform. The cerebral white matter is usually the most severely affected, with cerebellar and brain stem white matter better preserved. In some disorders peripheral myelin as well as central white matter is affected. Sampling of tissues at post mortem should therefore include peripheral nerves as well as spinal cord and brain. Fresh frozen cryostat blocks should be prepared from cerebral white matter and peripheral nerves, and further frozen samples need to be stored if biochemical

analyses are to be carried out. Clinical suspicion of a disorder of white matter is likely to be present at the time of death, and a CAT scan may have added weight to that suspicion. However, occasional cases present post mortem, and the pathologist should suspect the presence of one of these diseases from the peculiar feel of the brain after removal. The surface looks and feels normal, but a curious sensation is imparted of woody hardness inside, which is produced by the intense white matter gliosis. In occasional cases, in contrast, the white matter is unduly soft.

Lysosomal disorders

Metachromatic leucodystrophy

There are three forms of metachromatic leucodystrophy, all autosomal recessive disorders, but differing in the age of onset and rate of progression. In the commonest, late infantile, variety there is progressive motor disability and later dementia. Some adult cases have a clinical diagnosis of schizophrenia.

Post mortem the brain appears normal or only slightly atrophic externally, but feels very abnormal. On slicing it after fixation there is found to be undue firmness and discoloration of the cerebral white matter. Cavitation is sometimes seen in the region of the lentiform nuclei and internal capsules. Microscopic sections show loss of myelin, with relative sparing of axons, diffuse gliosis (Fig. 19.9), and infiltration by macrophages, which in routine paraffin sections appear PAS-positive, and in cryostat sections can

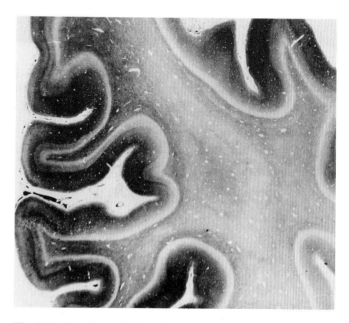

Fig. 19.9. Metachromatic leucodystrophy. Myelin-stained section of occipital cortex and white matter. The pale streak coincides with the 6th cortical layer. Most of the white matter myelin is lost, though some is preserved in the immediately subcortical layer.

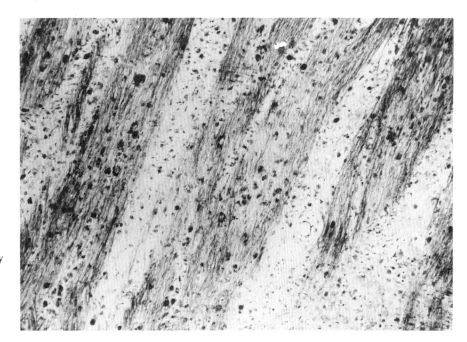

Fig. 19.10. Pontine bundles, showing partially preserved myelin sheaths, from a case of metachromatic leucodystrophy. The small, dark bodies are masses of metachromatic material. There are very few glial nuclei remaining. LBCV, ×130.

be shown to contain metachromatic, Alcian-blue-positive granules (Fig. 19.10), but no neutral fat. Although there is fibrillary gliosis, many neuroglial cell bodies disappear, imparting an air of desolation to the tissue. Metachromatic material (sulphatide) also accumulates in peripheral nerves and to some extent in the liver, gall bladder wall, and especially in the kidney. Deposits similar in nature to those found in the brain macrophages are also found in neurons in basal ganglia, brain stem and cerebellum, but not usually in cerebral cortex or peripheral ganglionic neurons. The ultrastructure of the stored cytoplasmic material is variable, but includes stacks of membranous discs, concentric or radial lamellae, paired membranes or zebra bodies. It consists chemically of sulphatide (cerebroside sulphate), and its accumulation is due to deficiency of arylsulphatase A. The diagnosis can be made by assaying the enzyme in blood leucocytes or cultured fibroblasts. A useful initial pointer to the diagnosis during life is provided by finding metachromatic granules in the urinary sediment.

Krabbe's leucodystrophy

This is a rare autosomal recessive disease with onset usually in early infancy, after normal development in the first few postnatal months. Neurological deficits are progressive, and epilepsy may occur. At post mortem the brain is usually small, and the white matter abnormally firm and discoloured (Figs 19.11 and 19.12). Microscopically there is severe myelin loss, with astrocytic gliosis and prominent collections of enlarged macrophages, including epithelioid and multinucleated globoid cells (Fig. 19.13 and Plate 7.3), but little or no neutral fat. Axons are relatively spared, but some are

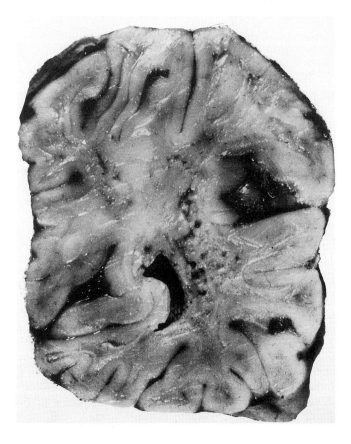

Fig. 19.11. Krabbe's leucodystrophy. Cerebral slice showing discoloration and central spongy degeneration of the white matter.

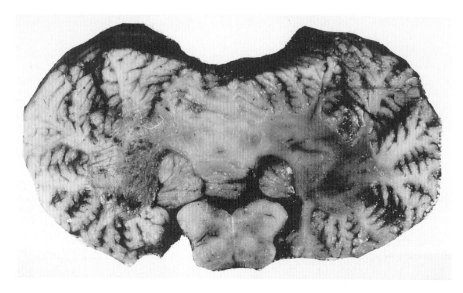

Fig. 19.12. Krabbe's leucodystrophy. Cerebellar hemispheres and medulla, showing white matter degeneration, and loss of the normal distinction between white and grey matter.

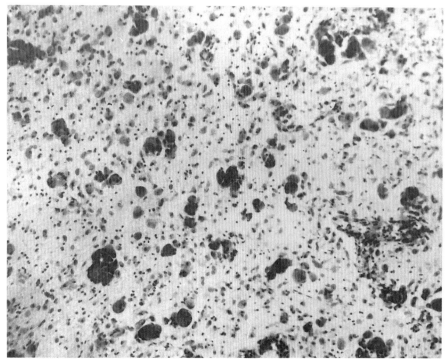

Fig. 19.13. Krabbe's leucodystrophy. Microscopic section of the white matter of the hippocampal gyrus, showing scattered and clustered epithelioid and globoid cells. PAS, ×250.

eventually lost, and oligodendrocytes disappear from the most severely affected parts of the white matter. Globoid cells are found chiefly in perivascular spaces. They are derived from macrophages and measure up to 50 μm across. Some are multinucleate. They contain PAS-positive cytoplasm, and in fresh-frozen sections are weakly sudanophilic, show no metachromasia and react strongly for acid phosphatase. EM of the stored material shows straight or curved tubular inclusions scattered or aggregated in globoid cell cytoplasm. Neurons do not contain obvious stored material, but there may be some neuron loss in dentate nuclei and among Purkinje cells of the cerebellum, and in some brain

stem nuclei, including the inferior olives. Peripheral nerves show segmental demyelination and increased acid phosphatase activity in Schwann cells but no collections of globoid cells. The enzyme which is deficient is lysosomal galactocerebroside-β-galactosidase. This can be assayed in blood leucocytes or cultured fibroblasts.

X-linked recessive leucodystrophies

Adrenoleucodystrophy

This is probably the most common form of sudanophilic leucodystrophy. Associated leucodystrophy and adrenal insufficiency in boys was its first recognized manifestation. There are now known to be infantile and adult varieties, not all sex-linked, as well as the juvenile form. Expression of the adrenal insufficiency is variable, and may occur only late in the course of the disease. Adult cases occur with cerebral disease or with a chronic myeloneuropathy, and females in affected families occasionally develop symptoms. In cases with cerebral disease the brain appears externally normal at post mortem, but on slicing shows diffuse white matter discoloration and firmness (Fig. 19.14). The most severe changes commonly occur in parieto-occipital and posterior temporal lobe white matter. Microscopically there is diffuse demyelination with relative, but far from complete, sparing of axons, and gliosis (Fig. 19.15). Macrophages containing sudanophilic material and reactive astrocytes are found in the affected white matter. There is also a prominent peri-vascular lymphocytic infiltrate, particularly at the sites of active myelin breakdown (Fig. 19.16.). In the spinal cord there may be loss of distal axons in pyramidal tracts and posterior columns, and these changes may be the only abnormality found in the nervous system in adrenomyelo-neuropathy (Fig. 19.17). Peripheral nerves show mild axonal loss. Macrophages in affected cerebral white matter and lymphoreticular tissue, Schwann cells in peripheral nerves, adrenal cortical cells and interstitial cells in the testis show typical ultrastructural cytoplasmic trilaminar inclusions (Fig. 19.18). The adrenal cortex is usually atrophic, and cortical cells have a fibrillary, or striated cytoplasmic appearance on microscopy. The enzyme defect has not been identified, but there is known to be an excess of very-long-chain fatty acids in serum and cultured fibroblasts, and assays of these allow a diagnosis to be made and heterozygotes to be identified. A non-X-linked form of the disease appears to be a peroxisomal disorder, and the same may be true of the X-linked form.

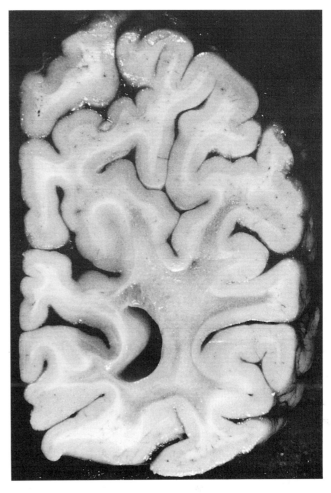

Fig. 19.14. Adrenoleucodystrophy. Granular discoloration of the parieto-occipital white matter.

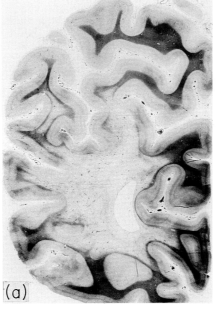

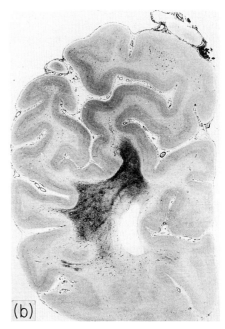

Fig. 19.15. Adrenoleucodystrophy. (a) Parieto-occipital white matter, extensively demyelinated. (b) Adjacent section, showing diffuse gliosis in the demyelinated white matter. (a) Myelin stain, (b) Holzer stain.

(a)

(b)

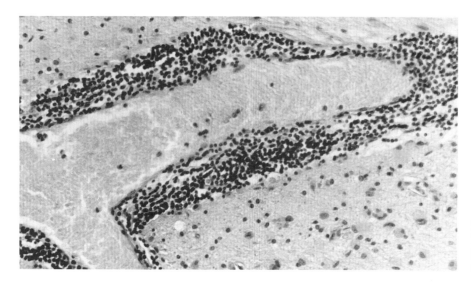

Fig. 19.16. Adrenoleucodystrophy. Prominent lymphocytic cuffing around a vein in the demyelinated white matter. Reactive astrocytes are seen bottom right. H&E, ×160.

Pelizaeus–Merzbacher disease

There are several recognized varieties of this rare disease, varying in age of onset and rate of progression. At post mortem examination the brain is frequently atrophic and the lateral ventricles dilated. White matter is discoloured and firm. Microscopically the white matter shows loss of myelin with some preservation of axons, reactive gliosis, but only rare macrophages which contain sparse sudanophilic material. The loss of myelin is not uniform, but shows characteristic preservation of myelin around blood vessels. Oligodendrocytes disappear from the demyelinated zones. Absence of proteolipid apoprotein has recently been demonstrated in the CNS in this disease. The peripheral myelin, which normally lacks this protein, is unaffected.

Other forms of sudanophilic leucodystrophy

Cases of diffuse and widespread myelin loss, apparently sporadic or familial, are seen from time to time in which no distinguishing features of diagnostic significance are present. Macrophages in areas of myelin breakdown contain neutral fat. Most such cases show no consistent abnormalities outside the CNS. Better characterization of these cases awaits biochemical analysis. The diagnosis is made largely by exclusion of other, better-defined diseases causing sudanophilic breakdown of CNS myelin, including the Schilder type of MS (Chapter 14).

Spongiform leucodystrophy (Canavan's type of diffuse sclerosis)

This is a rare familial disease affecting infants or children, who develop enlargement of the head, mental retardation and spastic weakness. The centrum semiovale is the most

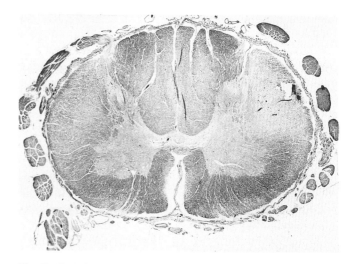

Fig. 19.17. Adrenoleucodystrophy. Transverse section of cervical spinal cord, showing pallor of myelin staining due to loss of fibres in lateral corticospinal tracts and posterior columns.

severely affected region, and it shows demyelination and a spongy state with vacuoles intersected by a meshwork of glial and axonal processes. The grey matter is relatively well preserved, but contains astrocytes with swollen, lobulated nuclei, similar to Alzheimer type 2 glia.

Cockayne's syndrome

This is an autosomal recessive disease commencing in late infancy, and characterized by dwarfism, cataracts, retinal pigmentation, optic atrophy, deafness, mental retardation, pyramidal and extrapyramidal motor disorders, ataxia and peripheral neuropathy. The skull is abnormally thick, and the brain small and covered in thickened leptomeninges. On slicing the brain there is a gritty texture due to extensive

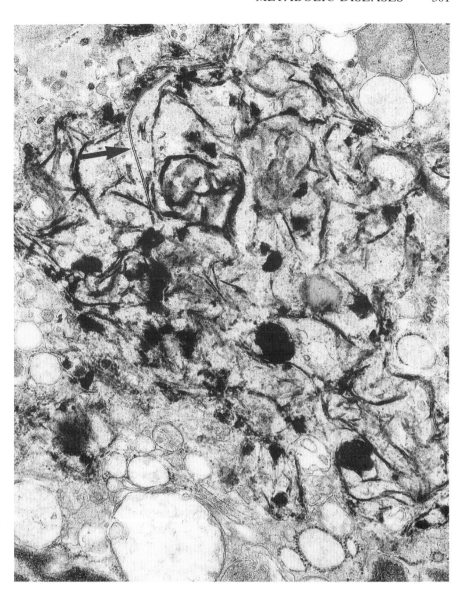

Fig. 19.18. Electron micrograph of the cytoplasm of a macrophage in the white matter in a cerebral biopsy from a case of adrenoleucodystrophy. There are characteristic trilaminar inclusions (arrowed). Uranyl acetate and lead citrate, ×43 000.

calcification of blood vessels, particularly in the basal ganglia. Both grey and white matter are reduced in amount, and the ventricles dilated in compensation for this. Microscopically, apart from the vascular calcification, there is patchy demyelination of cerebral white matter, and a deficiency of Purkinje and granule cells in the cerebellum. The pathogenesis of the disease is unknown.

Cerebrotendinous xanthomatosis

This is an autosomal recessive disease presenting in late childhood with progressive dementia and cerebellar ataxia. There is a defect in the synthesis of bile acid, and overproduction of cholesterol, which is converted to dihydrocholesterol, in which form it is deposited in tissues, including the brain. A pathological study reported softening and discoloration of the cerebellar white matter macroscopically,

and clefts resulting from dissolved cholesterol crystals in white matter accompanied by a macrophage and foreign-body giant-cell reaction microscopically.

Lipoprotein deficiencies

These are autosomal recessive conditions. Low-density lipoprotein deficiency (abetalipoproteinaemia, Bassen–Kornzweig syndrome) is characterized clinically by retinal degeneration, progressive neurological symptoms, acantho-cytosis and fat malabsorption. Demyelination has been described in long tracts of the spinal cord and peripheral nerves, with some loss of neurons in the motor cortex and anterior horns of the spinal cord. In high-density lipoprotein deficiency (Tangier disease) there may be a severe peripheral neuropathy, with axonal degeneration and accumulation of lipid-containing macrophages in nerves.

Sporadic metabolic diseases chiefly affecting grey matter

Non-wilsonian hepatic encephalopathy

In some patients dying of chronic or acute-on-chronic liver disease there are no naked-eye abnormalities in the brain other than a variable degree of generalized swelling. However, there are frequently microscopic changes attributable to liver disease. Astrocytes are increased in number and contain enlarged, lobulated vesicular nuclei (Alzheimer type 2 glia) (Fig. 19.3). These altered astrocytes are most frequently seen in the deep layers of the cerebral cortex, subcortical white matter, basal ganglia, thalamus, hypothalamus, and deep cerebellar grey and white matter. Some of these sites should be sampled for microscopy from cases of possible hepatic encephalopathy. There is also frequently a microcystic or spongy appearance in the deep cerebral cortex, with patchy necrosis and neuronal loss (Fig. 19.19), and widespread eosinophilic shrinkage of the cell bodies of some remaining neurons (Fig. 19.20). This change may proceed to necrosis in cortical layers 5 and 6, and may also involve subcortical white matter. Experimental work in animals has shown that the histological changes of hepatic encephalopathy can be produced by raising the blood ammonia level.

In addition to the cerebral changes, a peripheral neuropathy of predominantly demyelinating type has been described in hepatic failure. In practice, in an individual case of chronic liver disease due to alcoholism it is usually impossible to dissociate effects on peripheral nerves of thiamine deficiency from those due to liver disease.

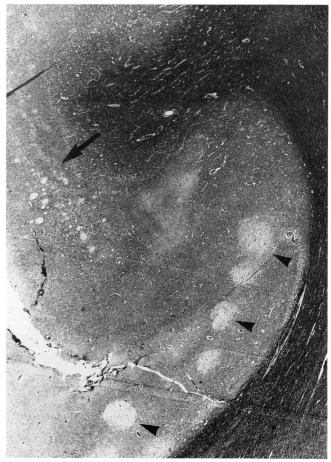

Fig. 19.19. Low-power view of cerebral cortex from a child with hepatic encephalopathy. There is patchy necrosis (arrow heads) and cortical oedema (arrowed). PTAH, ×2.5.

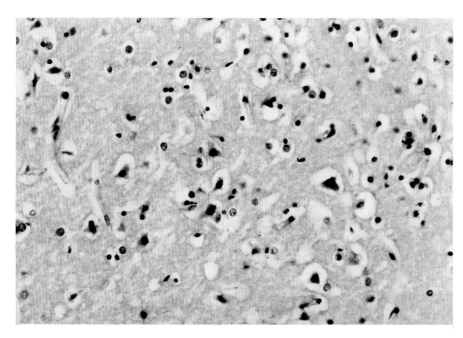

Fig. 19.20. Shrinkage of neurons, and oedema in the deep cortex from a case of hepatic encephalopathy. H&E, ×190.

Reye's syndrome

This is an acute disease of infants and children which should always be considered when performing a post mortem examination on a child who has died after a fulminating illness with epilepsy and coma. There is epidemiological evidence linking the disease to preceding acute viral infections, especially influenza or varicella, and with salicylate ingestion. In the course of the illness, liver function is abnormal and there is hyperammonaemia and hypoglycaemia. Post mortem there is panlobular, microvesicular fat deposited in liver hepatocytes, and a diffusely swollen brain, often with herniation. Microscopically the brain shows acute eosinophilic shrinkage of neurons in grey matter, sometimes affecting the cortex in a laminar distribution, and with associated oedema but no inflammation (Fig. 19.21). It is not clear whether the changes in the brain are wholly attributable to an acute derangement of liver function, hypoxia associated with swelling or hypoglycaemia, or whether there is also a primary metabolic brain abnormality. Mitochondrial structure has appeared abnormal in both neurons and hepatocytes in ultrastructural studies.

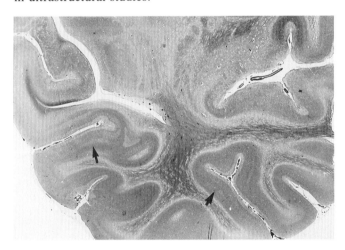

Fig. 19.21. Reye's syndrome. Low-power view of cortex and white matter, showing oedema of deep cortex and subcortical white matter, with some additional, patchy necrosis in more superficial layers of the cortex (arrowed). PTAH.

Hypoglycaemia

It is uncommon to find structural changes in the adult brain attributable to hypoglycaemia unless this has been profound and prolonged, as occurs after an overdose of insulin, or occasionally in patients with an insulin-producing islet cell tumour. Babies of low birth-weight may also suffer brain damage due to hypoglycaemia. In these circumstances the pathological changes in the brain are similar to those found in hypoxia (p.46). Neurons in the cerebral cortex, particularly in layers 3 and 5, are likely to show acute hypoxic

change, or to have disappeared, depending how much time has elapsed between the episode of hypoglycaemia and death. The hippocampus and deep grey matter may be similarly affected. Damage in the cortex tends to be worst at the depths of sulci (Fig. 7.5), as in hypoxia. The cerebellar Purkinje cells are only slightly less susceptible to hypoglycaemia than to hypoxia.

Calcification of the basal ganglia

A mild degree of calcification in the walls of blood vessels in the basal ganglia is a common incidental finding in elderly brains. Occasionally it is much more severe, occurs more widely in the brain and is associated with clinical disturbances, chiefly extrapyramidal movement disorders. This is seen mainly in patients who are suffering from hypoparathyroidism, but it is also seen in those with mitochondrial cytopathies, Albright's hereditary osteodystrophy, or Cockayne's syndrome (see above), and in some patients without a demonstrable endocrine disorder. Calcification, in all these cases, occurs most heavily in the basal ganglia, internal capsules, lateral thalamic nuclei and dentate nuclei of the cerebellum (Figs 19.22–19.24). Also affected are the cerebral and cerebellar cortex. It is apparent on slicing the brain, as it imparts a gritty resistance to the knife. Calcium deposits occur in the walls of capillaries as tiny calcospherites and more diffusely in larger vessel walls. The surrounding nervous tissue is destroyed but there is little glial or inflammatory reaction.

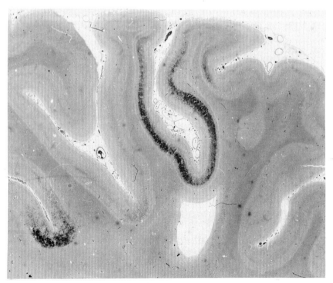

Fig. 19.22. Cerebral calcification, with deposits of calcium in the cortex appearing as dark streaks.

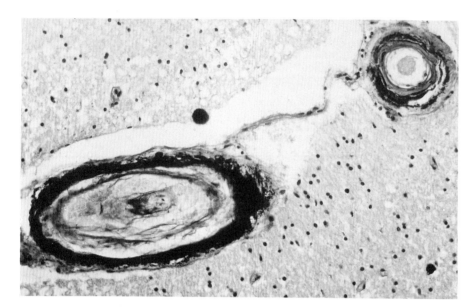

Fig. 19.23. Vascular calcification in a case of cerebral calcification with no predisposing factors. There is little cellular reaction. H&E, ×80.

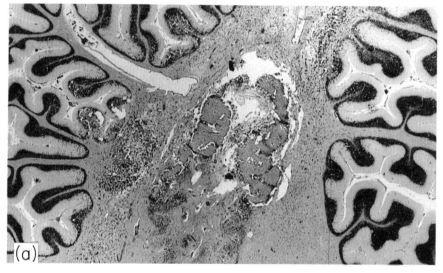

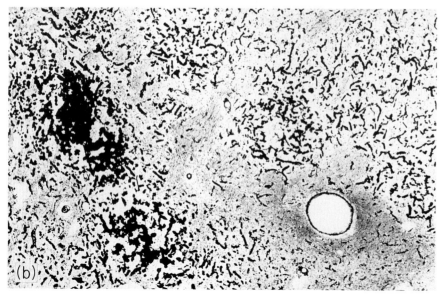

Fig. 19.24. Very extensive calcification in the dentate nucleus of the cerebellum: (a) low-power view; (b) higher power to show that small vessels are heavily affected. (a) H&E, ×9; (b) H&E, ×60.

Sporadic metabolic diseases chiefly affecting white matter

Alexander's disease

This is a rare, sporadic disease occurring in infants or children and presenting with progressive psychomotor retardation and epilepsy. At post mortem the brain tends to be larger than normal, and the cortical ribbon is relatively well preserved. The white matter is soft, almost jelly-like, and discoloured. Microscopically the white matter shows rarefaction with loss of myelin and of some of the axons. The brain stem is less severely affected. The distinctive feature is the presence of vast numbers of Rosenthal fibres (p.174), elongated, hyaline, eosinophilic structures, staining strongly with PTAH (Fig. 19.25). Many of these are oriented around blood vessels and pial and ependymal surfaces. The basic defect in this disease is not known.

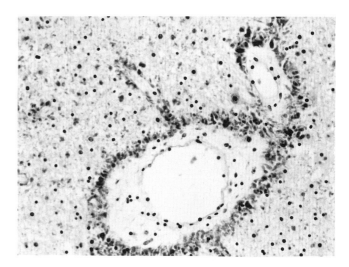

Fig. 19.25. Alexander's disease. Blood vessel in cerebral white matter, intensely rimmed with Rosenthal fibres. H&E, ×205.

Central pontine myelinolysis

This is a rare, sporadic disease affecting adults who are alcoholics or are suffering from a variety of other disorders such as carcinoma, severe malnutrition or chronic renal, pulmonary or hepatic disease. Symptoms and signs of a pontine lesion have usually been present for a few days before death. The lesion consists of a circumscribed zone of demyelination in the central part of the upper pons, involving the pontine nuclei and white matter of the base of the pons, but sparing the subpial and periventricular regions (Fig. 19.26). In the affected area there is loss of myelin with preservation of axons and neuron cell bodies, an important distinction from pontine infarcts. Cases that have survived several days may show softening in the centre of the lesion, and macrophages containing neutral fat infiltrating the area. Oligodendrocytes are lost, but astrocytes survive, and appear reactive. A rapid rise in plasma sodium following treatment to correct an initially low level is thought to play a key role in the development of this lesion.

Marchiafava—Bignami disease

This is a disorder described occasionally in chronic alcoholics, most of them heavy drinkers of red wine. A sharply circumscribed band of demyelination is present in the corpus callosum in this disease. It sometimes extends to the neighbouring white matter of the centrum ovale. Axons are relatively, but not completely, spared, and there is reactive gliosis and vascular proliferation in the area affected. Other white-matter tracts besides the corpus callosum are occasionally involved, such as the anterior commissure or the middle cerebellar peduncles. A toxic contaminant of red wine has been suspected of being the cause, but this has not been confirmed.

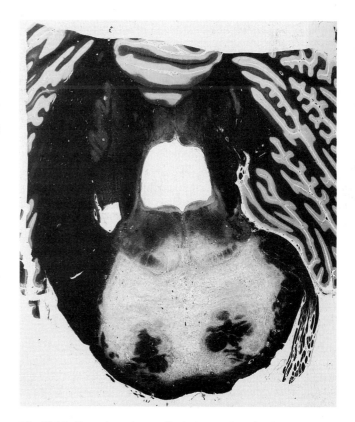

Fig. 19.26. Central pontine myelinolysis. Myelin-stained section of the pons, demonstrating extensive loss of myelin from the central region of the base of the pons. The myelin sheaths in the corticospinal tract bundles are less affected than the transversely running fibre bundles.

Further reading

Becker LE, Yates A. 1985. Inherited metabolic disease. In Davis RL, Robertson DM (Eds) *Textbook of Neuropathology*. Williams and Wilkins, Baltimore, pp. 372–402.

Lake BD. 1983. Metabolic disorders of the central and peripheral nervous systems. In Felipe MI, Lake BD (Eds) *Histochemistry in Pathology*. Churchill Livingstone, Edinburgh, pp. 53–69.

Lake BD. 1984. Lysosomal enzyme deficiencies. In Adams JH, Corsellis JAN, Duchen LW (Eds) *Greenfield's Neuropathology*, 4th edn. Edward Arnold, London, pp. 491–572.

Schutgens RBH, Heymans HSA, Wanders RJA *et al.* 1986. Peroxisomal disorders: a newly recognized group of genetic diseases. *Eur J Pediatr* **144**, 430–40.

Watts, RWE, Gibbs DA. 1986. *Lysosomal Storage Diseases: Biochemical and Clinical Aspects*. Taylor and Francis, London.

Chapter 20
Intoxications and Nutritional Diseases of the Nervous System

Intoxications

Puzzling cases of neurological disease, particularly peripheral neuropathies, often raise the possibility of a toxic cause for the patient's condition. It is always worth while examining the clinical notes to find out about possible exposures to toxic chemicals, including social and therapeutic drugs, in any case of undiagnosed neurological disease. No harm will be done if samples of liver, kidney, hair, urine and serum are taken at the time of post mortem and preserved deep-frozen in case the need arises at a later stage of investigation for biochemical assays.

It can be frustratingly difficult to pin down a toxic cause for neurological disease. In many instances the alterations produced by toxins on the nervous system, particularly in acute poisoning, are non-specific and of little diagnostic value. Furthermore, some exert an effect on the nervous system only indirectly. Valproate, for example, may cause liver damage and present with hepatic encephalopathy. Even so, some toxins produce pathological changes which are at least suggestive, and which may encourage further exploration of the circumstances of the patient's illness, and enable a toxic cause to be uncovered. The potential sources of exposure to toxins are perpetually increasing with alterations in social habits, drug prescribing and the manufacture of new chemicals and drugs, so that a constant awareness of the possibility of toxic damage to the nervous system needs to be maintained. Advice on the effects of toxins on the nervous system may be obtained from regional poisons centres (see Appendix 2 for some addresses). Detailed neuropathological studies of some commonly fatal toxic disorders which clearly affect the nervous system clinically are surprisingly sparse. It is important that such changes as

do occur should be carefully documented, particularly in newly described intoxications.

The pathologist may be called upon to answer two different types of question regarding cases of possible toxic nervous system disease. Firstly, a patient may have had a neurological disease of uncertain cause, and the question arises: could this be due to a poison? Secondly, the patient may be known to have been exposed to a particular poison, and the question to be answered is: does the nervous system show the expected changes caused by that poison? To answer questions of the first type it is necessary to scan the brain and the rest of the nervous system macroscopically and microscopically for lesions and, depending on the pattern of changes found, suggest possible causes for them. Of course, causes other than toxins will also need to be considered. If macroscopical lesions are not apparent, it is important to examine microscopically sections from several different parts of the nervous system: cerebral cortex and white matter, deep cerebral grey matter, brain stem, cerebellum (vermis and hemisphere), spinal cord, peripheral nerves and muscles. Tables 7.1, 15.2 and 22.1 should be referred to when trying to identify possible toxic causes of specific lesions that may be discovered in attempting to answer questions of the first type. When tackling the second type of question, in which a specific toxin is implicated, it is important to be aware of how toxic substances affect nervous tissue, and their often special selectivity for certain regions or systems. Sections for microscopy should be prepared from sites known to be at risk of damage. Table 20.1 summarizes the chief sites of damage in the various conditions considered in this chapter.

Many toxins produce their effects on cells by impairing their energy production. Neurons with very long axons are particularly dependent on a continuous supply of energy to

Table 20.1. Summary of lesions found in the nervous system in some intoxications

Toxin (and context in which intoxication seen)	Nervous system lesions
Acrylamide (industrial exposure)	*Peripheral neuropathy* with axonal degeneration and argyrophilic axonal swellings containing neurofilaments
Alcohol (ethyl) (excess intake)	Most effects probably due to associated nutritional deficiency, especially thiamine deficiency, *Wernicke's encephalopathy* (p.316); *cerebellar degeneration* (p.317); *peripheral neuropathy* with axonal degeneration (p.317); excess maternal intake may cause *fetal alcohol syndrome* (p.310). Rare complication: *Marchiafava–Bignami disease* (p.305), *central pontine myelinolysis* (p.305). Also risk of *repeated head injuries, cerebrovascular accidents* and *hepatic encephalopathy*
Amiodarone (treatment of arrhythmias)	*Peripheral neuropathy* with segmental demyelination and secondary axonal loss; presence of lipid-containing dense bodies in Schwann cells, perineurial and endothelial cells
Aluminium (renal dialysis)	No specific structural changes in 'dialysis dementia'; possible relationship to Alzheimer's disease (p.271) under investigation.
Arsenic (trivalent) (suicide, homicide)	Acute: no specific changes; chronic: distal sensorimotor *peripheral neuropathy* with predominant axonal degeneration (p.310)
Arsenic (pentavalent) (treatment of trypanosomiasis)	*Haemorrhagic encephalopathy*; occasional predominant motor *peripheral neuropathy* (p.310)
Botulinum toxin (ingestion of contaminated canned or bottled foods)	Preterminal nerve sprouting at motor end-plates in experimental animals (p.310)
Buckthorn toxin (fruit of desert plant)	Motor *peripheral neuropathy* with predominant segmental demyelination
Carbon monoxide (intentional or accidental exposure to gas produced by incomplete burning of fuel under conditions of inadequate ventilation)	*Cystic necrosis of inner segment of globus pallidus*; hypoxic change in cerebral cortex hippocampus and Purkinje cells; white matter damage (p.310)
Carbon disulphide (industrial exposure)	*Peripheral neuropathy* with giant axonal neuropathy
Chloroquine (treatment of malaria or autoimmune disease)	*Peripheral neuropathy* (rare) with axonal degeneration and lysosomal inclusions; also myopathy
cis-platinum (treatment of cancer)	Sensory *peripheral neuropathy* with axonal degeneration
Clioquinol (treatment of diarrhoea)	*SMON (subacute optic nerve degeneration), myelopathy and peripheral neuropathy* (p.311)
Cyanide (acute: suicide, homicide; chronic: diet high in cassava, possible effect of tobacco)	Acute: *haemorrhagic encephalopathy*; chronic: *myelopathy and peripheral neuropathy* (p.311)
Diphtheria toxin (synthesized by some phage-infected strains of *Corynebacterium diphtheriae*)	Predominant motor *peripheral neuropathy* with segmental demyelination; also heart arrhythmias (p.312)
Disulphiram (Antabuse) (treatment of alcoholism)	Distal *peripheral neuropathy* with axonal degeneration
Gold salts (treatment of rheumatoid arthritis)	*Peripheral neuropathy* with segmental demyelination and axonal degeneration
Hexacarbon solvents (glue sniffers)	*Peripheral neuropathy* with giant axonal neuropathy (p.312)
Hexachlorophane (antiseptic used in nurseries)	*Encephalopathy* with white matter oedema (p.312)
Isoniazid (treatment of tuberculosis)	*Peripheral neuropathy* with axonal degeneration (p.312)
Lathyrism (diet of chick peas during famine)	*Myelopathy* with degeneration of distal corticospinal tracts and posterior columns (p.313)
Lead (formerly industrial exposure; also in soft water in lead pipes; ingested by infants in paint; low levels in petrol)	Acute: *encephalopathy* with cerebral oedema; chronic: motor *peripheral neuropathy*, segmental demyelination, axonal degeneration, and endoneurial oedema (p.313)
Manganese (occupational exposure in miners)	*Encephalopathy* with neuron loss and gliosis in striatum, and other deep grey matter (p.313)

Table 20.1. (*continued*)

Toxin (and context in which intoxication seen)	Nervous system lesions
Mercury (inorganic) (formerly in proprietary medicines)	*Peripheral neuropathy* with axonal degeneration, or damage to cerebellar cortex (p.313)
Mercury (organic) (contamination of food)	*Encephalopathy* with damage to small neurons in visual, auditory and somatosensory cortex and granule cells of cerebellum; also *peripheral neuropathy* with axonal degeneration
Methotrexate (treatment of cancer, if combined with cranial irradiation)	*Encephalopathy* with white matter necrosis (p.313)
Methyl alcohol (contaminant of ethyl alcohol)	*Encephalopathy* with cerebral oedema and petechial haemorrhages; sometimes necrosis of retinal ganglion cells, putamen and all layers of cerebellar cortex (p.313)
Metronidazole (treatment of infections)	*Peripheral neuropathy* with axonal degeneration
MPTP (contamination of opiates)	*Subacute encephalopathy* with loss of cells in substantia nigra (p.314)
Nitrofurantoin (antibacterial drug)	*Peripheral neuropathy* with axonal degeneration
Opiates (drug abusers)	Usually no specific changes
Organophosphorus compounds (mainly contamination of food; also industrial exposure)	*Peripheral neuropathy* with axonal degeneration and *myelopathy* (p.314)
Perhexiline (treatment of angina pectoris)	*Peripheral neuropathy* with predominant segmental demyelination and variable axonal loss
Tetanus toxin (soil contamination of skin wounds, umbilical stump)	Vacuolation of lower motor neurons and intermediolateral column neurons; preterminal motor nerve sprouting in experimental animals (p.315)
Thallium (ingestion of rodent and ant pesticides; homicide)	*Peripheral neuropathy* with axonal degeneration and loss of sensory ganglion cells; hair loss (p.315)
Toluene (glue sniffers)	Clinical evidence of *encephalopathy*. No pathology described
Trichloroethylene (dry cleaning agent, former anaesthetic agent)	*Encephalopathy* with damage to cranial nerves and nuclei (p.315)
Triethyl tin (contamination of proprietary medicine)	*Encephalopathy*; white matter oedema in experimental studies (p.316)
Vincristine (treatment of cancer)	*Peripheral neuropathy* with axonal degeneration and hyaline neurofilamentous inclusions in sensory ganglion and CNS neurons

maintain their very extensive cytoplasmic and surface membrane structure. It is frequently the structural integrity of these neurons that is most at risk from the effects of toxins. Because the blood–brain barrier often restricts entry of toxins to the CNS, large neurons here may be to some extent protected from their effects, so that it is the large peripheral sensory neurons (whose cell bodies in sensory ganglia are not protected by any vascular barrier) and motor axons that are most commonly affected by many toxins. Some of the toxins that solely affect the nervous system in this selective way are listed in Table 15.2, but most of these toxins are not further considered in the text. Some assistance when dealing with cases affected in this way may be obtained by consulting Chapter 22, and the section on nerve biopsies in Chapter 4. It should be noted that many toxins selectively affect *distal* peripheral nerves, and it is therefore essential that these are sampled if the pathology is to be identified. The rest of this chapter provides an alphabetical summary of other common toxins known to exert an adverse effect on the nervous system.

Alcohol

Effects of chronic excess alcohol on the nervous system are largely attributable to deficiencies, particularly thiamine (vitamin B_1) deficiency, to which alcoholics are peculiarly susceptible (see below). This gives rise to Wernicke's encephalopathy and possibly to the cerebellar degeneration found in some alcoholics. Alcoholic peripheral neuropathy is also due to nutritional deficiency. These deficiencies are due partly to an inadequate diet, partly to the increased need for thiamine that metabolism of alcohol demands, and possibly to a reduced absorption of thiamine from the gut in patients with gastritis. No specific neuropathological changes have been found in the cerebral cortex in alcoholics, although reversible 'atrophy' has been described in CAT scans.

Patients with cirrhosis of the liver may develop the clinical and pathological features of hepatic encephalopathy (p.302). Exceptionally, the changes of Marchiafava–Bignami disease (p.305) are found. Central pontine myelinolysis (p.305) is occasionally found in alcoholics but may have other causes. Amblyopia in smokers and alcoholics has been attributed to chronic cyanide intoxication (see below). Alcoholics are also at extra risk from head injuries (Chapter 5) and cerebrovascular accidents (Chapter 7).

In the *fetal alcohol syndrome*, from which infants exposed *in utero* may suffer, there is a characteristic facial appearance with short palpebral fissures, flattened nose and maxilla, and wide mouth. Various brain malformations (Chapter 16) are encountered in this syndrome. These include microencephaly, hydrocephalus, grey matter heterotopias, agenesis of the corpus callosum, schizencephaly and cerebellar malformations.

For the effects of methyl alcohol intoxication see p.313.

Aluminium

Encephalopathy with dementia occurs in some renal dialysis patients who are treated with dialysis water containing high levels of aluminium. No specific neuropathological changes occur in such cases, though non-specific features of neuronal shrinkage and reactive astrocytosis in white matter are described.

There is considerable interest in the possible involvement of aluminium in the pathogenesis of Alzheimer's disease (p.271). Aluminosilicates have been described in the cores of the argyrophilic plaques which develop in the cortex in that disease, and in neuronal nuclei, but it is not certain whether these deposits have a primary role in the disease or occur as a secondary consequence of the degenerative changes. Aluminium salts by direct injection have been experimentally shown to cause abnormal accumulation of neurofilaments in neuron cell bodies, but these do not have the ultrastructural characteristics of the neurofibrillary tangles of Alzheimer's disease.

Arsenic

Chronic trivalent arsenic intoxication causes a peripheral sensory neuropathy with a minor motor component. Peripheral nerves show predominant wallerian degeneration, especially in the distal limb nerves. Pentavalent organic arsenic, used formerly to treat syphilis and still employed against trypanosomiasis, may cause an acute encephalopathy in which petechial haemorrhages and foci of haemorrhagic necrosis occur. In some cases the changes found were thought to be identical to those of acute haemorrhagic leucoencephalitis (p.154). Occasionally there is also a predominantly motor neuropathy resembling acute inflammatory polyneuropathy (Guillain–Barré syndrome) (p.337). These

manifestations of toxicity are probably related to the development of an Arthus-type hypersensitivity response.

Botulinum toxin

This exotoxin of *Clostridium botulinum* is occasionally ingested in contaminated food, and causes paralysis by blocking release of acetylcholine at neuromuscular junctions. Structural changes in motor end-plates in humans have not been described, perhaps because death occurs too rapidly for these to occur, but in experimental animals the toxin produces sprouting of terminal motor axons.

Carbon monoxide

Sources of carbon monoxide in the environment are numerous, and relate chiefly to the burning of fuel under conditions of insufficient ventilation and incomplete combustion. Poisoning is seen in subjects exposed to motor vehicle exhaust in a closed environment, improperly ventilated household heaters, and burning buildings and furniture. If acute carbon monoxide poisoning is suspected, a blood sample should be sent for analysis of the carboxyhaemoglobin content. In acute carbon monoxide poisoning, the brain, along with other viscera, muscle and skin are a deep pink–red colour and the leptomeninges are congested. Petechial

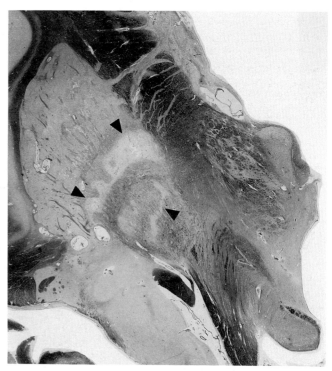

Fig. 20.1. Low-power view of the basal ganglia from a case of acute carbon monoxide poisoning. Irregular areas of necrosis are detectable as pallor in the outer segment and, to a lesser extent, the inner segment of the globus pallidus (arrow heads). At a later stage these areas might have been expected to become cystic. Myelin stain.

or larger haemorrhages are common, particularly in the cerebral white matter. There are characteristic alterations in the basal ganglia, which take at least 24 hours to become apparent, that take the form of well-circumscribed softenings, most commonly lying in the inner segment of the globus pallidus; they are usually bilateral (Fig. 20.1). Laminar cortical necrosis and acute hypoxic change (p.46) are frequently seen in the cerebral cortex, hippocampus and Purkinje cell layer of the cerebellum. White matter lesions are also common, and may accompany the grey matter changes or occur independently of them. They consist of microscopic foci of demyelination, mainly perivascular in distribution, or occurring as larger plaques or diffuse areas of myelin loss in cerebral white matter. Axons are relatively spared in some cases, and there is an associated astrocytic reaction. Old lesions are well demarcated from surrounding white matter.

Clioquinol

Used for treatment of 'travellers' diarrhoea', clioquinol has been found, when given in excessively large doses, to be responsible for a serious neurological disease with peripheral neuropathy, visual disturbances and an acute encephalopathy with prominent amnesia (subacute myelo-optico neuropathy, SMON). Pathological studies, chiefly from Japan, have shown grey matter oedema and white matter astrocytosis with, in the spinal cord, symmetrical posterior column fibre loss, some degeneration of spinocerebellar fibres and loss of distal corticospinal tract fibres (Fig. 20.2). In the peripheral nervous system there is degeneration of sensory and autonomic ganglion cells, secondary increase in satellite cells in ganglia, and axonal degeneration in posterior roots and peripheral nerves (Fig. 20.3). The optic tracts show loss of axons, particularly distally, close to the lateral geniculate bodies (Fig. 20.4). Neurons in the inner ganglion cell layer of the retina are selectively damaged.

Cyanide

In acute cyanide poisoning there is congestion of the brain with occasional petechial haemorrhages. If death is delayed, there may be small white matter haemorrhages and loss of cerebellar Purkinje cells and cortical neurons, with associated reactive gliosis.

Chronic cyanide poisoning has been suggested as an explanation of some cases of tropical neuromyelopathy in communities whose staple diet is cassava, a plant which contains cyanogenetic glycosides. Pathological studies of the CNS in such cases are not available.

Amblyopia associated with smoking and alcoholism in western countries and with cassava-eating in the tropics has also been attributed to chronic cyanide poisoning. Severe cases show loss of myelin in central parts of the optic nerves and of ganglion cells in the retina.

Diphenylhydantoin (phenytoin, Epanutin)

Loss of Purkinje cells and gliosis in the cerebellum have been ascribed to the effects of prolonged treatment of epilepsy with this drug. Others regard it as more likely that the cerebellar damage is a consequence of the epilepsy itself, or of hypoxia occurring during the fits. It is also possible that all these factors contribute to the Purkinje cell loss, which undoubtedly occurs in epileptics on Epanutin (see also Chapter 18). Phenytoin administration to animals has not resulted in Purkinje cell damage.

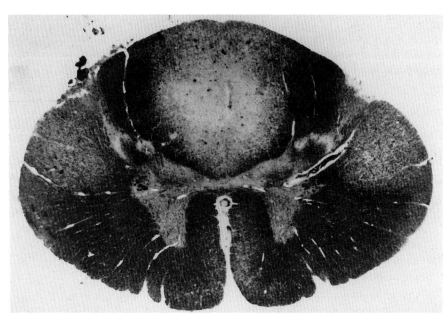

Fig. 20.2. Clioquinol intoxication. Transverse section of the cervical spinal cord showing degeneration in posterior columns (chiefly the gracile tracts), and crossed and uncrossed corticospinal tracts. Myelin stain. (Courtesy of Prof. H. Shiraki.)

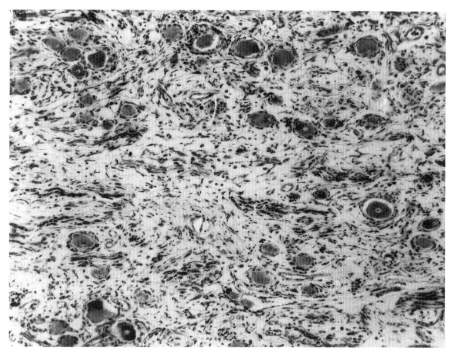

Fig. 20.3 (*above*). Clioquinol intoxication. Appearance of a sensory ganglion in which there is loss of ganglion cells and proliferation of satellite cells. H&E, ×108. (Courtesy of Prof. H. Shiraki.)

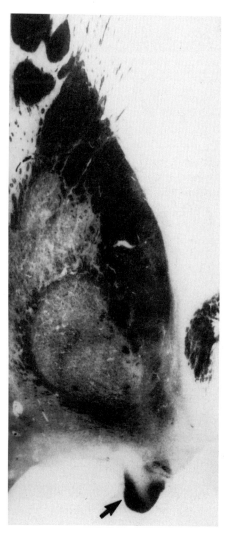

Fig. 20.4 (*right*). Clioquinol intoxication. Section showing loss of staining for myelinated axons in part of the optic tract (arrowed). (Courtesy of Prof. H. Shiraki.)

Diphtheria toxin

This is a toxin elaborated under certain conditions by a phage which infects some strains of *Corynebacterium diphtheriae*. It produces a predominantly motor neuropathy with characteristic segmental demyelination of peripheral nerves, sensory ganglia and nerve roots. During natural infection the early effects are often confined to the cranial nerves, but later may also become more generalized. The conducting system of the heart may be affected, rendering it susceptible to arrhythmias, bundle branch block or heart block.

Glue or solvent sniffing

This unwholesome habit entails exposure to organic solvents such as hexacarbons including toluene (see below). A very chronic peripheral neuropathy has been described as a result of some forms of *hexacarbon solvent* intoxication, in which distal axonal degeneration and marked axonal swel-

lings containing neurofilaments occur. These are likely to be found if peripheral nerves are examined post mortem. Affected fibres are intensely argyrophilic, as well as swollen, and many of the swellings can be shown, in teased fibre preparations, to lie proximal to the nodes of Ranvier. CNS lesions have rarely been described.

Hexachlorophane

This antiseptic has caused an encephalopathy in which there was marked white matter oedema, appearing as a spongy state with intramyelin oedema. This change was most obvious in the brain stem. Premature infants were those most frequently affected, when the antiseptic was used in maternity wards.

Isoniazid

A side-effect of this drug is the development of a painful sensory neuropathy with axonal degeneration. Some pro-

tection against this is afforded by pyridoxine supplements. It is thought that the drug may cause a local depletion of pyridoxal phosphate in axons. Acute ingestion of a high dose of isoniazid causes CNS symptoms, including fits and psychosis, with the development of intramyelin oedema. It may prove fatal.

Lathyrism

This condition, due to excessive consumption of chick peas during times of famine, is characterized by spastic paraparesis, with symmetrical loss of the distal corticospinal tract fibres. It has recently been suggested that the toxic factor involved is a potent neuro-excitatory amino acid, beta-N-oxylamino-L-alanine.

Lead

Adult poisoning with lead is an occupational hazard, associated with the breaking up of old batteries, or occurs as a result of exposure in homes. Childhood cases relate mainly to ingestion of lead-containing paint. In children lead tends to cause an acute encephalopathy, while occupational exposure in adults results in a chronic, predominantly motor, peripheral neuropathy. In acute cases with encephalopathy the brain is swollen and congested, and may show a few petechial haemorrhages. Microscopy shows widespread vascular abnormalities with capillary dilatation, endothelial cell swelling and necrosis, and perivascular protein exudates associated with damage to glia, axons and neurons.

In the peripheral neuropathy both axonal degeneration and segmental demyelination were described in the older literature. It is now rarely encountered. One suggested mechanism of the peripheral nerve changes is from damage to endothelium, as in the CNS, with leakage of fluid into the endoneurium and an increase in endoneurial fluid pressure.

Organic lead compounds

Tetraethyl lead, present in petrol, has been described as causing an acute encephalopathy with cerebral oedema and capillary haemorrhages, or foci of neuronal loss in the hippocampus (Sommer sector) and cerebellum (Purkinje cells and dentate nuclei). Similar cerebral swelling caused by intramyelin oedema may occur from intoxication by triethyl tin compounds used in industry, or accidentally contaminating medicines.

Manganese

Manganese poisoning has been described from India and Peru, where it is largely confined to workers mining the ore. Clinical presentation has many parkinsonian features. Pathological lesions in chronic intoxication are described in the striatum, globus pallidus and subthalamic nucleus, where there is neuron loss and gliosis. In some cases, other sites, including the red nucleus and thalamus, are affected.

Inorganic mercury compounds

Infant 'teething powders' and calomel, formerly used as a remedy for constipation, have in the past given rise to poisoning with mercurous salts. Infants affected developed a peripheral neuropathy with axonal degeneration ('pink disease'), and adults with chronic intoxication have shown diffuse loss of granule cells and a few Purkinje cells in the cerebellum. Metallic mercury or mercuric salts may occasionally cause intoxication which is manifested by tremor and psychological changes ('hatters' shakes'). No post mortem cases have been described.

Organic mercury compounds

Methyl mercury intoxication has occurred from the ingestion of contaminated fish and cereals. Paraesthesiae around the mouth and in the extremities, ataxia and tunnel vision are the characteristic clinical manifestations. Pathological studies have shown focal neuronal loss principally in the primary visual (calcarine) cortex of the occipital lobe, primary auditory cortex and postcentral somatosensory cortex, involving small granular cells in layers 2 and 3 particularly, and with accentuation of damage at the depths of sulci. In the cerebellar cortex there is loss of granule cells and to a lesser extent of Purkinje cells. Peripheral nerve lesions also occur but are less constant. They involve loss of sensory neurons, with secondary degeneration of fibres in the posterior columns of the spinal cord.

Methotrexate

When given as a chemotherapeutic agent intrathecally or intravenously, in combination with cranial irradiation, methotrexate may cause an encephalopathy in which there is damage to cerebral white matter. Extensive necrotic or demyelinating foci, with surrounding oedema and astrocytosis, occur mainly in the centrum semiovale (Fig. 20.5). Axons in the areas affected appear swollen but are not all destroyed. Inflammation is absent and vascular changes are inconstant.

Methyl alcohol

In acute methanol intoxication the brain is swollen and congested and there may be petechial haemorrhages. The cerebellar cortex is liable to undergo necrosis involving all three layers, and the putamen to undergo bilateral cystic necrosis. Retinal ganglion cells are also destroyed, and the optic nerves show loss of axons and astrocytic gliosis.

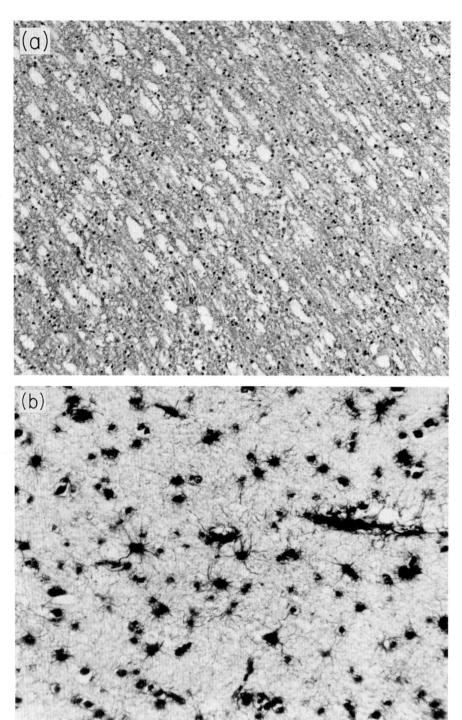

Fig. 20.5. Methotrexate intoxication. Diffuse spongy change associated with pallor of myelin staining in the cerebral white matter (a), with a marked astrocytic reaction (b). (a) H&E, ×300; (b) PTAH, ×150. (Courtesy of Dr F. Cruz-Sanchez.)

MPTP (1-methyl-4-phenyl-1,2,5,6-tetrahydropyridine)

MPTP is a relatively simple purine-type compound which has recently been found to cause a severe form of acute parkinsonian syndrome. Affected individuals have been industrial chemists exposed to the substance, or heroin users who have used synthetic heroin analogues contaminated with MPTP. Post mortem studies have shown severe loss of neurons in the substantia nigra without formation of Lewy bodies (cf. Parkinson's disease, p.240).

Organophosphorus compounds

These compounds, widely used in insecticides, as petrol additives and plasticizers, and in nerve gases, have caused occasional large outbreaks of toxic paralytic disease, usually

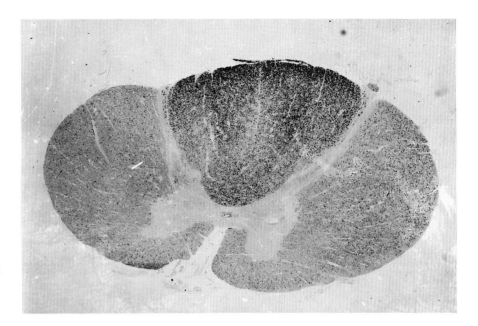

Fig. 20.6. Thallium poisoning. Transverse section of cervical cord stained by the Marchi method which demonstrates marked degeneration in the posterior columns. ×10. (Courtesy of Prof. J. Cavanagh.)

as a result of contamination of cooking oil or drinks ('ginger jake paralysis'). The more reactive alkyl compounds used in nerve gases and insecticides produce acute effects due to inhibition of acetylcholinesterase as well as delayed peripheral neuropathy. These compounds produce distal wallerian-type degeneration of long axons in both the peripheral nerves and long tracts of the spinal cord. Axonal degeneration in *distal* peripheral nerves only is found, together with loss of fibres in the gracile tracts of the spinal cord, maximal at the cervical level. There is also degeneration of pyramidal tract fibres at the lower end of the spinal cord, and spinocerebellar fibres entering the cerebellum.

Tetanus

Tetanus toxin, the exotoxin of *Clostridium tetani*, causes spasms in skeletal muscles due to inhibition of the firing of inhibitory interneurons acting on lower motor neurons in the spinal cord. The toxin reaches the CNS by retrograde transport in axons and then spreads trans-synaptically to the interneurons. Non-specific vacuolation of lower motor neurons and intermediolateral column neurons in the spinal cord is seen in some fatal cases. The toxin also damages motor nerve endings in skeletal muscle and stimulates pre-terminal motor nerve sprouting in experimental animals.

Thallium

Thallium, an ingredient of rat and insect poisons, is sometimes administered to humans with murderous intent. It produces gastrointestinal disturbance and a distal peripheral neuropathy, mainly sensory at first, but with later motor involvement and progression to affect cranial and respiratory nerves in severe cases (Figs 20.6 and 20.7). This is ac-

companied by a skin rash and later loss of hair. Peripheral nerves show wallerian degeneration, most severe in distal parts of the limbs.

Toxic oil syndrome

An unidentified contaminant in rapeseed oil caused an outbreak of disease with both muscle and peripheral nerve damage in Spain in 1981. Pathological studies showed an inflammatory infiltrate in peripheral nerves followed by fibrosis of the perineurium and degeneration and loss of myelinated nerve fibres as part of a general fibrotic reaction, with vascular occlusion due to fibrosis of small vessels.

Trichloroethylene

This is a solvent which has been used in dry-cleaning, and as an anaesthetic. In a few cases of poisoning severe axonal

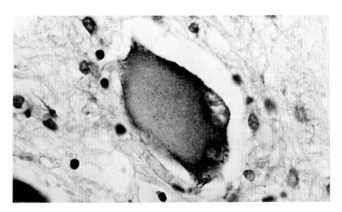

Fig. 20.7. Thallium poisoning. Chromatolytic anterior horn cell. Nissl, ×390. (Courtesy of Prof. J. Cavanagh.)

degeneration in cranial nerves, particularly the trigeminal nerve, has been described. In one fatal case with detailed pathological examination there was loss of neurons in the trigeminal motor nucleus and some other brain stem motor nuclei. The toxic effect of trichloroethylene has been frequently accompanied by an orofacial patch of herpes simplex infection, and this observation, as well as the curious distribution of the associated cranial nerve damage, suggests that reactivation of latent herpes simplex virus may be involved.

Triethyl tin

Organic tin compounds have many industrial and agricultural uses. Human poisoning has occurred through contamination of proprietary medicines. Triethyl tin causes an acute encephalopathy with striking cerebral oedema and prominent vacuole formation related to myelin sheaths, visible histologically in cerebral white matter.

Trimethyl tin intoxication has led to acute encephalopathy with nerve cell loss from the hippocampal formations.

Nutritional disorders

There are few well-defined nervous system diseases in humans that are recognized as being due to altered nutrition, and most of these are due to vitamin deficiencies. More general effects of under-nutrition, particularly in infancy, have not been studied adequately in humans, though experimental work leaves no doubt that permanent alterations in brain structure can occur if malnutrition is severe and occurs at a critical stage of brain growth, e.g. in kwashiorkor. Deficiency of a single vitamin is rare, but if the effects of malnutrition are compounded by high intake of a toxic substance, the result may be a disease attributable to an isolated

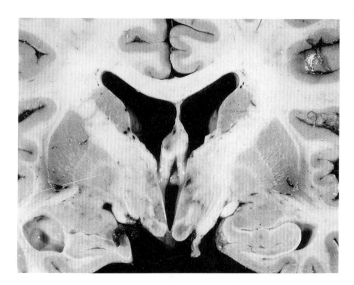

Fig. 20.8. View of the mamillary bodies in Wernicke's encephalopathy. They show brown discoloration and feel abnormally soft.

deficiency, as occurs in alcoholics who develop Wernicke's encephalopathy (see below). Selective gastrointestinal malabsorption may also cause an isolated vitamin deficiency, for instance of vitamin B_{12}, and the vitamin E deficiency that can accompany prolonged fat malabsorption.

Thiamine (vitamin B_1) deficiency

Wernicke's encephalopathy is the best-known condition affecting the CNS which results from thiamine deficiency. The lesions of Wernicke's encephalopathy are frequently encountered in chronic alcoholics. They are found in the subependymal regions around the third ventricle and aque-

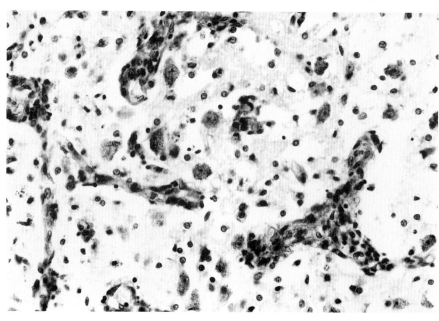

Fig. 20.9. Wernicke's encephalopathy. Subacute lesion with capillary congestion, oedema and endothelial cell hypertrophy in the mamillary body. Note the survival of healthy-looking neurons. PAS, ×170.

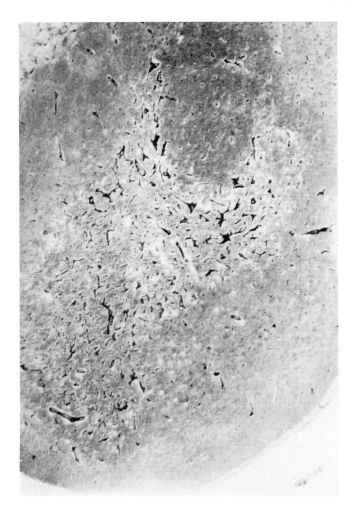

Fig. 20.10. Wernicke's encephalopathy. Chronic lesion in mamillary body, with scarring and pericapillary fibrosis. Reticulin stain, ×22.

duct, in the floor of the fourth ventricle and, most characteristically, in the mamillary bodies in the hypothalamus. They may be visible macroscopically as foci of congestion and haemorrhage, or at a later stage as foci of brown discoloration and softening (Fig. 20.8). However, the lesions cannot be excluded without microscopy, as they are not always visible with the naked eye. Many cases of Wernicke's encephalopathy are not clinically diagnosed. It is therefore recommended that the pathological lesion should be sought in all chronic alcoholics, if cases are not to go undiagnosed. Microscopy shows, in the acute stage, focal capillary dilatation, congestion and endothelial swelling (Fig. 20.9). Petechial haemorrhages and a few perivascular macrophages are also common. In the later stages capillary proliferation and pericapillary fibrosis are prominent (Fig. 20.10) and there are frequently accompanying macrophages containing haemosiderin and some fibrillary gliosis. Neurons are relatively spared, though they may be shrunken. In the thalamus there may be neuronal shrinkage without the capillary changes described above. The dorsomedial thalamic nucleus is the one most commonly affected.

Thiamine deficiency also causes peripheral neuropathy, which is seen not only in alcoholics but also, in the form of beriberi, in victims of malnutrition and starvation. Peripheral nerves show a predominantly distal axonal degeneration with some sensory ganglion cell loss and degeneration of fibres in the posterior columns of the spinal cord.

In addition to the lesions of Wernicke's encephalopathy, thiamine deficiency is thought to be responsible for the cerebellar lesions often found in alcoholics. These consist of loss of Purkinje cells and to a lesser extent of granule cells from the cerebellar cortex, particularly in the superior vermis, at the crowns of the folia (Fig. 20.11). In severe

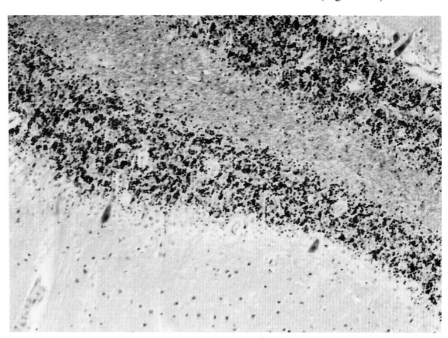

Fig. 20.11. Low-power view of the cerebellar cortex from a chronic alcoholic. Purkinje cells are reduced in number, and there is a proliferation of astrocytes in the molecular and Purkinje cell layers. H&E, ×100.

cases most of the anterior parts of the anterior lobes of the hemispheres are also affected. Secondary loss of neurons caused by retrograde degeneration may also be seen in the inferior olives.

Pyridoxine deficiency

Deficiency of pyridoxal phosphate (vitamin B_6) in experiments in animals results in a peripheral neuropathy with axonal degeneration, but there has been no convincing demonstration that isolated deficiency of this vitamin causes a peripheral neuropathy in man.

Nicotinic acid deficiency

Deficiency of this vitamin, one of the B group, or of its amino acid precursor tryptophan, causes pellagra. Most cases seen now are alcoholics or vegans. Morphological changes in the nervous system have been described in chronic deficiency, the most consistent being chromatolysis of neurons, particularly Betz cells in the motor cortex, pontine neurons in the brain stem and anterior horn cells. Degeneration is also described in peripheral nerves and long tracts in the spinal cord, principally in the posterior columns but also in the lateral columns

Riboflavin deficiency

Deficiency of this member of the B group of vitamins causes a peripheral neuropathy with axonal degeneration, and skin lesions around the mouth.

Vitamin B_{12} deficiency

Vitamin B_{12} deficiency causes pernicious anaemia and a myelopathy known as *subacute combined degeneration of the cord*. This is primarily a myelinopathy, but it is almost always accompanied by axonal loss in human cases if allowed to last long. The characteristic finding is of discontinuous foci of demyelination not conforming with anatomical or functional divisions, but situated mainly in lateral- and posterior-column white matter (Fig. 20.12). The thoracic level of the cord is usually the worst affected. The mildest lesions consist of patches of myelin sheath swelling and dissolution. In severe cases there is destruction of almost all the white matter around mid-thoracic cord level and extension of lesions upward in anterolateral and posterior columns and downward in lateral columns. In affected areas the tissue is spongy and has a honeycomb-like appearance in transverse sections of the cord (Fig. 20.12). The brain usually appears normal, but may show small perivascular areas of demyelination in the cerebral white matter.

Peripheral nerves are also damaged in vitamin B_{12} deficiency, though there are few pathological studies. A biopsy study showed demyelination in the anterior tibial nerve, and earlier, post mortem studies showed wallerian degeneration in peripheral nerves.

Vitamin E (α-tocopherol) deficiency

Vitamin E is a fat-soluble vitamin, deficiency of which has recently been recognized as the cause of neurological disease in subjects with prolonged impairment of fat absorption. Such cases show a dying-back type of axonal degeneration in peripheral sensory and motor axons, and particularly in central axons, sometimes with loss of neurons in brain stem sensory and motor nuclei.

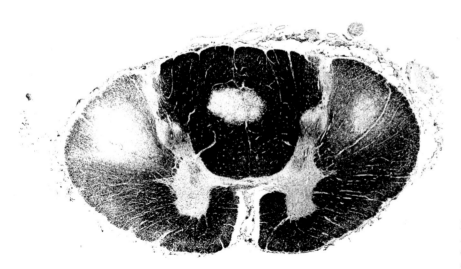

Fig. 20.12. Vitamin B_{12} deficiency. Appearance of myelin-stained section of the cervical cord showing foci of spongy myelin degeneration in lateral and posterior columns. (Courtesy of Prof. D. Graham.)

Further reading

Cavanagh JB. 1985. Mechanisms of damage by chemical agents. In Swash M, Kennard C (Eds) *Scientific Basis of Clinical Neurology*. Churchill Livingstone, Edinburgh, pp. 631–45.

Duchen LW, Jacobs JM. 1984. Nutritional and metabolic disorders. In Adams JH, Corsellis JAN, Duchen LW (Eds) *Greenfield's Neuropathology*, 4th edn. Edward Arnold, London, pp. 573–626.

Jacobs JM, Le Quesne PM. 1984. Toxic disorders of the nervous system. In Adams JH, Corsellis JAN, Duchen LW (Eds) *Greenfield's Neuropathology*, 4th edn. Edward Arnold, London, pp. 627–98.

Schochet SS. 1985. Exogenous toxic-metabolic diseases, including vitamin deficiency. In Davis RL, Robertson DM (Eds) *Textbook of Neuropathology*. Williams and Wilkins, Baltimore, pp. 372–402.

Spencer PS, Schaumberg HH. (Eds) 1980. *Experimental and Clinical Neurotoxicology*. Williams and Wilkins, Baltimore.

Victor M. 1976. The Wernicke–Korsakoff syndrome. In Vinken PJ, Bruyn GW (Eds) *Handbook of Clinical Neurology*. Elsevier, Amsterdam, **28**, 243–70.

Chapter 21
Neuropathology of the Very Young

General recommendations about post mortem examination

A careful examination of the nervous system, and particularly of the brain, may form an important part of many post mortems following death in infancy. Cerebral pathology is responsible for many such deaths and even in cases in which death is due to disease outside the nervous system, such as congenital heart disease, it is common to find secondary pathology in the brain. In another large group of infant deaths, sudden unexplained death, it is also advisable to examine the brain with care since primary cerebral pathology is occasionally demonstrable. It is preferable in all such cases to fix the brain before slicing it. However, before this is done thought should be given to whether there is a need to remove fresh samples for microbiological or biochemical investigation, the former if pre- or postnatal infection is considered possible, and the latter if a metabolic disease is suspected. CSF and serum samples are also worth collecting from such cases; even if they are not examined immediately, they can be stored deep-frozen for subsequent investigation when the diagnostic possibilities have been narrowed down.

Removal of the infant brain from the skull must be performed with great care, since its soft consistency at this age makes it more fragile than the adult brain (p.2). Special procedures have been described on p.8 that may be employed in cases of hydrocephalus in infancy. The infant brain can be conveniently removed by incising the sutures and reflecting the parietal and frontal bones outwards. In some cases the spinal cord should also be removed and fixed for later examination. These include cases of suspected malformations, hydrocephalus, metabolic and toxic diseases and inflammatory disease. Cases of suspected neuromuscular disease require removal of the spinal cord and samples of nerves and muscles. Frozen blocks should be prepared from some of these samples if histochemical stains are to be employed, for example for enzymes in muscle and metachromatic material in nerves.

The maturity of an infant brain may be assessed by weighing it, and by examining the state of development of the cerebral gyri and the extent of myelination. All show a wide range of individual variation, however. Weights of the developing fetal brain are given in Table 21.1. Gyral patterns at various stages of fetal development are illustrated in Fig. 21.1. All main and secondary gyri are normally present at term. There is probably little or no nerve cell division or

Table 21.1. Brain weights related to gestational age (data from Friede (1975), with permission

Gestational age (weeks/days)	Brain weight (g)	Body weight (g)
23/5 +/− 2/3	70 +/− 18	500
26/0 +/− 2/6	107 +/− 27	750
27/5 +/− 3/1	143 +/− 34	1000
29/0 +/− 3/0	174 +/− 38	1250
31/3 +/− 2/3	219 +/− 52	1500
32/4 +/− 2/6	247 +/− 51	1750
34/6 +/− 3/2	281 +/− 56	2000
36/4 +/− 3/0	308 +/− 49	2250
38/0 +/− 3/2	339 +/− 50	2500
39/2 +/− 2/2	362 +/− 48	2750
40/0 +/− 2/1	380 +/− 55	3000
40/4 +/− 1/6	395 +/− 53	3250
40/4 +/− 1/5	411 +/− 55	3500
40/6 +/− 2/3	413 +/− 55	3750
41/4 +/− 1/3	420 +/− 62	4000
41/2 +/− 2/1	415 +/− 38	4250

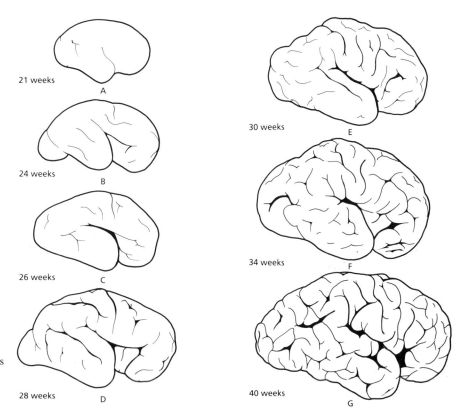

Fig. 21.1. Gyral patterns on the lateral aspects of the cerebral hemispheres during fetal development. (Redrawn from *Gray's Anatomy*, 36th edn, with permission.)

migration after birth except in the cerebellum, where the external layer of granule cells is still present at birth, the cells migrating through the molecular and Purkinje cell layers to augment the granule cell population of the cerebellar cortex during the first postnatal year (Fig. 21.2). There is little myelination of the brain until the second half of the second trimester of pregnancy. Thereafter, myelin is laid down at different rates and at different times depending on the site. The extent of myelination can be assessed with the naked eye, or microscopically in myelin-stained sections. The first white matter tract to myelinate is the medial longitudinal fasciculus (Fig. 2.26) This tract is more or less fully myelinated by about the end of the second trimester, and it provides a useful standard with which to compare the

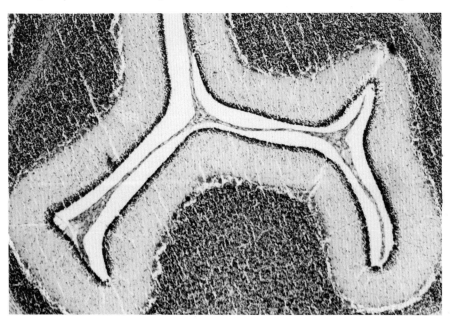

Fig. 21.2. Low-power view of a section of an infant's cerebellum, showing the presence of the external granular layer visible as the dark line at the leptomeningeal surface of the cerebellar cortex. H&E, ×50.

extent of myelination in other tracts in the brain and spinal cord. The approximate order and time of appearance of myelin at some easily identified sites are indicated in Table 21.2. If intrauterine development is impaired, there may be considerable delay in myelination. For detailed recommendations on assessment of the degree of myelination we refer the reader to Chapter 12 of Gilles, Leviton & Dooling's *The Developing Human Brain* (1983). These authors recommend taking six blocks from the brain for this purpose: three brain stem levels (medulla, pons and midbrain), and three cerebral blocks containing, respectively, the optic radiation at the level of the lateral geniculate body, the posterior limb of the internal capsule and optic tract, and the hippocampus and parahippocampal gyrus, also at the level of the lateral geniculate body. These blocks contain the tracts marked with asterisks in Table 21.2. To locate those in the brain stem reference may be made to Figs 2.26 and 2.29.

When selecting blocks for microscopy from infant brain slices areas of naked-eye abnormality are an obvious choice for inclusion, together with areas known to be at risk in the condition that is suspected to be present. If naked-eye lesions are hard to discern and the diagnosis is unclear, the following blocks are useful for initial routine evaluation: a coronal section through one cerebral hemisphere at or just behind the mamillary body, midbrain, pons, mid-medulla,

and cerebellum in a slice through the vermis close to the midline and in an oblique section through one cerebellar hemisphere that includes the dentate nucleus. Blocks from infant brains at term or after can generally be satisfactorily processed into paraffin wax, but those from preterm infants profit from celloidin embedding, which makes the sections easier to handle.

When examining infant skeletal muscle from cases of suspected neuromuscular disease the muscle fibre diameters should be measured and compared with those found in normal muscle from the same site and at the same age (Table 23.1)

For convenience the conditions considered in this chapter are divided into (i) those associated with birth trauma, (ii) those associated with perinatal asphyxia, (iii) other conditions peculiar to infancy and not considered elsewhere, and (iv)

Table 21.2. Times of attainment during gestation of approximately full myelination in at least 80% of fetuses at selected CNS sites (data from Gilles, Leviton & Dooling (1983)

Tract	Gestational age (weeks)	Blocks among those recommended by Gilles *et al*.
*Medial longitudinal fasciculus	23	Pons
Spinal cord tracts (excluding lateral corticospinal tracts)	24–29	
*Inferior cerebellar peduncle	27	Medulla
*Medial lemniscus	29	Medulla
*Lateral lemniscus	30	Pons
*Superior cerebellar peduncle	34	Pons
*Optic tract	35	Cerebrum
*Posterior limb of internal capsule	36	Cerebrum
*Anterior optic radiation	40	Cerebrum
*Pyramid	40	Medulla
*Medial and lateral thirds of cerebral peduncle	After birth	Midbrain
Corpus callosum	After birth	Cerebrum

* Tracts recommended for block-taking to assess the degree of myelinaton.

Table 21.3. Summary of pathological conditions encountered in the very young and considered elsewhere in this book

Malformations	Chapter 16
Hydrocephalus	Chapter 8
Metabolic diseases	Chapter 19
Toxic conditions, especially	
Tetanus	p.315
Botulism	p.310
Lead poisoning	p.313
Fetal alcohol syndrome	p.310
Hexachlorophane poisoning	p.312
Diphtheritic neuropathy	p.312
Tumours, especially	
Gliomas	p.172
Meningiomas	p.201
Meningeal sarcomas	p.208
Choroid plexus papillomas	p.190
Neuroblastoma	p.192
Teratomas	p.220
Epilepsy	Chapter 18
Infections	
Bacterial	Chapter 9
Parasitic, viral	Chapter 10
Neuromuscular diseases	
Werdnig–Hoffmann disease	p.239
Poliomyelitis	p.147
Neonatal and congenital myasthenia	p.362
Congenital muscular dystrophy	p.362
Congenital myotonic dystrophy	p.356
Mitochondrial myopathies	p.360
Arthrogryposis	p.353
Type II glycogenosis (Pompe's disease)	p.358
Central core disease	p.353
Nemaline rod myopathy	p.366
Myotubular myopathy	p.353
Congenital fibre type disproportion	p.354

conditions to look out for in stillbirths. Many other conditions found in infants, but not confined to that age group, are considered in other chapters, as indicated in Table 21.3. It should also be pointed out that some of the diseases considered below do not invariably cause death in infancy and their sequelae may be encountered both in children and adults who survived the acute insult.

Lesions associated with birth trauma

Infants with a history of a traumatic birth often suffer from intracranial haemorrhage. The falx and tentorium are liable to be torn, and this can give rise to bleeding from venous sinuses. Subdural haematomas occur as a result of deforming the cranium during delivery and tearing of superficial cortical veins (Fig. 21.3). Cerebellar haematomas also occur following birth trauma. Trauma may also be associated with asphyxia (see below).

Despite the frequency of intracranial haemorrhage in infants, severe herniations of brain tissue are uncommon because of the distensibility of the infant skull vault, which allows it to expand when intracranial pressure rises.

Perinatal asphyxia

Perinatal asphyxia is a major cause of death or of later severe disability. Preterm infants are particularly at risk. Asphyxia can result in both haemorrhagic and non-haemorrhagic lesions in the brain. The acute forms are found in infants dying shortly after birth. Late consequences, particularly periventricular white matter loss, and cell loss and gliosis in deep grey matter, are commonly found in children and adults dying after a long history of 'cerebral palsy' (Figs 8.7 and 8.8).

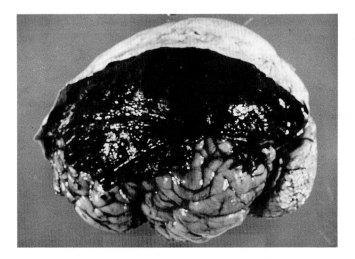

Fig. 21.3. Acute subdural haematoma in an infant dying shortly after a difficult birth.

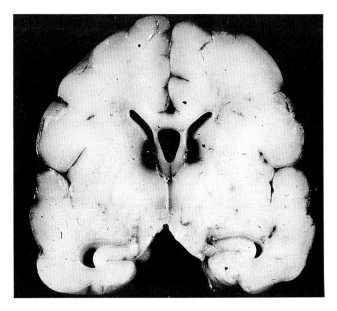

Fig. 21.4. Mid-cerebral coronal slice through the brain of a premature infant dying shortly after birth. There are bilateral germinal matrix haemorrhages over the heads of the caudate nuclei.

Haemorrhagic lesions

Haemorrhagic lesions in the brain are particularly common in preterm infants suffering perinatal asphyxia and respiratory distress. The most characteristic site for these haemorrhages is the subependymal germinal matrix in the lateral wall of the lateral ventricles, chiefly at the level of the head of the caudate nucleus. Haemorrhages may be multiple and bilateral (Fig. 21.4). They are frequently small, but can be large, and may rupture into the ventricles (Fig. 21.5), or extend into adjacent cortex. Even small periventricular haemorrhages produce destruction of the surrounding germinal matrix. Intraventricular haemorrhages occasionally originate in the choroid plexus.

The cause of germinal matrix and choroid plexus haemorrhages is thought to be cerebral hypoxia and hypercapnia, particularly associated with respiratory distress in preterm infants. This leads to reactive vasodilatation, increased cerebral blood flow and raised cerebral arterial pressure, resulting in haemorrhage from the sinusoidal capillaries and congested, poorly supported, veins of the germinal matrix region (Wigglesworth 1984). A different sequence of events with the same results occurs if systemic hypotension develops as a consequence of birth asphyxia and causes ischaemic damage to periventricular regions, including the germinal matrix. Subsequent re-perfusion of this vascular bed when the blood pressure is restored may then cause haemorrhages in the same region. Under these circumstances periventricular haemorrhages and infarcts coexist.

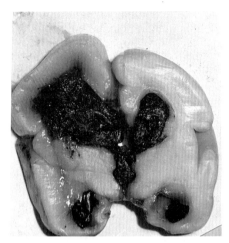

Fig. 21.5. Intracerebral haemorrhage in a premature infant, arising from periventricular haemorrhage. (Courtesy of Dr A.L. Sheehan.)

Subependymal and intraventricular haemorrhages are much less common in full-term than preterm infants. This is probably due to the disappearance of the germinal matrix after 36 weeks' gestation.

Other sites for haemorrhage associated with birth asphyxia are the subarachnoid space and the subpial region of the superficial cerebral or cerebellar cortex, where haemorrhages are usually small and frequently multiple (Fig. 21.6). Larger amounts of subarachnoid blood collect in the basal cisterns in the posterior fossa as a consequence of intraventricular haemorrhage. Hydrocephalus is a common sequel in the survivors of such events. Larger, often multiple, cerebellar haemorrhages are common in preterm infants and are usually seen near the tentorial surface or over the lateral aspects of the hemispheres.

Non-haemorrhagic lesions

Non-haemorrhagic cerebral lesions are common findings in full-term or preterm infants subjected to prolonged labour, or with respiratory distress or cyanotic congenital heart disease. The lesions may predominate in grey or white matter, or occur in both, the site to some extent depending on maturity.

The white matter lesions consist initially of multiple, irregular or rounded, circumscribed patches of coagulative necrosis appearing white or yellow and measuring a few millimetres across (Fig. 21.7). Later these areas become softened or cystic (Fig. 21.8). Microscopically they show features of acute infarction (p.106) (Fig. 21.9), and show up well with PAS and Luxol fast blue stains. A few days later there is infiltration of the area by lipid phagocytes, and breakdown of the parenchyma with formation of axon retraction bulbs at the margins. Small haemorrhages may be found in affected areas at the acute stage, and later there may be haemosiderin and mineral deposition. Gliosis occurs during the healing phase. The centrum ovale is the most vulnerable site for development of these lesions, which are sometimes referred to as *periventricular leucomalacia*. It has been suggested that this vulnerability is due to poor perfusion of the region. The late effects are loss of white matter and gliosis in periventricular regions, with thinning of the corpus callosum and compensatory enlargement of the lateral ventricles, which, in coronal sections, have a characteristic squared-off shape to their lateral margins (Fig. 8.6).

Lesions in grey matter may be found in the thalamus, basal ganglia or cerebral cortex (Fig. 21.10). The distribution of damage in deep grey matter is patchy and unpredictable, but in the cortex tends to occur at the depths of sulci and at the boundary zones between the major arterial territories. The acute lesions are often ill-defined and inconspicuous. In the deep grey matter they consist of patchy foci of neuron

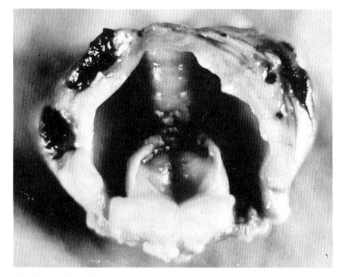

Fig. 21.6. Superficial haemorrhages in the subpial tissue of the cerebral hemispheres in an asphyxiated infant.

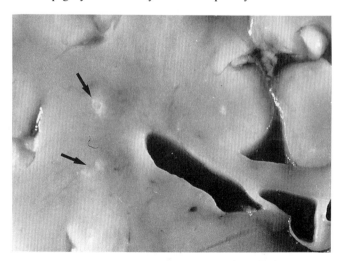

Fig. 21.7. Multiple, small focal areas of necrosis (arrowed) in periventricular white matter of the brain from a premature infant.

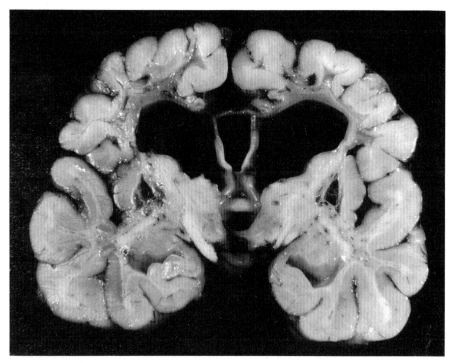

Fig. 21.8. Late consequences of perinatal asphyxia in the brain of a 4-year-old child with 'cerebral palsy'. There is marked dilatation of the bodies of the lateral ventricles and extensive loss of cerebral white matter. In addition, there is cystic change in the white matter and basal ganglia. The septum is split open. (See also Figs 8.7 and 8.8.)

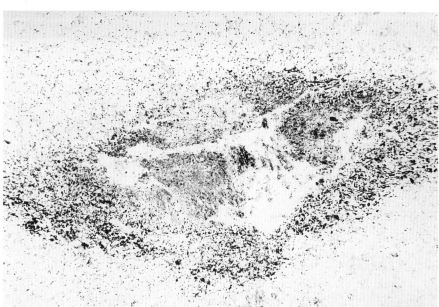

Fig. 21.9. Microscopic appearance of a focus of periventricular necrosis, such as that illustrated in Fig. 21.7. LBCV, ×150.

pallor with nuclear pyknosis, and eosinophilic staining of the cytoplasm. Affected cerebral cortex at the depths of sulci contains poorly-stained, ghost-like or eosinophilic neuron cell bodies and spongy oedema of the parenchyma in a laminar distribution, chiefly in layers 3 and 5 (Figs 21.10 and 21.11). More distinctive are the residual lesions seen months or years later in either deep grey matter or cortex or both. In deep grey matter there are prominent bundles of aberrant myelinated glial fibres which appear to the naked eye as white streaks or spots (Fig. 21.12) (*état marbré*). This may be present bilaterally in subjects with a history of choreo-athetosis from early infancy. Affected areas of cortex show shrivelling in the depths of the sulci, with relative preservation of the crowns of the gyri, a condition known as *ulegyria* (see p.261 and Fig. 16.14). Different patterns of distribution of ulegyria are observed. Most commonly affected are the arterial boundary zones on both sides, but on occasion the gyri within an arterial territory are predominantly affected. Extensive hypoxic/ischaemic damage to the cerebral cortex gives rise to later retrograde atrophy of the ipsilateral thalamus and sometimes to contralateral cerebellar atrophy (Figs 16.6 and 16.7).

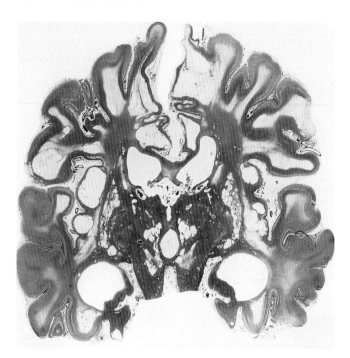

Fig. 21.10. Mid-coronal section through the cerebrum of an infant dying 37 days after suffering severe intrapartum asphyxia. Gross cystic necrosis is evident in putamen, thalamus, subthalamic nucleus and substantia nigra. In the cortex there is laminar necrosis and developing ulegyria. The white matter shows cystic necrosis in subcortical regions, and the lateral ventricles are grossly dilated.

Cerebellar lesions attributable to perinatal hypoxia and circulatory collapse are less common than cerebral lesions, but cerebellar folia can be affected, giving rise to late gliosis with depletion of neurons, most commonly in the boundary zones between arterial territories. As in the cerebral cortex, the worst damage is to regions around the depths of the sulci, giving rise to cerebellar ulegyria.

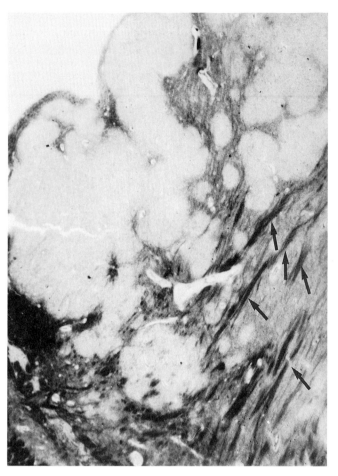

Fig. 21.12. Myelin-stained section of the pulvinar of the thalamus from a 4-year-old girl who had suffered from severe choreoathetosis following a difficult birth. Dark-stained bundles (arrowed) consist of aberrant, myelinated glial fibres. Areas of pallor are sites where almost total neuron loss has occurred. LBCV, ×20.

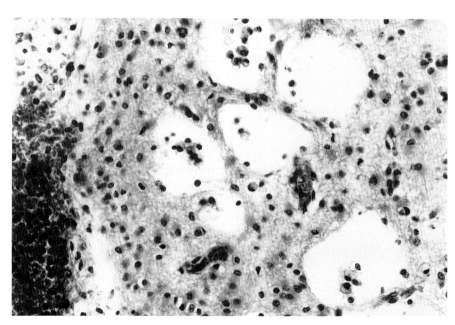

Fig. 21.11. Cystic necrosis and virtually complete neuron loss in the cerebral cortex of the brain shown in Fig. 21.10. Most of the nuclei present are those of reactive astrocytes, which have survived in the non-cystic areas. Cortical surface and congested leptomeningeal vessels left. PTAH, ×200.

Other sites vulnerable to neuronal loss in infants with respiratory insufficiency or hypotension and hypoxia include the pontine and other brain stem nuclei, the subiculum, and the granule cells, Purkinje cells and dentate nuclei of the cerebellum. The brain stem nuclei of infants are much more sensitive than those of adults to hypoxic damage.

Other central nervous system pathology in infants

Kernicterus

Heavy bilirubin staining associated with selective damage to certain parts of the brain in deeply jaundiced infants is known as kernicterus (Plate 7.4). It is much less common now than previously in countries where active steps are taken to prevent effects of rhesus incompatibility. Most of the bilirubin staining and neuronal loss with later gliosis occur in subthalamic, lateral thalamic and lentiform nuclei,

cranial nerve nuclei, gracile and cuneate nuclei, inferior olives and dentate nuclei of the cerebellum. In some cases the hippocampus and the mamillary bodies are also affected.

Infections

Pathogens known to cause intrauterine or perinatal infection of the brain include cytomegalovirus (CMV), rubella virus, herpes simplex type 2 virus, varicella virus, HIV (AIDS virus), the spirochaete *Treponema pallidum*, and the protozoan *Toxoplasma gondii*. Consequences vary, depending on the stage of development at which the infection occurs and on the severity of the infection. Frequently the brain is maldeveloped following intrauterine infections, showing microencephaly, hydrocephalus or polymicrogyria (p.260), as well as destructive lesions attributable to the infection. Table 21.4 summarizes the common cerebral and extra-

Table 21.4. Summary of intrauterine and congenital infections associated with cerebral pathology in infants

Organism	Type of cerebral pathology	Extracerebral pathology	Diagnostic samples
Cytomegalovirus (exposure during pregnancy or birth)	Microencephaly, gyral malformations, foci of calcification, especially in periventricular regions, meningoencephalitis with nuclear inclusion bodies	Hepatitis, chorioretinitis, cardiovascular and skeletal malformations, purpura. Large inclusion-bearing cells in affected organs (often present in kidney); may be stillborn	Softened brain and kidney tissue for culture and IPX staining for viral antigen
Rubella virus (1st trimester infection)	Microencephaly, hydrocephalus, agenesis of corpus callosum, cerebral cysts and mild calcification. Very rarely progressive rubella syndrome	Cataracts, other ocular defects, deafness due to inner ear disease, cardiac abnormalities, liver disease, abnormalities of bone development, haematological abnormalities	Serum for IgM-specific antibody
HIV (AIDS) virus (exposure during pregnancy or birth)	Microencephaly, encephalitis, multinucleated giant cells, white matter degeneration and gliosis, vascular calcification	Thymic atrophy and lymphoid tissue depletion, disseminated infections with, e.g., atypical mycobacteria, CMV, fungi. Pneumocystitis in lungs	Serum for specific antibody, fresh brain samples for nucleic acid hybridization
Herpes simplex type II virus (exposure usually during birth)	Diffuse acute encephalitis. Inclusion bodies may be seen in glial and neuronal nuclei	Necrotic foci in lungs, liver and adrenal glands	Softened brain tissue for culture and IPX staining for herpes simplex antigen
Varicella virus (exposure in 1st trimester)	Microencephaly, meningoencephalitis or myelitis, occasionally cerebral malformations	Chorioretinitis, necrotic, scarred skin lesions and muscle atrophy in segmental distribution	Serum for specific antibody level
Treponema pallidum (2nd trimester onwards)	Leptomeningitis, hydrocephalus, vascular lesions associated with arteritis. Later in childhood there may be dementia due to loss of neurons in cerebral cortex and cerebellum with gliosis	Stillbirths, placental infiltration with spirochaetes which are also present in the liver, lungs, heart and bones	Serum and CSF for fluorescent treponemal antibody test; stain for spirochaetes in tissues
Toxoplasma gondii (especially end of 1st and during 2nd trimester)	Hydrocephalus, foci of calcification scattered throughout the brain, meningoencephalitis with necrotic foci. Free organisms and cysts in lesions	Chorioretinitis, hepatitis; may be stillborn; placenta infected also	Serum for IgM-specific antibody; detection of organisms or cysts in brain and placenta

IPX   immunoperoxidase.

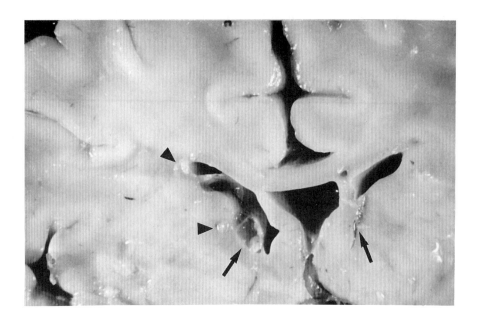

Fig. 21.13. Coronal slice through the cerebrum of an infant with congenital cytomegalovirus (CMV) infection. There are small foci of calcification (arrow heads), and areas of periventricular necrosis (arrowed).

cerebral lesions associated with the chief pathogenic organisms, and contains recommendations on samples to take for diagnostic purposes.

CMV infection produces multiple scattered foci of necrosis and has a particular predilection for the periventricular regions of the brain (Fig. 21.13). Microscopically the lesions show variable inflammation, reactive gliosis and typical, though sometimes sparse, CMV inclusion bodies in nuclei of neurons, glial cells and endothelial cells (Fig. 21.14). Foci of calcification are common in the necrotic parenchyma and nearby vessel walls (Fig. 21.15). There is usually evidence of infection with CMV in other organs besides the brain.

Rubella virus infection of the brain *in utero* may cause a variety of changes: microencephaly, chronic meningitis with a mild degree of hydrocephalus, and developmental delay, or dense perivascular mononuclear inflammatory cells in the brain and leptomeninges. The brain may show scattered small foci of necrosis detectable microscopically, with associated vascular calcification and intimal proliferation. The virus cannot be demonstrated in the brain lesions, which are probably vascular in origin. Exceptionally, a progressive subacute encephalitis may develop after congenital or perinatal rubella infection (see p.149).

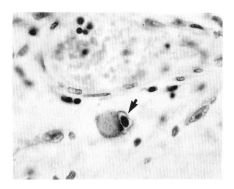

Fig. 21.14 (*above*). Intranuclear inclusion body in the spinal cord from an infant with congenital CMV infection (arrowed). H&E, ×320.

Fig. 21.15 (*right*). Low-power view of a section of periventricular and septal areas in an infant with congenital CMV infection. Irregular periventricular foci of calcification are present. H&E, ×10.

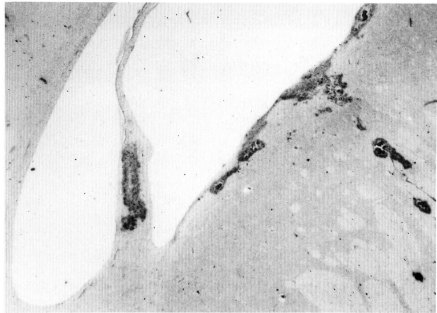

Herpes simplex type 2 infection of the brain occurs during passage through an infected birth canal. The virus infects other organs such as the liver and adrenal glands and reaches the brain via the bloodstream. In the brain the virus causes a severe encephalitis with widespread macroscopic areas of softening, particularly in grey matter. If death occurs at the acute stage of the infection, viral antigen can be demonstrated in the brain in glial cells and neurons using immunohistological techniques on paraffin sections.

The AIDS virus, HIV, produces changes in the brain in congenitally infected infants. Brain weights are abnormally low, and an encephalopathy with white matter degeneration and gliosis has been described (Sharer *et al.* 1986). Variable inflammatory cell infiltrates, multinucleate giant cells and vascular calcification, particularly in the basal ganglia, are also found. Infection with opportunistic organisms may additionally be found in the brain and elsewhere.

Varicella infection *in utero* occasionally produces damage to the nervous system. This may take the form of necrosis in a segmental distribution in the spinal cord. Muscles and other tissues innervated by the destroyed neural segment(s) are atrophic, and the skin may be necrotic and scarred.

Toxoplasma gondii can cause a congenital meningo-encephalitis which is usually manifest in the first few weeks of life. Lesions may be evident on inspection of the external surface of the brain, and consist of scattered, necrotic, yellowish areas a few millimetres in diameter. On slicing the brain there may be evidence of an ependymitis and hydrocephalus, and in addition further necrotic foci may be found scattered throughout the cerebrum and brain stem. The spinal cord may also be affected. Microscopically the lesions consist of foci of intense infiltration with mixed inflammatory cells, which include neutrophils and eosinophils as well as mononuclear cells. Prominent reactive gliosis, capillary proliferation and calcification are also present in and around the lesions. Organisms 2−3 μm long and 1.5−2 μm wide are found lying singly or in cysts (Fig. 10.47).

Congenital syphilis may affect the nervous system and typically produces scattered infiltrates of mononuclear inflammatory cells, chiefly lymphocytes and plasma cells, in the leptomeninges and Virchow−Robin spaces. Numerous spirochaetes can be demonstrated with appropriate stains in the leptomeninges and superficial parts of the brain.

Sudden infant death ('cot death')

Occasional cases of sudden death in infants are found to have a primary neurological disease as the cause of death. These include meningitis, encephalitis and Leigh's encephalopathy. In most cases of sudden unexplained death in infancy the brain is described as normal or showing agonal hypoxic changes only. However, a few reports suggest that in some cases there may be detectable developmental abnormalities in the brain, though they may require use of special techniques for their detection. For example, Quattrochi *et al.* (1985) describe abnormal retention of dendritic spines on neurons of brain stem nuclei involved in cardiovascular and respiratory regulation in the majority of a series of cases of unexplained sudden infant death, and others have described brain stem gliosis in some cases.

Non-traumatic postnatal vascular lesions

Major cerebral infarction is rare in infants, and if present is usually associated with an abnormality outside the nervous system, such as congenital heart disease, or a coagulopathy. Another cause is the rare inherited disease, homocystinuria. The internal carotid artery territory is the most common site involved. The infarcts produced are usually haemorrhagic. Venous thrombosis is another rare cause of haemorrhagic cerebral infarction in infants. Occasional haemorrhages in infants and children occur from ruptured arterial aneurysms and arteriovenous malformations, or in association with a blood-clotting defect.

Traumatic postnatal lesions

Haemorrhages, often multiple, occur at a variety of sites in and around the brain in accidental and non-accidental injury after birth (see Chapter 5).

Alpers' disease

Alpers' disease is a rare, progressive neurological disorder with clinical features that include epilepsy, spastic weakness and, in children, progressive dementia. The cerebral cortex is selectively affected, and at death cortical atrophy is readily appreciable to the naked eye (Fig. 21.16). The cerebral white matter shows secondary atrophy, with myelin pallor and sometimes cystic change. Microscopy shows very severe neuron loss in the cerebral cortex, affecting all cell layers. Spongy change may be evident in a laminar distribution, mainly in layers 3 and 4 (Fig. 21.17). Astrocytic gliosis is also clearly evident in cortex and white matter. The basal nuclei, thalamus, brain stem and cerebellum are relatively well preserved, showing only secondary tract degeneration or additional mild changes similar to those of the cerebral cortex in grey matter. There is some doubt as to whether all cases described as suffering from Alpers' disease have the same affliction. Some cases have had a familial occurrence and in others liver disease has been described. Some cases may be due to a mitochondrial enzyme deficiency.

Effects of whooping cough immunization

It might be thought that the importance of monitoring the possible deleterious effects of immunization procedures is obvious. Nevertheless, there is a dearth of information on the pathological changes underlying the cerebral damage which some have ascribed to the effects of whooping cough immunization. This is despite experimental evidence that *pertussis* can act as a powerful adjuvant in the production of allergic encephalomyelitis (Levine & Wenk 1967). In a careful review of the literature, and a study of 29 identified cases, Corsellis *et al.* (1983) concluded that, although a variety of cerebral abnormalities were found in cases of brain damage alleged to be associated with whooping cough vaccination, there were no consistent features that could be accepted as a specific reaction to the whooping cough vaccine. Post mortem examination should be undertaken on any such infants who die. We recommend, most emphatically, that the brain be preserved for detailed neuropathological examination.

Neuropathological examination of stillbirths

Careful examination of the nervous system should be undertaken on as many stillbirths as possible. Although maceration may frustrate attempts to define the pathology in all cases, there are many that are likely to reveal significant CNS pathology. This is also the case in some pregnancy terminations, since some of these now follow detection of CNS malformations by imaging techniques early in pregnancy. We have seen examples of hydrocephalus due to aqueduct stenosis, obstruction produced by periventricular

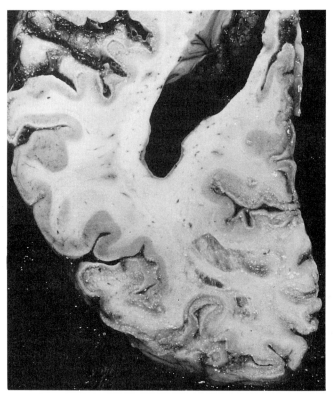

Fig. 21.16. Horizontal slice through the left occipital lobe from a 12-year-old boy with Alpers' disease, who was blind and demented. The occipital cortex is necrotic and the white matter cystic. Further forward the cortex is better preserved. The occipital horn of the ventricle is dilated.

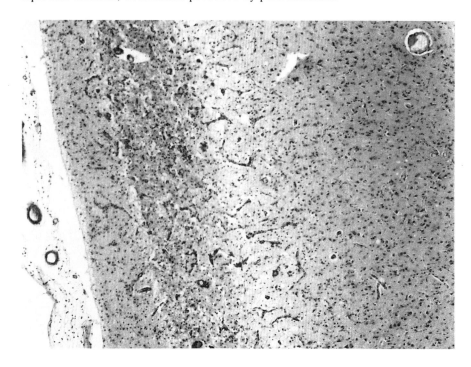

Fig. 21.17. Low-power view of a section of cortex from the occipital lobe of the case shown in Fig. 21.16. Neurons have disappeared from layers 2 and 3, leaving pale, spongy tissue containing small vessels and fibrous astrocytes. PAS, ×90.

masses possibly associated with tuberous sclerosis, and intrauterine CMV infection. Stillbirths in late pregnancy may show periventricular or intraventricular haemorrhages, or neuron loss with gliosis in a pattern suggesting cerebral hypoxia as the cause. These features may be associated with poor uteroplacental perfusion, or, following major trauma or illness in the mother, particularly if these caused severe maternal circulatory collapse.

In conclusion, to end this chapter we would urge paediatric pathologists and neuropathologists to cooperate closely in the investigation of infant deaths.

Further reading

Corsellis JAN, Janota I, Marshall AK. 1983. Immunisation against whooping cough: a neuropathological review. *Neuropathol Appl Neurobiol* **9**, 261–70.

Friede RL. 1975. *Developmental Neuropathology*. Springer, Berlin.

Gilles F, Leviton A, Dooling E. 1983. *Development of the Human Brain*. John Wright, Guildford, USA.

Keeling JW (Ed). 1987. *Fetal and Neonatal Pathology*. Springer, Berlin.

Larroche J-C. 1984. Perinatal brain damage. In Adams JH, Corsellis JAN, Duchen LW (Eds) *Greenfield's Neuropathology*, 4th edn. Edward Arnold, London, pp. 451–90.

Levine S, Wenk EJ. 1967. Hyperacute allergic encephalomyelitis: lymphatic system as site of adjuvant effect of pertussis vaccine. *Amer J Pathol* **50**, 465–83.

Quattrochi JJ, McBride PT, Yates AJ. 1985. Brain stem immaturity in sudden infant death syndrome: a quantitative rapid Golgi study of dendritic spines in 95 infants. *Brain Res* **325**, 39–48.

Rorke LB. 1982. *Pathology of Perinatal Brain Injury*. Raven Press, New York.

Sharer LR, Epstein LG, Cho E-S *et al*. 1986. Pathologic features of AIDS encephalopathy in children. *Hum Pathol* **17**, 271–84.

Volpe JJ. 1981. *Neurology of the Newborn*. WB Saunders, Philadelphia.

Wigglesworth JS. 1984. Central nervous system. In Wigglesworth JS (Ed) Perinatal pathology. Vol. 15 of *Major Problems in Pathology*. Bennington JL (Series Ed). WB Saunders, Philadelphia, pp. 243–88.

Wigglesworth JS, Pape KE. 1987. *Perinatal Brain Injury*. Blackwell Scientific Publications, Oxford.

Chapter 22
Diseases of Peripheral Nerves

This chapter reviews diseases of peripheral nerves and their parent cell bodies other than those due to deficiency or metabolic diseases or toxic states, which are considered in Chapters 19 and 20 respectively. Discussion of the handling of nerve biopsies can be found on pp.85−6.

When performing a post mortem examination on a case of peripheral nerve disease more time is required than for the average case so that careful attention can be given to removal of all necessary specimens. These should include examples of distal and proximal, upper and lower limb, cranial and autonomic nerves, samples of skeletal muscle, sensory and autonomic ganglia and the spinal cord. In dealing with post mortem specimens of peripheral nerve it is seldom worth while expending much time and effort on EM examination of samples unless the delay between death and post mortem is very short. However, glutaraldehyde fixation with resin embedding of samples is recommended in order to prepare 1 μm sections for light microscopy. Routine sections are also usually prepared of transverse and longitudinally orientated blocks of paraffin-embedded material, and these can be stained for axons (e.g. with Holmes' or Palmgren's stains), myelin (e.g. with Page's or Weil's stains), and with H&E and van Gieson's stain. A Gomori trichrome stain shows both myelin (pink) and fibrous tissue in the same section, and Appendix 1 describes a useful stain that combines the Palmgren stain for fibres with a red myelin stain. Thick frozen sections stained with Schofield's technique demonstrate nerve terminations clearly (Fig. 4.38). Samples should also be set aside for teasing and osmicating in order to look for segmental demyelination and remyelination in individual nerve fibres. Appearances of a normal sural nerve using these various techniques are illustrated in Figs 4.35 and 4.36 and Plates 3.3 and 3.4.

The range of reactions in peripheral nerves to a wide variety of disease processes is somewhat limited, and although the pathologist can describe these, it may not always be possible to identify the cause of neuropathy from these changes. These reactions will be described first and then those that are found in particular diseases will be summarized. We shall also refer to quantitative changes that occur in peripheral nerves, since these can also help to narrow the diagnostic possibilities. Numbers and proportions of nerve fibres of different diameters in nerve fascicles can be measured and compared with those for the same nerve from a normal subject of approximately the same age (since some alterations occur with advancing age). Semi-automatic image analysis systems are well equipped to assist with carrying out the necessary measurements, and software to enable this to be done is now available. Measurements are best carried out on resin-embedded sections. With semi-automatic image analysis systems measurements are made by drawing outlines of the fibres at high power with the microscope image projected on to the measuring pad, or from photographs placed on the pad. There are difficulties in assessing total nerve numbers in a fascicle from their density, since this will be influenced by alterations in the volume of the endoneurial space, which may be expanded by oedema or by artefact. It is important to note alterations to the shape of the nerve fascicles in transverse section. In most cases with axonal loss the normal, rounded outline is replaced by an irregular 'collapsed' appearance (compare Plate 3.3 and Fig. 22.1). Unmyelinated fibres cannot be satisfactorily assessed by light microscopy and need to be examined in electron micrographs. Also, by light microscopy it is difficult to distinguish normal small-diameter nerve fibres from regenerating fibres. Because of large vari-

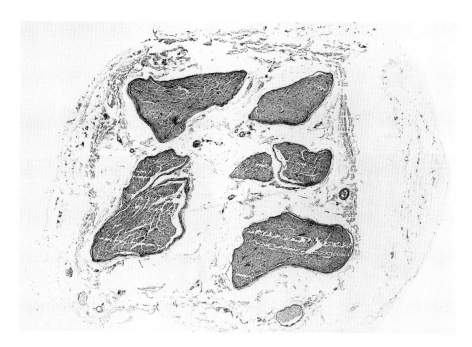

Fig. 22.1. Transverse section of peripheral nerve from a case of peripheral neuropathy with axonal degeneration. Note the collapsed shape of the nerve fascicles (cf. Plate 3.3). Holmes, ×33.

ations between normal subjects, deviation from 'normal' figures has to be fairly gross to be significant. Figure 22.2 is a histogram showing the diameters of nerve fibres in the normal sural nerve, the nerve that is most frequently examined quantitatively.

Pathological reactions in peripheral nerves are divided into (i) those that primarily affect the axon, and (ii) those that affect the myelin sheath. In practice it is frequently found that features of both types of reactions are present in any given case (Table 22.1).

Primary axonal degeneration

An axon cut off from its parent cell body undergoes wallerian degeneration. This change is seen with traumatic nerve injury, and in some forms of peripheral nerve disease. The axons develop irregular swellings and then break into fragments which eventually become resorbed (Fig. 22.3). At the same time the myelin sheath around the axon is destroyed and digested, chiefly by macrophages (Fig. 22.4). Schwann cells proliferate in the surviving endoneurial tubes, and

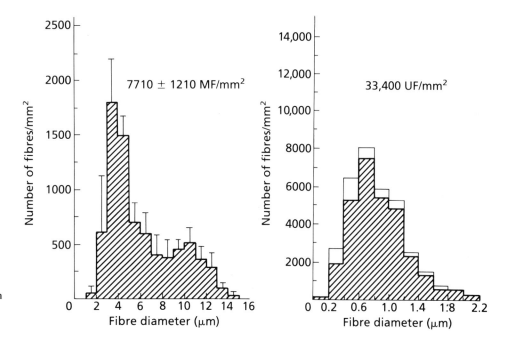

Fig. 22.2. Histograms of myelinated (left) and unmyelinated (right) nerve fibres in normal sural nerve. Non-hatched areas relate to Schwann cells in an immature pattern. (Redrawn from Asbury & Johnson 1978, with permission.)

Table 22.1. Summary of some principal causes of peripheral nerve damage (commoner conditions in bold)

Neuropathy with 'dying-back' axonal pathology

Acrylamide toxicity	Porphyria (p.294)
Arsenic (trivalent) toxicity (p.310)	Pyridoxine deficiency (p.318)
Carbon disulphide toxicity	Riboflavin deficiency (p.318)
Chloroquine toxicity	Thallium toxicity (p.315)
Cis-platinum toxicity	**Thiamine (vit B₁) deficiency** (p.316)
Hexacarbon toxicity (p.312)	Tocopherol (vit E) deficiency (p.318)
Isoniazid toxicity (p.312)	
Metronidazole toxicity	Vincristine/vinblastine toxicity
Nitrofurantoin toxicity	
Organophosphorus compounds (p.313)	

Neuropathy with wallerian-type degeneration

Adrenomyeloneuropathy (p.298)	**Leprosy** (p.340)
Alcohol (p.309)	**Malignant disease** (p.160)
Amyloidosis (p.338)	Organic mercury toxicity (p.313)
Clioquinol toxicity (p.311)	Nicotinic acid deficiency (p.318)
Cyanide toxicity (p.311)	**Pressure palsies and entrapment neuropathies** (p.342)
Disulphiram toxicity	
Fabry's disease (p.292)	Toxic oil syndrome (p.315)
Friedreich's ataxia (p.244)	Uraemia (chronic) (p.342)
Hereditary axonal neuropathies (p.338)	
Herpes zoster (segmental) (p.339)	
Lead toxicity (p.313)	

Neuropathies with segmental demyelination
(may be accompanied by axonal degeneration as well)

Acute inflammatory polyneuropathy (Guillain–Barré syndrome) (p.337)	Ischaemia (p.340)
	Lead (chronic) toxicity (p.313)
Acromegaly (p.337)	Krabbe's leucodystrophy (p.297)
Arsenic (pentavalent) (p.310)	Paraproteinaemias (p.341)
Amiodarone toxicity	Perhexilene toxicity
Buckthorn toxicity	Pressure palsies due to inherited susceptibility (p.342)
Cyanide (chronic) toxicity (p.311)	Refsum's disease (p.339)
Diabetes mellitus (p.338)	**Rheumatoid arthritis** (p.342)
Diphtheria toxin (p.312)	**Sarcoidosis** (p.342)
Gold salts	Uraemia (acute) (p.342)
Hypertrophic hereditary neuropathies (p.338)	Vitamin B₁₂ deficiency (p.318)

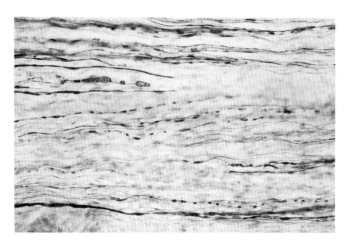

Fig. 22.3. Axonal degeneration with beading of axonal fragments. Schofield, ×140.

axonal sprouts generated at the proximal nerve stump slowly grow into these tubes and acquire new myelin sheaths (Fig. 22.5), though this process of regeneration can be frustrated by the development of scar tissue and may be far from complete. The cell body of the severed axon undergoes a series of morphological changes (chromatolysis), which are more evident if the axon is severed close to the parent cell body (Plate 1.6, p.47). Chromatolysis is more evident in motor than in sensory neurons. Wallerian-type degeneration is seen in human diseases which destroy lower motor neurons or sensory neurons and their axons. If sensory neurons are affected, the central fibres in the posterior columns of the spinal cord may degenerate as well as the distal fibres in peripheral nerves, though degeneration of the central and peripheral processes of sensory neurons do not always go hand in hand. Sensory cell loss is accompanied by focal satellite cell proliferation in the ganglion, the resulting groups of satellite cells sometimes being referred to as nodules of Nageotte (Fig. 22.6). If motor neurons and their axons degenerate, there is denervation atrophy of the muscles they innervate (see Chapter 23). The histological changes found in a peripheral nerve from a subject with a disease that produces wallerian-type degeneration will depend on the stage reached and the tempo and severity of the disease. They are likely to include some or all of the following: axons undergoing fragmentation, with non-segmental disintegration of the myelin sheaths, presence of some infiltrating macrophages, and increased collagen deposition; axonal sprouts lying in clusters (Fig. 22.5); loss of nerve fibres; and, in distal axons, fusiform swellings along the course of regenerating fibres and growth cones at the tips. A severed nerve may result in the formation of a traumatic neuroma, which consists of a nodule of haphazardly arranged interlacing bundles of nerve fibres intermingled with dense scar tissue (Figs 22.7 and 22.8).

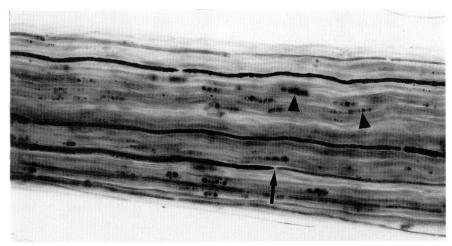

Fig. 22.4. Osmicated and teased preparation of a sural nerve biopsy. Fat droplets mark the sites where fibres have undergone wallerian degeneration (arrow heads). A partially demyelinated internode is seen between the arrow and the edge of the photograph. ×250.

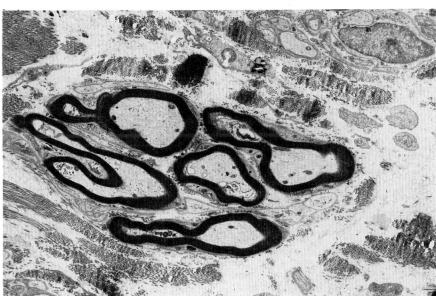

Fig. 22.5. Low-power electron micrograph showing a cluster of small myelinated axons indicating previous axonal sprouting in response to axonal damage. Uranyl acetate and lead citrate, ×3630.

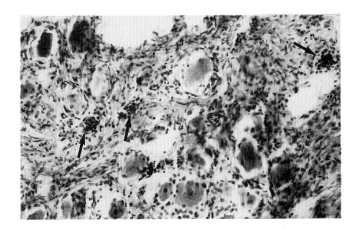

Fig. 22.6. Fibrotic sensory ganglion from which ganglion cells have disappeared, and focal proliferation of satellite cells at these sites has occurred (nodules of Nageotte) (arrowed). The section is from a case of sensory neuropathy associated with oat-cell carcinoma of the lung. H&E, ×80.

'Dying-back' processes in axons

In many peripheral as well as some CNS diseases there is a tendency for the damage to axons to be manifest first, and most severely at the distal ends of long axons — a condition referred to as *'dying back'*. Distal cutaneous and intra-muscular nerve branches and the gracile tract fibres at the cervical level of the spinal cord are the first to be affected if sensory nerve fibres are involved, and intramuscular motor endings if motor fibres are affected. In some diseases both motor and sensory fibres are affected, though not necessarily to the same extent. For example, in isoniazid toxicity the distal peripheral fibres are more affected than the centrally projecting fibres, possibly owing to the exclusion of the drug from the CNS by the blood–brain barrier. Parts of fibres affected by a dying-back process show similar mor-phological changes to those seen in wallerian degeneration (p.333). Unmyelinated fibres, like myelinated ones, can be affected by wallerian-type degeneration, but more com-

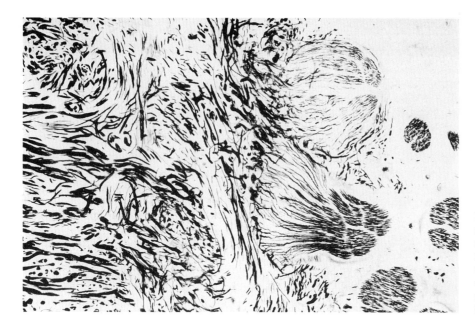

Fig. 22.7. Schofield preparation of a traumatic neuroma. Intact nerve bundles are seen (right), fibres in two of which are seen to enter the neuroma (left). Nerve bundles in the traumatic neuroma are not arranged in ordered, uniformly-orientated fascicles, but run in disorganized, intermingled groups (left). ×25.

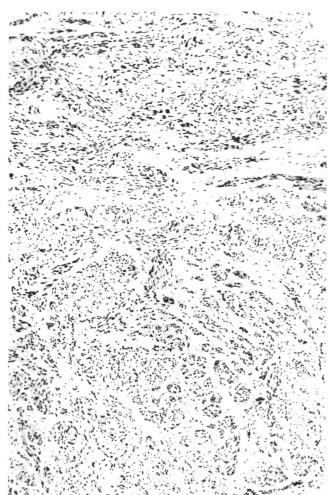

Fig. 22.8. Appearance of a traumatic neuroma in an H&E-stained section. Randomly orientated nerve bundles lie in dense connective tissue. ×33.

monly there is evidence of their loss, which results in the presence of small Schwann cells, lacking any contained axons.

Segmental demyelination

Demyelinating diseases of peripheral nerves cause loss of myelin sheaths but initially leave axons intact. The pattern of myelin loss in primary demyelinating diseases is characteristically discontinuous along the length of the axon. Individual internode lengths of myelin, maintained by one Schwann cell, are destroyed, commencing close to a node, and the result is a patchy loss of myelin with surviving stretches of myelin in between. This is best appreciated in teased nerve fibre preparations, in which long stretches of a single axon can be traced more reliably than in a section of embedded nerve (Fig. 4.36). The destroyed myelin sheaths of each internode are replaced by myelin supplied by two or more Schwann cells, rather than a single one, and each cell therefore remyelinates a shorter internode. Repeated, frustrated attemps at remyelination in chronic demyelinating diseases eventually result in Schwann cell hyperplasia and the formation of concentric Schwann cell processes known as 'onion bulbs' (Fig. 22.9). The whole affected nerve becomes enlarged or hypertrophic. Features found in demyelinating neuropathies are therefore segmental demyelination, remyelinated axons with thin myelin sheaths and shortened internodes, Schwann cell hyperplasia and onion bulb formation. With long-standing demyelination, loss of axons and fibrosis also occur.

In addition to features of axonal degeneration and segmental demyelination microscopy of peripheral nerves may show other changes, some of which are of diagnostic value. At the light microscope level these include inflammation,

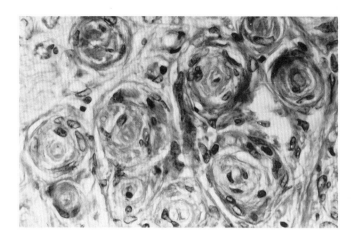

Fig. 22.9. Transverse section of peripheral nerve from a case of relapsing/remitting polyneuropathy containing 'onion bulb' formations composed of proliferated Schwann cells with their cytoplasmic processes wrapped concentrically. H&E, ×560.

vasculitis, granuloma formation, and amyloid deposition. At the EM level Schwann cell inclusions, or axonal swellings containing neurofilaments, may be detectable.

Individual neuropathies

In Table 22.1 some principal causes of the main types of histological reactions in peripheral nerves are summarized, while listed alphabetically below are the histological changes that occur in specific diseases.

Acromegaly

Entrapment neuropathies occur in acromegaly and some cases also show a peripheral neuropathy with segmental demyelination and an increase in endoneurial interstitial tissue (see pressure palsies and entrapment neuropathies below).

Acute inflammatory polyneuropathy (Guillain–Barré syndrome)

Onset of symptoms of this uncommon disease often occurs within one or two weeks of recovery from an acute, febrile illness, or immunization. It is also seen in those with HIV infection. Numbness, paraesthesiae and weakness of the limbs develop rapidly, and may progress to respiratory failure requiring assisted ventilation. Some cranial nerves may be affected. Recovery frequently starts after one to several weeks, but may be incomplete. A few cases pursue a relapsing/remitting course. In the classical, acute form of the disease the predominant pathological change is segmental demyelination, which is seen in nerve roots and peripheral nerves in a patchy distribution (Figs 22.10 and 22.11). In addition there are usually, though not invariably, mononuclear inflammatory cells present in affected parts of the nerves. These consist mainly of lymphocytes and macrophages. In cases that follow a relapsing/remitting course peripheral nerves show Schwann cell hyperplasia and variable, sometimes severe, axonal degeneration as well as inflammation and demyelination. The disease is thought to have an immunopathological basis, but immunohistochemical investigations at present do not have any diagnostic value. There are close similarities between this disease and experimental allergic neuritis as discussed by, among others, Leibowitz & Hughes (1982).

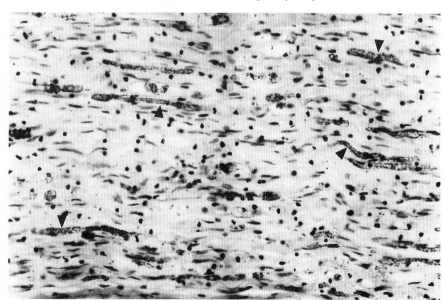

Fig. 22.10. Acute inflammatory polyneuropathy (Guillain–Barré syndrome). Longitudinal section stained for myelin and cells. Only short stretches of myelinated internodes remain (arrow heads), and a diffuse scattering of lymphocyte nuclei is visible. Weil's stain, ×150.

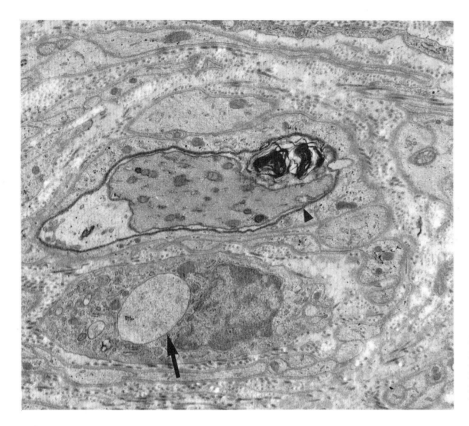

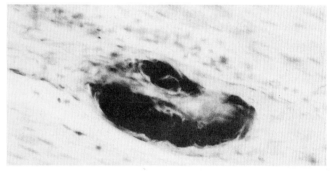

Fig. 22.11. Electron micrograph from a patient with acute inflammatory polyneuropathy. Completely (arrow) and partially (arrow head) demyelinated axons are present. Uranyl acetate and lead citrate, ×13 100.

Amyloidosis

Peripheral neuropathy may form a prominent feature of both sporadic and familial types of amyloidosis. Clinical presentation and age of onset vary, but the pathology is similar in all forms, except that the protein deposited as amyloid, which can in some cases be determined immuno-histochemically, varies. In hereditary amyloidosis it is a form of prealbumin, and in most cases of sporadic amyloid polyneuropathy it is light chains of immunoglobulin, despite the usual absence of evidence of a plasma cell dyscrasia. Affected peripheral nerves contain deposits of amyloid in the form of irregular clumps in the endo- and perineurium, and in the walls of the vasa nervorum (Fig. 22.12). Loss of large and small myelinated and unmyelinated nerve fibres occurs, and some cases may also show segmental demyeli-nation. Occasionally isolated involvement of the trigeminal nerve by amyloid deposition has been described in cases of trigeminal neuralgia or neuropathy.

Diabetes mellitus

Peripheral neuropathy in diabetes mellitus is accompanied by the pathological changes of segmental demyelination and remyelination, Schwann-cell hyperplasia, axonal degeneration and axonal loss (Fig. 22.13). Perineurial and endoneurial capillaries show luminal narrowing and basal

Fig. 22.12. Deposit of amyloid in a perineurial vessel in the femoral nerve from an 80-year-old woman with severe, progressive peripheral neuropathy. No predisposing condition associated with amyloid deposition was found at post mortem examination. Congo Red, ×180.

lamina thickening and reduplication of a degree sufficient to suggest that chronic ischaemia plays a part in producing the nerve damage (Fig. 22.14).

Hereditary neuropathies

Familial dysautonomia (see p.370)

Hypertrophic neuropathies

Inheritance in the hypertrophic form of Charcot−Marie−Tooth disease is recessive; in Déjerine−Sottas disease it is dominant. In both these diseases there is thickening of the

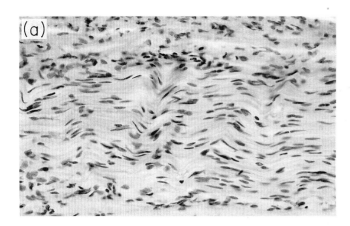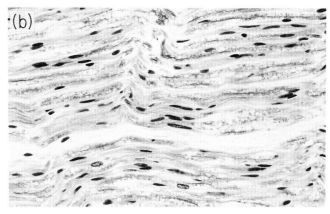

Fig. 22.13. A longitudinal section of nerve from a long-standing diabetic (a). In comparison with (b) (normal), there is marked hyperplasia of Schwann cells, and virtual disappearance of myelinated fibres. (a) & (b): H&E, ×200.

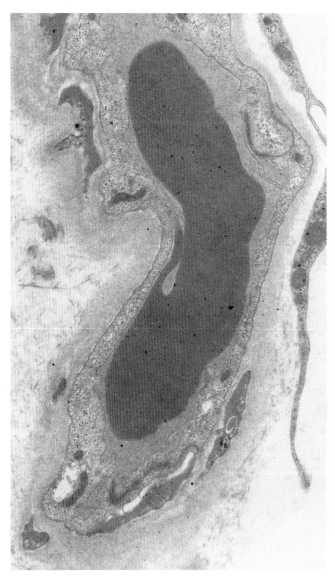

Fig. 22.14. Diabetes mellitus. Intramuscular capillary with basement lamina thickening. Uranyl acetate and lead citrate, ×15 600.

peripheral nerves. Individual nerve fascicles are thickened, but contain fewer nerve fibres than normal. Large myelinated fibres are particularly reduced in number. Teased fibre preparations show segmental demyelination, and abnormally short internodes, and embedded preparations show 'onion bulbs' (Fig. 22.9). Metachromatic ground substance in the endoneurium may be increased. In Déjerine–Sottas disease, in which there is marked sensory loss clinically, spinal sensory ganglia are depleted of neurons, and satellite cells are increased. Posterior column fibres in the spinal cord are also depleted.

Axonal neuropathy (see p.248)

Refsum's disease

This rare autosomal recessive disease presents in late childhood or early adult life. Clinical features include ataxia, retinal degeneration, a sensorimotor neuropathy and sometimes nerve deafness. There is an excess of the long-chain fatty acid, phytanic acid, in the serum, and fibroblasts are deficient in the enzyme phytanic acid oxidase. The chief neuropathological feature is a hypertrophic, demyelinating neuropathy, with evidence of remyelination and Schwann-cell hyperplasia, often taking the form of 'onion bulbs'. There is also an increased amount of acid mucopolysaccharide ground substance in the endoneurium, and a considerable loss of myelinated nerve fibres. The leptomeninges are thickened and show some infiltration with lipid phagocytes.

Herpes zoster (see also p.145)

Herpes zoster is due to reactivation of varicella zoster virus from a site of latency in sensory ganglia. It produces a severe ganglionitis and neuritis of the affected spinal segmental or cranial nerve, with, in some cases, milder inflammation in the CNS at the same segmental level. Adjacent ipsilateral ganglia may also be mildly affected. In the main ganglion involved there is intense congestion, inflammation and often a vasculitis with fibrinoid necrosis of vessel walls. Many neurons are destroyed. Viral antigen may be demonstrable in the ganglion and nerve in the first few days from the onset. In the segmental nerve there is wallerian degeneration and inflammation with axonal loss and fibrosis. (See also p.145, and for advice about locating and removing the trigeminal (gasserian) ganglion, p.3.)

Hirschsprung's disease

In this congenital disorder of the distal colon there is a lack of ganglion cells in the affected part of the bowel wall and an increase in number and abnormal clustering of unmyelinated nerve fibres. The affected portion of the bowel may be resected surgically, and biopsies from the upper and lower resected margins sent for microscopy to check that ganglion cells are present in the retained ends of the anastomosed bowel.

Hypothyroidism

A mild sensory neuropathy has been described in some patients with hypothyroidism. Sural nerve biopsies have shown an excess of mucopolysaccharide ground substance in the endo- and perineurium in such cases.

Ischaemic neuropathy

Combined features of both segmental demyelination and axonal degeneration are seen in nerves damaged by patho-

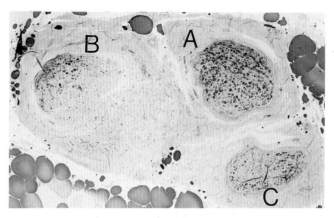

Fig. 22.15. Ischaemic neuropathy. Three fascicles of the sural nerve, showing reasonably good preservation of axons in fascicle A, but severe, focal depletion in B and C. (Compare with Fig. 4.35.) All fascicles show some fibrosis of the perineurium. Toluidine blue, ×80.

logical processes associated with ischaemia. Axonal degeneration tends to predominate (Fig. 22.15). These features are seen in polyarteritis nodosa and in some cases of systemic lupus erythematosus and rheumatoid arthritis. In such cases vasculitis is likely to be present in the nerves affected (Fig. 22.16). Since the vascular supply to several different nerves is liable to be affected, the clinical picture is frequently that of *mononeuritis multiplex*.

Leprosy

This disease, caused by infection with *Mycobacterium leprae*, manifests itself chiefly as a disease of skin and peripheral nerves. Nerves are damaged in all forms of the disease, the varieties of which are attributable to variation

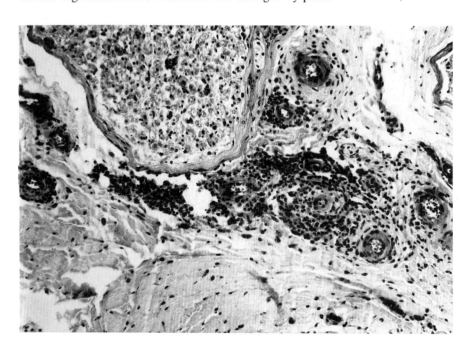

Fig. 22.16. Polyneuropathy associated with polyarteritis nodosa. Inflamed perineurial arterioles. H&E, ×160.

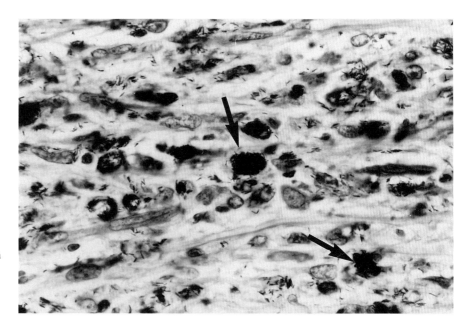

Fig. 22.17. Lepromatous leprosy. Section of a small dermal nerve containing scattered and aggregated clumps of bacilli in macrophages (arrowed). Fite-Farraco, ×600. (Courtesy of Dr C. McDougall.)

in the immune response to the organism. In lepromatous leprosy, in which the cell-mediated immune response is low, there are innumerable organisms spread throughout the skin in macrophages and in Schwann cells of peripheral nerves (Fig. 22.17). In tuberculoid leprosy, which is associated with a strong cell-mediated immune response, the organisms are scanty and associated with the formation of granulomas, centred mainly on peripheral nerves including those of the dermis. Intermediate forms between these polar types also commonly occur. In lepromatous leprosy nerves show loss of axons and myelin, and an increase in number of Schwann cells, with some infiltrating macrophages containing numerous organisms, detectable with the

Fite-Farraco stain. Few, if any, lymphocytes are seen in the nerves. Some axonal sprouting may be present, indicating attempts at regeneration. In tuberculoid leprosy there are scattered granulomas in nerves containing lymphocytes, epithelioid cells and a few multinucleate giant cells (Fig. 22.18). There may be central caseation, which can completely destroy all the nerve fibres in the affected fascicle. The oedema and inflammation, localized to the endoneurial compartment, cause further damage to axons by compressing them, particularly at sites where nerves lie in fibro-osseous tunnels. In the healing phase of all types of leprosy there is intense fibrosis in the affected nerves.

Neuropathy associated with malignant disease (see p.160)

Neuropathy associated with paraproteinaemia

There is a relatively common association between paraproteinaemia and polyneuropathy. Peripheral nerves from such cases usually show combined features of segmental demyelination and axonal degeneration. In some of these cases it has recently been shown that there is a circulating IgM antibody which reacts specifically with a myelin component, myelin-associated glycoprotein. Segmental demyelination is a prominent part of the pathology; in some cases IgM can be shown to be present on the surface of many of the remaining myelin sheaths by immunofluorescence. Complement components are not usually present. Diagnosis in such cases can be made by screening patients' serum on frozen sections of normal nerve for reactivity with myelin sheaths, followed by immunoassay for antibody to myelin-associated glycoprotein. At the ultrastructural level there is found to be an increased periodicity of the outer lamellae of some myelin sheaths in affected cases.

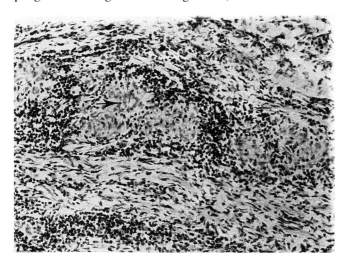

Fig. 22.18. Tuberculoid leprosy. Biopsy from the radial cutaneous nerve of a 10-year-old girl with extensive thickening and tenderness of limb nerves. There is destruction of most of the nerve bundles and heavy infiltration with mononuclear inflammatory cells, with a few giant cells (arrowed). H&E, ×110. (Courtesy of Prof. D. Dastur.)

Pressure palsies and entrapment neuropathies

Damage can be inflicted on peripheral nerves through the direct effect of pressure and through impairment of blood supply when a nerve is compressed. Although in experimental studies the first change is swelling of myelin sheaths and intussusception of paranodal myelin leading to demyelination, in human cases there is usually more severe damage with additional axonal degeneration or loss. A common finding in peripheral nerve samples, taken from sites where they are routinely subject to some compression (e.g. the median nerve at the wrist), is the presence of Renaut bodies (Fig. 22.19). These are subperineurial clumps of polysaccharide-like material. They are more common and numerous in some neuropathies, but are not a specific pathological feature, and may be found in normal subjects. Some individuals are particularly susceptible to the development of pressure palsies. Sural nerve biopsies from these subjects show evidence of demyelination and remyelination with curious sausage-shaped swellings in the myelin sheaths. At the ultrastructural level redundant loops or an excess number of lamellae are found in the myelin sheaths.

Rheumatoid neuropathy

Peripheral nerves may be damaged in rheumatoid arthritis by a number of mechanisms. There may be nearby focal granulomas, entrapment of nerves passing over damaged and deformed joints, or a vasculitis producing ischaemic damage to nerves. Patchy segmental demyelination and axonal degeneration are both described. Gold salts used in the treatment of rheumatoid arthritis may cause similar changes.

Sarcoidosis

Granulomas can occur in sarcoidosis in peri- or endo-neurium. Both segmental demyelination and axonal degeneration are found in the nerves involved.

Scleroderma

Fibrous thickening of the epi- and perineurium occurs as part of the generalized collagen deposition in scleroderma. Vasculitis may also be found. Affected nerves usually show evidence of both segmental demyelination and axonal degeneration.

Uraemia

In acute renal failure segmental demyelination may occur in peripheral nerves. In chronic renal failure axonal degeneration and loss of axons, particularly distal ones, is the usual finding in neuropathy associated with uraemia. Some patients treated with renal dialysis develop amyloidosis, which may be accompanied by a peripheral neuropathy. In these cases the amyloid has been shown to consist of β2 microglobulin.

Further reading

Asbury AK, Johnson PC (Eds). 1978. *Pathology of Peripheral Nerve.* WB Saunders, Philadelphia.

Cajal SR. 1959. *Degeneration and Regeneration in the Nervous System.* Hafner, New York. (Originally published, 1928.)

Dyck PJ, Thomas PK, Lambert EH, Bunge R (Eds). 1984. *Peripheral Neuropathy* (2 vols). WB Saunders, Philadelphia.

Leibowitz S, Hughes RAC. 1982. *Immunology of the Nervous System.* Edward Arnold, London.

Thomas PK, Landon DN, King RHM. 1984. Diseases of the peripheral nerves. In Adams JH, Corsellis JAN, Duchen LW (Eds) *Greenfield's Neuropathology*, 4th edn. Edward Arnold, London, pp. 807–920.

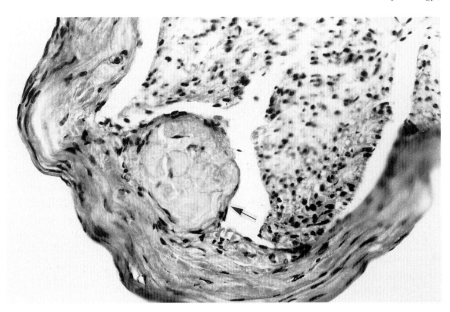

Fig. 22.19. Transverse section of a fascicle from the median nerve showing the appearance of a Renaut body (arrowed) adjacent to the perineurium. H&E, ×180.

Chapter 23
Diseases of Muscle

While diseases of peripheral nerves fall clearly within the scope of the neuropathologist, it is not as obvious why muscle pathology should do so when retinal pathology, on the other hand, does not. The reason for this is historical rather than logical; ophthalmology developed as an independent speciality early on in many medical centres, with its own specialized pathology services. Muscle disease has always been the responsibility of neurologists, general physicians and rheumatologists, and muscle pathology naturally came to fall within the province of pathologists with whom these clinicians had dealings. Some muscle pathology used to be, and in some places still is, dealt with by general pathologists, an arrangement that it is quite acceptable provided they have the facilities to undertake histochemistry and EM on muscle biopsies. Discussion of the handling of muscle biopsies

will be found in Chapter 4, and recommendations for collection of post mortem muscle samples in Chapter 1 (p.6). In either case it is important to obtain accurately orientated transverse and longitudinal sections.

Some aspects of normal skeletal muscle structure need to be recalled when examining muscle for pathological changes (Plate 5; Figs 4.38 and 4.39). Precise longitudinal and transverse sections are essential for proper evaluation of muscle. In longitudinal sections the transverse striations should be visible in normal muscle, and the nuclei should be found lying close to the sarcolemma. Fewer than 5% of fibres should contain centrally placed nuclei. There is a single end-plate on each fibre which lies near to the mid-length of the fibre (Fig. 4.38). In transverse section normal muscle fibres from adults have a polygonal outline (Fig. 23.1), though in

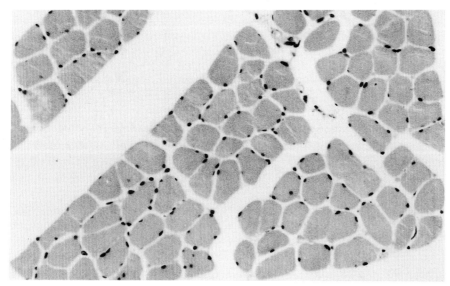

Fig. 23.1. Transverse section of normal muscle. Points to note for comparison with pathological specimens are the polygonal shape of most fibres, the slight variation in fibre width, the subsarcolemmal position of the myonuclei and the absence of easily detectable endomysial collagen between the fibres. H&E, ×100.

children they appear more rounded. Their size varies with age during development (Table 23.1), and to some extent according to training and use. Each adult muscle has a normal range of fibre diameters which differ slightly between the sexes (Table 23.2). Measurement of muscle fibre diameters is often important in the evaluation of muscle. It can be undertaken easily with semi-automatic image analysis systems which require simply that the outlines of fibres are traced on the digital pad. This should be carried out for at least 100 randomly selected fibres of each histochemical type (see below).

Table 23.1. Variation in normal muscle fibre mean diameters with age during childhood

Age (years)	Diameter (μm)	Age (years)	Diameter (μm)
3/12	12	8	30
1	17	10	38
2	17	12	48
4	18	14	53
6	29		

Standard deviations less than 0.25 of the value of the mean diameter

Table 23.2. Mean diameters and proportions of the main fibre types in normal adult muscle (from Dubowitz 1985, with permission)

	Type 1 Male	Type 1 Female	Type 2A Male	Type 2A Female	Type 2B Male	Type 2B Female
Mean diameter (μm)	61	53	69	52	62	42
Mean percentage of total fibres	36	39	24	29	40	32

Standard deviations less than 0.25 of the value of the mean diameter and usually less than 10 μm.
Normal range of fibre diameters: male 40−80 μm; female 30−70 μm.

Another point to note about normal muscle is that very little collagen is detectable in the endomysium between the individual fibres of each muscle fascicle.

Histochemical reactions for enzymes, performed on snap-frozen cryostat sections of muscle, show two main types of muscle fibres which differ in their histochemical properties (Table 23.3). Normally the two types are closely intermingled, giving a checkerboard pattern in transverse sections (Plates 5.3 and 5.4). Type 2 fibres give strong reactions for glycolytic enzymes and glycogen, and weak reactions for oxidative enzymes and neutral fat. They can be subdivided into two main types, and a third that is intermediate between the two. However, for most purposes the type 2 fibres can be regarded together, and for details of their subdivisions

Table 23.3. Histochemical reactions in the two main fibre types

	Type 1 fibres	Type 2 fibres
Mitochondrial enzymes	Strong	Weak
Myosin ATPase (pH 9.4)	Weak	Strong
Phosphorylase	Weak	Strong
Glycogen	Weak	Strong
Neutral fat	Strong	Weak

and their significance the reader should consult one of the monographs devoted to muscle disease which are listed at the end of this chapter. Type 1 fibres contain more fat and less glycogen than the type 2 fibres, and give weak reactions for glycolytic enzymes and strong ones for oxidative enzymes. Histochemical reactions are better carried out on biopsy than post mortem samples of muscle, but they can be used on both.

Muscle spindles are seen from time to time in muscle biopsies and will of course be encountered in post mortem samples of muscle. They are easy enough to recognize in transverse sections of muscle when their surrounding connective tissue sheath is clearly visible (Fig. 23.2). In longitudinal sections intrafusal fibres should not be mistaken for regenerating fibres. Muscle spindles survive relatively unscathed in many denervating and myopathic conditions and in end-stage muscle disease appear increased in numbers owing to the disappearance of many of the extrafusal muscle fibres. However, they are affected in dystrophia myotonica (p.356).

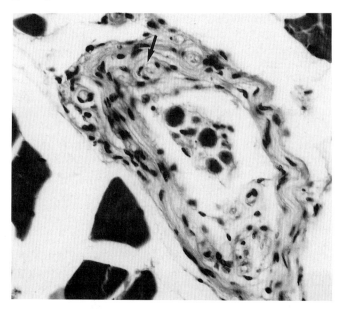

Fig. 23.2. Transverse section of a muscle spindle. Note small and large intrafusal fibres and the fibrous tissue capsule in which several nerve fibres run (arrowed). All the intrafusal fibres are smaller than the extrafusal muscle fibres. H&E, ×170.

Effects of denervation on skeletal muscle

Maintenance of normal skeletal muscle structure and metabolism is closely dependent on the motor innervation. Diseases that destroy motor neurons or their axons give rise to characteristic changes in the skeletal muscle they innervate. These changes reflect both the loss of nerve supply and a compensatory reaction of remaining intact motor axons, which attempt to re-innervate the denervated muscle fibres.

The structural consequence of loss of the motor nerve supply to a muscle fibre is atrophy, which occurs gradually and progressively until eventually the fibre may disappear altogether or be represented by a clump of myonuclei (Fig. 23.3). However, if healthy neighbouring motor nerve endings remain, re-innervation occurs by sprouting from preterminal nerve fibres and formation of a new motor end-plate (Fig. 23.4a). The muscle fibre then regains its normal size

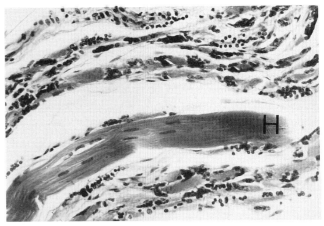

Fig. 23.3. Longitudinal section of denervated muscle. There is a single, slightly hypertrophied fibre (H), with atrophic fibres containing clumps of myonuclei above and below it. H&E, ×110.

(a)

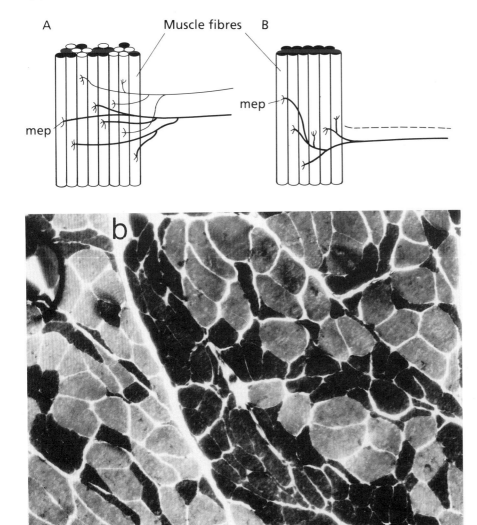

Fig. 23.4. (a) The normal pattern of innervation in muscle (A), and the altered pattern produced by denervation followed by reinnervation (B). (b) Grouping of type 2 fibres is seen in the centre of the figure. Some type 2 fibres are also atrophied. The clinical diagnosis was motor neuron disease. ATPase reaction at pH 9.4, ×180.

and assumes the metabolism and histochemical characteristics imparted by the new nerve supply. Slowly progressive or short-lived denervating processes give opportunities for extensive re-innervation, and this results in the establishment of large motor units in which muscle fibres of one histochemical fibre type come to lie side by side, a condition referred to as *type grouping* (Fig. 23.4b). Further denervation of this group of fibres, all innervated by the same motor nerve fibre, results in a large group of atrophic fibres (Fig. 23.5). Progressive denervation which outstrips the ability to re-innervate gives rise to muscles in which groups of atrophic fibres differ in the severity of their atrophy, reflecting differing lengths of time of denervation. This is found, for example, in motor neuron disease (p.238). A single episode of denervation, such as occurs in acute poliomyelitis, produces atrophic fibres all of much the same size. It should be emphasized that *small* groups of atrophic fibres are not specific for denervation and similarly small groups of fibres all of the same histochemical type are not a reliable indication of re-innervation — the groups have to be quite large to be used as a sound basis for the diagnosis of denervation.

Histological preparations which demonstrate the terminal motor innervation of muscle, such as the Schofield silver stain (Fig. 4.38), nicely display the preterminal sprouting involved in re-innervation (Figs 23.6–23.8).

Another feature seen in re-innervated muscle fibres is the presence of a pale central zone in histochemical preparations for oxidative enzymes. Fibres with this appearance are called *target fibres*, and they appear similar to all the type 1 fibres in central core disease (p.353) (Fig. 23.21).

Demyelination, in contrast to axonal degeneration of motor nerve fibres, does not result in denervation of skeletal muscle.

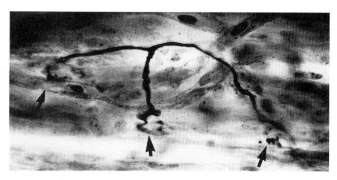

Fig. 23.6. Preterminal sprouting of the nerve fibre seen here has resulted in the formation of three motor end-plates (arrowed). Schofield, ×360.

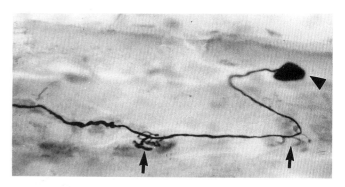

Fig. 23.7. Preterminal motor nerve fibre sprouting with formation of multiple end-plates (arrowed). The fibre terminates in an expanded growth cone (arrow head). Schofield, ×360.

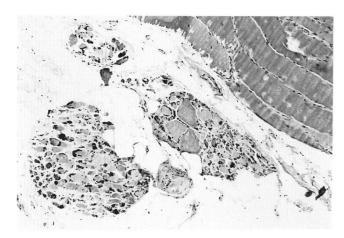

Fig. 23.5. Group atrophy of muscle, characteristic of denervation. The larger of the two transversely sectioned fascicles is entirely denervated, and the smaller one contains a few innervated fibres. Top right, normally innervated fibres sectioned longitudinally. H&E, ×90.

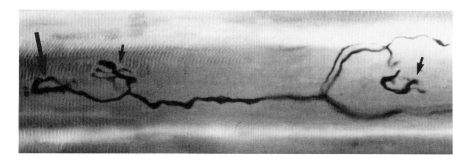

Fig. 23.8. Preterminal motor nerve fibre sprouting with formation of multiple end-plates (arrowed). Schofield, ×360.

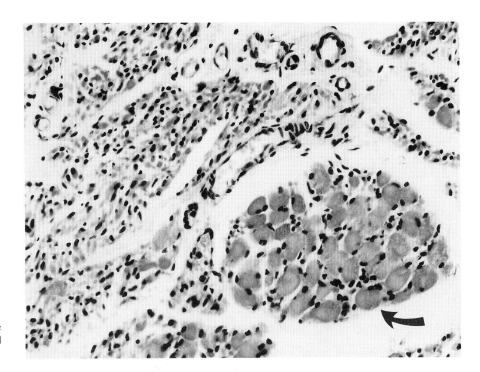

Fig. 23.9. Muscle biopsy appearance in Werdnig–Hoffmann disease. Most of the muscle fibres are severely atrophied, but one group of fibres is, by contrast, hypertrophied (arrowed). H&E, ×200.

Hereditary denervating diseases (see also Chapter 15)

There are a number of forms of progressive denervating disease due to loss of lower motor neurons which are inherited and present in infancy, childhood or adult life. The infantile form, Werdnig–Hoffmann disease, is the most severe, often causing death within the first two years of life (p.239). Its onset is before, at or just after birth. In muscle biopsies from such cases there is smallness of many muscle fibres and conspicuous compensatory hypertrophy in a few islands of fibres (Fig. 23.9). Myelinated intramuscular nerves are greatly reduced in number. Later forms of inherited denervating disease are classified as *spinal muscular atrophy*. They are slowly progressive and tend to show prominent type grouping of muscle fibres as well as group atrophy. Like Werdnig–Hoffmann disease these also spare the upper motor neurons.

Primary muscle diseases

Apart from the changes described above, which are characteristic of denervation, other pathological changes found in muscle usually indicate the presence of a myopathy. Occasionally evidence is seen in a muscle biopsy of both denervation and a myopathy. This occurs in some cases of collagen diseases in which the disease process may simultaneously damage both nerve and muscle. Many myopathic changes are not pathognomonic of one disease. Clinical as well as pathological features should always be taken into account in reaching a diagnosis.

Pathological changes occurring in the myopathies

Some of the commoner pathological changes encountered in skeletal muscle are listed in Table 23.4 along with their diagnostic significance. They are considered in a little more detail below.

Excess inequalities in muscle fibre size

Atrophy of muscle fibres has already been mentioned as a characteristic consequence of denervation. Some myopathic conditions also cause fibre atrophy, whose distribution differs from that found in denervation. In most myopathic conditions atrophy, if present, occurs in randomly scattered fibres, though in some forms of myositis and in scleroderma it affects the fibres at the edges of the muscle fascicles (Fig. 23.10). Regenerating muscle fibres are also small, but can be distinguished from atrophic fibres by their basophilic cytoplasm and characteristically prominent nuclei (see below), and in transverse section by their rounded outline, compared to the angular shape of many atrophic fibres (Fig. 23.11). In some myopathic conditions atrophy selectively affects one histochemical fibre type; for example, selective atrophy of type 2 fibres is a very common and non-specific finding observed in association with poor general health (Fig. 23.12).

Muscle fibres may also undergo hypertrophy. This may occur to compensate for atrophy in other fibres, for example in a partially denervated muscle, or as a physiological response to increased work. It also occurs in primary muscle

Table 23.4. Commoner causes of some pathological features found in muscle

Pathological feature	Distinguishing characteristics	Cause
Abnormalities of muscle fibre size	Scattered atrophy; one or both main fibre types affected	Myopathy
	Scattered atrophy and marked hypertrophy of fibres	Dystrophy
	Groups of atrophic fibres; both main fibre types usually affected	Neurogenic atrophy
	Perifascicular atrophy	Dermatomyositis
	Selective atrophy of one fibre type	See under abnormal histochemistry below
Muscle fibre necrosis	Scattered	Myopathy, myositis, dystrophy
	Grouped	Infarct, as in PAN
Internal nuclei in more than 5% of fibres	Small to moderate numbers of fibres affected	Myopathy, dystrophy, denervation (uncommon)
	Numerous fibres affected	Myotonic dystrophy (also seen following 'muscle trauma)
	Large, vesicular nuclei with prominent nucleoli	Regeneration, as in myositis or early dystrophy
	Single, large nucleus in most fibres	Myotubular myopathy
Pyknotic nuclei in clumps		Chronic denervation, occasionally chronic dystrophy
Muscle fibre splitting		Myopathy or dystrophy, especially myotonic dystrophy
Abnormal muscle spindles		Myotonic dystrophy
Ring fibres (spiral annulets)		Chronic dystrophy, especially myotonic dystrophy
Inflammation	Focal or diffuse, variable in severity	Myositis
	Focal, mild	Some dystrophies, especially facio-scapulo-humeral type, or myopathies
	Forming granulomas	Sarcoidosis
Endomysial fibrosis	Mild/moderate, diffuse	Myopathy
	Mild/moderate, related to areas with group atrophy	Denervation
	Severe, with many muscle fibres still present	Dystrophy
	Severe, with increased adipose tissue and collagen and few remaining muscle fibres	Late effect, usually of dystrophy or denervation
Abnormal histochemistry	Target fibres, with central cores lacking reaction product for mitochondrial enzyme reactions	Central core disease; similar appearances may be seen with denervation and re-innervation
	Scattered fibres containing excess reaction product for mitochondrial enzyme reactions	Mitochondrial myopathy (occasionally non-specific)
	Atrophy of type 1 fibres	Congenital fibre type disproportion and some other congenital myopathies; myotonic dystrophy
	Atrophy of type 2 fibres	Non-specific feature; seen in e.g. disuse, 'collagen' diseases, malignancy
	Excess glycogen	Glycogen storage myopathy; occasionally non-specific if mild
	Excess fat droplets	Lipid storage myopathy
	Type grouping of muscle fibres	Denervation with re-innervation
	Predominance of type 1 fibres	Myopathy

PAN   polyarteritis nodosa.

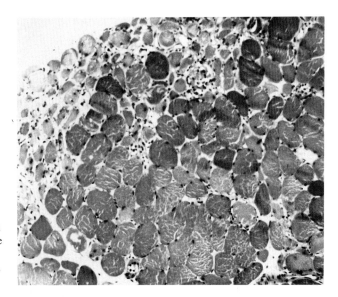

Fig. 23.10. Transverse section of muscle from a case of scleroderma. The muscle fibres at the edge of the fascicle (top left) are atrophied, while the remainder are of normal size. H&E, ×90.

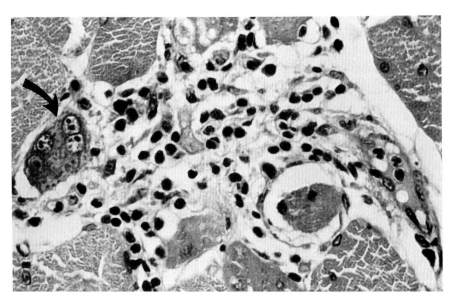

Fig. 23.11. Regenerating muscle fibre (arrowed) in transverse section, with surrounding inflammatory cells, from a case of polymyositis. Note rounded outline and prominent, vesicular nuclei with nucleoli in the regenerating fibre. H&E, ×350.

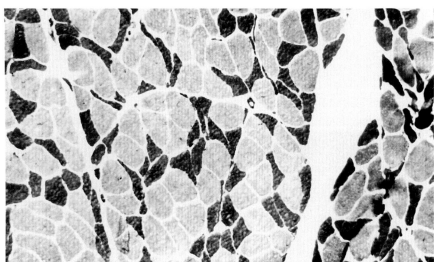

Fig. 23.12. Selective type 2 fibre atrophy. ATPase reaction at pH 9.4, ×110.

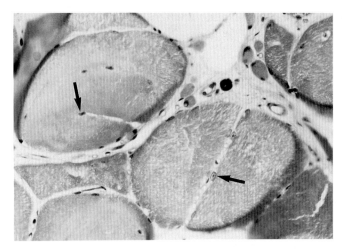

Fig. 23.13. Muscle fibres undergoing splitting from a case of limb girdle dystrophy. Nuclei are seen along the cleavage line of two fibres (arrowed). H&E, ×400.

diseases, most notably muscular dystrophy. As an abnormal feature hypertrophy is usually more extreme than when it occurs in healthy fibres. For example, diameters of over 100 μm are rarely found except in pathological conditions. Abnormally large fibres frequently contain *central or internal nuclei*, and may show evidence of *splitting*, when myonuclei are seen lying to either side of a cleft separating the two parts of the fibre (Fig. 23.13).

Muscle fibre necrosis

Necrosis in muscle fibres usually involves a segment or segments of their lengths (Fig. 23.14). The affected area may appear hyaline or glassy, lacking striations (Fig. 23.15), floccular (Fig. 23.14) or vacuolated. Sarcolemmal nuclei disappear from the necrotic zone, and macrophages infiltrate and phagocytose the remnants (Fig. 23.14), following which

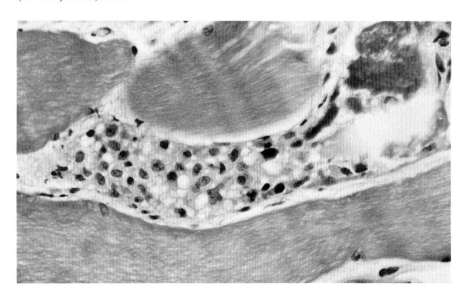

Fig. 23.14. Muscle fibre undergoing segmental floccular degeneration (top right). The same sarcolemmal sheath is filled with phagocytes which have removed the debris from this adjacent degenerate segment. H&E, ×440.

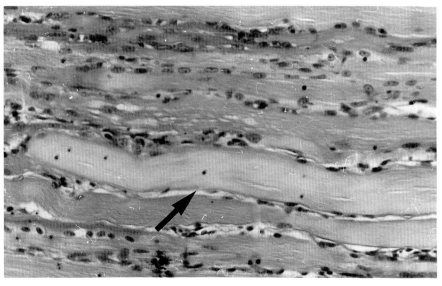

Fig. 23.15. Muscle fibre undergoing hyaline degeneration (arrowed) from a case of polymyositis. The affected fibre is swollen and its sarcoplasm structureless. An adjacent fibre (above) shows vacuolar degeneration. H&E, ×220.

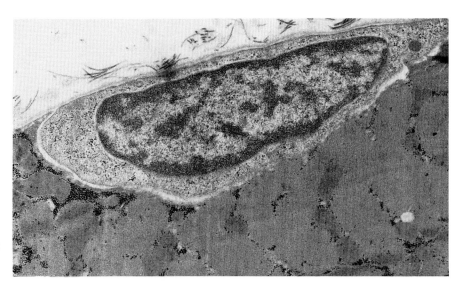

Fig. 23.16. Satellite cell lying between the basal lamina and plasmalemma of the adjacent muscle fibre. Uranyl acetate and lead citrate, ×16 430.

regeneration is attempted. Focal necrosis of muscle fibres may occur non-specifically, for example in severe systemic infections.

Regeneration of muscle

The presence of regenerating fibres in muscle implies previous necrosis. Frequently a muscle will show evidence of both necrosis and regeneration. Satellite cells are the source of cells that proliferate and differentiate to produce muscle regeneration. These cells are not distinguishable by light microscopy, but can be seen lying outside the plasmalemma and inside the basal lamina of muscle fibres by EM (Fig. 23.16). Regenerating muscle fibres appear small, with basophilic cytoplasm and chains of prominent large, centrally placed, vesicular nuclei with clearly visible nucleoli (Fig. 23.11).

Alterations in muscle fibre architecture

Ring fibres (Ringbinden, spiral annulets) and sarcoplasmic masses. Ring fibres, *Ringbinden*, or spiral annulets, are myofibrils spirally wrapped around the inside of otherwise normally orientated, longitudinal muscle fibres (Fig. 23.17). Their striations can be seen in transverse sections of the fibre. Sarcoplasmic masses are accumulations of structureless material within the sarcolemma.

Vacuoles. Vacuoles of various types may occur in otherwise normal-looking muscle fibres. Some contain stainable material, most commonly glycogen. Others contain autophagic debris. Some contain fluid, and represent dilatations of the sarcoplasmic reticulum or T tubules.

Nemaline rods. These are short, rod-like structures, visible in a modified trichrome stain as red bodies, measuring up to

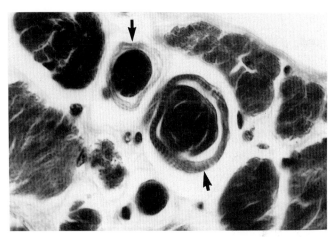

Fig. 23.17. Ring fibres, *Ringbinden*, or spiral annulets from a case of dystrophia myotonica. Transverse striations are seen in the spirally directed myofibrils situated at the margins of two transversely sectioned fibres (arrowed). H&E, ×400.

5 μm in length and 1.5 μm in width (Fig. 23.18). They consist of Z-band material.

Whorled fibres. A disorderly swirling arrangement of myofibrils is sometimes seen in histochemical preparations. Neighbouring fibres may appear 'moth-eaten'.

Ragged red fibres. These are muscle fibres showing coarse intermyofibrillar granular material and irregular marginal zones which stain red with the modified Gomori trichrome stain. These regions consist of abnormal clumps of mitochondria, and they give an excessively strong reaction for oxidative enzymes (Fig. 23.19).

Further architectural distortions of muscle fibres are detectable by EM, but are seldom visible by light microscopy. Details of altered ultrastructure are not described here but can be found in the textbooks of muscle disease listed at the end of the chapter.

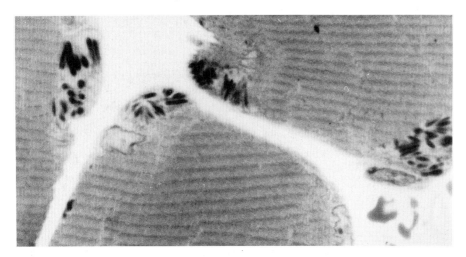

Fig. 23.18. Clusters of nemaline rods lying in a subsarcolemmal position close to myonuclei. Toluidine blue, ×940.

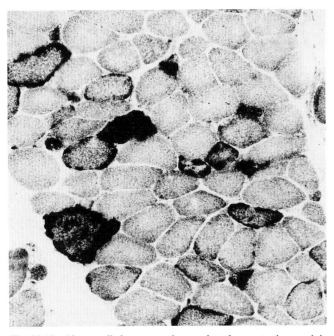

Fig. 23.19. Abnormally heavy reaction product demonstrating succinic dehydrogenase activity in some muscle fibres throughout their fibre width, and in other fibres just beneath the sarcolemma, in a case of mitochondrial myopathy. ×160.

Alterations in histochemical reactions and stored metabolites

Excessive storage material can be found in some diseases in otherwise normal muscle fibres. Glycogen or neutral fat can accumulate in this way in occasional fibres as a non-specific abnormality in diseases unrelated to storage disorders. In the latter diseases there are usually many fibres containing abnormal amounts of the stored material. There are also usually alterations in enzyme activity relevant to the stored material, e.g. absence of myophosphorylase activity with excess glycogen deposition in McArdle's disease (type 5 glycogenosis).

Alteration in distribution and proportions of different histochemical fibre types

This change is common in muscle disease. In addition to type grouping, which occurs in denervating conditions, there may be predominance of one fibre type. In many myopathic disorders there is predominance of type 1 fibres, but in small biopsies this can be difficult to distinguish from type grouping, or from physiological alterations in fibre proportions which can to some extent be influenced by training and physical exercise. In isolation it is, therefore, not a reliable indication of a myopathy.

Alterations in interstitial tissues

Abnormalities of interstitial structures may be of considerable diagnostic value when examining muscle. There may be an arteritis affecting intramuscular arteries, as in polyarteritis nodosa (Fig. 23.20), or reduced numbers of capillaries. Endomysial and perimysial fibrosis is very common in muscle disease, and as an early feature can have diagnostic value, particularly in the muscular dystrophies. Adipose tissue replacement of muscle is also a common late change occurring in many primary muscle or denervating diseases, but is particularly common and severe in muscular dystrophy. Amyloid is occasionally deposited in intramuscular connective tissue in systemic amyloidosis. Inflammatory cells are not normally found in muscle, and their presence in a focal or diffuse distribution is valuable evidence of muscle disease, particularly myositis.

Individual muscle diseases

Particular constellations of the changes outlined above are relatively, though seldom absolutely, specific for particular muscle diseases, as indicated alphabetically below. Table 23.4 summarizes some causes of the main types of pathological change.

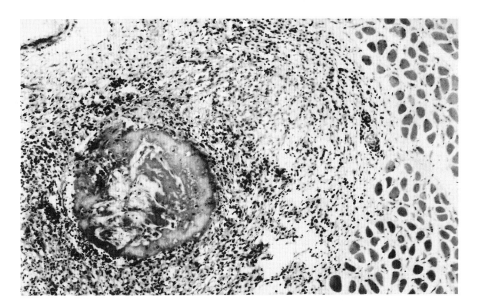

Fig. 23.20. Polyarteritis nodosa. Fibrinoid necrosis and intense inflammation in and around the walls of a small intramuscular artery. H&E, ×80.

Acute necrotizing myopathy

In this rare condition, which may cause massive myoglobinuria resulting in acute renal failure, there is extensive acute necrosis of many, often the majority of, muscle fibres in skeletal mucles. This necrosis is reflected in a high level of the creatine phosphokinase activity in the serum. Depending on the time that has elapsed since the onset, the muscle examined may contain macrophages infiltrating the dead muscle fibres, and there may be evidence of early regeneration. Inflammation is lacking. The causes are varied, but include damage secondary to viral infection (by a mechanism unknown), massive ischaemia of muscle (when it is limited to the ischaemic region), an acute episode of metabolic malfunction, a remote effect of carcinoma and the effect of certain toxins.

Arthrogryposis

The presence of limb joint deformities and associated contractures is referred to as arthrogryposis. This occurs in a number of neuromuscular diseases arising in early life and causing muscle weakness, such as Werdnig–Hoffmann disease, congenital muscular dystrophy, congenital myotonic dystrophy, central core disease and congenital fibre type disproportion. It is also sometimes found when there is a disease or malformation of the CNS which results in abnormal limb tone or movement. In some cases of arthrogryposis there may be no other abnormalities and in these cases microscopical examination of affected muscle usually reveals only non-specific abnormalities such as mild fibrosis or atrophy. This abnormality is thought to reflect abnormal positioning of the affected limb *in utero*.

Carcinomatous myopathy

The most common finding in weakness that is associated with the presence of a carcinoma is selective atrophy of type 2 fibres. In patients with severe, acute or subacute weakness there may be myositis or acute necrotizing myopathy. Patients with malignant disease also commonly develop weakness due to peripheral nerve disease resulting from direct invasion of nerve roots by tumour, or from a remote effect of carcinoma on the nervous system (p.160).

Central core, multicore or minicore disease

These conditions produce weakness, usually mild and non-progressive, from childhood onward. Microscopy shows abnormal central regions in the type 1 muscle fibres, seen best in preparations for oxidative enzyme reactions (Fig. 23.21). These areas, or cores, extend the full length of the affected fibres in central core disease, but in multi- or minicore disease many small foci are seen in each affected fibre. EM studies show disruption of myofibrillar architecture in the region affected, with an absence of mitochondria (Fig. 23.22).

Centronuclear (myotubular) myopathy

There are several variants of this inherited myopathy which differ in age of onset, severity and pattern of inheritance. In the severe infantile form the extrafusal muscle fibres are small and most have centrally placed nuclei with myofibril-free sarcoplasm around the nuclei (Fig. 23.23). Milder forms show atrophy of type 1 fibres, type 1 fibre predominance and some central nuclei.

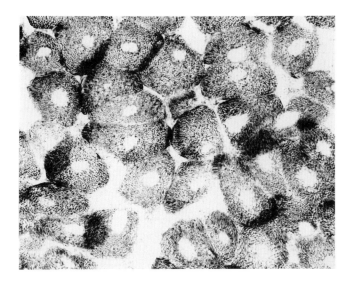

Fig. 23.21. Central core disease. Succinic dehydrogenase reaction on a transverse section of muscle, demonstrating an absence of reaction product in the centres of the fibres. ×270.

Congenital fibre-type disproportion

This condition causes floppiness and delay in achieving motor milestones in infancy. In histochemical preparations of muscle it can be seen that the diameter of the type 1 fibres is unusually small, while the diameter of the type 2 fibres is normal or slightly increased (Fig. 23.24).

Cramps

In most subjects complaining of severe muscle cramps no morphological abnormalities are found in muscle. However, cramps may be a manifestation of muscle disease, particularly metabolic disease. A few cases have shown excess tubular aggregates on EM.

Distal myopathy

This is a rare autosomal dominant disease which causes a clinically fairly distinctive, slowly progressive weakness of

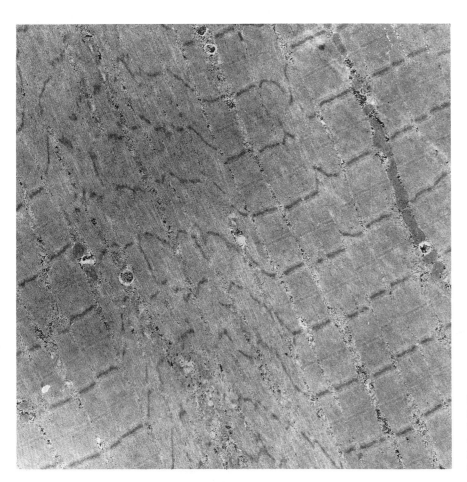

Fig. 23.22. Ultrastructure of a central core running from top left to bottom, midline. In the core region the sarcomeres are disorganized and mitochondria (seen top right between intact myofibrils) are absent. Uranyl acetate and lead citrate, ×10 560.

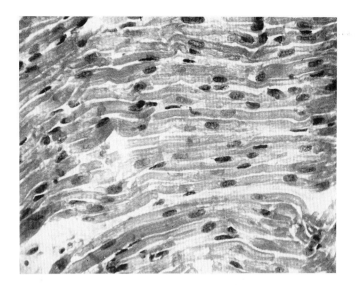

Fig. 23.23. Longitudinal section of muscle from an infant with centronuclear myopathy. The nuclei are large, occupying much of the diameter of the fibres, and are often centrally situated. ×300.

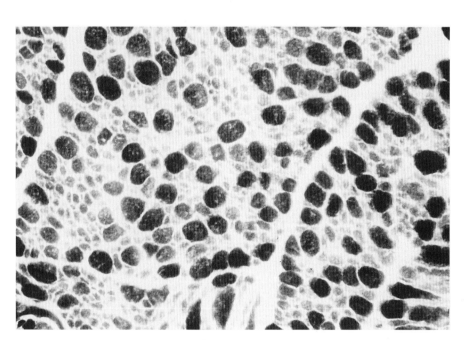

Fig. 23.24. Congenital fibre-type disproportion. ATPase reaction at pH 9.4 showing large type 2 fibres (dark) and abnormally small type 1 fibres (pale). ×280.

the hands and feet in middle-age or later. Muscle biopsies show non-specific myopathic changes, including excess variation in fibre size, internal nuclei, occasional necrosis of segments of muscle fibres and endomysial fibrosis. Autophagic vacuoles have been described with EM.

Drug-induced and toxic myopathies

Alcohol

There are acute and chronic forms of alcoholic myopathy. Acutely there may be a necrotizing myopathy or less widespread but similar features of scattered segmental necrosis,

often with associated vacuolar change, phagocytosis and regeneration. In the chronic phase there are scattered atrophic fibres, internal nuclei and variable fibrosis.

Carbon monoxide poisoning

This may cause an acute necrotizing myopathy.

Chloroquine

High doses of chloroquine occasionally cause a severe myopathy with vacuolar necrosis particularly affecting the type 1 fibres. By EM the vacuoles can be seen to contain autophagic debris.

Clofibrate

High doses of this drug may cause a painful myopathy with segmental muscle fibre necrosis, phagocytosis and regeneration.

ε-aminocaproic acid (EACA)

This antifibrinolytic drug occasionally causes a myopathy with segmental necrosis of muscle fibres, phagocytosis and regeneration.

Penicillamine

This drug occasionally causes a myasthenic syndrome or a vasculitis which may involve intramuscular, among other, vessels.

Snake venom

Some snake venoms (Australian mulga snake, tiger snake and sea snake) cause an acute necrotizing myopathy.

Steroids

A painless proximal myopathy may complicate treatment with steroids or occur in subjects with Cushing's disease. Muscle microscopy shows selective atrophy of type 2 fibres.

Dystrophia myotonica

There are congenital and adult forms of this dominantly inherited disease which causes weakness and myotonia in varying proportions. Congenital myotonic dystrophy, in which weakness predominates, occurs in infants of affected mothers. There is smallness of muscle fibres, particularly the type 1 fibres, and internal nuclei (Fig. 23.25). Sarcoplasmic masses and ring fibres may also be seen. Ultrastructurally the muscle fibres contain a rim of peripheral sarcoplasm which lacks myofibrils. In adult cases type 1 fibres are usually small but type 2 fibres may be hypertrophic. Nuclear clumps are frequently present. An increased number of internal nuclei is always found, and these characteristically form long chains (Fig. 23.26). Ring fibres and sarcoplasmic masses are also common (Fig. 23.17). There are occasional foci of necrosis and regeneration and endomysial collagen is increased. Adipose tissue replaces muscle at a late stage and muscle spindles tend to have increased numbers of intrafusal muscle fibres (Fig. 23.27).

Endocrine myopathies

Acromegaly

Proximal muscle weakness occurs in some acromegalic subjects. Muscle biopsies have shown non-specific changes of excess variation in fibre size and occasional segmental necrosis in such cases.

Cushing's disease

Selective type 2 fibre atrophy is the usual finding in cases of myopathy associated with Cushing's disease.

Hyperthyroidism

Thyrotoxic patients may have a proximal myopathy, but there are usually no structural changes found on muscle

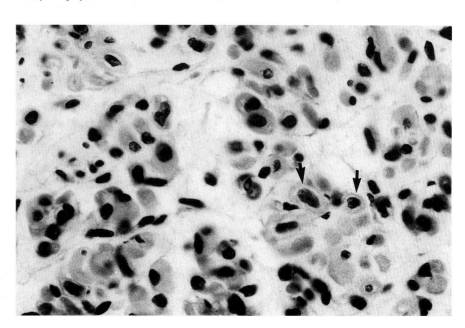

Fig. 23.25. Congenital dystrophia myotonica. Section of muscle showing small muscle fibres with relatively large, central nuclei, in some fibres surrounded by a clear rim of sarcoplasm (arrowed). H&E, ×400.

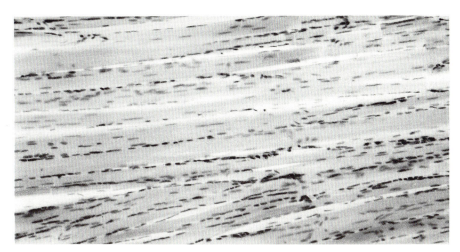

Fig. 23.26. Longitudinal section of muscle from a case of adult dystrophia myotonica. There are increased numbers of myonuclei, many of them arranged in chains. H&E, ×130.

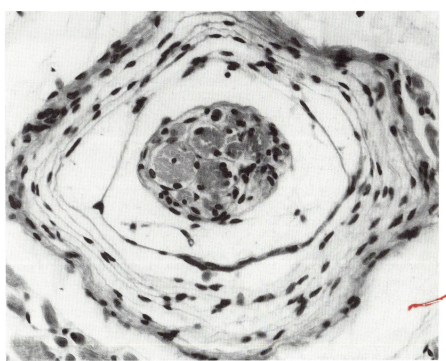

Fig. 23.27. Muscle spindle from a case of adult dystrophia myotonica showing increased numbers of intrafusal muscle fibres (cf. Fig. 23.2). H&E, ×350.

biopsy. Exophthalmos in thyrotoxicosis is due to severe oedema causing swelling of extraocular muscles and adjacent adipose tissue. There is also lymphocytic infiltration and segmental necrosis of extraocular muscle fibres.

Hypothyroidism

Mild type 2 atrophy and prominent collections of subsarcolemmal glycogen are described in hypothyroid patients with myopathy.

Eosinophilic fasciitis

In this condition inflammatory infiltrates are found in the deep fascia and immediately adjacent muscle fascicles. There may also be some segmental muscle fibre necrosis and regeneration. Eosinophils are sometimes prominent in the inflammatory infiltrates.

Fingerprint body myopathy

This is a rare congenital myopathy in which inclusions reminiscent of fingerprints are seen by EM of muscle.

Ischaemic myopathy

Ischaemic changes in muscle are seen commonly in lower limb muscles of subjects with severe atheroma or diabetes mellitus. They are also seen following acute interruption of the blood supply to a muscle, as can occur after trauma or as a result of prolonged, heavy pressure on a muscle, for example in deeply comatose subjects. Small muscle infarcts are also seen in muscle in polyarteritis nodosa. Microscopic appearances vary according to the age of the infarct. Initially there is acute necrosis affecting a sharply defined group of muscle fibres or fascicles, with loss of myonuclei. This is followed by phagocytosis and attempts at regeneration, but much of the healing in large infarcts is by scar formation.

Malignant hyperpyrexia

Occasionally apparently normal subjects react to certain anaesthetic agents, particularly succinyl choline or halothane, by developing a rise in temperature which may prove fatal. The tendency so to react is inherited in a dominant fashion. Muscle biopsy is occasionally undertaken to try to detect this tendency. Pharmacological and biochemical tests are much more useful for this purpose than is microscopy; so it is important that arrangements for these to be carried out are made before the biopsy is undertaken. There are no specific structural changes.

Metabolic myopathies

With glycogen storage

Acid maltase deficiency (type 2 glycogenosis). There is a severe infantile form and a milder adult form of this inherited disease. Affected infants have excessive deposits of glycogen in skeletal and cardiac muscle, and often die of cardiac failure. Cryostat sections of affected muscle show excess glycogen and acid phosphatase activity in the muscle fibres (Fig. 23.28). At the ultrastructural level some of this

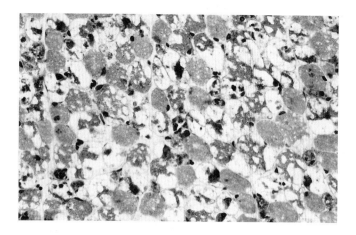

Fig. 23.28. Infantile acid maltase deficiency (glycogenosis type 2, Pompe's disease). Transverse cryostat section of muscle showing vacuoles and excess, residual, dark-staining glycogen deposits in type 2 fibres. Type 1 fibres, though vacuolated, are better preserved. PAS, ×220.

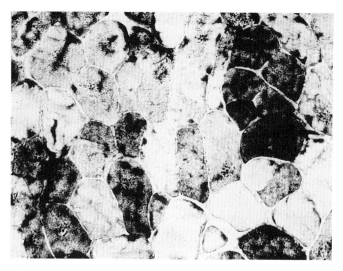

Fig. 23.29. Adult acid maltase deficiency. Heavy glycogen deposition in scattered type 2 fibres. PAS, ×250.

glycogen is seen to be membrane bound. Brain stem and spinal cord neurons can be shown at post mortem also to contain excess glycogen. The deficiency of acid maltase activity can be demonstrated in muscle, liver, blood leucocytes and cultured fibroblasts. In the adult form of the disease some muscle fibres contain a few vacuoles filled with glycogen and reacting positively for acid phosphatase (Fig. 23.29).

Debranching enzyme deficiency (type 3 glycogenosis). In this rare disease there may be muscle weakness and wasting and exercise intolerance in childhood. Skeletal muscle fibres contain multiple glycogen-filled vacuoles and some fibres are atrophic. Subsarcolemmal glycogen particles are also increased. The enzyme deficiency can be demonstrated in liver, muscle or leucocytes.

Branching enzyme deficiency (type 4 glycogenosis). This rare inherited disease causes fatal liver disease commencing in infancy. Skeletal muscle is affected along with many other tissues. It shows circumscribed deposits of granular amylopectin stainable with PAS, colloidal iron and iodine. Enzyme assays for the enzyme should be performed on liver or leucocytes.

McArdle's disease (type 5 glycogenosis). Pain and fatigability of muscles on exercise clinically characterize this rare inherited disease. Another finding is failure of the blood lactate level to rise on ischaemic exercise of the forearm. Cryostat sections of muscle show excess subsarcolemmal deposits of glycogen and an absence of phosphorylase activity. The glycogen deposits are also evident on ultrastructural examination of muscle (Fig. 23.30).

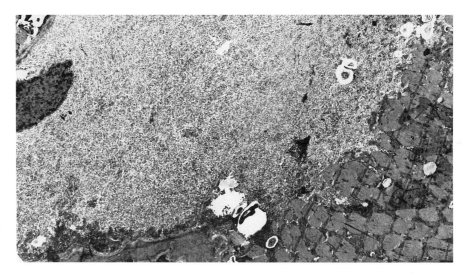

Fig. 23.30. McArdle's disease (glycogenosis type 5). Subsarcolemmal, granular deposits of glycogen (above and left). Uranyl acetate and lead citrate, ×3890.

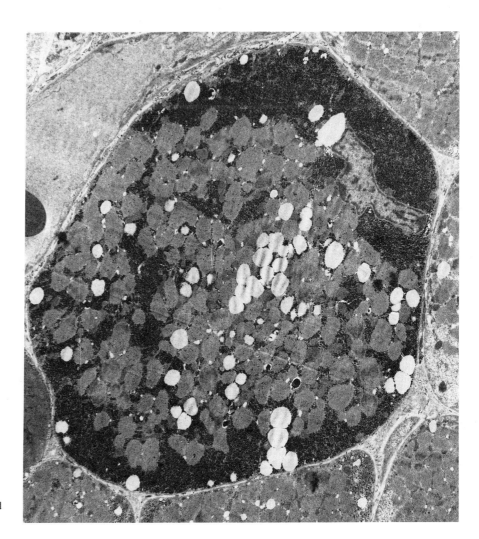

Fig. 23.31. Low-power electron micrograph showing excess fat droplets (pale) and glycogen (dark) in a transversely sectioned muscle fibre from an infant with a mitochondrial myopathy. Uranyl acetate and lead citrate, ×4490.

Phosphofructokinase deficiency (type 7 glycogenosis). Muscle pain and exercise intolerance from childhood onward occur in this inherited disease, and as in McArdle's disease there is a failure of the blood lactate level to rise after ischaemic exercise. Cryostat sections of muscle show excess subsarcolemmal deposits of glycogen, but phosphorylase activity is normal and phosphofructokinase deficiency can be demonstrated biochemically in muscle. Other rare enzyme deficiencies can give similar histochemical findings, details of which can be obtained from textbooks devoted to muscle disease.

With lipid storage

Metabolic disorders that influence oxidative metabolism are liable to give rise to excess storage of lipid which is a major source of energy in type 1 fibres. Carnitine deficiency produces increased storage of lipid droplets in muscle. Carnitine palmitoyl transferase deficiency may be, but is not always, associated with a slight increase in stored lipid; but it should be noted that there is a wide range of lipid stored in normal muscle. Disorders of mitochondrial metabolism can give rise to moderate storage of both fat and glycogen (Fig. 23.31). For the diagnosis of carnitine or carnitine palmitoyl transferase deficiency a sample of muscle should be deep-frozen and reserved for biochemical study.

With mitochondrial abnormalities

Mitochondrial myopathies are disorders in which symptoms of myopathy, often very slight, are found associated with morphological changes in the fine structure of mitochondria and with an excess of oxidative enzyme activity detected histochemically (Fig. 23.19). Affected fibres appear as 'ragged red' fibres. Some cases have symptoms of CNS disease that are much more serious than the manifestations of muscle disease, as occurs in the Kearns—Sayre syndrome (p.377), and they are better termed *mitochondrial cytopathies*. Clarification of the biochemical basis of a mitochondrial myopathy entails specialized studies of freshly isolated mitochondria. If this is contemplated it may be desirable to confirm a tentative clinical diagnosis by performing light microscopy, histochemistry and EM on a needle biopsy sample of muscle before proceeding to an open biopsy which will be necessary for the removal of tissue for mitochondrial studies. Ultrastructural changes in the mitochondria are variable, some cases showing enlarged mitochondria and other abnormalities in the arrangement of the cristae, or paracrystalline intramitochondrial inclusions (Fig. 23.32). Not all mitochondria are affected, however, and several muscle fibres may need to be examined ultrastructurally before abnormal forms are found. The presence or absence of other myopathic features, the

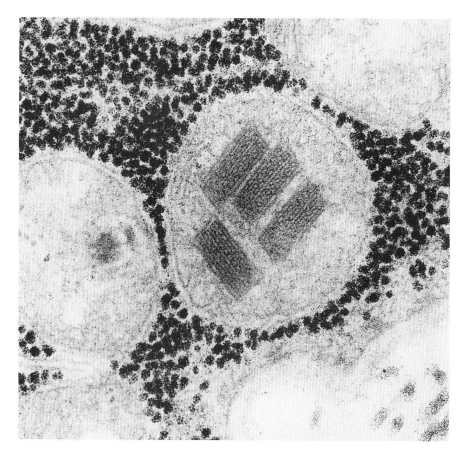

Fig. 23.32. Paracrystalline inclusions in abnormal mitochondria from a case of mitochondrial myopathy. Uranyl acetate and lead citrate, ×123 500.

clinical presentation and biochemical findings all need to be taken into account when a diagnosis of mitochondrial myopathy is made, as some alteration in mitochondrial numbers and structure can occur in other diseases, e.g. myositis.

Muscular dystrophy

Muscular dystrophies are genetically determined myopathies which share common structural abnormalities while differing in their age of onset and rate of progression. They all cause muscle weakness and, at some stage in the disease, an elevation in the serum level of creatine phosphokinase activity. This enzyme is present in high concentration in muscle, and is thought to leak out of muscle into the serum to produce the elevated levels seen in muscular dystrophy. Very recently it has been demonstrated that muscle from patients with muscular dystrophy lacks, or contains abnormally low quantities of, a recently discovered protein, *dystrophin* (Lancet 1988). Pathologically the similarities of the muscular dystrophies outweigh their differences and most pathologists are rightly hesitant about classifying a case of muscular dystrophy solely on the basis of the histopathological features. Very late in the course of muscular dystrophy appearances of the muscle can be indistinguishable from long-standing denervation.

The implied consequences for the patients and their families are so important that most clinicians rightly insist on obtaining pathological verification of the diagnosis of muscular dystrophy. Most of the pathological changes are detectable in routinely stained sections, and histochemistry adds no crucial information for the diagnosis of muscular dystrophy. The sections of muscle show excess variation in size of the fibres, with randomly scattered atrophic and hypertrophic fibres, an excess of internal nuclei, fibre splitting, foci of necrosis, generally sparse evidence of regeneration, and a marked excess of endoneurial collagen. In the late stages of the disease most muscle fibres disappear and are replaced to some extent by adipose tissue and collagen. Pathological features that are relatively pronounced in the various types of muscular dystrophy are summarized below.

Duchenne dystrophy

Inheritance of this X-linked, recessive form affects boys in early childhood after a normal infancy. Death usually occurs in the late teens or early twenties, and cardiac failure supervenes in many cases. Necrosis of muscle fibres, with prominent hyaline change, is evident early in the course of the disease, as is endomysial fibrosis (Figs 23.33 and 23.34). Regenerating fibres are seen early on, but regeneration tends to fall off as the disease progresses. Histochemical differentiation of fibre types is usually rather difficult to confirm. In the late stage there is preservation of muscle

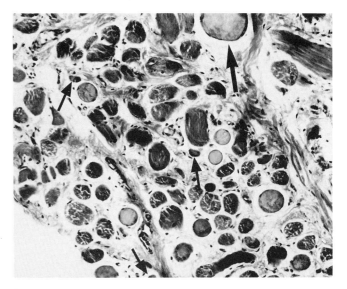

Fig. 23.33. Duchenne muscular dystrophy. Transverse section of muscle showing variation in fibre diameters, with abnormally large (large arrow) and small (small arrow) fibres, and endomysial fibrosis. H&E, ×90.

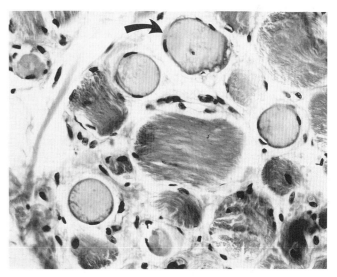

Fig. 23.34. Duchenne muscular dystrophy. Higher power view of a transverse section of muscle showing abnormally rounded and swollen, hyaline fibres, including one with an internal nucleus (arrowed). H&E, ×215.

spindles, intramuscular nerves and blood vessels, in sharp distinction from the virtually complete replacement of extrafusal muscle fibres by adipose tissue and collagen (Fig. 23.35). Ultrastructural studies have emphasized the frequent absence of stretches of the sarcolemma over regions of otherwise intact fibres, and reduplication of the basal lamina.

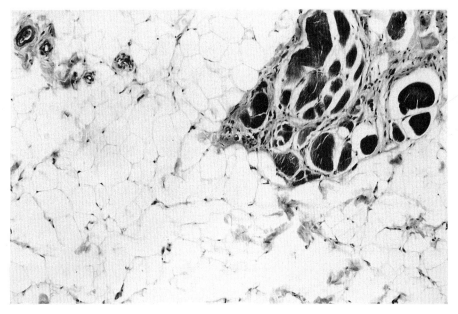

Fig. 23.35. Appearance of muscle late in the course of muscular dystrophy. Most of the muscle is replaced by adipose tissue. A small cluster of muscle fibres remains (top right), with excess surrounding collagen. At this stage the appearances of muscular dystrophy are similar to those of late-stage denervation atrophy. H&E, ×80.

Becker dystrophy

Pathological features resemble those of Duchenne dystrophy, but necrosis of muscle fibres tends to be less extensive, in keeping with the generally slower course of the disease.

Congenital muscular dystrophy

This form is less well defined than the other types of muscular dystrophy and is also unusual in showing little tendency to progress clinically. The main pathological features are excess variation in muscle fibre size, some necrosis and phagocytosis, and a marked excess of endomysial collagen.

Facio-scapulo-humeral dystrophy

Small angular-shaped fibres scattered singly or in small groups are a prominent feature in this very slowly progressive disease. Little necrosis is evident in biopsies, but 'moth-eaten' fibres are common.

Limb girdle dystrophy

This is a slowly progressive disease in which marked hypertrophy of muscle fibres and many internal myonuclei are prominent features. Atrophic fibres are also present, sometimes in small groups, and fibre splitting is also common. 'Moth-eaten' fibres may be seen, as in facio-scapulo-humeral dystrophy.

Oculopharyngeal dystrophy

Ophthalmoplegia, ptosis and dysphagia occur in this rare form of late-onset muscular dystrophy. Abnormalities in limb muscles are sparse and non-specific. A few 'ragged red' fibres may be present, together with mild atrophy and a few vacuolated fibres.

Myasthenia gravis

Routine microscopic examination of muscle is of little diagnostic value in myasthenia gravis and the various myasthenic syndromes. The diagnosis is usually made on the basis of the clinical features, backed up by a Tensilon test, electromyography and assay of serum for acetylcholine receptor antibody. That is not to say, however, that there are no features of interest in the microscopy and ultrastructure of myasthenic muscle. Examination of motor end-plates is of considerable interest, but requires that a motor point biopsy is taken to ensure that they are included in the sample. They can be detected easily at the light microscope level with the non-specific esterase enzyme reaction on cryostat sections (Fig. 4.39) and with silver stains such as the Schofield stain in fixed samples. Intravitam methylene blue staining is another way by which they can be displayed. The end-plate region tends to be more spread out than in normal muscle, but the specialized terminations are ill-formed and the preterminal nerve is irregular in calibre (Fig. 23.36). EM

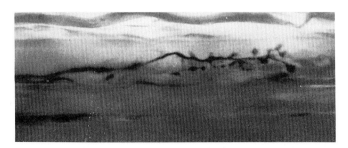

Fig. 23.36. Myasthenia gravis. Schofield-stained section showing a motor nerve terminal. The junctional area between terminal and muscle is expanded, abnormally branched and poorly formed. ×200.

shows widening of the synaptic clefts at the end-plates and loss of the secondary clefts in the postsynaptic membrane (Fig. 23.37). Elsewhere in the muscle small clusters of lymphocytes ('lymphorrhages') may be found between muscle fibres and there may be occasional foci of segmental necrosis. Occasionally in long-standing myasthenia, denervation atrophy or selective type 2 atrophy may be seen. Denervation of the tongue can be particularly severe, and associated with fatty pseudohypertrophy and marked proliferation of terminal nerve fibres (Fig. 23.38). The thymus is almost always abnormal in myasthenia, showing either hyperplastic features or the presence of a thymoma.

Myasthenic syndromes, which also give rise to fatiguability of muscle, occur usually in association with carcinoma. They do not have any distinctive microscopic pathology.

Myositis

Inflammatory change in muscle is relatively commonly encountered by pathologists regularly examining muscle biopsies. It can occur to a mild extent as a non-specific feature in cases with a myopathy or muscular dystrophy. This can give rise to diagnostic confusion, particularly as some cases of primary myositis may also show only mild

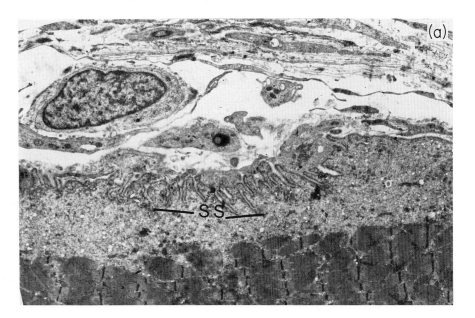

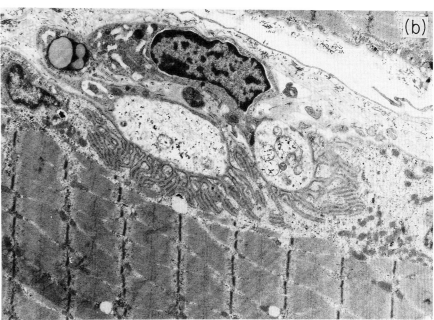

Fig. 23.37. Low-power electron micrographs of a myasthenic motor end-plate (a) and normal end-plate (b). In myasthenia the secondary synaptic clefts (SS) are irregular, widened and shallow, and the presynaptic nerve ending is not closely applied to the postsynaptic muscle membrane. Uranyl acetate and lead citrate, (a) ×4800; (b) ×6860.

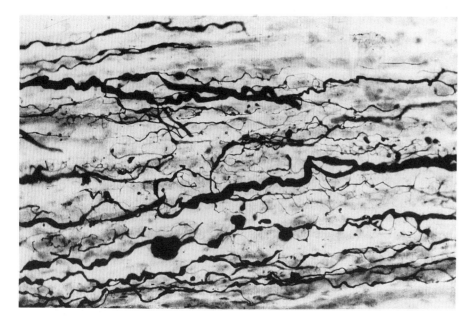

Fig. 23.38. Myasthenia gravis. Proliferation of nerve fibres, with abnormal branching and formation of numerous lateral and terminal expansions in the tongue. Schofield, ×190.

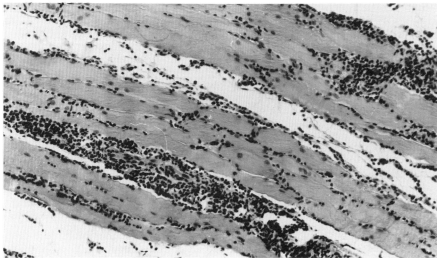

Fig. 23.39. Polymyositis. There is a predominantly lymphocytic inflammatory cell infiltrate among the muscle fibres. H&E, ×170.

inflammation. Macrophages infiltrating necrotic muscle fibres do not constitute a myositis. Various forms of myositis occur, of which the idiopathic (probably autoimmune), forms are the commonest.

Dermatomyositis and polymyositis

These idiopathic forms differ mainly according to whether or not there is a skin rash associated with the muscle disease, whose chief manifestation is muscle weakness. There are associations with rheumatoid arthritis and other collagen diseases and, particularly for dermatomyositis, with malignancy. The key pathological features are a mononuclear inflammatory cell infiltrate in and around the muscle fascicles, scattered segmental necrosis of muscle fibres and the

presence of regenerating fibres (Figs 23.11 and 23.39). The inflammatory cells consist chiefly of lymphocytes, many of them T-cells, macrophages and plasma cells. In childhood and some adult cases of dermatomyositis deposits of IgG and complement components C3 and C9 may be detectable in the muscle. In childhood myositis there is frequently atrophy of muscle fibres at the margins of the fascicles, thrombosis of vessels, loss of capillaries and relatively sparse inflammation. Scattered muscle fibre atrophy occurs in all forms of myositis, and there may be fibrosis of variable degree.

Granulomatous and giant cell myositis

Granulomas containing multinucleate giant cells, but without caseation, occur in muscle in some patients with sarcoidosis and others with a thymoma with or without accompanying myasthenia gravis. Occasionally extensive granulomatous myositis occurs as an isolated finding. In all these conditions the granulomas occur mainly in interstitial tissues between the muscle fibres, but occasionally they cause focal destruction of muscle fibres.

Inclusion body myositis

This rare condition is characterized pathologically by the presence of inclusion bodies visible by EM, which consist of collections of 15–18 nm filaments lying in muscle fibre cytoplasm or nucleus (Fig. 23.40). The muscle fibres may also contain small vacuoles and show foci of segmental necrosis with mild inflammation.

Parasitic myositis

Trichinosis, due to the ingestion of insufficiently cooked meat infected with *Trichinella*, produces multifocal inflammation at sites in the muscles where larvae are deposited. At these sites there is focal segmental necrosis of muscle fibres with a mixed inflammatory cell infiltrate including lymphocytes, plasma cells, macrophages, neutrophils and eosinophils. Encysted larvae may also be present. Other parasites may also invade muscle and cause a myositis. These include toxoplasma, sarcosporidium and cysticercus.

Pyogenic myositis

Myositis associated with gas gangrene due to *Clostridium welchii* infection may be seen complicating deep wounds. The infection produces extensive muscle necrosis and intense infiltration with neutrophils and other inflammatory cells.

Muscle abscesses from which *Staphylococcus aureus* can usually be grown are quite common in the tropics. Intense inflammation and an abscess cavity develop. The pathogenesis of the condition is not clear.

Myositis associated with viral infection

Viruses have been implicated as a cause of occasional cases of acute localized myositis, usually in children. Biopsies of affected muscle show oedema and an inflammatory cell infiltrate of neutrophils and lymphocytes with segmental necrosis of some muscle fibres. In occasional cases virus has been demonstrated in muscle. A non-inflammatory acute necrotizing myopathy is another rare complication of systemic viral infection.

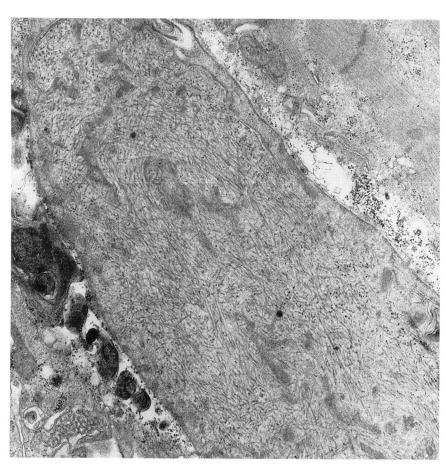

Fig. 23.40. Intranuclear filaments in a muscle fibre from a case of inclusion body myositis. Uranyl acetate and lead citrate, ×19 660.

Myositis ossificans

Bone and cartilage are deposited in deep connective tissue in this condition. Muscle is only secondarily affected. In one familial form there are repeated episodes of ectopic bone formation from childhood, usually with congenital anomalies of the fingers or toes. There is also a localized sporadic form. For details, a textbook of muscle pathology should be consulted.

Myotonia congenita

Clinical manifestations of this rare disease are muscle hypertrophy and myotonia. Histologically the muscles show increased fibre diameters, especially of the type 2 fibres. Some internal nuclei and scattered atrophic fibres are also present.

Nemaline rod myopathy

This may present as a childhood disorder with hypotonia and weakness, or in adults with slowly progressive proximal muscle weakness. Clusters of nemaline rods are found in the type 1 muscle fibres. These are composed of material resembling Z-bands. Many muscle fibres are slightly atrophic and there tends to be a predominance of type 1 fibres. The rods are visible with a modified Gomori trichrome stain as red bodies up to 5 μm long and 1.5 μm wide. They are readily visible as electron-dense inclusions by EM (Figs 23.18 and 23.41).

Osteomalacia

Atrophy of type 2 muscle fibres has been described in muscle weakness associated with osteomalacia.

Periodic paralysis

During attacks of paralysis there are vacuoles in the muscle fibres (Fig. 23.42). By EM these appear smooth walled and empty. They appear to communicate with the T tubules and there may also be proliferated T tubules or tubular aggregates present (Fig. 23.43). Between attacks of paralysis there are usually no abnormalities in muscle apart from occasional vacuoles.

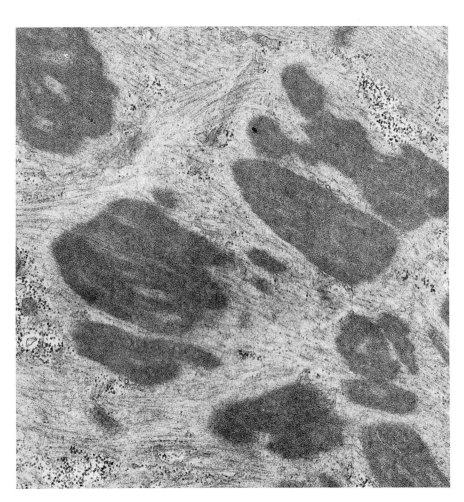

Fig. 23.41. Ultrastructural appearance of nemaline rods. Uranyl acetate and lead citrate, ×35 420.

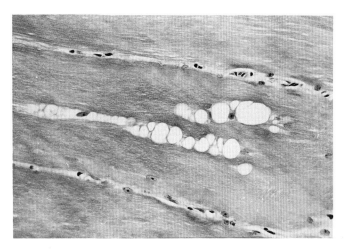

Fig. 23.42. Periodic paralysis. Vacuoles, and a few internal nuclei present in otherwise normal muscle fibres. H&E, ×340.

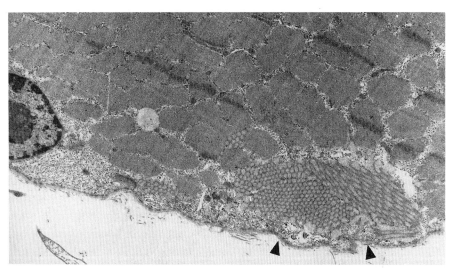

Fig. 23.43. Subsarcolemmal tubular aggregates (arrow heads) from a case of periodic paralysis in which many such aggregates were present. Uranyl acetate and lead citrate, ×8640.

Reducing body myopathy

This is a rare cause of severe muscle weakness commencing in childhood. Muscle fibres contain reducing bodies, so-called because they stain with a menadione nitro-blue tetrazolium stain. With H&E they appear reddish-pink and they show green autofluorescence. They have irregular margins, and large ones occupy the full diameter of the fibre.

Trauma to muscle

Mechanical trauma can itself directly damage muscle and it may interrupt the blood supply and thereby cause additional ischaemic damage. Denervation of muscle may also occur if the nerve supply is damaged. Mechanical damage results in acute necrosis, phagocytosis and attempts at regeneration often with scar formation. A ruptured muscle may fail to re-establish continuity with its tendon and under these circumstances may show a variety of myopathic features.

Further reading

Carpenter S, Karpati G. 1984. *Pathology of Skeletal Muscle*. Churchill Livingstone, Edinburgh.

Dubowitz V. 1985. *Muscle Biopsy, a Practical Approach*, 2nd edn. Baillière Tindall, London.

Harriman DGF. 1984. Diseases of muscle. In Adams JH, Corsellis JAN, Duchen LW (Eds) *Greenfield's Neuropathology*, 4th edn. Edward Arnold, London, pp. 1026−96.

Lancet. 1988. Dystrophin editorial **2**, 429−30.

Mastaglia FL, Walton J. 1982. *Skeletal Muscle Pathology*. Churchill Livingstone, Edinburgh.

Chapter 24
Assorted Malfunctions

In this chapter we consider various signs and symptoms of disordered working of the nervous system, and suggest procedures for the post mortem examination of affected patients. The list is, of course, far from complete. It is in alphabetical order.

Acromegaly and gigantism
Ageusia (loss of taste)
Agnosias, various
Akinetic mutism
Amnesia
Amusia
Anhidrosis: *see* Autonomic failure
Anosmia
Ataxia
Athetosis: *see* Involuntary movements
Autonomic failure
Bell's palsy: *see* Facial palsy
Blindness: *see* Visual disturbances
Brown-Séquard syndrome
Cerebral palsy: *see* Chapter 21
Chorea: *see* Involuntary movements
Coma: *see* Unconsciousness
Concussion: *see* Chapter 5
Cushing's syndrome
Deafness: *see* Hearing loss
Dementia: *see* Chapter 17
Diabetes insipidus
Diplopia
Disorientation: *see* Agnosias
Dysarthria: *see* Speech disorders
Dysautonomia: *see* Autonomic failure
Dysgraphia: *see* Speech disorders
Dyslexia: *see* Speech disorders
Dysphasia: *see* Speech disorders
Dystonia
Encephalopathies of uncertain origin
Epilepsy: *see* Chapter 18
Facial palsy
Flaccidity

Gigantism: *see* Acromegaly
Headache
Hearing loss
Hemianopia: *see* Visual disturbances
Hemiballism: *see* Involuntary movements
Hemiplegia
Horner's syndrome
Hyperalgesia: *see* Pain syndromes
Hypopituitarism
Impotence: *see* Autonomic failure
Incontinence
Insensitivity to pain: *see* Sensory loss
Involuntary movements
Irradiation
Korsakoff's syndrome: *see* Amnesia
Lateral medullary (Wallenberg's) syndrome
'Locked-in' syndrome
Memory loss: *see* Amnesia
Ménière's syndrome: *see* Hearing loss
Mental defect
Migraine: *see* Headache
Mongolism: *see* Chapter 16
Myasthenia: *see* Chapter 23
Myoclonus: *see* Involuntary movements
Myotonia: *see* Chapter 23
Narcolepsy: *see* Sleep disturbances
Nystagmus
Ophthalmoplegia
Orthostatic hypotension: *see* Autonomic failure
Pain syndromes

Paraplegia and paraparesis
Parkinsonism
Postural hypotension: *see* Autonomic failure
Precocious puberty
Pseudobulbar palsy
Psychosis
Rigidity
Riley–Day syndrome: *see* Autonomic failure
Schizophrenia: *see* Psychosis
Sensory loss
Sheehan syndrome: *see* Hypopituitarism
Shy–Drager syndrome: *see* Autonomic failure
Sleep disturbances
Spasticity
Speech and language disorders
Stiff man syndrome: *see* Rigidity
Thalamic syndrome: *see* Pain syndrome
Tic douloureux: *see* Pain syndromes
Tics: *see* Involuntary movements
Tremor
Trigeminal neuralgia: *see* Pain syndromes
Unconsciousness
Vertigo
Visual disturbances
Wallenberg's syndrome: see Lateral medullary syndrome
Weakness

Acromegaly and gigantism

It may be assumed that the cause is an eosinophil adenoma of the pituitary, which may be either pure or mixed with chromophobe tumour. The mixed tumours, in particular, may reach a considerable size, and cause extra trouble by compressing the optic tracts, the nerves in the walls of the cavernous sinus, or the hypothalamic region of the forebrain. A block of the sphenoid bone should be removed at post mortem (see p.3); after fixation, coronal sections, including the upper cranial nerves and internal carotid arteries, may be examined histologically. If it is intended to carry out histochemical or immunohistological studies on the tumour (see p.213), samples of the tumour are taken at post mortem.

Ageusia (loss of taste)

This is most commonly due to trauma, involving either an olfactory tract or a chorda tympani. In acceleration injuries, one or both olfactory bulbs are avulsed from the cribriform plates, with rupture of fibres arising from the olfactory mucosa (see anosmia, below). Fractures of the petrous temporal bone may cause compression of the facial nerve, including the chorda tympani, within the facial canal, causing ageusia on one side of the tongue. If the pathologist fails to execute a thorough examination of these structures, he is unlikely to arouse fierce criticism from his colleagues.

Agnosias, various

The term *agnosia* implies a failure of perception, with inability to make sense of incoming sensory data. In general, the relevant lesions are found either in the parietal cortex or in subcortical white matter, where they are thought to disconnect the receiving areas (which remain more or less intact) from other areas of cortex where information is, as they say, processed. Auditory agnosia, for instance, is caused by *bilateral* lesions behind the auditory cortex (Heschl's gyri, in the buried upper surfaces of the temporal lobes; see Fig. 24.5). Visual agnosia, which may be one-sided, depends on disconnection of visual cortex from the temporal and parietal cortex of *both* sides. Loss of spatial orientation and failure to understand spatial relationships are commonly associated with lesions of the right parietal lobe. Agnosias involving the use of language tend to occur with lesions of the left parietotemporal region.

Akinetic mutism

Patients, not in true coma, who yet lie inert, not speaking or making 'voluntary' movements, may belong to one of three or more groups. In the first, there is widespread diffuse damage to the cerebral white matter, such as occurs in leucodystrophies and in severe cases of demyelinating disease. Strich (1956) described a series of cases in which the damage was caused by acceleration injuries to the brain. In her view, their state was one of profound and irreversible dementia. In another group there is an expanding lesion in the vicinity of the third ventricle and aqueduct. Cases of this type have been described in which the state of akinetic mutism could be almost instantaneously reversed by surgical relief of intracranial pressure. Similar states, without associated lesions, are said to occur in the course of mental illness, or the use of hypnotic drugs, or a combination of these. If a case of this kind comes to post mortem, even if no naked-eye lesions are found, it is reasonable to examine sections of the thalamus, hypothalamus and temporal lobe with the microscope.

Further reading

Strich SJ. 1956. Diffuse degeneration of the cerebral white matter in severe dementia following head injury. *J Neurol Neurosurg Psychiat* **19**, 163–85.

Amnesia

The neural mechanisms through which memories are formed, established, recalled at will, and lost, constitute one of the most fascinating areas of neuropsychological physiology, in which research is advancing rapidly. Disturbances of these mechanisms produce a variety of clinical disabilities, a few of which can be traced to lesions in some part of the so-called fornix system (hippocampus/fimbria/fornix/mamillary body/anterior nucleus of thalamus/cingulate cortex/hippocampus; see p.43. In the past, over-enthusiastic attempts to treat epilepsy by bilateral temporal lobectomy, with removal of large amounts of hippocampus, have resulted in loss of the ability to form new memories, although old memories were retained. In Korsakoff's syndrome, there is a similar inability to form new memories, combined with a failure to sort old memories into their proper temporal order. The syndrome is most often a feature of Wernicke's encephalopathy (see p.316), in which bilateral lesions occur in the mamillary bodies and elsewhere in the periventricular grey matter. Simple forgetfulness, beyond what is accepted as permissible in the elderly, is an early presenting feature of Alzheimer's disease (see pp.270–3).

Amusia

This term should perhaps be discarded. Several quite different activities are involved in the performance, memorizing, recognition, recall and composition of music; it is therefore not surprising if there is no recognized 'musical centre' in the brain. It is to be doubted, in fact, whether there is much consistency among different subjects in the 'localization' of an activity so recently acquired in primate history as music-making. Loss of various musical abilities is sometimes, but not always, associated with aphasia. The subject is discussed, with a review of the literature, by Benton (1977).

Further reading

Benton AL. 1977. The Amusias. In Critchley M., Henson RA (Eds) *Music and the Brain*. William Heinemann, London, Chapter 22.

Anosmia

This is usually a temporary inconvenience caused by the common cold. Lasting anosmia results when the olfactory bulbs are torn away from the cribriform plate. This may be due either to acceleration injury to the head, or to retraction of the frontal lobes in the course of a surgical operation. Traces of the injury may be found in the form of yellow staining of the bulbs and surrounding cortex.

One-sided anosmia is also a feature of tumours in the floor of the anterior cranial fossa — in particular, olfactory groove meningiomas.

In Alzheimer's disease (pp.270–3) the sense of smell has recently been shown to be blunted early in the course of the illness. This may be related to the finding, in a number of cases of Alzheimer's disease, of numerous argyrophilic plaques and neurofibrillary tangles in the olfactory (peri-amygdaloid) cortex and in parts of the amygdaloid nucleus having intimate olfactory connections (corticomedial nuclei); also of neurofibrillary tangles and cell loss in the anterior olfactory nuclei.

Ataxia (see also Chapter 15, pp.244−7)

The term covers many manifestations of bad coordination of voluntary movements. Some of these have been given pleasing names such as dyssynergia and dysdiadochokinesis; for details, textbooks of neurology should be consulted. Most of them can be traced to lesions in the cerebellum and its connections; but in some cases the cerebellar network appears intact, and the relevant lesions are in some part of the sensory apparatus. The best-known example of a disease causing sensory ataxia is tabes dorsalis.

In examining a case of ataxia, if there is a suitably-placed lesion, apparent to the naked eye, such as a tumour, a haemorrhage or an infarct, there is little point in exploring the rest of the cerebellar and sensory systems. If, however, there is a history of progressive ataxia, and naked-eye inspection reveals nothing more than symmetrical shrinkage (associated, perhaps, with a palpable gliotic hardening), a system degeneration is the probable diagnosis; and multiple histological blocks are needed in order to determine the extent of the degeneration (see Chapter 15). When exploring the cerebellum, it should be borne in mind that lesions in a lateral lobe are associated with ataxia of the limbs on the same side of the body, whereas midline lesions are commonly associated with trunk ataxia.

Table 24.1 shows some sites where lesions bearing on ataxia may be found, along with the diseases in which such lesions are apt to occur. Anatomical relations are shown in Figs 2.26−2.28.

Autonomic failure

This term covers many functional disturbances, including anhidrosis (inability to sweat), retention of urine, impotence, orthostatic (or postural) hypotension, i.e. a tendency to faint in the upright posture, and other manifestations of defective vasomotor control. Four different types of morbid change have been implicated in autonomic failure:

1 Peripheral nerve diseases, of which by far the commonest is diabetic neuropathy (see p.338).
2 A group of rare genetic disorders, most of which involve both autonomic and sensory nerve fibres. Best known of these is familial dysautonomia (Riley−Day syndrome). For details, see Thomas *et al.* (1984). Most of the patients are children.
3 A group with destructive or expanding lesions in the region of the pituitary and hypothalamus.
4 In the most studied form of autonomic failure, the principal lesions are found in the CNS. The condition is progressive, affects middle-aged and elderly people, and is often associated with degenerative lesions in many parts of the CNS. It is discussed in Chapter 15, pp.241−3.

The clinical notes will usually indicate whether the main lesions should be looked for in the central or the peripheral nervous system. In any case, peripheral autonomic and

Table 24.1. Sites of lesions in diseases causing ataxia

Sites of lesions	Diseases
Sensory ganglia and roots	Disc protrusions; toxic and inflammatory neuropathies; tabes dorsalis; FA; CMTD; AT; spinal radiculitis; carcinoma; chronic meningitis
Cord; posterior columns	As above; MS; spinal tumours
Dorsal (Clarke's) nuclei	FA; various spinocerebellar degenerations
Spinocerebellar tracts	FA; MS; various degenerations
Gracile and cuneate nuclei	'Chain' degeneration from posterior column lesions
Medial lemnisci	As above; MS
Accessory cuneate nuclei	FA
Inferior olives	Retrograde degeneration from cerebellar cortex; MSA; Leigh's disease
Inferior cerebellar peduncles	Degeneration of spino-, cuneo- and olivocerebellar tracts; lateral medullary syndrome; MS; MSA; FA
Cerebellar white matter	Degeneration of cerebellopetal fibres and Purkinje axons; MS; MSA; CCD; infarction
Cerebellar Purkinje cells	Hypoxia; epilepsy; toxins (including alcoholism); MSA; CCD; AT; old age
Cerebellar granule cells	Hypoxia; haemosiderosis; AT; CJD
Pontine nuclei	MSA; Leigh's disease
Middle cerebellar peduncles	MSA; MS
Dentate nuclei	FA; DRPLA; PSP
Superior cerebellar peduncles	FA; DRPLA; PSP; MS; trauma
Red nuclei	DRPLA; PSP

AT   ataxia−telangiectasia.
CCD   cerebellar cortical degeneration.
CJD   Creutzfeldt−Jakob disease.
CMTD   Charcot−Marie−Tooth disease.
DRPLA   dentato-rubro-pallido-luysian degeneration.
FA   Friedreich's ataxia.
MS   multiple sclerosis.
MSA   multiple system atrophy.
PSP   progressive supranuclear palsy.

sensory ganglia should be examined. If the vertebral column has been taken, the sympathetic chains will be available in the thoracolumbar region; and if a deep dissection of the neck has been carried out, there are cervical sympathetic ganglia and the (parasympathetic) inferior (nodose) ganglion of the vagus. The coeliac plexus provides a rich source of distal autonomic ganglia. This lies in the connective tissue around the origins of the coeliac, superior mesenteric and renal arteries.

Cases of progressive autonomic failure fall into two groups: in the first, there are Lewy inclusion bodies in pigmented cells of the substantia nigra and locus ceruleus; in the second, there is multiple system atrophy (see pp.241–4) affecting the putamen and substantia nigra, and in many cases the pons, olives and cerebellar cortex. Cells of the intermediolateral columns, lying in the lateral horns of the thoracic cord, are depleted, sometimes devastated; but as their distribution is somewhat irregular, it is not safe to assess the degree of cell loss without examining five or more sections of thoracic cord and comparing these with sections of similar thickness from control material. Cell loss has recently been recorded from the intermediolateral columns of the sacral cord. These are the source of the sacral parasympathetic outflow. It has also been noted that cells are lost from the nucleus of Onufrowicz ('Onuf's nucleus'), a group of cells of somatic motor type, lying at the ventral edge of the anterior grey horn at level S2. These are believed to be the cells innervating the 'voluntary' sphincters of the anus and bladder neck. They are spared in motor neuron disease and in Werdnig–Hoffmann disease, even when the remaining sacral motor cells are devastated. For further discussion of the pathology of autonomic failure see Bannister (1988).

The histological examination in any case of autonomic failure should include samples of both central and peripheral nervous systems. In a middle-aged or elderly subject with a progressive history, the two likely diseases are (i) multiple system atrophy of striatonigral type, and (ii) Parkinson's disease. Areas of the CNS at risk in these diseases are indicated in Table 15.1 (p.236).

Further reading

Bannister R (Ed.). 1988. *Autonomic Failure*, 2nd edn. Oxford University Press, Oxford.
Thomas PK, Landon DN, King RHM. 1984. Diseases of the peripheral nerves. In Adams JH, Corsellis JAN, Duchen LW (Eds) *Greenfield's Neuropathology*, 4th edn. Edward Arnold, London, Chapter 18.

Brown-Séquard syndrome

This is characterized by paralysis, of upper motor neuron type, of one lower limb, with loss of position and vibration sensibility on the same side, and loss of painful and thermal sensibility on the opposite side. In its classical form it is due to hemisection of the spinal cord by a stab wound in the back. Other types of lesion may result in a more or less similar clinical picture. The neuropathologist's task is to identify the lesion, determine its segmental level, and observe, from sections taken a few centimetres above and below the lesion, the amount of upward and downward tract degeneration. In a 'classical' case, there will be a clear-cut myelin pallor and loss of axons in the pyramidal tract below the lesion, and in the gracile and spinocerebellar tracts above it. Upward degeneration of the so-called spinothalamic tract may be hard to appreciate, as the fibres in this group are mixed with others, many of them descending; but unless the lesion is very old, Marchi studies should reveal considerably more than can be seen by myelin staining. For cord tracts, see Fig. 2.28.

Cushing's disease

Cushing's disease, resulting from over-activity of the adrenal cortex, is sometimes due to excess production of ACTH by basophil cells in the anterior lobe of the pituitary. These may be scattered, or collected into a small discrete adenoma (for procedures, see pp.210, 215). Rarer causes are adenomas and carcinomas of the adrenal cortex and oat-celled carcinomas of the lung, mischievously secreting ACTH or an analogous hormone. In all cases, the adrenals should be weighed, and studied histologically.

Diabetes insipidus

In a case of diabetes insipidus the structures needing detailed examination are the paraventricular and supra-optic nuclei of the hypothalamus (see Fig. 24.1), their efferent pathway in the infundibulum and pituitary stalk, and the posterior lobe of the pituitary itself. Some cases are 'primary', i.e. due to unknown causes. A few are familial. Among the rest, the causes include trauma, tumours and chronic inflammations. For details of anatomy and histopathology, see Treip (1984).

Further reading

Treip CS. 1984. The hypothalamus and pituitary gland. In Adams JH, Corsellis JAN, Duchen LW (Eds) *Greenfield's Neuropathology*, 4th edn. Edward Arnold, London, Chapter 16.

Diplopia

An acquired diplopia may be due to mechanical displacement of one eyeball (for instance, by an orbital tumour) or by a lesion affecting one or more of cranial nerves III, IV and VI. Such lesions include: trauma involving the superior orbital fissure; compressing or infiltrating lesions in or near the lateral wall of the cavernous sinus, including pituitary

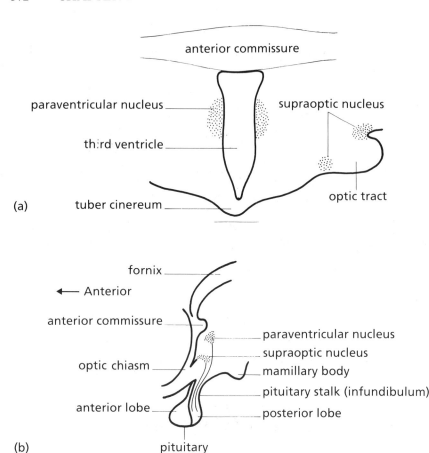

anterior commissure

paraventricular nucleus

supraoptic nucleus

third ventricle

optic tract

tuber cinereum

(a)

fornix

← Anterior

anterior commissure

optic chiasm

anterior lobe

(b)   pituitary

paraventricular nucleus
supraoptic nucleus
mamillary body
pituitary stalk (infundibulum)
posterior lobe

Fig. 24.1. Innervation of the neurohypophysis (posterior lobe of the pituitary). (a) Coronal section of the hypothalamus at the level of the anterior commissure, showing the position of the paraventricular and supraoptic nuclei. (b) Midline section, showing projections of the paraventricular and supraoptic nuclei on the wall of the third ventricle, and their efferent pathway to the neurohypophysis.

tumours, craniopharyngiomas, meningiomas, aneurysms of the internal carotid artery; meningitis; and a variety of brain stem disturbances (see below, under ophthalmoplegia.) Refractive errors giving rise to double vision in one eye lie outside the neuropathologist's province.

Dystonia

Disturbances of muscular tone are of several types, three of which are considered below, under the headings Flaccidity, Rigidity and Spasticity. Some are associated with involuntary movements (see under this heading below). Others are features of primary muscular and neuromuscular diseases, of which the pathology is discussed in Chapters 22 and 23. These include *myotonia*, i.e. slowness of relaxation following a muscular contraction (note that 'amyotonia' does not mean 'absence of myotonia'; it is merely a fancy synonym for 'flaccidity' or 'floppiness'). At post mortem on patients described as 'dystonic' it is prudent to take not only the brain and spinal cord, but also samples of nerve and muscle.

Encephalopathies of uncertain origin

The word encephalopathy means no more than 'something wrong with the brain'. Some patients die with a clinical diagnosis no more precise than this, or (which comes to the same thing) with a string of alternative diagnoses. Junior neurologists have been heard to murmur 'Some sort of brain-rot, I suppose'. From the neuropathologist's point of view, these are often the most fascinating and instructive cases. They may turn out to be unfamiliar manifestations of well-known conditions such as tuberculosis, sarcoidosis, MS, PML, congophilic angiopathy, Creutzfeldt–Jakob disease, lymphoma, normal pressure hydrocephalus (the list is long; we are merely enumerating a few cases of 'brain-rot' from our own experience; for children, the list is even longer). Some cases are merely examples of a very rare disease. No general principles can be given for dealing with these post mortems, except that the spinal cord, as well as the brain, should be taken; and it must be remembered that the combined effects of two or more diseases can be very puzzling, especially if one is trained to make unitary diagnoses.

Facial palsy

Two types are distinguished, according to whether the responsible lesion lies above or below the facial nucleus in the lower pons (see Fig. 2.26). When the lesion is above this, there are usually other hemiplegic disturbances. The lesion may be sought in the lower part of the opposite postcentral gyrus; in the internal capsule, behind the genu; or in the middle of the crus cerebri, still on the side opposite the palsy. Lesions of the nerve itself may be reflected in chromatolytic changes (p.47; Plate 1.6) in the motor cells of the facial nucleus on the damaged side. The nucleus may be affected by intrinsic tumours — gliomas or secondary deposits — and its rather convoluted emerging root may be involved in a plaque of multiple sclerosis, or an area of traumatic damage. Having emerged, it may be compressed by a tumour — notably an acoustic schwannoma. Using older surgical techniques, the operation for removal of an acoustic nerve tumour commonly converted a partial facial palsy to a complete one. A fracture of the petrous temporal bone may cause compression by blood or oedema within the facial canal; and branches of the nerve may be involved in tumours within the parotid gland. If the neck has been dissected in the manner suggested on pp.5–6, the posterior belly of the digastric muscle may be examined for signs of denervation. In most cases of Bell's palsy — the commonest form of facial paralysis — the pathology remains uncertain.

Flaccidity

Flaccid paralysis ensues when a muscle is deprived of its motor nerve supply. This may happen when motor neurons are destroyed by intrinsic tumours of the brain stem or spinal cord; by infarction; by the expansion of a syrinx; by poliomyelitis; or in the course of a degenerative disease such as motor neuron disease (amyotrophic lateral sclerosis), Werdnig–Hoffmann disease, or variants of these (see pp. 238–9). A reversible, flaccid paralysis may result from nerve injuries or nerve compression, or from a variety of toxic, metabolic and inflammatory neuropathies (see Chapter 22). In infantile hypotonia (the 'floppy baby' syndrome) it is said that in about half the cases the disease is benign, and muscle tone returns to normal within a year. These are said to have *amyotonia congenita*. The pathology is not known. Most of the rest are suffering from Werdnig–Hoffmann disease, and do not live many months.

Control of muscular tone by the brain is poorly understood, and the effects of focal brain lesions cannot be predicted from first principles. Infarcts involving the motor cortex commonly cause a flaccid hemiplegia in the first instance, with spasticity coming on later. Surgical section of the corticospinal tracts at midbrain level (Bucy *et al.* 1964) has produced an immediate flaccid hemiplegia, with recovery of power after several months, but with lasting hypotonia. In Huntington's chorea, where the most conspicuous lesions are in the striatum (caudate nucleus and putamen), all the limbs are hypotonic. Lesions of a cerebellar hemisphere are commonly associated with hypotonia of the limbs on the same side.

Further reading

Bucy PC, Keplinger JE, Siqueira EB. 1964. Destruction of the pyramidal tract in man. *J Neurosurg* 21, 385–98.

Headache

When headache is prominent in the clinical history, one should look for (i) an expanding lesion in the cranial cavity, (ii) subarachnoid blood, and (iii) signs of acute or chronic meningitis. Expanding lesions include obstructive hydrocephalus. Subarachnoid bleeding does not have to be of large extent to cause headache; post-concussion headaches, for instance, are probably due to the relatively trivial bleeding associated with minor head injuries. In migraine sufferers, there are usually no distinct pathological findings, but it is worth searching the cerebral cortex for infarcts, such as have been seen in cases of hemiplegic migraine; and the pituitary fossa and cavernous sinus should be explored, as unruptured aneurysms of an internal carotid artery are known to be responsible for some cases of 'symptomatic' migraine. Severe headaches are a feature of temporal, or giant-celled, arteritis. This condition comes to the notice of the neuropathologist in the form of temporal artery biopsies more often than in post mortem material. The histological features are mentioned in Chapter 7.

Further reading

Dalessio DJ. 1984. Headache. In Wall PD, Melzack R (Eds) *Textbook of Pain*. Churchill Livingstone, Edinburgh, pp. 277–92.

Hearing loss

The parts of the auditory system lying within the petrous temporal bone are well within the territory of neuropathological interest; but apart from centres where an ENT surgeon has a lively interest in acoustic pathology, neuropathologists are seldom called on to explore this region. Where such interest exists, blocks of petrous temporal bone should be removed with the vibrating saw at post mortem and fixed in formalin. The subsequent dissection can be planned and carried out after consultation between the clinician and the pathologist. Conditions in which such dissections may be informative include Ménière's disease, and a number of rare disorders discussed by Konigsmark (1975), in which sudden onset of deafness occurs, from unexplained causes.

Destructive lesions of an acoustic nerve will be reflected in myelin loss and, with time, gliosis, in the dorsal and ventral cochlear nuclei (see Fig. 15.8). The pathways from these to the inferior colliculi may be involved in vascular lesions or diffuse gliomas; but there are no well-defined clinical syndromes associated with particular lesions of the superior olives or trapezoid body. The input from each ear is relayed to both inferior colliculi (mainly to the contralateral one), and thence via the medial geniculate bodies to Heschl's gyri on the upper, buried surfaces of the temporal lobes. Lesions at these levels do not cause deafness unless they are bilateral.

In a case examined in this department there were bilateral temporal lobe infarcts, sparing a small amount of Heschl's gyrus on one side. The lesions were reflected in a severe retrograde loss of cells in the medial geniculate bodies. The patient was not deaf, but suffered from auditory agnosia, i.e. what he heard conveyed no meaning to him.

Further reading

Konigsmark BW. 1975. Hereditary diseases of the nervous system with hearing loss. In Vinken PJ, Bruyn GW (Eds) *Handbook of Clinical Neurology*. Elsevier, Amsterdam, **22**, Chapter 23.

Hemiplegia

By far the commonest causes of hemiplegia are vascular accidents, occlusive or haemorrhagic, affecting the territory of a middle cerebral artery, with cerebral tumours in third place. Intracerebral haemorrhage is discussed in Chapter 6, infarction in Chapter 7, and tumours in Chapters 12 and 13. Causes of *hemiparesis* are varied: they include migraine, MS and trauma. In exploring the brain of a hemiplegic patient it is worth noting that the position of the corticospinal tract in the internal capsule is well behind the position commonly assigned to it in textbooks of anatomy. It occupies the middle third of the crus cerebri, and the entire medullary pyramid. The decussation is at the junction of medulla and cord; thus the tract degeneration is contralateral to the paralysis in the brain and ipsilateral in the cord (Figs 2.26 and 2.28).

Horner's syndrome

This consists in unilateral ptosis and enophthalmos, with pupillary constriction and relative flushing and dryness of the same side of the face. It is due to interruption of the sympathetic pathway which runs from the medulla via the lateral white column of the cervical cord to the intermedio-lateral cell column at the upper end of the thoracic cord. Here the upper sympathetic fibres end, and the second-order sympathetic pathway begins. Its fibres run, via a white ramus communicans, to the sympathetic chain, ending in the superior cervical ganglion. The third-order fibres reach the face and eye by way of the carotid plexus, and thence via a multitude of little vessels and nerves. Clearly, interruption of the pathway may occur at many points. Here we will mention only a few such points. First, there is the lower medulla, where occlusion of the posterior inferior cerebellar artery may produce the lateral medullary (Wallenberg's)

syndrome, which is discussed on p.375. In the cervical cord, a syrinx may destroy the upper sympathetic fibres. Injury to the lower cervical spine may sever an upper thoracic root; and a malignant tumour in the neck may destroy the upper stretches of the sympathetic chain.

Hypopituitarism

This term is generally taken to mean depression of anterior lobe functions — most conspicuously, sexual functions. The two best known causes are infarction and compression of the gland. The latter occurs with expanding lesions within or above the pituitary fossa, in particular chromophobe adenomas, craniopharyngiomas and meningiomas. With chromophobe adenomas, doubts have been expressed on whether in some cases depression of anterior lobe function is due more to excessive prolactin secretion than to mechanical compression. In *Sheehan's syndrome*, infarction is said to be due to massive blood loss, with resulting arterial hypotension, during the puerperium.

Hypopituitarism may also result from fracture of the base of the skull, or traumatic tearing of the pituitary stalk. Inflammatory processes within the sella include tuberculosis and sarcoidosis. Examination of the region is best carried out on a block of sphenoid bone removed as described on p.3.

Incontinence

In many cases, the causes of incontinence of urine and/or faeces are obvious to the clinicians, and there is no need for the pathologist to strain his energies laying bare the structural changes responsible for it. In other cases, this is not so; for example, many an innocent prostate has been surgically assaulted in cases of progressive autonomic failure. Leaving aside the mechanical and psychiatric causes of incontinence, the post mortem examination should concentrate on the spinal cord. Plaques of MS are among the commoner causes of failure of sphincter control: but other parts of the CNS may be involved. In the heyday of prefrontal leucotomy, it was said that the operation seldom achieved its intended effect unless it rendered the patient incontinent for at least a few days.

Involuntary movements

The commonly-used clinical terms, in alphabetical order are: *athetosis* (slow, writhing movements of head, trunk and limbs), *ballism* (or hemiballism: sudden wild flinging movements, commonly affecting one or two limbs on one side of the body), *chorea* (jerky movements, affecting many parts of the body), *clonus* and *myoclonus* (rhythmic or periodic contractions of a muscle or of a group of muscles), *tics* (irregular localized movements, to some extent under

Table 24.2. Some diseases associated with involuntary movements

Type of movement	Diseases	Sites of lesions
Athetosis	Wilson's disease (p.293)	Striatum, etc; liver
	Perinatal hypoxia (pp.323−7)	
	Kernicterus (p.327)	Scattered in brain
	DRPLA (p.248)	Pallidum, etc.
Ballism	Vascular disease	Subthalamic nucleus
	DRPLA (p.248)	Subthalamic nucleus, etc.
Chorea	Sydenham's chorea (rheumatic fever)	? Basal ganglia
	Huntington's disease (p.247)	Striatum
	Wilson's disease (p.293)	Striatum, etc; liver
	DRPLA (p.248)	Pallidum, etc.
Myoclonus	Lafora body disease (p.285)	Scattered in brain
	Creutzfeldt−Jakob disease (pp.274−6)	Striatum, etc.
	SSPE (p.149)	Scattered in brain
Tremor	Paralysis agitans (pp.240−1)	Substantia nigra; nucleus basalis
	'Senility'; multi-infarct dementia (pp.276−7)	Thalamus; basal ganglia

DRPLA   dentato-rubro-pallido-luysian atrophy; SSPE   subacute sclerosing parencephalitis.

voluntary control), and *tremor*. Table 24.2 shows some of the CNS afflictions associated with abnormal movements, and sites where lesions may be found.

Irradiation

It sometimes happens, in the course of X-ray treatment of a tumour situated in the head, neck or back, that part of the CNS receives an intolerable dose of irradiation. When such a case comes to post mortem, the precise geometry of the area of radionecrosis and of its surroundings is (or should be) of intense interest to the radiotherapist, and the pathologist should be prepared to supply detailed information on this.

The lesions may take weeks, or months, or over a year to develop. Characteristically they consist of coagulative necrosis, with hyaline or fibrinoid necrosis of vessels. According to one view, which we find plausible, the primary effect of the X-rays is exerted on vascular endothelium, which loses its ability to regenerate, and the parenchymal changes are attributable to ischaemia. The observation that white matter tends to be worse affected than grey matter may be related to the relatively poor blood supply of white matter (see Duchen 1984).

The effects of irradiation on the tumours themselves are discussed by Russell and Rubinstein (1977). A special case is the medulloblastoma, which is said to be one of the most radiosensitive of all malignant tumours. It has repeatedly been observed that 10 days or so after treatment the tumour is transformed into a highly pleomorphic tissue, with bizarre giant cells, indistinguishable from a giant-celled glioblastoma.

Occasionally, after a long delay, irradiation causes a tumour to develop at the irradiated site. Sarcomas have developed in the suprasellar region following irradiation of a benign pituitary adenoma, and in the meninges after irradiation of gliomas. In the past, irradiation of the scalp for tinea capitis has resulted in the late development of brain tumours, including both gliomas and meningiomas.

Further reading

Duchen LW. 1984. Effects of irradiation on the nervous system. In Adams JH, Corsellis JAN, Duchen LW (Eds) *Greenfield's Neuropathology*, 4th edn. Edward Arnold, London, pp. 42−5.

Russell DS, Rubinstein LJ. 1977. *Pathology of Tumours of the Nervous System*, 4th edn. Edward Arnold, London.

Lateral medullary (Wallenberg's) syndrome

This syndrome, well loved by teachers of neuro-anatomy, is caused by an infarct in the territory of the PICA, which includes a variable amount of cerebellum and an area in the dorsolateral quadrant of the lower medulla (see Fig. 7.11). The syndrome consists of cerebellar ataxia, palatal palsy, Horner's syndrome and loss of pain and temperature sense over the face, all on the side of the lesion, and loss of pain and temperature sense on the other side of the body. The accompanying diagram is intended to show how this combination of disturbances is produced (Fig. 24.2)

After identifying and mapping the infarct, it remains to discover its cause. In some cases there is an occlusive thrombus in the vertebral artery, blocking the origin of the PICA; in others, the same effect is produced by atheroma,

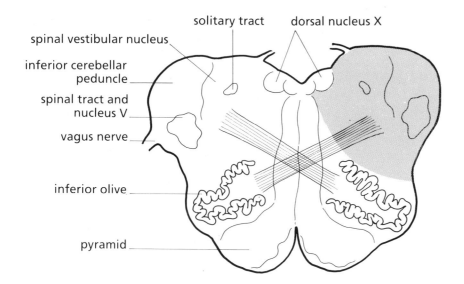

spinal vestibular nucleus

inferior cerebellar peduncle

spinal tract and nucleus V

vagus nerve

inferior olive

pyramid

solitary tract   dorsal nucleus X

Fig. 24.2. Area of the medulla commonly supplied by the posterior inferior cerebellar artery (stippled). Structures involved in the lateral medullary syndrome include: the inferior cerebellar peduncle, containing the dorsal spinocerebellar tract and olivocerebellar fibres from the opposite side; the spinal (descending) vestibular tract and nucleus; emerging and entering fibres of the vagus nerve; the spinal (descending) trigeminal tract and nucleus; and a mixture of ascending and descending pathways, continuous with the anterolateral columns of the cervical cord, including the spinothalamic and spinoreticular (sensory) pathways and the upper sympathetic fibres running from the hypothalamus to the intermediolateral columns of the spinal cord.

without thrombosis. In a few cases the vertebral artery is patent, but the PICA itself is thrombosed. A rare cause, which we have encountered, is a mechanical buckling of a loop of the PICA as it passes between the medulla and cerebellum. The course, size and territory of the artery are all variable, and the clinical syndrome varies accordingly.

'Locked-in' syndrome

Patients who, though alert, are unable to carry out any voluntary movements except of the eyes and eyelids are said to suffer from the 'locked-in' syndrome. The lesion responsible is one that interrupts descending tracts in the pons, or occasionally in the midbrain. This is usually due to infarction associated with occlusion of the basilar artery; but a few cases are due to the effects of trauma, tumour, or demyelination.

Mental defect

This is distinguished from dementia in being (in most cases, at least) congenital and non-progressive. Examination of the cerebral hemispheres of severe mental defectives usually reveals naked-eye abnormalities. When none are found, and the histology appears normal, the pathologist may well conclude that the subject simply lay at the left-hand end of the normal distribution curve for intelligence, or was autistic.

Most of the recognized lesions responsible for mental defect fall into one of three categories: (i) *developmental anomalies*, which are discussed in Chapter 16; (ii) *perinatal vascular mishaps*, discussed in Chapter 21; and (iii) *metabolic disorders*, discussed in Chapter 19. Examples of these are (i) tuberous sclerosis, (ii) cerebral palsy, and (iii) lipidosis. More rarely, the defect is traceable to intrauterine or perinatal infections, for instance, by cytomegalovirus, *Treponema pallidum* or *Toxoplasma* (Chapters 9 and 10).

Some metabolic disorders, e.g. phenylketonuria, are identifiable biochemically, but have no recognized histopathology. For the most part they cause progressive dementia rather than congenital mental defect.

Nystagmus

The physiology of the various types of nystagmus is discussed in considerable detail by Brodal (1981). In general, the lesions associated with it are to be found in the labyrinth, in the vestibular nerves and the nuclei in the lower brain stem to which they project, or in the connections between the vestibular nuclei and (i) the cerebellum, and (ii) the nuclei of the third, fourth and sixth cranial nerves, including the medial longitudinal fasciculus (see Fig. 2.26). Diseases in which such lesions occur include acute labyrinthitis, Ménière's disease, posterior fossa tumours (in particular acoustic schwannomas), occlusion of a posterior inferior cerebellar artery, brain stem gliomas and MS.

Further reading

Brodal A. 1981. *Neurological Anatomy in Relation to Clinical Medicine*, 3rd edn. Oxford University Press, Oxford.

Ophthalmoplegia

Unilateral oculomotor palsy may be caused by: intra-orbital tumours, pseudotumours and granulomas; trauma, including difficult birth; or by an expanding lesion — tumour or internal carotid aneurysm — in or near the cavernous sinus. Isolated nerve palsies occur in both acute and chronic forms of meningitis, meningeal carcinomatosis and sarcoidosis, and may also be a feature of diphtheritic neuropathy.

Bilateral ocular palsy may be due to a variety of myopathies and neuropathies. The myopathies, discussed by Harriman (1984), include the Kearns—Sayre syndrome ('ophthalmoplegia plus'), a slowly progressive disease of childhood, in which ocular palsy is associated with retinitis pigmentosa, mental defect, and deafness. The characteristic finding is of 'ragged red' fibres, containing abnormal mitochondria (see p.360).

In cases labelled *progressive external ophthalmoplegia*, the clinical diagnosis between myopathy and neuropathy is often difficult and dependent upon finding evidence of one or the other condition elsewhere in the body. The histological diagnosis from a tiny, often damaged, biopsy specimen is likewise difficult. In the post mortem examination it is important to be aware of the differences between normal external ocular muscle and skeletal muscle elsewhere in the body. Silver preparations of normal eye muscles show a wide scatter of fibre calibres, including groups of small fibres, and a bewildering tangle of irregular branching nerve fibres.

In system degenerations of the CNS causing denervation of muscle elsewhere in the body, the oculomotor (III, IV and VI) nuclei are very rarely involved. An exception is *progressive supranuclear palsy*, which is discussed on p.248.

In the condition *exophthalmic ophthalmoplegia*, met with in some cases of thyrotoxicosis, the ocular palsy appears to be due largely to mechanical factors.

Further reading

Harriman DGF. 1984. Diseases of muscle. In Adams JH, Corsellis JAN, Duchen LW (Eds) *Greenfield's Neuropathology*, 4th edn. Edward Arnold, London, Chapter 21.

Pain syndromes

Cases of severe persistent or episodic pain (other than headache) which call for post mortem examination by a neuropathologist tend to belong to one of four categories: (i) 'central' pain (see Pagni 1984), including the *thalamic syndrome*; (ii) cases that have undergone *surgery* on the CNS for the relief of pain; (iii) cases of *tic douloureux* (trigeminal neuralgia); and (iv) cases of *post-herpetic neuralgia*.

1 *Thalamic syndrome.* In its classical presentation, the lesion is an infarct or haemorrhage involving the posterolateral area of the thalamus, which results in a condition of *hyperpathia* or *hyperalgesia* on the opposite side of the body. Thresholds for common sensation are raised, and normal stimuli evoke a spreading, slowly subsiding, discomfort which the patient may describe as 'agonizing'. In all such cases the thalamus should be examined in multiple sections, and the damaged area mapped. If no lesion is found in the thalamus, the search should include the sensory pathways from the brain stem to the parietal white matter and cortex.

2 The commonest surgical procedures for the relief of pain include *anterolateral chordotomy* and *posterior rhizotomy*. The post mortem examination has two aims: first, to give the surgeon accurate information on the extent of the lesion; and, second, to trace the resulting tract degeneration in the CNS. Even if it is decided not to pursue the second aim, the material should be kept for the benefit of colleagues with neuro-anatomical interests.

3 In cases of *trigeminal neuralgia*, whether or not they have undergone surgical attack on the affected nerve root or its ganglion, these should be preserved and carefully dissected after fixation (see p.3 and Fig. 1.3 for details of removal at post mortem). There are published reports of apparently successful operations for this condition in which abnormal relations of the nerve with the surrounding dura have been observed. Trigeminal neuralgia is said to be unduly frequent in patients with MS; and small plaques have repeatedly been seen in the trigeminal root entry zone (Fig. 2.26, level E) in such cases (see Loeser 1984).

4 In cases of *post-herpetic neuralgia*, the suspected dorsal root ganglion (or trigeminal ganglion) should be examined histologically; likewise one or two spinal ganglia above and below the suspected one. It has been suggested (Noordenbos 1959) that pain ensues when there is selective destruction of large myelinated nerve fibres. To prove this point, many controlled fibre counts would be necessary. If such counts are contemplated, portions of ribs may be taken at post mortem, and intercostal nerves dissected out after fixation. The fifth intercostal nerve, for instance, is found in the costal groove on the under-surface of the fifth rib.

The pathology of *causalgia* is discussed by Schott (1986).

Further reading

Loeser JD. 1984. Tic douloureux and atypical facial pain. In Wall PD, Melzack R (Eds) *Textbook of Pain*. Churchill Livingstone, Edinburgh, pp. 426—34.
Noordenbos W. 1959. *Pain: Problems Pertaining to the Transmission of Nerve Impulses which give rise to Pain*. Elsevier, Amsterdam.
Pagni CA. 1984. Central pain due to spinal cord and brainstem damage. In Wall PD, Melzack R (Eds) *Textbook of Pain*. Churchill Livingstone, Edinburgh, pp. 481—95.
Schott GD. 1986. Mechanisms of causalgia and related conditions. *Brain* **109**, 717—38.

Paraplegia and paraparesis

Paralysis of both lower limbs is usually due to a transverse lesion of the spinal cord; less often, to compression of the roots of the cauda equina. In the former (except perhaps for a few days following a back injury) the paralysis is of spastic type, with pathologically brisk tendon reflexes; in the latter it is flaccid, with loss of reflexes, and eventually with wasting of muscles. For obvious reasons it is desirable, where possible, to remove the vertebral column at post mortem in cases of paraplegia.

Causes of paraplegia include:

1 MS.

2 Expanding lesions in the spinal canal.

3 Spinal deformity causing compression of the cord.

4 Spinal trauma.

5 Infarction of a length of spinal cord, which may in turn be due to:

(a) atheroma of the abdominal aorta;

(b) malignant infiltration of, or accidental damage to, a major radicular artery;

(c) arteriovenous malformation ('angioma of the spinal cord'; see p.31).

The term *transverse myelitis* is freely used by clinicians to denote any acute ailment causing blockage of conduction in the long tracts of the spinal cord with a definite sensory level. It does not refer to any specific pathological process. In most of the cases thus labelled the cause is either a vascular disorder or an acute demyelinating process.

Whatever the cause of the paraplegia, the blood supply of the affected stretch of cord should be examined. The lesion itself is of interest; the amount of glial and fibrous scarring, and the extent of invasion of the necrotic tissue by sprouting of peripheral fibres from the central processes of sensory ganglion cells, are all worth looking at; and sections should be taken from above and below the lesion, to determine whether *any* nerve fibres, ascending or descending, were getting through. In cases of cauda equina compression, the lumbosacral cord should be examined for central chromatolysis in motor cells and wallerian degeneration in the posterior columns. When the lesion is recent, Marchi preparations may be more informative than myelin stains.

Parkinsonism

Patients who have responded well to L-dopa are almost certainly cases of *Parkinson's disease*, which is discussed on p.240. Where this is not the case, especially if there were also cerebellar or autonomic disturbances, one may suspect the striatonigral variety of *multiple system atrophy* (pp. 241–3). Rigid muscles are a feature of *progressive supranuclear palsy* (p.248). Tremor and bradykinesia are common in elderly patients, and may be related to scattered rarefactions in the thalamus and lentiform nuclei, which are generally attributable to atheroma of the basal arteries. This, we feel, is probably the pathological basis of the 'arteriosclerotic parkinsonism' spoken of in textbooks of neurology. The other parkinsonian syndrome discussed in the textbooks — the *post-encephalitic* type — is becoming increasingly rare, as survivors from the 1920s outbreak of encephalitis lethargica die off. The lesions to be looked for consist in massive loss of pigmented cells in the substantia nigra, which to the naked eye may be totally depigmented; and scattered gliotic foci, shown up in Holzer or PTA preparations, throughout the basal grey matter (hypothalamus, subthalamic area and tegmentum); and neurofibrillary tangles in nerve cells in a similar distribution. Whether this picture can be produced by other virus infections is at present unknown. These tangles, unlike those seen in Alzheimer's disease, are not particularly well displayed in silver impregnations, but show up well enough in H&E and van Gieson preparations. Cases are occasionally met with having the histological stigmata of post-encephalitic parkinsonism but no history of encephalitis.

After Parkinson's disease, the commonest type of parkinsonism is probably an effect of *phenothiazine drugs*. Clear evidence on the pathology of this condition is still lacking. Another toxic state which sometimes gives rise to a parkinsonian syndrome is *carbon monoxide poisoning*. The principal lesion here is usually bilateral necrosis of the globus pallidus. This involves not merely the cells of the pallidum but also most of the outflow from the putamen.

Precocious puberty

This has repeatedly been found associated with gliomas or hamartomas involving the hypothalamus. It affects boys more often than girls; but the patient in Fig. 24.3 was a woman.

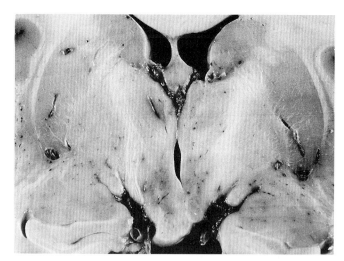

Fig. 24.3. Hamartoma of hypothalamus in a woman of 24, with epilepsy since the age of 4 and precocious puberty since the age of 8. There is a normal mamillary body on the right. The left hypothalamus is expanded by a mass of ectopic grey matter, with no evidence of neoplasia.

Pseudobulbar palsy

This is a term used by clinicians when bilateral weakness of muscles supplied by cranial nerves is attributed to vascular lesions in the cerebral hemispheres. The affected muscles do not undergo atrophy. Post mortem, the diagnosis is confirmed by finding lesions in the hemispheres and none in the brain stem. Plaques of MS should be looked for, if infarcts are not present; and progressive supranuclear palsy (p.248) should be borne in mind as a possible diagnosis.

Psychosis

Psychotic behaviour, sometimes closely resembling schizophrenia, may occur in a number of organic brain diseases — frontal gliomas, for instance, and Huntington's chorea — in the absence of positive neurological signs. Transient psychosis due to various drugs is exceedingly common. Outbursts of *maniacal behaviour* may occur in hypoglycaemic attacks due either to an overdose of insulin or to a secreting islet-cell adenoma. In a case examined in this department, a middle-aged man, in good health, suddenly went mad. After about two hours of maniacal behaviour he lapsed into coma and stayed there, undiagnosed, for six months. At post mortem he was found to have multiple necrotic foci in the brain, and diffuse hyperplasia of islet cells in the pancreas. Serious mental disturbances associated with excessive consumption of alcohol include *Korsakoff's psychosis*, most commonly associated with Wernicke's encephalopathy (p.316), and the *Marchiafava—Bignami syndrome*, discussed on p.305.

Infections causing madness are dealt with in Chapters 9 and 10. The best documented of these is *chronic syphilitic encephalitis* (also known as general paralysis of the insane; see p.276). Since the introduction of penicillin, the full-blown pathology described in the older literature is very rarely seen, but it is still worth looking for in suspect cases. In general, the cruder and more easily recognizable brain diseases are apt to cause dementia rather than madness.

In a typical case of *schizophrenia*, with onset after puberty, the disease is idiopathic, i.e. utterly mysterious. There are no gross changes in the brain, and there is no general agreement about the various fine histological changes which have been reported from time to time. The subject is reviewed by Kovelman & Scheibel (1986). The fact that the manifestations of the disease can be modified by drugs suggests that the basic disorder may be a biochemical one; and a public-spirited pathologist will preserve the brains of schizophrenic patients in a deep refrigerator, and hand them over to colleagues in centres where the neurochemistry and neuropharmacology of madness are studied. The same applies for cases of 'idiopathic' manic-depressive psychosis. Some addresses are given in Appendix B.

Further reading

Kovelman JA, Scheibel AB. 1986. Biological substrates of schizophrenia. *Acta Neurol Scand* **73**, 1—32.

Rigidity

The commonest form of muscular rigor is *cramp*, of the type that afflicts many elderly people, most commonly in the legs and feet. The physiological disorder in this condition is unknown. In *miner's cramp* and *tetany*, on the other hand, electrolyte imbalance is given the blame. The second commonest is the rigidity of hemiplegic limbs following a stroke. Since pure lesions of the corticospinal tracts do not cause rigidity, this is presumably due to interruption of extra-pyramidal pathways which inhibit reflex muscular contractions. The same principle may apply to so-called *decerebrate rigidity*, and to the 'cog-wheel' and 'lead pipe' rigidity of parkinsonism. There have been reports of intense, painful muscular rigidity in which the responsible lesion appears to have isolated groups of motor neurons from descending inhibitory influences; and we have encountered a case of rigid hemiplegia in a patient with selective infarction of the striatum, with intact corticospinal tracts.

There is no recognized pathology for the so-called *Stiff man syndrome*. Indeed, some sceptical clinicians regard it as an hysterical behaviour pattern.

Sensory loss

From the pathologist's point of view, the simplest cases are those with peripheral nerve lesions. When there is a localized area of anaesthesia, reference to a textbook of anatomy will usually indicate where to look for the lesion, and the clinical notes should make it plain whether the cause of the lesion is leprosy, a slipped disc, a glass splinter or a horse's hoof. More generalized disturbances call for procedures outlined in Chapter 22, to determine whether the neuropathy is of toxic, metabolic or inflammatory origin. To these three categories one may add a fourth, namely 'idiopathic', i.e. 'having no apparent cause'. Some would add a fifth: neurotic.

Dulling of sensation in the limbs is a regular feature of some diseases of the CNS — in particular, MS. In this condition, numbness is commonly associated with *paraesthesiae*, among them *Lhermitte's sign* — a sensation like an electric shock running down the back when the neck is flexed. When this is known to have occurred, the cervical cord should be carefully examined. MS is the commonest but not the only disorder causing this symptom.

Cases of *congenital indifference to pain* have been found to show a deficiency of sensory ganglion cells. We have no experience of such cases. They are discussed by Thomas, Landon & King (1984).

Cases of *dissociated sensory loss* (the dissociation being between 'posterior column' and 'spinothalamic' sensibility) usually offer a good ratio of reward to effort. In most cases the lesion lies in the spinal cord; less often in the brain stem; rarely elsewhere, e.g. in the thalamus. Interruption of a sensory tract will produce a sensory *level*, with sensation normal above, and impaired below. An exception to this rule occurs in some cases of syringomyelia, in which the decussation of the 'spinothalamic' pathway is destroyed over a few segments. Thermal and noxious stimuli are ignored over the relevant segments, but felt normally above and below.

Further reading

Thomas PK, Landon DN, King RHM. 1984. Diseases of the peripheral nerves. In Adams JH, Corsellis JAN, Duchen LW (Eds) *Greenfield's Neuropathology*, 4th edn. Edward Arnold, London, Chapter 18.

Sleep disturbances

Most disorders of sleep patterns occur as part of the rough-and-tumble of life — anxiety, pain, air travel, intoxication, banal feverish illnesses and so forth. In such cases it is generally assumed that the disturbances are caused by variations in the discharge of impulses in the *brain stem reticular formation* — a convenient term used to cover numerous scattered small groups of nerve cells whose connections are difficult to trace, but which exert profound influence upon our normal physical and mental functions, including waking and sleeping. Indeed, sleep disturbances are among the common features of cases of MS and brain stem glioma. They also occur with lesions of the hypothalamus. Von Economo (1931) observed that in fatal cases of 'sleeping sickness' lesions affecting the posterior hypothalamus and upper midbrain were usually associated with excessive sleep, while lesions in the anterior hypothalamus often resulted in insomnia; and the examination of the hypothalamus and its immediate surroundings remains the first requirement when a sleep disturbance figures large in the clinical history. The anatomy and physiology of the subject are reviewed by Moruzzi (1963) and Brodal (1981).

In fatal cases of *sleeping sickness* due to infection by *Trypanosoma gambiense*, a diffuse meningoencephalitis is described. Since much of the hypothalamus lies exposed at the base of the brain, the disturbance of sleep may be due to its involvement in the inflammatory process.

Further reading

Brodal A. 1981. *Neurological Anatomy*, 3rd edn. Oxford University Press, Oxford.
von Economo C. 1931. *Encephalitis Lethargica. Its Sequelae and Treatment*. Oxford University Press, Oxford.
Moruzzi G. 1963. Active processes in the brain stem during sleep. *Harvey Lectures*, Academic Press, New York, **58**, 233–97.

Spasticity

We understand this term to denote increased muscular tone, resistance to passive stretch, and enhanced tendon reflexes. Spastic paralysis is conventionally attributed to lesions of 'upper motor neurons' (UMNs). If UMNs are taken to include non-pyramidal descending pathways and their cells of origin, this is probably correct; if it refers only to the corticospinal (pyramidal) tracts, it is not. The clearest evidence on this is the report by Bucy *et al.* (1964) on a case of incapacitating hemiballismus, treated by transection of the outer two-thirds of one crus cerebri. The resulting hemiplegia, without ballismus, delighted the patient. A few months later, power returned to the affected limbs, along with control of fine finger movements. The Babinski sign was positive, and reflexes were slightly brisker. Tone was normal. The patient died of a malignant lymphoma. Post mortem showed almost total degeneration of the medullary pyramid on the side of the operation.

Spasticity is usually associated with weakness or paralysis of the affected limbs, whether the lesion lies in a cerebral hemisphere or in the brain stem or spinal cord. In the cerebrum, vascular accidents and tumours are the commonest lesions; in the brain stem, MS; and in the spinal cord, MS and compressing lesions. In none of these conditions is the corticospinal tract affected in isolation from other descending pathways.

Obviously, the corticospinal tracts should be examined in cases of spastic paralysis; and if the pathologist's interests lie elsewhere, he need do little more than that. Our justification for introducing unsolved problems in motor physiology into a practical treatise is that a careful examination may provide useful general information, if it is not hampered by traditional myths, repeated through successive editions of medical textbooks.

Further reading

Bucy PC, Keplinger JE, Siqueira EB. 1964. Destruction of the pyramidal tract in man. *J Neurosurg* **21**, 385–98.

Speech and language disorders

Two areas of cerebral cortex are concerned with speech functions. The better known, and less important, of these is *Broca's area* — a small patch at the hind-end of the left inferior frontal convolution. The main 'speech centre' is *Wernicke's area*, which includes the posterior third of the left superior temporal convolution, and a certain amount (there is disagreement about how much) of neighbouring temporal and parietal cortex (Fig. 24.4). Regarding this disagreement, it has been pointed out (Bogen & Bogen 1976) that whereas Broca's area is clearly defined anatomically while its function remains uncertain, Wernicke's area is *defined* as the main centre for the organization of language functions, but there is no agreement about its *extent*. Regarding function, it is a suggestive fact that Broca's area is very close to the motor area for the face, while the 'speech

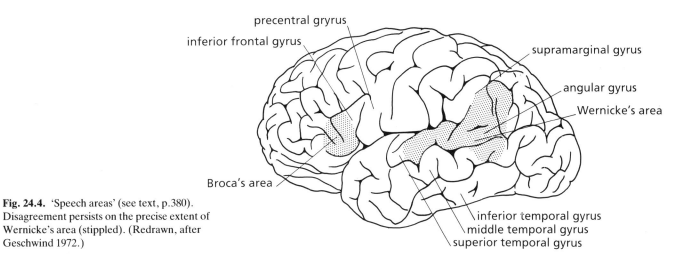

Fig. 24.4. 'Speech areas' (see text, p.380). Disagreement persists on the precise extent of Wernicke's area (stippled). (Redrawn, after Geschwind 1972.)

area' of the temporal lobe lies immediately behind the auditory receiving area in the transverse (Heschl's) gyri (Fig. 24.5). In conformity with this, clinicians sometimes speak of 'Broca's dysphasia' in cases with a predominantly motor, or expressive, disability, and of 'Wernicke's dysphasia' for the rest of the dysphasic syndromes — word deafness, word blindness, dyslexia, dysgraphia, and so forth.

Human language is a recently evolved faculty; it is therefore not surprising that it has no hard-and-fast, genetically determined, cerebral localization. In some people, dysphasic disorders result from lesions in the right hemisphere. Children with congenital or acquired lesions of the left hemisphere nevertheless learn to talk, read and write. The area

in the right hemisphere responsible for the take-over in such cases is not known.

Language 'centres', if they are to be of any use, must be adequately connected with other 'centres' — for hearing, vision, thought, memory, and so on. Geschwind (1965, 1972) drew attention to various *'disconnection' syndromes*, in which the important lesion lies not in this or that area of cortex, but in the white matter connecting these. From what has been said, it follows that the examination of the brain from a case of aphasia or dysphasia may involve more than the inspection of the 'speech centres' of the left hemisphere.

By definition, *dysphasia* implies a defect in the use of language, either on the receptive side, in the understanding of spoken or written words, or on the expressive side, in the choice of words and phrases. *Dysarthria*, on the other hand, implies defective utterance. Lesions responsible for dysphasia are assumed to lie in the cerebrum — most commonly in the left hemisphere. *Dysarthria* may be due to lesions in many places, including motor cortex (strokes, tumours, etc.), basal ganglia (as in Huntington's and Parkinson's diseases), pathways in the brain stem (commonly affected in MS), motor nuclei (motor neuron disease, bulbar polio), the cerebellum and its connections; not to mention the effects, which may be transitory, of various neuropathies and myopathies. Dysarthria is also an effect of congenital deafness. Careful reading of the clinical notes, plus appropriate histology, will usually elucidate the cause of dysarthria; of dysphasia, not so often.

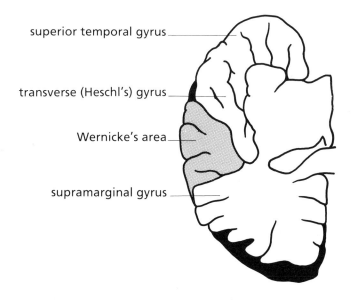

Fig. 24.5. Drawing to show the upper surface of the left temporal lobe. The Sylvian fissure has been opened up, and the frontal lobe removed. Wernicke's area (stippled) lies immediately behind the transverse (Heschl's) gyrus, which is the auditory area, receiving its main input from the medial geniculate body. (Redrawn, after Geschwind 1972.)

Further reading

Bogen JE, Bogen GM. 1976. Wernicke's region — where is it? *Ann NY Acad Sci* **280**, 834–43.

Brain WR. 1965. *Speech Disorders*. Butterworth, London.

Geschwind N. 1965. Disconnexion syndromes in animals and man. *Brain* **88**, 237–94, 585–644.

Geschwind N. 1972. Language and the brain. *Sci Am* **226**, 76–83.

Luria AR. 1970. *Traumatic Aphasia: its Syndromes, Psychology and Treatment*. Mouton & Co, New York.

Tremor

A mild tremor, occurring at rest, with a frequency around 10 per second, and unassociated with known lesions in the brain, is commonly referred to as physiological tremor. A somewhat coarser tremor, seen particularly in elderly people with atheroma, has been attributed to multiple rarefactions in the lentiform nuclei and thalamus. In Parkinson's disease and striatonigral degeneration coarse resting tremor of the limbs may become a fairly violent flapping movement. This is still sometimes relieved by stereotactic operations aimed at the ventrolateral nucleus of the thalamus (less often, the globus pallidus) on one side or both. In the post mortem examination, it is worth mapping the precise extent of the resulting lesion, if only to reassure the surgeon as to the accuracy of his technique.

Intention tremor — that is, tremor not present at rest, but coming into play in the course of voluntary movements, especially of the hands — is generally associated with disease involving the cerebellum and its connections. It is commonly seen in cases of MS.

Unconsciousness

Neuropathologists are seldom asked to explain why a particular patient was unconscious at the time of his death. They may, however, be moved by curiosity as to why, of two patients with similar lesions, one was conscious and the other not. This question arose when one of us was looking for microscopic lesions in the brain following head injury. One of the patients was a man of 66 who was knocked down by a motor scooter and suffered multiple rib fractures. He was concussed, but was fully conscious 20 minutes later. He died of a chest infection 13 days later. The brain, which was macroscopically normal, was found to contain microglial clusters, characteristic of acceleration injury, in all areas, including the brain stem. The other case was of a 19-year-old girl who drove a car into a telegraph pole, and was deeply unconscious, responding to painful stimulation with 'decerebrate' movements, until her death 5 days later. There were naked-eye lesions in the cerebral hemispheres, but no tentorial hernia, and the brain stem looked normal apart from some bruising around the aqueduct. Sections of the brain stem resembled those in the previous case, except for a concentration of microscopic lesions in the periaqueductal grey matter.

Descartes placed the soul in the pineal body, apparently because this lies at the geometrical centre of the brain. It may seem equally childish to imagine that the 'centre' for consciousness lies about a centimetre below the site of Descartes' soul, but it is scarcely less childish to speak of 'centres' for sleep a centimetre in front of this. It may be recalled that one of the cardinal signs that the upper brain stem is being compressed by a transtentorial hernia is a progressive lowering of the level of consciousness.

When death has been preceded by a period of *coma*, the cause of the coma is usually made fairly clear by the clinical history, signs and investigations. The commoner causes of progressive clouding of consciousness include *cerebral hypoxia* (which in very many instances results from impaired lung function, as in pneumonia), *toxic and metabolic disorders*, and *space-occupying lesions* causing transtentorial herniation (see Chapters 7, 11, 19 and 20). Regarding toxic states, it hardly needs stressing that if there is the least suspicion of coma and death being due to drugs, self-administered or otherwise, the coroner will be displeased if the pathologist has not taken the stomach contents and samples of blood. Similarly, in a case of acute encephalopathy of unknown nature, the possibility of an infection should be kept in mind, and appropriate specimens taken for bacteriological and virological examination. It should also be remembered that two factors may be working together to produce coma; for instance, a diabetic may lapse into ketosis when assailed by pneumonia or meningitis; and either the infection or the ketosis may have been missed in the ward. Again, hypoglycaemic coma due to an overdose of insulin in a fasting diabetic will usually be spotted; but when it is due to a sudden release of insulin from an islet-cell tumour, it may be missed.

Prolonged coma following a head injury is sometimes attributable to brain stem damage. It may also result from a combination of cerebral trauma and cerebral hypoxia — due, for example, to aspiration of vomit during a period of concussion (see Table 5.1). There is also a state referred to as *vigil coma* or *persistent vegetative state*, in which the patient remains inert and unresponsive for months or even years; yet appears, from movements of the eyes, to have periods of alternating sleep and waking.

Vertigo

True vertigo, as opposed to dizziness due to circulatory disturbances, is attributed to lesions in the vestibular system. These may be peripheral, as in Ménière's disease and acute labyrinthitis, or due to nerve damage by, for instance, an acoustic schwannoma, or central, involving the vestibular nuclei and their connections in the brain stem and cerebellum, as in the lateral medullary syndrome. Vertigo is nearly always associated with *nystagmus* (see above).

Visual disturbances

The common disorders of vision which may call for investigation by a neuropathologist include: loss of acuity in one eye or both, up to the point of total blindness; loss of vision in a particular visual field in one eye or both; loss of stereoscopic vision; double vision; and loss of the ability to interpret what one sees (visual agnosia), which is sometimes confined to loss of reading ability.

For a crude map of the visual pathways see Fig. 2.30, and p.42. The retina, which is developmentally a part of the brain, lies outside the usual scope of neuropathology. Not so the optic nerves, which should be taken in all cases of optic atrophy, from whatever cause, and in all cases with a history of optic neuritis or in which the diagnosis of MS has been suggested. In cases of double vision not attributable to congenital squints, the cause may be found to be an orbital tumour displacing the eyeball, or interfering with the third, fourth or sixth cranial nerves, or more proximally in the nuclei of these nerves (see Fig. 2.26), or in their intracranial course. The commonest site for such interference is probably in the side walls of the pituitary fossa, where they are at risk from tumours and from aneurysms of the internal carotid arteries. The optic nerves themselves are likewise at risk in this area, which is best explored by dissection, after fixation, of a block of the sphenoid bone, removed as described on p.3. Figure 24.6 and Plate 2.4 show two uncommon causes of blindness from trouble in this region.

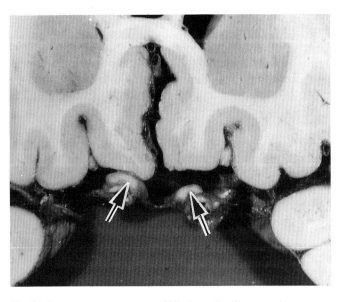

Fig. 24.6. An uncommon cause of blindness, in a hypertensive woman aged 83, with severe calcifying atheroma of the cerebral arteries. Both optic nerves (arrowed) are compressed by calcified anterior cerebral arteries.

Causes of *bitemporal field loss* are to be looked for just in front of, or just behind, the optic chiasm. They are nearly always neoplastic. Causes of *homonymous field loss* are found on the side opposite the field defect, anywhere between the chiasm and the visual cortex. Causes of the various forms of *visual agnosia* are commonly due to vascular or neoplastic lesions in the white matter connecting the visual cortex with other parts, in particular the cortex of the parietal and temporal lobes (for a discussion of 'disconnection syndromes' see Geschwind 1965).

The raw material, so to speak, of vision is processed and re-processed in the retinae, in the lateral geniculate bodies, and in the striate cortex. Physiological research has revealed a certain amount about the further stages involved in *seeing* — that is, making sense of the visual input; but at present there is no more than a vague hope that neuropathology can contribute to the understanding of such disorders as colour anomia and visual agnosia. All we can suggest is that material which might in future be used to throw light on these subjects should be carefully preserved. For the anatomy of the visual system see Polyak (1957).

Further reading

Geschwind N. 1965. Disconnexion syndromes in animals and man. *Brain* **88**, 237–94, 585–644.
Polyak S. 1957. *The Vertebrate Visual System*. University of Chicago, Chicago.

Weakness

Weakness of limbs, trunk and cranially-innervated muscles is a common affliction in neurological practice. In searching for the pathological cause of weakness it is helpful to discover from the clinical notes whether it is generalized or restricted to one side of the body or to one limb; and whether it is accompanied by spasticity and hyper-reflexia, or by flaccidity and reduced or absent reflexes. Spastic weakness and involvement of one side of the body usually point to damage to motor pathways in the CNS, while if weakness is flaccid and generalized there is usually damage in the periphery, in nerves or in the muscles themselves. Flaccid weakness is often accompanied by wasting of muscles. In motor neuron disease (p.236) both upper and lower motor neurons are affected, and the relative severity of damage to each will determine whether weakness is predominantly spastic (upper motor neuron damage) or flaccid (lower motor neuron damage), but both need to be examined at post mortem together with samples of muscles. In other cases of spastic weakness the causes are varied, and can be found anywhere from the cerebrum to the spinal cord. If a lesion such as a cerebral infarct is found that will account for the weakness experienced during life, there is no indication to examine peripheral nerves and muscles. Cases in which there is generalized flaccid weakness are likely to have suffered from one of the diseases discussed in Chapters 22 and 23, and require examination of spinal cord and samples of peripheral nerves and muscles. If eye muscles were clinically affected, these and their innervating nerves should be taken for histological examination (see also ophthalmoplegia, above).

Chapter 25
Other Matters

A neuropathologist runs little risk of developing *folie de grandeur*. He needs only to remind himself that, whereas his clinical colleagues can manage quite nicely without his help, he is lost without theirs. They, of course, need someone to examine their patients' blood, pus, urine and CSF; but in many — perhaps most — centres these tasks are carried out by other kinds of pathologist. On the whole, the clinician, assisted by the radiologist, can judge for himself what kind of tumour he is dealing with, whether the patient is losing his motor neurons, and what he finally dies of. The diagnostic neuropathologist, on the other hand, cannot function without his raw materials, which are either supplied directly, as biopsy specimens, or steered in his direction after the patient's death, by clinicians. His pronouncements are generally not treated as oracles, but taken into consideration in conjunction with the rest of the available evidence.

Relations with clinicians

Ideally, the relation between pathologist and clinician is a kind of symbiosis, or, using another analogy, a mystical brotherhood, reinforced by periodical 'love-feasts' in the form of slide-showing sessions and brain cuttings. These ceremonies are supposed to enable the clinicians to compare their previous guesses with the truths revealed by the microscope. In practice, they have a slightly different function — that of allowing the clinicians to recollect their patients in tranquillity, and to discuss with one another the merits of different lines of treatment. The pathologist may grow impatient with these debates, and may wish to recall attention to his carefully assembled slices and slides; but it is unwise to show this too openly. It is a still greater mistake to stress the point in cases where the clinician has got the diagnosis

wrong. The pathologist who appears to exult in his superior cleverness is not quickly forgiven.

'Brain cuttings'

'Brain cuttings' is a term in general use for demonstrations of post mortem material. These are of two types. In the first, the pathologist, robed in a protective apron and armed with a long knife, listens to the clinical history, and the general discussion of possible diagnoses, before displaying the fixed brain and/or spinal cord and proceeding with the dissection and slicing of the specimens. Sometimes the diagnosis, previously in doubt, becomes clear at this point. At other times, it does not. Somebody says 'It will be interesting to see what the histology shows', and the discussion turns to the next case. In the second type, the brain and cord are cut up in the laboratory; blocks are taken, sections are stained, mounted, photographed, and reported on. Six months or more after the post mortem the case is demonstrated. The proceedings tend to begin with the query, 'Does anybody remember this case?'

Avoidance of delay

Delays of this magnitude can generally be avoided. The irreducible minimum is about three weeks — the time taken for fixation of the brain. In an interesting and complicated case, multiple blocks, and multiple stains, may be needed before the case can be adequately reported on; but for the simple purpose of making a diagnosis, a few may suffice. These few may be hurried through along with the current surgical specimens. Histological details may be demonstrated either with the aid of a projector — still better, if it can be afforded, by a closed-circuit television unit — or in the form of colour transparencies. Delays greater than about two months between post mortem and demonstration are rarely necessary.

A situation in which delay should be kept to a minimum is when the patient is a child with an undiagnosed progressive encephalopathy. A number of such patients turn out to have been suffering from a genetically determined disease — Leigh's encephalopathy, for instance, or a lipidosis, or a leucodystrophy. One of the authors has more than once suffered remorse, having let some months elapse between making the diagnosis and issuing his report, only to learn that by the time the news reached the family doctor the child's mother was already pregnant again.

Reporting

In a letter to the General Assembly of the Church of Scotland in the year 1650, Oliver Cromwell is said to have written: 'I beseech you, in the bowels of Christ, think it possible you may be mistaken'. This admonition is as applicable to diagnostic pathology as it is to politics and religion. From time to time the pathologist receives a polite letter referring to one of his previous reports, giving details of the patient's subsequent progress, and enquiring whether, in the light of these, the pathologist would care to modify his earlier opinion. The response to such an enquiry should not be distorted by personal vanity. A rather more delicate situation arises when the pathologist is asked to review another pathologist's report. Here again the response should not be coloured either by loyalty or by malice. In any case, the author of the previous report should be told what the response has been.

Regarding biopsy reports, it is important that the pathologist should know what are the questions which the clinician wants answered. For instance, most surgeons will not be very interested in whether a particular meningioma is of syncytial or transitional type, but would like to know whether the tumour shows signs of transgressing its capsule and invading the brain.

Relations with other pathologists

In centres where neuropathologists and general pathologists work in close proximity, the importance of maintaining friendly relations between the two need hardly be stressed. If each pathologist is aware of the research interests of each of his colleagues, exchanges of pathological material bring both scientific and social rewards. Often the question of shared post mortems arises, and it is important to avoid demarcation disputes by having agreed conventions about these. Situations where coroners' fees may be involved — in post mortems on cases of fatal head injury, for example — may call for some diplomatic delicacy.

It is also important to maintain good communications with pathologists in neighbouring areas. In the Oxford region, for example, there are a dozen or so hospitals with pathology departments, but only one teaching hospital with a department of neuropathology, associated with departments of clinical neurology, neurosurgery, neuroradiology, neurophysiology, and the rest. Clinicians from the centre pay regular visits to other hospitals in the region; patients are transferred to the centre for investigation and treatment, and subsequently returned to the regional hospital. If a patient dies, the clinicians in both places are likely to be interested in the outcome of the post mortem. This may be arranged in various ways: for instance, the body may be transported to the centre, where the neuropathologist carries out the post mortem, and the body is returned; or the neuropathologist drives out to the regional hospital, where he shares the post mortem with the local pathologist; or the local pathologist does the post mortem, and keeps the relevant material, fixed in formalin, for the neuropathologist to deal with. This last is a good arrangement, but very dependent on good communication; in particular, on the local pathologist's knowledge of the neuropathologist's requirements in a particular type of case, and readiness to satisfy them. In a case diagnosed clinically as Friedreich's ataxia or motor neuron disease, the brain, unaccompanied by the spinal cord, is not really adequate. In return, the neuropathologist must be ready to display his findings in a form which evokes the interest of the pathologist and his clinical colleagues. Failing this, a detailed histological report should be sent out with the least possible delay.

In this context, it is worth stressing the advantages of the practice of taking the spinal cord within the vertebral column, as described on p.4. Not only does this give access to spinal ganglia, roots, and sympathetic chain, it also preserves the cord from the hazards of unskillful dissection, and the further hazards of storage and transit. Besides, it involves the pathologist in less expense of time and effort than would the careful removal of the cord at post mortem.

It is hardly necessary to stress the importance to research of close communications between neuropathologists in their own and in other countries, and of awareness of what lines of research are being pursued at many different centres. One hears growls of criticism directed against the self-advertising antics observed at international congresses, but the value of the conversations over cups of inferior coffee in the intervals between sessions should not be underestimated.

Relations with laboratory staff

The pathologist should never forget how much his own success depends on good rapport with the laboratory staff. This involves being aware of the factors which may diminish that rapport. Perhaps the most important of these is the temptation to take their work for granted. The production of consistently good histological preparations requires not merely the application of an acquired technique, but the willingness to try again, with modifications of the technique, if it does not work well the first time. This willingness cannot be taken for granted; it has to be earned. In other words, the pathologist must show that he really cares about the result, and share the technician's delight when the result is good. Conversely, he must not let it be thought that he asks for sections to be cut, stained and mounted which he does not require, and which he does not trouble to examine. In practice, some skilled technicians are concerned about the aesthetic merits of their work rather than about the information derived from it, while others are keenly interested in pathological interpretations. Appreciation in the first case, and explanation in the second, will not be wasted. Finally, and most important, technicians' worries about health hazards must be taken very seriously. These may arise, for instance, over the handling of material from suspected cases of Creutsfeldt–Jakob disease, or about the toxic effects of exposure to aniline (used in the Holzer technique) or xylol (xylene), which is widely used as a clearing agent.

Behaviour in court

At this point we feel that for the sake of completeness we ought to make some recommendations to pathologists on how to behave in a court of law, including the coroner's court. As witnesses, we are enjoined, on oath, to tell the truth, the whole truth, and nothing but the truth; but this injunction cannot be taken literally. In general, the truth is an elusive thing, and what we are being asked for is our opinions. If we set out to tell the whole truth, we should only succeed in being tedious, irrelevant, and in most cases unintelligible to our audience. We do not favour telling downright untruths — for instance, that the cause of death in a case of closed head injury was a fractured skull; on the other hand, giving 'foraminal herniation' as a cause of death is not likely to enlighten a coroner's jury. We can only advocate the use of common sense, and of extreme wariness in answering a barrister's questions.

Indexing

A word is needed about the tedious but necessary business of indexing. We do not know how many different systems are in use, and are not in a position to recommend one rather than another. We are, however, in no doubt about what the system should achieve: in a word, accessibility. For our own convenience, we need an indexing system which gives each case a departmental (as opposed to hospital) number, assigned as soon as the material is received, which from then on will lead us to the jar in which the material is stored, the case notes and/or diagnostic report, the stored histological preparations, the black-and-white negatives and prints and colour transparencies of the case, and any correspondence relating to it. For dealing with enquiries from outside the department, we need an index of patients' names, with initials, ages and dates, with hospital and departmental numbers.

For research based on series of cases of particular conditions, a diagnostic index, though not essential, is extremely useful, and saves time in the long run. For this purpose many laboratories have adopted the classification of disease compiled by the American Medical Association (SNOMED: systematized nomenclature of medicine) as a basis. This index can be maintained either by the pathologists themselves, or by the departmental secretary. In the past we have tried it both ways, and are in no doubt that it is far better if the pathologists do the work themselves. This is particularly so for half-remembered, peculiar 'one-off' findings in old cases. The same applies to the indexing of photographs; one needs to know where to look for pictures illustrating particular points; and having found a suitable print, where to find the negative. Last and not least, there is the job of instructing each new departmental secretary in the intricacies of the different filing systems, and imparting a general understanding of what it is all about. Rapport with the secretary is hardly less important than rapport with the technicians.

The neuropathologist's role

In our undoubtedly biased opinion, biology is the most interesting province of natural science. We think that animals are more interesting than plants, and that the most interesting thing about animals is their behaviour, and the complex of mechanisms giving rise to their behaviour. Doubtless, because we are ourselves human, we think that man is the most interesting animal of all. As matters stand, neurology and psychology are separate fields, and those who cultivate these two fields use different conceptual models and different terminologies. Yet both groups know that animal behaviour, including thinking and talking, depends on the functioning of a nervous system. They know that in theory their fields overlap, although in the present state of ignorance, the overlap — that is, the area sometimes referred to as neuropsychology — is pathetically small. At the same time it constitutes what we regard as one of the most enthralling parts of biological science. Working on his own, or even in collaboration with practitioners in the clinical parts of these fields, there is little that the neuropathologist can do to enlarge the area of overlap. We hope that in future there will be more and better facilities for cooperative work involving psychologists, anatomists, physiologists, chemists, pharmacologists and molecular biologists, with clinicians and pathologists playing their part.

The pleasures of problem-solving

The world will have to wait for answers to the really big questions in biology; in the meantime, there are thousands of little questions, a few of which lie within the power of neuropathologists to answer. For most of us, solving puzzles is fun. And the fun is enhanced if the solution — unlike the solution of a crossword puzzle — leads one on to further puzzles, calling for further solutions. Furthermore, there is the chance that the solution of little puzzles may in time contribute to the solution of bigger, and yet bigger, puzzles. We end, therefore, by wishing our readers fun, in the form of successful problem-solving.

Acid phosphatase (Gomori lead acetate method):

Solutions:

0.1 M acetate buffer pH 5.0 — 5 ml.
0.008 M lead acetate — 5 ml.
Sodium β-glycerophosphate — 31.5 mg.
10% ammonium sulphide diluted with distilled water.

Technique:
1 Dissolve sodium β-glycerophosphate in 5 ml 0.1 M acetate buffer.
2 Slowly add and mix 5 ml 0.008 M lead acetate.
3 Incubate slides face down at 37°C for 30 min.
4 Wash in tap water for 30 sec.
5 Immerse in diluted ammonium sulphide for 30 sec.
6 Wash well in tap water.
7 Light haematoxylin counterstain.
8 Wash in tap water (blue).
9 Mount in glycerin jelly.

Results:
Acid phosphatase activity   dark down
   NB Sodium β-glycerophosphate must be dissolved in acetate buffer before slowly adding lead acetate, mixing well.
Glassware must be very clean.
Acetate buffer at pH 5 may be stored at 4°C.
Lead acetate may be stored at room temperature.

Myelin

Methods: Klüver-Barrera (Luxol fast blue, with cresyl fast violet) (1, 2, 3, 4), Loyez (1, 2, 3, 4), Page (sometimes called the solochrome cyanin method) (1, 3, 4), and Weil (1, 3, 4). Page's method works well with peripheral nerves. The Gomori one-step trichrome stain (1, 4) gives good results, staining myelin red. The use of 2% brilliant crystal scarlet, used in combination with Holmes' silver technique, or a toned Palmgren for axons, will also produce a pleasant, delicately-stained myelin counterstain, particularly in peripheral nerves (see below).

Fixation: Formalin.

Sections: Paraffin.

Technique:
1 Cut sections at 5—10 μm.
2 Stain with either Holmes or Palmgren (toned) for axons.
3 Wash in distilled water.
4 Stain in 2% brilliant crystal scarlet (2 g bcs in 100 ml distilled water, with 2.5 ml glacial acetic acid) for 30 min.
5 Rinse in distilled water.
6 Differentiate with 1% phosphotungstic acid until good

differentiation is apparent between myelin and connective tissue.
7 Wash.
8 Dehydrate, clear and mount.

Results:
Axons   black
Myelin   orange red

For displaying myelin breakdown products before they are cleared away by phagocytes, a fat stain may be used on frozen sections. More detailed pictures can be obtained with the Marchi method (1, 2, 3, 4). Note that this method entails the use of osmium tetroxide (OsO_4), which is (a) very expensive and (b) the source of a highly toxic vapour. Its use must be confined to a fume cupboard. The vapour, which is given off both by the solid and by the solution, attacks the eyes, the entire respiratory tract, and the skin. Gloves must be worn.

Nerve biopsies

In our laboratory tissue is routinely processed for EM, paraffin, frozen, semi-thin and teased preparations.

Procedure for teased nerve preparations

A stretch of nerve 3—4 mm long is fixed for one hour in 0.1 M phosphate-buffered 3.6% glutaraldehyde. After two 15-min buffer washes, the nerve is immersed in 0.1 M phosphate buffered 2% osmium tetroxide for 4—6 hours. Following two further washes, the tissue is placed in 66% glycerin in water for at least 12 hours. In practice we find that formalin fixation followed by immersion in 1% osmium tetroxide after several changes of distilled water is quite adequate. The nerve may be stored in 100% glycerin for several months. Nerves may be teased after 12 hours or more immersion in 66% glycerin.

Method: Using a dissecting microscope the nerve is stripped of its softened epineurium by using fine syringe needles. Individual fibres or small bundles of fibres may then be carefully separated. The glycerin may serve as a mounting medium, using either molten wax or nail varnish as a sealant.

Procedure for semi-thin sections

Technique:
1 Fix in EM fixative at 4°C.
2 Phosphate buffer at 4°C for at least 3 hours.
3 1% osmium tetroxide for 3 hours at room temperature in fume cupboard.
4 Distilled water — two washes over a period of 10 min.

The pleasures of problem-solving

The world will have to wait for answers to the really big questions in biology; in the meantime, there are thousands of little questions, a few of which lie within the power of neuropathologists to answer. For most of us, solving puzzles is fun. And the fun is enhanced if the solution — unlike the solution of a crossword puzzle — leads one on to further puzzles, calling for further solutions. Furthermore, there is the chance that the solution of little puzzles may in time contribute to the solution of bigger, and yet bigger, puzzles. We end, therefore, by wishing our readers fun, in the form of successful problem-solving.

Acid phosphatase (Gomori lead acetate method):

Solutions:

0.1 M acetate buffer pH 5.0 — 5 ml.
0.008 M lead acetate — 5 ml.
Sodium β-glycerophosphate — 31.5 mg.
10% ammonium sulphide diluted with distilled water.

Technique:
1   Dissolve sodium β-glycerophosphate in 5 ml 0.1 M acetate buffer.
2   Slowly add and mix 5 ml 0.008 M lead acetate.
3   Incubate slides face down at 37°C for 30 min.
4   Wash in tap water for 30 sec.
5   Immerse in diluted ammonium sulphide for 30 sec.
6   Wash well in tap water.
7   Light haematoxylin counterstain.
8   Wash in tap water (blue).
9   Mount in glycerin jelly.

Results:
Acid phosphatase activity   dark down
   NB Sodium β-glycerophosphate must be dissolved in acetate buffer before slowly adding lead acetate, mixing well.
Glassware must be very clean.
Acetate buffer at pH 5 may be stored at 4°C.
Lead acetate may be stored at room temperature.

Myelin

Methods: Klüver-Barrera (Luxol fast blue, with cresyl fast violet) (1, 2, 3, 4), Loyez (1, 2, 3, 4), Page (sometimes called the solochrome cyanin method) (1, 3, 4), and Weil (1, 3, 4). Page's method works well with peripheral nerves. The Gomori one-step trichrome stain (1, 4) gives good results, staining myelin red. The use of 2% brilliant crystal scarlet, used in combination with Holmes' silver technique, or a toned Palmgren for axons, will also produce a pleasant, delicately-stained myelin counterstain, particularly in peripheral nerves (see below).

Fixation: Formalin.

Sections: Paraffin.

Technique:
1   Cut sections at 5—10 μm.
2   Stain with either Holmes or Palmgren (toned) for axons.
3   Wash in distilled water.
4   Stain in 2% brilliant crystal scarlet (2 g bcs in 100 ml distilled water, with 2.5 ml glacial acetic acid) for 30 min.
5   Rinse in distilled water.
6   Differentiate with 1% phosphotungstic acid until good

differentiation is apparent between myelin and connective tissue.
7   Wash.
8   Dehydrate, clear and mount.

Results:
Axons   black
Myelin   orange red

For displaying myelin breakdown products before they are cleared away by phagocytes, a fat stain may be used on frozen sections. More detailed pictures can be obtained with the Marchi method (1, 2, 3, 4). Note that this method entails the use of osmium tetroxide (OsO_4), which is (a) very expensive and (b) the source of a highly toxic vapour. Its use must be confined to a fume cupboard. The vapour, which is given off both by the solid and by the solution, attacks the eyes, the entire respiratory tract, and the skin. Gloves must be worn.

Nerve biopsies

In our laboratory tissue is routinely processed for EM, paraffin, frozen, semi-thin and teased preparations.

Procedure for teased nerve preparations

A stretch of nerve 3—4 mm long is fixed for one hour in 0.1 M phosphate-buffered 3.6% glutaraldehyde. After two 15-min buffer washes, the nerve is immersed in 0.1 M phosphate buffered 2% osmium tetroxide for 4—6 hours. Following two further washes, the tissue is placed in 66% glycerin in water for at least 12 hours. In practice we find that formalin fixation followed by immersion in 1% osmium tetroxide after several changes of distilled water is quite adequate. The nerve may be stored in 100% glycerin for several months. Nerves may be teased after 12 hours or more immersion in 66% glycerin.

Method: Using a dissecting microscope the nerve is stripped of its softened epineurium by using fine syringe needles. Individual fibres or small bundles of fibres may then be carefully separated. The glycerin may serve as a mounting medium, using either molten wax or nail varnish as a sealant.

Procedure for semi-thin sections

Technique:
1   Fix in EM fixative at 4°C.
2   Phosphate buffer at 4°C for at least 3 hours.
3   1% osmium tetroxide for 3 hours at room temperature in fume cupboard.
4   Distilled water — two washes over a period of 10 min.

5 35% alcohol (4°C) for 20 min (two washes of 10 each).
6 70% alcohol (4°C) 12−24 hours or overnight.
7 95% alcohol (room temperature) — 30 min.
8 Methcol — two changes of 30 min each.
9 Absolute alcohol — two changes of 15 min each.
10 Propylene oxide — 15 min.
11 Propylene oxide — 30 min.
12 Propylene oxide and embedding resin (equal part 90 min.
13 Embedding resin — 1½−2 hours at room temperat
14 Embed in mould containing embedding resin at overnight.

Buffer:
0.1 M Na_2HPO_4 3.55 g/250 ml distilled water — 8 par
0.1 M KH_2PO_4 3.4 g/250 ml distilled water — 3 parts.

Embedding resin:

TAAB embedding resin	10 ml
TAAB DDSA	10 ml
TAAB DMP-30	0.3 ml
TAAB dibutyl phthalate	0.6 ml

Mix well. This solution may be stored at 4°C for sev days or for 2 days at room temperature.

When sufficiently hardened the embedding resin b may be broken out of its mould and sections cut on an u microtome at 1 μm thickness. The sections are colle onto a drop of water on a clean microscope slide and dried on, by placing them on a hot plate set to al 50−60°C. When dried, a drop of 1% toluidine blue in borax is placed on the section. At the first sign of dr back, remove the slide and wash off excess stain in run water. Differentiate, controlling microscopically, in alcohol. Because of the danger of wrinkling when moun it is our practice to leave the mounting to the last mom Any synthetic resin mounting medium will do, but we RAL mountant (now supplied by BDH), which has a viscosity, and appears to penetrate more quickly.

Note that this procedure involves the use of osm tetroxide, which gives off a toxic vapour (see note Marchi technique above). It must be carried out in a fu cupboard.

Neurofibrillary tangles

Methods: Bielschowsky (1, 2, 4), von Braunmühl's met (4), and Cross's modification of Palmgren (Cross I 1982. Demonstration of neurofibrillary tangles in para sections: a quick and simple method using a modificatio Palmgren's method. *Medical Laboratory Science* **39**, 67−

The pleasures of problem-solving

The world will have to wait for answers to the really big questions in biology; in the meantime, there are thousands of little questions, a few of which lie within the power of neuropathologists to answer. For most of us, solving puzzles is fun. And the fun is enhanced if the solution — unlike the solution of a crossword puzzle — leads one on to further puzzles, calling for further solutions. Furthermore, there is the chance that the solution of little puzzles may in time contribute to the solution of bigger, and yet bigger, puzzles. We end, therefore, by wishing our readers fun, in the form of successful problem-solving.

Acid phosphatase (Gomori lead acetate method):

Solutions:

0.1 M acetate buffer pH 5.0 — 5 ml.
0.008 M lead acetate — 5 ml.
Sodium β-glycerophosphate — 31.5 mg.
10% ammonium sulphide diluted with distilled wa

Technique:

1 Dissolve sodium β-glycerophosphate in 5 m
acetate buffer.
2 Slowly add and mix 5 ml 0.008 M lead acetate
3 Incubate slides face down at 37°C for 30 min.
4 Wash in tap water for 30 sec.
5 Immerse in diluted ammonium sulphide for 30
6 Wash well in tap water.
7 Light haematoxylin counterstain.
8 Wash in tap water (blue).
9 Mount in glycerin jelly.

Results:

Acid phosphatase activity   dark down
  NB Sodium β-glycerophosphate must be diss
  acetate buffer before slowly adding lead acetate
  well.
Glassware must be very clean.
Acetate buffer at pH 5 may be stored at 4°C.
Lead acetate may be stored at room temperature.

Myelin

Methods: Klüver-Barrera (Luxol fast blue, with cr
violet) (1, 2, 3, 4), Loyez (1, 2, 3, 4), Page (someti
ed the solochrome cyanin method) (1, 3, 4), and
3, 4). Page's method works well with peripheral ner
Gomori one-step trichrome stain (1, 4) gives good
staining myelin red. The use of 2% brilliant crysta
used in combination with Holmes' silver techniq
toned Palmgren for axons, will also produce a
delicately-stained myelin counterstain, particu
peripheral nerves (see below).

Fixation: Formalin.

Sections: Paraffin.

Technique:

1 Cut sections at 5–10 μm.
2 Stain with either Holmes or Palmgren (toned) fc
3 Wash in distilled water.
4 Stain in 2% brilliant crystal scarlet (2 g bcs ir
distilled water, with 2.5 ml glacial acetic acid) for
5 Rinse in distilled water.
6 Differentiate with 1% phosphotungstic acid ur

The pleasures of problem-solving

The world will have to wait for answers to the really big questions in biology; in the meantime, there are thousands of little questions, a few of which lie within the power of neuropathologists to answer. For most of us, solving puzzles is fun. And the fun is enhanced if the solution — unlike the solution of a crossword puzzle — leads one on to further puzzles, calling for further solutions. Furthermore, there is the chance that the solution of little puzzles may in time contribute to the solution of bigger, and yet bigger, puzzles. We end, therefore, by wishing our readers fun, in the form of successful problem-solving.

Acid phosphatase (Gomori lead acetate method):

Solutions:

0.1 M acetate buffer pH 5.0 — 5 ml.
0.008 M lead acetate — 5 ml.
Sodium β-glycerophosphate — 31.5 mg.
10% ammonium sulphide diluted with distilled water.

Technique:
1 Dissolve sodium β-glycerophosphate in 5 ml 0.1 M acetate buffer.
2 Slowly add and mix 5 ml 0.008 M lead acetate.
3 Incubate slides face down at 37°C for 30 min.
4 Wash in tap water for 30 sec.
5 Immerse in diluted ammonium sulphide for 30 sec.
6 Wash well in tap water.
7 Light haematoxylin counterstain.
8 Wash in tap water (blue).
9 Mount in glycerin jelly.

Results:
Acid phosphatase activity   dark down
   NB Sodium β-glycerophosphate must be dissolved in acetate buffer before slowly adding lead acetate, mixing well.
Glassware must be very clean.
Acetate buffer at pH 5 may be stored at 4°C.
Lead acetate may be stored at room temperature.

Myelin

Methods: Klüver-Barrera (Luxol fast blue, with cresyl fast violet) (1, 2, 3, 4), Loyez (1, 2, 3, 4), Page (sometimes called the solochrome cyanin method) (1, 3, 4), and Weil (1, 3, 4). Page's method works well with peripheral nerves. The Gomori one-step trichrome stain (1, 4) gives good results, staining myelin red. The use of 2% brilliant crystal scarlet, used in combination with Holmes' silver technique, or a toned Palmgren for axons, will also produce a pleasant, delicately-stained myelin counterstain, particularly in peripheral nerves (see below).

Fixation: Formalin.

Sections: Paraffin.

Technique:
1 Cut sections at 5—10 μm.
2 Stain with either Holmes or Palmgren (toned) for axons.
3 Wash in distilled water.
4 Stain in 2% brilliant crystal scarlet (2 g bcs in 100 ml distilled water, with 2.5 ml glacial acetic acid) for 30 min.
5 Rinse in distilled water.
6 Differentiate with 1% phosphotungstic acid until good differentiation is apparent between myelin and connective tissue.
7 Wash.
8 Dehydrate, clear and mount.

Results:
Axons   black
Myelin   orange red

For displaying myelin breakdown products before they are cleared away by phagocytes, a fat stain may be used on frozen sections. More detailed pictures can be obtained with the Marchi method (1, 2, 3, 4). Note that this method entails the use of osmium tetroxide (OsO_4), which is (a) very expensive and (b) the source of a highly toxic vapour. Its use must be confined to a fume cupboard. The vapour, which is given off both by the solid and by the solution, attacks the eyes, the entire respiratory tract, and the skin. Gloves must be worn.

Nerve biopsies

In our laboratory tissue is routinely processed for EM, paraffin, frozen, semi-thin and teased preparations.

Procedure for teased nerve preparations

A stretch of nerve 3—4 mm long is fixed for one hour in 0.1 M phosphate-buffered 3.6% glutaraldehyde. After two 15-min buffer washes, the nerve is immersed in 0.1 M phosphate buffered 2% osmium tetroxide for 4—6 hours. Following two further washes, the tissue is placed in 66% glycerin in water for at least 12 hours. In practice we find that formalin fixation followed by immersion in 1% osmium tetroxide after several changes of distilled water is quite adequate. The nerve may be stored in 100% glycerin for several months. Nerves may be teased after 12 hours or more immersion in 66% glycerin.

Method: Using a dissecting microscope the nerve is stripped of its softened epineurium by using fine syringe needles. Individual fibres or small bundles of fibres may then be carefully separated. The glycerin may serve as a mounting medium, using either molten wax or nail varnish as a sealant.

Procedure for semi-thin sections

Technique:
1 Fix in EM fixative at 4°C.
2 Phosphate buffer at 4°C for at least 3 hours.
3 1% osmium tetroxide for 3 hours at room temperature in fume cupboard.
4 Distilled water — two washes over a period of 10 min.

The pleasures of problem-solving

The world will have to wait for answers to the really big questions in biology; in the meantime, there are thousands of little questions, a few of which lie within the power of neuropathologists to answer. For most of us, solving puzzles is fun. And the fun is enhanced if the solution — unlike the solution of a crossword puzzle — leads one on to further puzzles, calling for further solutions. Furthermore, there is the chance that the solution of little puzzles may in time contribute to the solution of bigger, and yet bigger, puzzles. We end, therefore, by wishing our readers fun, in the form of successful problem-solving.

Appendix A
Neurohistological Staining Methods

Most of the staining methods referred to in this book are described in the following commonly used textbooks of histopathological techniques.

1 Drury RAB, Wallington EA. 1980. *Carleton's Histological Technique*, 5th edn. Oxford University Press, Oxford.
2 Culling CFA. 1985. *Handbook of Histopathological Techniques*, 4th edn. Butterworth, London.
3 Bancroft JD, Stevens A. 1982. *Theory and Practice of Histological Techniques*, 2nd edn. Churchill Livingstone, Edinburgh.
4 Ráliš HM, Beesley RA, Ráliš ZA. 1973. *Techniques in Neurohistology*. Butterworth, London. (A useful neurohistological textbook, unfortunately out of print at the time of writing.)

In what follows, details are given of a number of neurohistological techniques which are in common use in our laboratory. When a technique is already well known in general pathology, it is referred to with numbers (1, 2, 3 or 4) indicating which of the textbooks listed above contain details of the method. For some methods which have not yet reached the standard textbooks, references are given for published articles in journals.

Amyloid

Method: Congo Red.

Fixation: Not critical; formalin is satisfactory.

Sections: Paraffin or frozen, 10 μm.

Technique:
1 Take sections down to 70% alcohol.
2 Stain in Congo Red in 0.2% potassium hydroxide in 80% alcohol for 25 min.
3 Wash in tap water.
4 Counterstain lightly with haematoxylin.
5 Blue.
6 Dehydrate, clear and mount.

Results:
Amyloid   pink
Nuclei   blue

Astrocytes

Methods: Cajal's gold sublimate; Holzer; Mallory's phosphotungstic acid/haematoxylin (PTAH) (all 1, 2, 3, 4). When using the PTAH method with surgical specimens we get better results by pre-mordanting in a solution of equal parts of potassium dichromate and acetic acid, as follows:

Fixation: Usually formalin.

Sections: Paraffin, 5–10 μm.

Technique:
1 Take sections down to water.
2 Incubate in a 60°C oven for 60 min in a solution of equal parts of 5% acetic acid and 5% potassium dichromate.
3 Wash well in tap water to remove residual chromate.
4 Oxidize with 0.5% potassium permanganate for 3 min. NB This time must not be exceeded.
5 Remove potassium permanganate with 2% oxalic acid.
6 Wash well in tap water.
7 Stain for 5–6 hours in PTAH or overnight if PTAH is not fresh.

Results:
Glial fibres, myelin and astrocytes   slaty blue
Nerve cell bodies   pink

Axons

Methods:
Palmgren (1, 3, 4).
Schofield (1, 4).
Holmes (1, 2, 3, 4).
Marsland, Glees and Erikson (1, 2, 3, 4).
Palmgren, Holmes, and Marsland, Glees and Erikson methods are suitable for demonstrating axons in both CNS and PNS material. Schofield's is the method of choice for the demonstration of axons and nerve endings in muscle and other peripheral tissues.

Fat

The technique preferred in our laboratory is as follows:

Technique:
1 Cut frozen formalin-fixed sections at 10 μm.
2 Mount on gelatinized slides or free-float.

3 Stain in 0.5% Oil red O in 60% triethyl phosphate for 15 min.
4 Wash in tap water.
5 Lightly counterstain with haematoxylin.
6 Blue.
7 Mount in glycerin jelly.

Results:
Fat   red
Nuclei   blue
Myelin   pale pink

Fungi

Methods:
Periodic acid−Schiff reaction (PAS) (1, 2, 3).
Grocott (1, 3).

Glial fibres

Methods:
Holzer (1, 3, 4).
PTAH (1, 2, 3, 4).
NOTE: in the Holzer method a frequent problem is the deposition on the section of granules of dark blue stain. If during differentiation under the microscope such deposits become visible, allow the section to dry completely. When it is dry, flood the section with pure aniline. The deposits are dissolved by the aniline, and can be seen to disperse. This step may be repeated if necessary. Differentiation is then continued as before.

NB Because of the use of aniline and chloroform, this technique should be performed only in a fume cupboard. Aniline is toxic in contact with skin, and gives off a poisonous vapour. (Threshold limiting volume (TLV) 5 p.p.m.). Inhalation or absorption causes headache, drowsiness and other troubles.

Inclusion bodies in Parkinson's disease

Method: Lendrum's phloxine tartrazine (1, 2, 3, 4).

Melanin

Methods: Masson−Fontana (1, 2, 3, 4).

Muscle biopsy

The muscle biopsy should be received in the laboratory as soon as possible after removal from the patient, to prevent the loss of labile enzymes. We find that we can still attain good results after 30 min. For best results, ideally the specimen should measure about $3 \times 1 \times 1$ cm with muscle fascicles running in the long axis. We cut the muscle, where

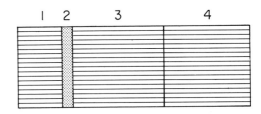

possible, into segments, as shown in the above figure. The shaded area (2) is reserved for EM. This area should have escaped surgical damage. Portions (1) and (4) are placed on a stiff card for about 10 min. The muscle will dry onto the card, and so avoid distortion. The card with the muscle attached is placed in formalin to fix. Portion (3) is placed on a cork disc in a small amount of Tissue Tek and then orientated, using a dissecting microscope if required, so that the fibres may be sectioned transversely. The cork disc is then placed on a freezing microtome chuck with a blob of Tissue Tek to hold it in place. The whole is then held by forceps in iso-pentane, which has been cooled with liquid nitrogen until it is viscous. This will prevent the formation of ice-crystal artefact, which sometimes occurs if muscle is placed directly into liquid nitrogen, owing to the production of an insulating pocket of nitrogen gas. 10−15 sec immersion should be sufficient: too short a period will allow ice-crystal artefact to form; too long may cause cracking. Sections are then cut in a cryostat at not more than 10 μm. If ice crystals have formed, they can be removed by allowing the tissue to come up to room temperature and then refreezing in chilled iso-pentane. The disadvantage of thawing and refreezing is that the muscle fibres swell and become more rounded. They do, however, keep their relative proportions and are easily identifiable. The histochemistry also appears to be unaltered.

Methods:
Routinely, we use the following:
Haematoxylin and eosin.
Fat — see above.
PAS.   ⎫
PAS with glycogen digestion. ⎬ 0.25% celloidinized slides.
ATP pH 9.4.   ⎭
NADH.
Gomori one-step trichrome pH 3.4 (1, 4).
Acid phosphatase (Gomori lead acetate method) — see below.

With the exception of the lead acetate method for acid phosphatase, all the other methods may be found in: Dubowitz V. 1985. *Muscle Biopsy, a Practical Approach*, 2nd edn. Baillière Tindall, London.

Acid phosphatase (Gomori lead acetate method):

Solutions:

0.1 M acetate buffer pH 5.0 — 5 ml.
0.008 M lead acetate — 5 ml.
Sodium β-glycerophosphate — 31.5 mg.
10% ammonium sulphide diluted with distilled water.

Technique:
1 Dissolve sodium β-glycerophosphate in 5 ml 0.1 M acetate buffer.
2 Slowly add and mix 5 ml 0.008 M lead acetate.
3 Incubate slides face down at 37°C for 30 min.
4 Wash in tap water for 30 sec.
5 Immerse in diluted ammonium sulphide for 30 sec.
6 Wash well in tap water.
7 Light haematoxylin counterstain.
8 Wash in tap water (blue).
9 Mount in glycerin jelly.

Results:
Acid phosphatase activity   dark down
   NB Sodium β-glycerophosphate must be dissolved in acetate buffer before slowly adding lead acetate, mixing well.
Glassware must be very clean.
Acetate buffer at pH 5 may be stored at 4°C.
Lead acetate may be stored at room temperature.

Myelin

Methods: Klüver-Barrera (Luxol fast blue, with cresyl fast violet) (1, 2, 3, 4), Loyez (1, 2, 3, 4), Page (sometimes called the solochrome cyanin method) (1, 3, 4), and Weil (1, 3, 4). Page's method works well with peripheral nerves. The Gomori one-step trichrome stain (1, 4) gives good results, staining myelin red. The use of 2% brilliant crystal scarlet, used in combination with Holmes' silver technique, or a toned Palmgren for axons, will also produce a pleasant, delicately-stained myelin counterstain, particularly in peripheral nerves (see below).

Fixation: Formalin.

Sections: Paraffin.

Technique:
1 Cut sections at 5–10 μm.
2 Stain with either Holmes or Palmgren (toned) for axons.
3 Wash in distilled water.
4 Stain in 2% brilliant crystal scarlet (2 g bcs in 100 ml distilled water, with 2.5 ml glacial acetic acid) for 30 min.
5 Rinse in distilled water.
6 Differentiate with 1% phosphotungstic acid until good

differentiation is apparent between myelin and connective tissue.
7 Wash.
8 Dehydrate, clear and mount.

Results:
Axons   black
Myelin   orange red

For displaying myelin breakdown products before they are cleared away by phagocytes, a fat stain may be used on frozen sections. More detailed pictures can be obtained with the Marchi method (1, 2, 3, 4). Note that this method entails the use of osmium tetroxide (OsO_4), which is (a) very expensive and (b) the source of a highly toxic vapour. Its use must be confined to a fume cupboard. The vapour, which is given off both by the solid and by the solution, attacks the eyes, the entire respiratory tract, and the skin. Gloves must be worn.

Nerve biopsies

In our laboratory tissue is routinely processed for EM, paraffin, frozen, semi-thin and teased preparations.

Procedure for teased nerve preparations

A stretch of nerve 3–4 mm long is fixed for one hour in 0.1 M phosphate-buffered 3.6% glutaraldehyde. After two 15-min buffer washes, the nerve is immersed in 0.1 M phosphate buffered 2% osmium tetroxide for 4–6 hours. Following two further washes, the tissue is placed in 66% glycerin in water for at least 12 hours. In practice we find that formalin fixation followed by immersion in 1% osmium tetroxide after several changes of distilled water is quite adequate. The nerve may be stored in 100% glycerin for several months. Nerves may be teased after 12 hours or more immersion in 66% glycerin.

Method: Using a dissecting microscope the nerve is stripped of its softened epineurium by using fine syringe needles. Individual fibres or small bundles of fibres may then be carefully separated. The glycerin may serve as a mounting medium, using either molten wax or nail varnish as a sealant.

Procedure for semi-thin sections

Technique:
1 Fix in EM fixative at 4°C.
2 Phosphate buffer at 4°C for at least 3 hours.
3 1% osmium tetroxide for 3 hours at room temperature in fume cupboard.
4 Distilled water — two washes over a period of 10 min.

5   35% alcohol (4°C) for 20 min (two washes of 10 min each).

6   70% alcohol (4°C) 12–24 hours or overnight.

7   95% alcohol (room temperature) — 30 min.

8   Methcol — two changes of 30 min each.

9   Absolute alcohol — two changes of 15 min each.

10   Propylene oxide — 15 min.

11   Propylene oxide — 30 min.

12   Propylene oxide and embedding resin (equal parts) — 90 min.

13   Embedding resin — 1½–2 hours at room temperature.

14   Embed in mould containing embedding resin at 60°C overnight.

Buffer:
0.1 M Na_2HPO_4 3.55 g/250 ml distilled water — 8 parts.
0.1 M KH_2PO_4 3.4 g/250 ml distilled water — 3 parts.

Embedding resin:

TAAB embedding resin	10 ml
TAAB DDSA	10 ml
TAAB DMP-30	0.3 ml
TAAB dibutyl phthalate	0.6 ml

Mix well. This solution may be stored at 4°C for several days or for 2 days at room temperature.

When sufficiently hardened the embedding resin block may be broken out of its mould and sections cut on an ultra-microtome at 1 µm thickness. The sections are collected onto a drop of water on a clean microscope slide and then dried on, by placing them on a hot plate set to about 50–60°C. When dried, a drop of 1% toluidine blue in 1% borax is placed on the section. At the first sign of drying back, remove the slide and wash off excess stain in running water. Differentiate, controlling microscopically, in 70% alcohol. Because of the danger of wrinkling when mounted, it is our practice to leave the mounting to the last moment. Any synthetic resin mounting medium will do, but we use RAL mountant (now supplied by BDH), which has a low viscosity, and appears to penetrate more quickly.

Note that this procedure involves the use of osmium tetroxide, which gives off a toxic vapour (see note on Marchi technique above). It must be carried out in a fume cupboard.

Neurofibrillary tangles

Methods: Bielschowsky (1, 2, 4), von Braunmühl's method (4), and Cross's modification of Palmgren (Cross RB. 1982. Demonstration of neurofibrillary tangles in paraffin sections: a quick and simple method using a modification of Palmgren's method. *Medical Laboratory Science* **39**, 67–9).

Method: Von Braunmühl.

Fixation: Formalin.

Technique:

1   Cut frozen sections at 10–30 µm

2   Wash in distilled water.

3   Impregnate with 20% silver nitrate at 60°C for 30 min.

4   Transfer, without washing, to 50 ml distilled water* containing 20 drops of ammonia.

5   Wash in distilled water.

6   Reduce in 10% formalin in *tap* water until sections are grey.

7   Wash in distilled water.

8   Tone in 0.2% gold chloride.

9   Wash in distilled water.

10   Fix in 5% sodium thiosulphate.

11   Wash in distilled water, float onto a gelatinized slide, blot, dehydrate, clear and mount.

Results:

Neurofibrils	black
Senile plaques	black
Background	pale grey

Cross's modification of Palmgren

This method has the advantages (i) of using solutions already made up for routine use in Palmgren's method, and (ii) the use of paraffin sections.

Fixation: Formalin.

Technique:

1   Cut paraffin sections at 10 µm.

2   Take down to water.

3   Place in 1% ammonia in distilled water for 5 min.

4   Wash in two changes of distilled water.

5   Impregnate with Palmgren's silver solution for at least 15 min (myelin goes brown). Longer times may be required if the silver solution is not freshly made.

6   Without washing, pour on previously warmed (37°C) Palmgren's reducer. Agitate the slide to ensure even impregnation. When the section goes brown, wash in distilled water.

7   Tone with 0.2% gold chloride until sections are grey.

8   Wash in distilled water.

9   Fix with 5% sodium thiosulphate.

10   Dehydrate, clear and mount.

---

* We find that using 50 ml of 1% silver nitrate to which 20 drops of ammonia have been added will give more even impregnation.

Results:

Neurofibrillary tangles	black
Senile plaques	black
Background	grey to purple

NB Untoned sections will show senile plaques rather better than toned.

Nerve cells

Methods:
Nissl (cresyl fast violet, etc.) (1, 2, 3, 4).
Bielschowsky (1, 2, 3, 4).
Golgi (1, 3, 4).

Oligodendroglia and microglia

Method: Weil and Davenport (1, 2, 3, 4). An advantage of this method is that by changing the concentration of formalin and silver nitrate either oligodendroglia or microglia may be enhanced selectively, thus:
10% silver nitrate for microglia.
15% silver nitrate for oligodendroglia.
10% formalin for microglia.
15% formalin for oligodendroglia.

Pituitary

Method: PAS/Orange G (1, 2, 3, 4).

Results:

Eosinophil cells and red blood cells	yellow
Basophil cells	pink to red

Senile plaques

Methods:
Von Braunmühl (4): see above.
Cross's modification of Palmgren: see above.

Immunohistological techniques

Peroxidase antiperoxidase (PAP) technique using rabbit polyclonal antisera

1   Paraffin sections are dewaxed and taken to alcohol.
2   Transfer to acid alcohol (1% HCl in 70% alcohol) for 30 min to block endogenous peroxidase.
3   Wash twice in Tris saline.*

4   Transfer to wet tray and incubate in normal swine serum diluted 1:5 with Tris saline for 15 min.
5   Swine serum is drained off and replaced with suitably diluted primary antibody for 30 min.
6   Wash three times with Tris saline for total of 10 min.
7   Incubate in swine anti-rabbit serum diluted 1:20 with Tris saline for 30 min.
8   Wash three times with Tris saline for total of 10 min.
9   Incubate in PAP diluted 1:50 with Tris saline for 30 min.
10   Wash twice with Tris saline for at least 5 min.
11   Treat with DAB (60 mg in 100 ml Tris saline plus 1 drop 100 vol hydrogen peroxide) for 4−6 min.
12   Wash in running water for 5 min.
13   Lightly counterstain with haematoxylin, blue, dehydrate, clear and mount.

All antisera are diluted with Tris saline and all washes use Tris saline at pH 7.6.

Indirect peroxidase technique for mouse monoclonal antibodies

If cryostat sections are used, these are cut and air-dried, then fixed in acetone for 10 min. Cryostat sections can be stored at −20°C wrapped in foil until stained. Paraffin sections are dewaxed, taken through descending alcohols and transferred to Tris saline.

1   Primary antibody, suitably diluted with Tris saline, is incubated for 45 min.
2   Wash three times with Tris saline for 10 min.
3   Incubate with peroxidase conjugated rabbit anti-mouse serum, diluted 1:50 with normal human serum, diluted 1:20 with Tris saline for 30 min.
4   Wash twice with Tris saline for at least 5 min.
5   Treat with DAB (60 mg in 100 ml Tris saline plus 1 drop 100 vol hydrogen peroxide) for 4−6 min.
6   Wash in running water for 5 min.
7   Lightly counterstain with haematoxylin, blue, dehydrate, clear and mount.

* Tris buffer is made by dissolving 60.57 g Tris (hydroxymethyl) methylamine (BDH) in 500 ml distilled water and adding 1N HCl to pH 7.6 (approx. 300−400 ml usually needed). Make up to 1 litre with distilled water. Tris saline is made freshly each time it is used by diluting Tris buffer 1:10 with normal saline. DAB (3, 4, 3′, 4, tetra-aminobiphenyl hydrochloride) used is from BDH. The swine anti-rabbit and PAP are purchased from DAKO.

Appendix B
Useful Addresses

Alzheimer's Disease Society, 3rd Floor, Bank Buildings, Fulham Broadway, London SW6 1EP.
Tel: 01-381-3177.

COMBAT, the Association to combat Huntington's Chorea, 34A Station Road, Hinckley, Leics LE10 1AP.
Tel: 0455-615558.

Foundation for the Study of Infant Deaths, Cot Death Research and Support, 15 Belgrave Square, London SW1X 8PS.
Tel: 01-235-1721/0965.

LINK, the Neurofibromatosis Association, D15, London House, 26-40 Kensington High Street, London W8 4PF.
Tel: 01-938-2222.

Medical Research Council Head Office (for information about brain banks supported by the Council), 20 Park Crescent, London W1N 4AL. Tel: 01-636-5422.

Medical Research Council Toxicology Research Unit, Woodmansterne Road, Carshalton, Surrey SM5 4EF.
Tel: 01-643-8000.

Motor Neuron Disease Society, 61 Derngate, Northampton NN1 1VE. Tel: 0604-22269/250505.

Multiple Sclerosis Society of Great Britain and Northern Ireland, 25 Effie Road, London SW6 1EE.
Tel: 01-736-6267.

Muscular Dystrophy Group of Great Britain, Nattrass House, 35 Macaulay Road, London SW4 OQP.
Tel: 01-720-8055.

Parkinson's Disease Society, (Brain Bank), Department of Neurology, Institute of Neurology, 1 Wakefield Street, London WC1N 1PG. Tel: 01-837-8370.

National Poisons Information Service
Belfast 0232-40503
Cardiff 0222-569200
Dublin 0001-745588
Edinburgh 031-229-2477
London 01-635-9191 or 01-407-7600

Research Trust for Metabolic Diseases in Children, 9 Arnold Street, Nantwich, Cheshire CW5 5QB.
Tel: 0270-629782.

Schizophrenia Brain Bank, Division of Psychiatry, Clinical Research Centre, Northwick Park Hospital, Watford Road, Harrow, Middx HA1 3UJ. Tel: 01-864-0180.

Schizophrenia National Fellowship, 79 Victoria Road, Surbiton, Surrey KT6 4NS. Tel: 01-390-3651/2/3.

Index

Page numbers in *italic* refer to figures, those in **bold** refer to tables

DEPARTMENT OF PATHOLOGY

THE ROYAL INFIRMARY

WORCESTER.